Essential Atlas of

HEART DISEASES

Third Edition

Essential Atlas of
HEART DISEASES
Third Edition

Editor-in-Chief
Eugene Braunwald, MD, MD (Hon), ScD (Hon)

Distinguished Hersey Professor of Medicine
Harvard Medical School
Faculty Dean for Academics
Brigham and Women's Hospital
Massachusetts General Hospital
Vice President for Academic Programs
Partners Heathcare System
Boston, Massachusetts

With 174 Contributors

Developed by Current Medicine, LLC.
Philadelphia

CM CURRENT MEDICINE

Current Medicine LLC

400 Market Street, Suite 700

Philadelphia, PA 19106

Director of Editoral, Design, Production	Wendy Vetter
Senior Developmental Editor	Elizabeth Rexon
Commissioning Supervisor Books	Annmarie D'Ortona
Cover Design	William Whitman, Jr.
Design and Layout	Christine Keller-Quirk
Illustrators	Marie Dean, Theresa Englehart, Matthew Holmes, Wieslawa Langenfeld, Maureen Looney, Deborah Lynam, John McCullough, William Whitman, Jr.
Assistant Production Manager	Margaret La Mare
Indexer	Holly Lukens

Credits for cover photographs:
   Figure 8-25D from Chapter 8 edited by Dr. Rahimtoola
   Figure 2-10A from Chapter 2 edited by Dr. Califf
   Image courtesy of Dr. Yuzo Hirota
   Figure 9-4A from Chapter 9 edited by Dr. Freedom

Library of Congress Cataloging-in-Publication Data

Essential atlas of heart diseases / editor-in-chief, Eugene Braunwald ; with 130 contributors.-- 3rd ed.
      p. ; cm.
      Includes bibliographical references and index.
      ISBN 1-57340-214-1 (hardcover)
   I. Heart--Diseases--Atlases.
   [DNLM: 1. Cardiovascular Diseases--Atlases. WG 17 E78 2005] I. Braunwald, Eugene, 1929- III. Title.

   RC682.E85 2005
   616.1'2--dc22

                                                            2004065676

ISBN 1-57340-214-1

Printed in Thailand by Imago

10 9 8 7 6 5 4 3 2

Although every effort has been made to ensure that drug doses and other information are presented accurately in this publication, the ultimate responsibility rests with the prescribing physician. Neither the publishers nor the author can be held responsible for errors or for any consequences arising from the use of the information contained therein. Any product mentioned in this publication should be used in accordance with prescribing information prepared by the manufacturers. No claims or endorsements are made for any drug or compound at present under clinical investigation.

PREFACE

Disorders of the cardiovascular system are the most common causes of death and serious morbidity in the industrialized world. In 2003, more than 40% of all deaths in the United States were attributed to cardiac and vascular diseases. These conditions accounted for almost 5 million years of potential life lost. Cardiovascular disease is rising in a staggering manner in the developing world as well. The World Health Organization has predicted that cardiovascular disease will be the most common cause of death worldwide by 2020.

Despite these sobering statistics, progress in cardiovascular medicine has been immense, and is, in fact, accelerating. Our understanding of the pathobiology of most forms of heart disease has advanced steadily and there have been enormous advances in the diagnosis, treatment, and prevention of cardiovascular disorders. For example, during just one decade, from 1993 to 2003, the overall death rates from cardiovascular disease declined by 26% and death rates from acute myocardial infarction and stroke declined by 32%. Similar progress has been made in other major cardiovascular disorders, including hypertension, valvular and congenital heart disease, congestive heart failure, and the arrhythmias.

Physicians responsible for the care of patients with cardiovascular disease—both primary care physicians and specialists—now have available numerous publications for obtaining up-to-date information, including excellent journals and textbooks of every conceivable size, scope, and depth. In developing new strategies for transmitting information about these conditions, it is important to consider that cardiovascular medicine is the most "visual" of medical specialties. Cardiovascular diagnosis is based on the recognition and understanding of a variety of graphic waveforms, images, decision trees, and microscopic sections. Treatment increasingly involves the intelligent use of algorithms, which are most effectively portrayed visually. Likewise, mechanical correction of cardiovascular disorders, whether catheter-based or surgical, can best be described pictorially. This *Essential Atlas of Heart Diseases* has been designed to provide a detailed and comprehensive visual exposition of all aspects of cardiovascular medicine. The *Essential Atlas* should be especially useful to primary care physicians as well as to specialists. The most important images from each volume in the *Atlas of Heart Diseases* series, accompanied by detailed captions written by the expert authors, were reviewed by their respective volume editors, who serve as chapter authors in this *Essential Atlas*.

Many people deserve credit for the successful completion of this ambitious effort. The expertise and hard work of the contributors and the devoted efforts of the volume editors naturally form the foundation of the *Essential Atlas of Heart Diseases*. Great credit is also due to Abe Krieger, President of Current Medicine, who conceived the project, and to Kathryn Saxon, who coordinated the efforts in my office.

All of us who have been engaged in this project hope that this *Essential Atlas* will be useful to physicians of all specialties who are responsible for the care of patients with cardiovascular disorders, to investigators and teachers of cardiovascular medicine, and ultimately to the millions of patients worldwide with disorders of the heart and circulation.

Eugene Braunwald, MD

CONTRIBUTING EDITORS

Kenneth L. Baughman, MD
Professor
Department of Medicine
Harvard Medical School;
Director, Advanced Heart
  Disease Section
Brigham and Women's Hospital
Boston, Massachusetts

George A. Beller, MD
Professor of Cardiology
Department of Internal Medicine
University of Virginia Health System
Charlottesville, Virginia

Robert M. Califf, MD
Professor of Medicine
Duke University School of Medicine;
Director
Duke Clinical Research Institute
Durham, North Carolina

Wilson S. Colucci, MD, FACC, FAHA
Professor of Medicine
Boston University
  School of Medicine;
Chief, Cardiovascular Medicine
Boston University Medical Center
Boston, Massachusetts

Vasken Dilsizian, MD
Professor
Departments of Medicine
  and Radiology
Director of Nuclear Cardiology
  and Cardiac PET
The University of Maryland
  Medical Center
Baltimore, Maryland

Robert M. Freedom, MD
Professor of Pediatrics, Pathology,
  and Medical Imaging
University of Toronto;
Director Emeritus, Division
  of Cardiology
Hospital for Sick Children
Toronto, Ontario
Canada

Samuel Z. Goldhaber, MD
Associate Professor
Department of Medicine
Harvard Medical School;
Director, Venous Thromboembolism
  Research Group
Director, Cardiac Center's
  Anticoagulation Service
Staff Cardiologist
Brigham and Women's Hospital
Boston, Massachusetts

Norman K. Hollenberg, MD, PhD
Professor of Medicine
Department of Medicine
Harvard Medical School;
Director of Physiologic Research
Brigham and Women's Hospital
Boston, Massachusetts

David R. Holmes, Jr., MD
Professor of Medicine
Department of
  Cardiovascular Disease
Mayo Medical School;
Consultant, Cardiovascular Diseases
Mayo Clinic
Rochester, Minnesota

Byron K. Lee, MD
Assistant Professor
Department of Medicine
University of California
  San Francisco Medical Center
San Francisco, California

Verghese Mathew, MD
Assistant Professor of Medicine
Mayo Medical School;
Consultant, Division of
  Cardiovascular Diseases
  and Internal Medicine
Mayo Clinic
Rochester, Minnesota

Jagat Narula, MD, PhD
Professor and Chief
Department of Cardiology
University of California Irvine
Medical Center
Orange, California

Shahbudin H. Rahimtoola, MB, FRCP, MACP, MACC, DSc (Hon)
Distinguished Professor/George C.
  Griffith Professor of Cardiology
Department of Cardiology
Keck School of Medicine
University of Southern California
Los Angeles, California

Melvin M. Scheinman, MD
Professor of Medicine
Department of Medicine
University of California
  San Francisco
San Francisco, California

Peter W.F. Wilson, MD
Professor
Department of Endocrinology,
Diabetes, and Metabolic Genetics
Medical University of
  South Carolina;
Program Director, General
  Clinical Research Center
Charleston, South Carolina

CONTENTS

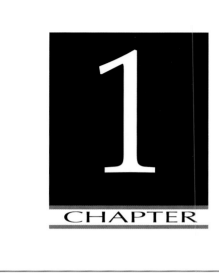

1

CHAPTER

ATHEROSCLEROSIS: RISK FACTORS AND TREATMENT

Edited by Peter W.F. Wilson

G.M. Anantharamaiah, H. Bryan Brewer, Jr., Alan Chait, David W. Garber, Don P. Giddens, Seymour Glagov, Michael B. Gravanis, Jeffrey M. Hoeg, Andreas R. Huber, Donald B. Hunninghake, Ngoc-Anh Le, Sampath Parthasarathy, Michael E. Rosenfeld, Marschall S. Runge, Jere P. Segrest, Christopher K. Zarins

FORMATION OF THE ATHEROSCLEROTIC PLAQUE

EARLY EVENTS IN THE INITIATION OF ATHEROSCLEROTIC LESIONS

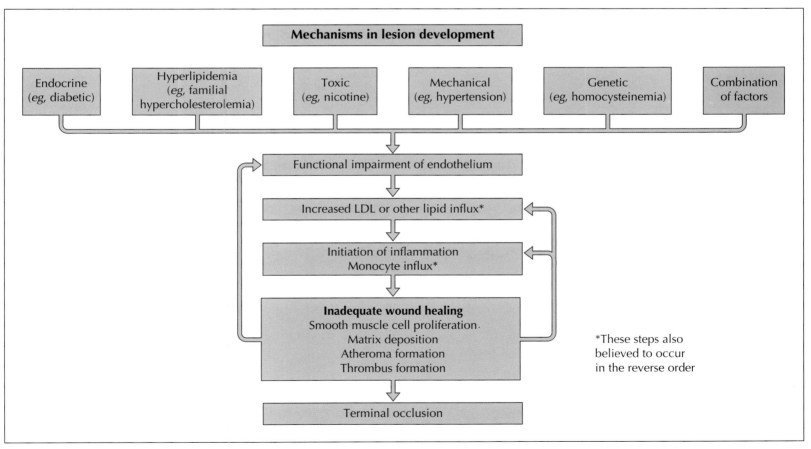

FIGURE 1-1. Mechanisms in arteriosclerotic lesion formation. Multiple risk factors and pathologic states have been correlated with early lesion formation and lesion progression. It is hypothesized that these factors all induce functional impairment of the arterial endothelium resulting in either increased lipid influx or initiation of an inflammatory vessel wall response. This process is propagated by additional accumulation of inflammatory cells such as monocytes within the vessel wall. Consequently, under persistence of the noxious agent(s), chronic inflammation persists, leading to inadequate wound healing. Ultimately terminal occlusion of the vessel by a thrombus occurs. LDL—low-density lipoprotein.

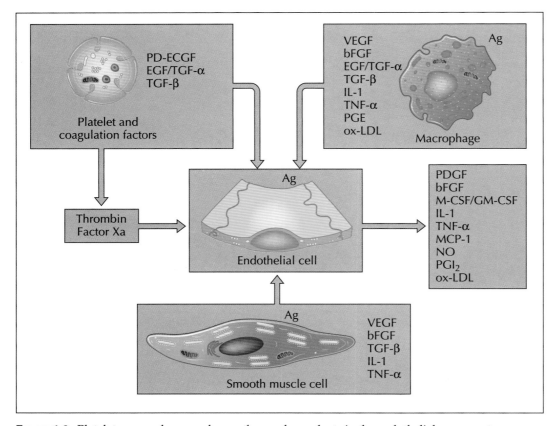

FIGURE 1-2. Platelet, macrophage, and smooth muscle products in the endothelial response to vascular injury. During atherogenesis, the endothelium interacts with macrophages, platelets, smooth muscle cells, and T lymphocytes. These interactions result in the expression and secretion of several potential mediators of vascular lesion formation. Macrophages produce endothelial mitogens including vascular endothelial growth factor (VEGF), fibroblast growth factor (FGF), interleukin-1 (IL-1), and transforming growth factor-α and -β (TGF-α, TGF-β). IL-1 and both TGF-α and TGF-β can inhibit endothelial proliferation and induce secondary gene expression by the endothelium of such growth factors as platelet-derived growth factor (PDGF) and other potential regulators of vascular lesion formation. TGF-β also induces synthesis and secretion of connective tissue by the endothelium.

The endothelium and macrophages can produce oxidized low-density lipoprotein (ox-LDL), causing further injury to endothelial cells. Platelets produce TGF-α, TGF-β, and platelet-derived endothelial cell growth factor (PD-ECGF), a potent mitogen. A procoagulant state of the endothelium can be stimulated by thrombin and factor Xa, present in plasma. Several of the same molecules formed by macrophages and platelets are also generated in the artery wall or in atherosclerotic lesions underlying the endothelium by smooth muscle cells. Endothelial cells in injured vessels express several growth-regulatory molecules, including those that cause connective tissue to proliferate (PDGF, bFGF, TGF-β) and those that induce secondary gene expression for PDGF in smooth muscle and endothelial cells. Further, endothelial cells produce macrophage colony stimulating factor (M-CSF), granulocyte macrophage-colony stimulating factor (GM-CSF), and ox-LDL, which are mitogenic and activating factors for underlying macrophages. Endothelial cells also provide potent chemotactic factors that affect leukocyte chemotaxis, including ox-LDL and monocyte chemotactic protein-1 (MCP-1), and modulate vasomotor tone through the formation of nitric oxide (NO) and prostacyclin (PGI$_2$).

Thus, multiple interactions among platelets, macrophages, and smooth muscle cells have been documented and are likely to provide the inflammatory and growth-promoting milieu necessary for repair of vascular injury. In abnormal arteries, it is likely these same mechanisms stimulate formation of pathologic vascular lesions. Ag—antigen; EGF—epidermal growth factor; PGE—prostaglandin E; TNF—tumor necrosis factor. (*Adapted from* Ross [1].)

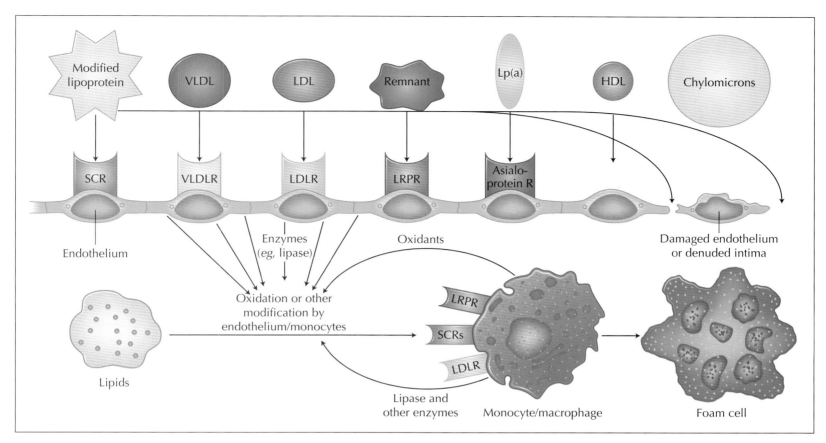

FIGURE 1-3. Postulated lipid entry mechanisms into macrophages. Many lipoproteins have been associated with arteriosclerosis. Foremost low-density lipoprotein (LDL), modified (*eg*, oxidized) LDL, lipoprotein (a) (Lp[a]), and other substances in the blood can be detected at high levels within the damaged vessel wall segments. Accumulation in the vessel wall may occur through diffusion either interjunctionally or in areas of denudation. In addition, a functionally impaired endothelium could mediate increased lipoprotein uptake via specific receptor-coupled pathways. To date, at least five lipoprotein receptors have been characterized in detail, including the two or more scavenger receptors (SCRs), LDL receptor (LDLR), very LDL receptor (VLDLR), LDL receptor related protein (LRPR), and asialoprotein receptor (R). Furthermore, lipoproteins captured in the subendothelial intimal space may be modified by oxidants or enzymes derived from either endothelial cells, monocytes, or smooth muscle cells leading to increased uptake into monocytes via the SCRs and, possibly, other receptors. With time, monocytes will develop into foam cells. HDL—high-density lipoprotein.

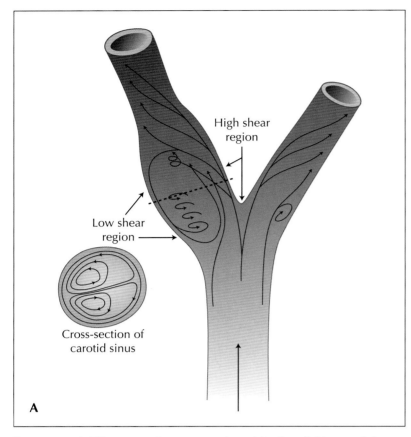

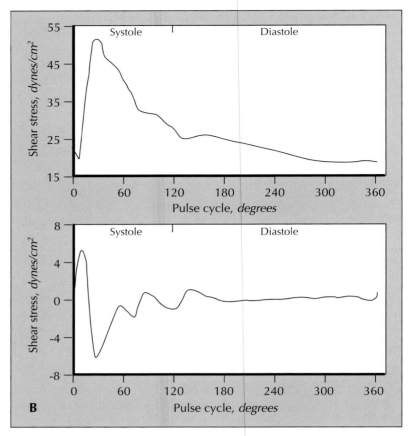

FIGURE 1-4. A, Diagrammatic representation of the flow field around the carotid bifurcation [2]. **B,** Graphic representation of the quantitative estimates of wall shear stress obtained from *in vitro* model studies [2]. Wall shear stress is high and flow is laminar and unidirectional at the flow divider side (*top*); plaques do not form initially or predominantly in this location. In the region opposite the flow divider, however, a zone of flow separation occurs, the flow profile is complex, and wall shear stress is relatively low and reverses in direction during the downstroke of systole (*bottom*). (*Adapted from* Ku *et al.* [2].)

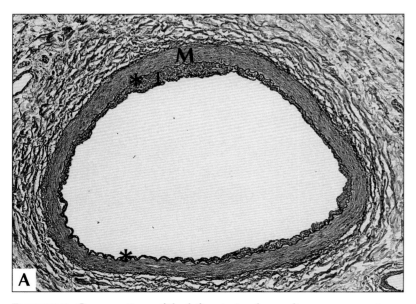

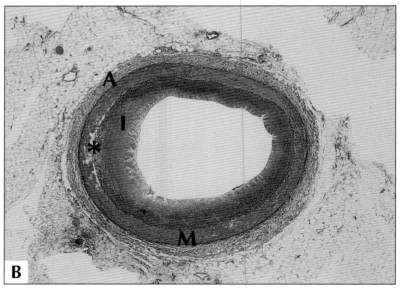

FIGURE 1-5. Cross-sections of the left anterior descending coronary artery from a 2-year-old girl (**A**; Verhoeff–van Gieson elastic stain, original magnification, ×80), and from a 41-year-old man (**B**; Verhoeff–van Gieson elastic, original magnification, ×40; **C**; hematoxylin and eosin, original magnification, ×200). (*continued*)

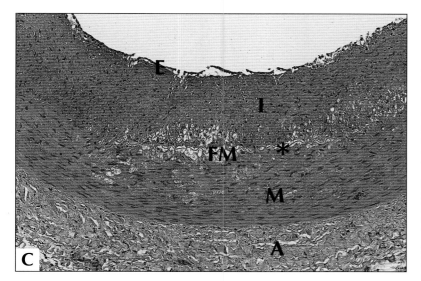

FIGURE 1-5. (*continued*) Both subjects died from noncardiac causes. The photomicrographs reveal an intimal thickening that is rather limited in *A*, but circumferential and of considerable thickness in *B* and *C*.

The interna elastica (*asterisks*) appears to be intact except in the sections from the adult in which a focal area between the intima (I) and media (M) where foam cell infiltration is present and the interna elastica appears fragmented or absent. Diffuse intimal thickening is characterized by

proliferation of myointimal cells (smooth muscle cells) with subsequent synthesis of collagen, elastin, and proteoglycans. An intriguing similarity exists between this vascular reaction in atherosclerosis and the lesions observed in the allograft heart, the so-called accelerated atherosclerosis, in post-angioplasty restenosis, and the intimal proliferation observed in saphenous vein grafts. The underlying pathogenetic mechanisms leading to the intimal reaction in these different settings, however, are quite dissimilar, reaffirming the dictum that vascular injury—regardless of its nature or its precise localization (intima, media, or adventitia [A])—will eventually manifest as an intimal reaction. According to many investigators [3], the intimal smooth muscle masses (cushions) found near arterial branch sites are more likely to predispose to the development of atherosclerotic plaques. Thus, there is a good correlation between focal smooth muscle masses seen early in life and arteriosclerotic lesions observed later. However, lipid accumulation leads the smooth muscle cell mass to progress into an advanced atherosclerotic lesion.

According to one hypothesis, atherogenesis begins early in life as fibroblastic intimal thickening into which necrotic cores later appear. Furthermore, fibrocellular proliferation in the intima may foster lipid deposition, probably because of stimulation of smooth muscle cells by growth factors resulting in expression of additional low-density lipoprotein receptors by smooth muscle cells. With increasing age when the thick fibroproliferative intima approaches a threshold of about 150 μm, atherosclerosis occurs. The biologic threshold, therefore, appears to be determined by the product of two measured variables such as age and fibroplasia [3]. E—endothelium; FM—foamy macrophage.

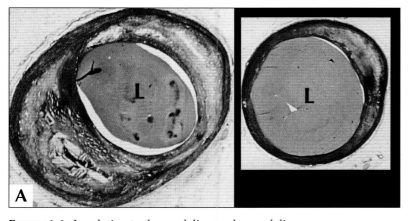

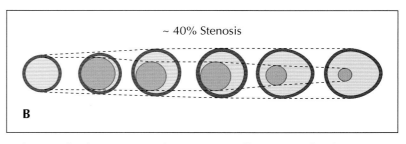

FIGURE 1-6. In relation to the modeling and remodeling processes described, arteries appear to enlarge initially as plaques form, tending to preserve a lumen of adequate cross-section even in the presence of relatively large intimal plaques [4,5]. **A,** Postmortem sections of the left anterior descending coronary artery taken at the same level in two individuals. The lumen cross-sectional area (L) is approximately the same for each individual, although the lesion area is vastly different. If the artery on the left had not enlarged to compensate for the large plaque that formed, the lumen would have been totally occluded. That artery enlargement is a consequence of plaque formation is indicated by the fact that in any given artery segment lumen cross-sectional area is often similar for involved

and uninvolved segments. Enlargement usually occurs only where plaques are forming.

B, Diagram of artery enlargement with plaque formation based on a study of the human left main coronary artery [4]. Although plaque formation may be arrested at any stage, lumen stenosis appears to be evident on the average when 40% or more of the potential lumen area (as defined by the area encompassed by internal elastic lamina) is occupied by plaque. Plaque enlargement is mainly associated with outward bulging of the artery wall beneath the lesion. (*Adapted from* Glagov *et al.* [4].)

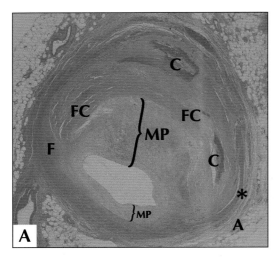

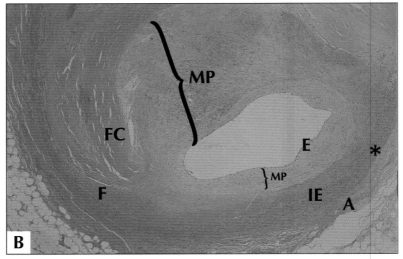

FIGURE 1-7. Lesion progression in a fibrofatty plaque in the left anterior descending coronary artery of a 52-year-old man who died from a cardiac ischemic episode. The eccentric fibrofatty calcified plaque occupies approximately two thirds of the arterial circumference. Luminal to the plaque, there is a concentric, relatively cellular proliferation of fibromuscular tissue that stains lighter than the underlying plaque. Similar fibromuscular tissue is also recognized extending between the fibrous cap of the original plaque (FC) and the media (*asterisks*) through an obvious fissure (F) of the FC at the shoulder region. Besides being the site of growth (recruitment of monocytes), the plaque "shoulders" also show significant neovascularization (angiogenesis). Mechanical transmural shearing forces, secondary to the cardiac cycle, are likely to be maximal at these sites, probably due to differences in compliance of the diseased versus nondiseased segment of the arterial wall. Plaques in which the lipid core is situated eccentrically are also associated with fissuring [6].

Arterial wall reaction to fissuring of a plaque may contribute to the growth of the lesion by either a neointimal proliferation or organization of a thrombus formed at the site of plaque fissuring. In the sections shown, fingerprints of a preceded thrombotic episode (hemosiderin deposition, neovascularity) are lacking. The "thrombogenic" or "encrustation" hypothesis proposes that fibrin deposition and thrombus organization on an atheromatous plaque may play a role in plaque development. Evidence that thrombus incorporation contributes to the plaque progression has been demonstrated with monoclonal antibodies, which have identified fibrin, fibrinogen, and their split products [7].

This case clearly demonstrates that the atheromatous plaque is not a static structure, but is subject to either growth or dynamic modification and remodeling process (**A**; hematoxylin and eosin, original magnification, ×40; **B**; original magnification, ×80). A—adventitia; C—calcification; E—endothelium; IE—interna elastica; MP—myofibroblastic proliferation.

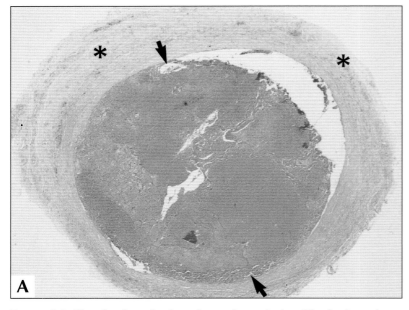

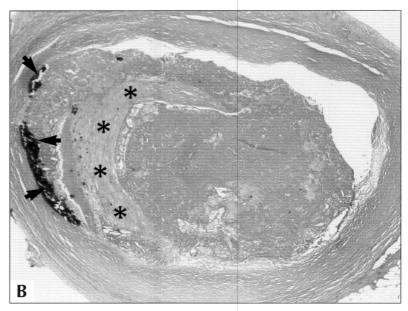

FIGURE 1-8. Vascular thrombosis and vascular occlusion. The final step in myocardial infarction is often thrombus formation with occlusion of the vessel lumen. However, it is distinctly unusual for a thrombus to form in the normal artery. **A,** Thrombotic occlusion of an epicardial coronary artery in a patient who died of myocardial infarction. The erythrocyte-rich thrombus (*arrows*) virtually occludes the entire lumen of this vessel. Close inspection of this light micrograph indicates that this vessel had been subject to numerous prior insults that resulted in the presence of proliferative vascular lesions and of cholesterol plaque (*asterisks*). Clinicians recognize that coro-

nary heart disease is episodic in its symptomatic manifestations, and often the episodic nature of the disease is also evident pathologically [8]. For example, thrombus formation may occur on many occasions in the life cycle of an artery. **B,** Coronary artery in which thrombus formation (*arrows*) followed by proliferative lesion formation (*asterisks*) occurred in several discrete stages over time. In both *A* and *B*, thrombus formation most likely occurred spontaneously, following disruption of the fibrous cap of an atherosclerotic plaque with exposure of plaque contents to the bloodstream. (*Courtesy of* M. B. Gravanis, MD, Emory University, Atlanta, GA.)

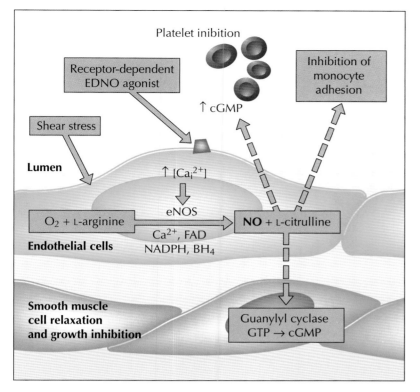

FIGURE 1-9. Endothelium-derived nitric oxide (EDNO) synthesis and action. In endothelial cells, a constitutive membrane-associated nitric oxide (NO) synthase (eNOS) catalyzes the conversion of the amino acid l-arginine to NO and l-citrulline. eNOS cofactors include FAD (flavin adenine dinucleotide), NADPH (nicotinamide adenine dinucleotide phosphate), BH4 (tetrahydrobiopterin), and calcium. Endothelial synthesis of NO is tightly controlled and linked to changes in ionized calcium concentration. Several agonists, including acetylcholine, bradykinin, substance P, and platelet-derived serotonin, act on specific membrane receptors that trigger cytosolic calcium release and eNOS activation. Increased shear stress from enhanced blood flow also serves as an important stimulus for NO production. NO modulates basal vascular tone, and exerts a relaxant effect on vascular smooth muscle through activation of soluble guanylyl cyclase and consequent increase in intracellular cyclic guanosine monophosphate (cGMP), which also mediates NO-dependent inhibition of platelet activation. Individuals with coronary risk factors or atherosclerosis demonstrate impaired shear stress- and agonist-induced endothelium-dependent vasodilation. Other actions of NO include inhibition of monocyte adhesion and smooth muscle cell proliferation. GTP—guanosine 5'-triphosphate. (*Adapted from* Gokce *et al.* [9].)

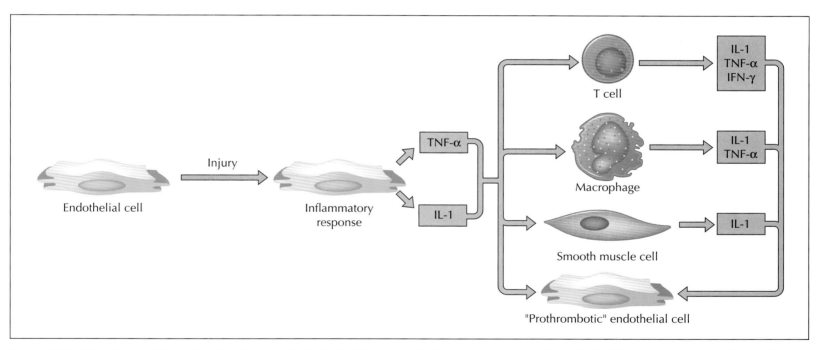

FIGURE 1-10. The role of cytokines in atherothrombosis. Endothelial injury, or exposure to atherogenic stimuli, triggers endothelial cell inflammatory responses leading to recruitment of leukocytes and release of cytokines, including tumor necrosis factor-a (TNF-α), interleukin-1 (IL-1), and interferon gamma (IFN-γ). These cytokines, in addition to amplifying the immune response, alter endothelial cell function towards a prothrombotic phenotype, characterized by increased production of plasminogen activator inhibitor-1, tissue factor expression (and activation of the extrinsic coagulation pathway), and release of platelet-derived growth factors (PDGF). (*Adapted from* Dobroski *et al.* [10].)

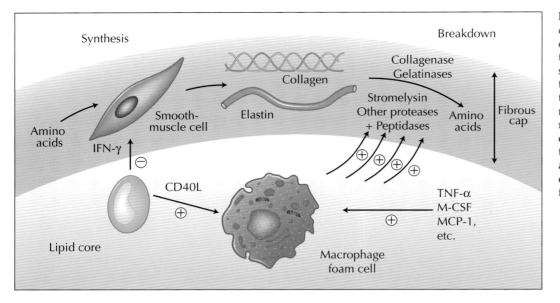

Figure 1-11. Matrix metabolism and integrity depends on the balance of synthesis and breakdown products in the fibrous cap, especially at the shoulder regions. T lymphocytes provide signals via interferon gamma, (IFN-γ), leading to decreased collagen formation. Aggravating these effects is the action of interleukin-1, tumor necrosis factor-a (TNF-α), MCP-1, and macrophage colony-stimulating factor (M-CSF) on macrophages, leading to increased production of collagenases, gelatinases, stromelysin, and other proteases and peptidases that break down and limit accretion of collagen in the fibrous cap [3]. (*Adapted from* Libby [11].)

HYPERLIPOPROTEINEMIAS

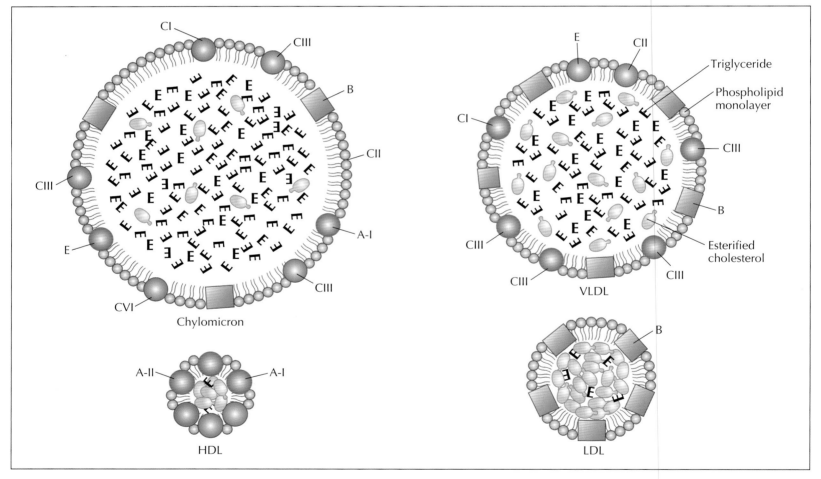

Figure 1-12. The oil-drop or mixed micelle model of lipoprotein structure is presented for chylomicron, very low-density lipoprotein (VLDL), low-density lipoprotein (LDL), and high-density lipoprotein (HDL). Apos in the outer phospholipid membrane are designated by letters. The major differences between the different lipoproteins are in the size of the neutral lipid (triglyceride and esterified cholesterol) core, the lipid composition in the core, and the apo composition. Although not shown, unesterified cholesterol is found predominantly in the phospholipid monolayer. (*Adapted from* Oberman *et al.* [12].)

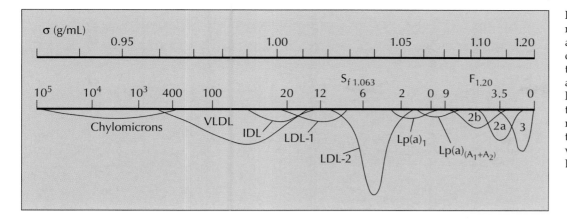

FIGURE 1-13. A summary of lipoprotein components subfractionated and characterized by analytic ultracentrifugation. The determination of both lipoprotein flotation coefficient distribution and refractometric concentration can be achieved by analytic ultracentrifugation. The lipoprotein (a) [Lp(a)] generally occurs at relatively low concentrations and normally is not resolved. IDL—intermediate-density lipoprotein; LDL—low-density lipoprotein; VLDL—very low-density lipoprotein. (*Adapted from* Lindgren [13].)

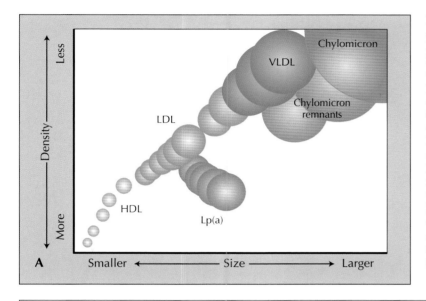

FIGURE 1-14. A, Size and density of lipoproteins. Although lipoproteins are similar in their basic structure, they differ in size and density. **B,** Very low-density lipoprotein (VLDL) structure. VLDL is a triglyceride-rich lipoprotein secreted directly by the liver. It possesses high levels of triglycerides and some esterified cholesterol in its core; its surface lipids are predominantly phosphatidylcholine and unesterified cholesterol. There are many apolipoproteins (apos) on the surface, including apos B-100, E, C-I, C-II, and C-III. the carboxy-terminal G amphipathic helix is the domain of apo C-II that activated lipoprotein lipase; lipoprotein lipase hydrolyzes triglycerides to produce VLDL remnants called *intermediate-density lipoprotein* (IDL). Further metabolism produces low-density lipoprotein (LDL). During this process, excess surface remnants are removed by apo A-I-containing high-density lipoprotein (HDL) particles to produce remnant HDL particles that contain the apos C-I, C-II, and C-III. The schematic model for VLDL shown here is simplified to contain only one copy of apos C-I, C-II, C-III, and E; there may be up to 20 molecules of apo E per VLDL particle, for example. Apo B-100 is shown in a more extended conformation than that shown for LDL. (*Adapted from* Segrest *et al.* [14].)

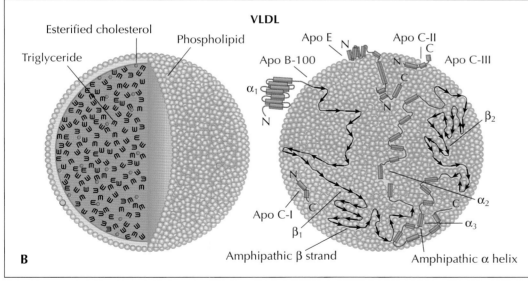

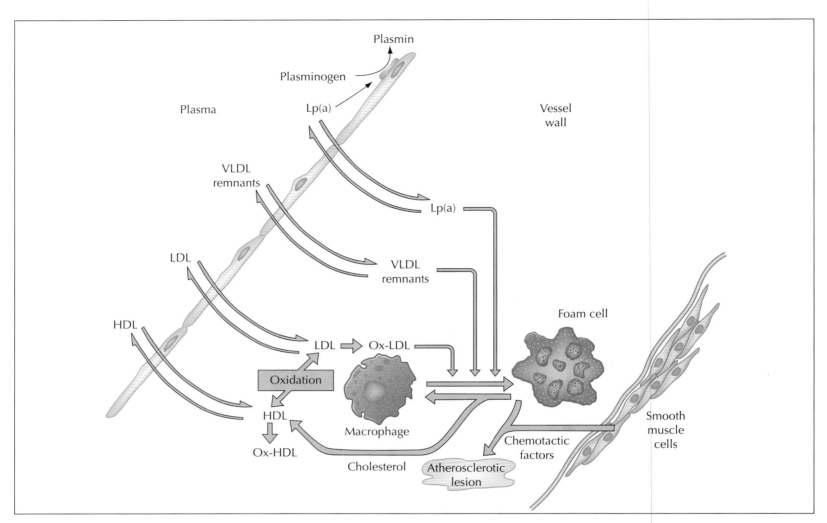

FIGURE 1-15. Role of the plasma lipoproteins in the development of the atherosclerotic lesion. The development of the atherosclerotic lesion involves the interaction of lipoproteins with macrophages with the formation of foam cells, which are characteristic of early atherosclerosis. Elevated levels of three major classes of plasma lipoproteins—low-density lipoprotein (LDL), very LDL (VLDL) remnants, and lipoprotein (a) (Lp[a])—have been associated with an increased risk of early cardiovascular disease. Increased plasma concentrations of these lipoproteins are associated with increased diffusion into the vessel wall. The major atherogenic lipoprotein, LDL, requires oxidative modification to be taken up by the macrophage with the formation of foam cells. Elevated intimal levels of Lp(a) are also associated with foam cell formation. Lp(a) may also contribute to the development of atherosclerosis by competition with plasminogen for the plasminogen receptor [15]. Thus, the atherogenic potential of Lp(a) may result from both uptake by the macrophage with foam cell formation and its thrombotic potential as a competitor of plasminogen. Foam cell formation, macrophage activation, lipid oxidation, and endothelial cell injury all lead to the release of chemotactic factors that contribute to the development of the atherosclerotic lesion. The major antiatherogenic lipoprotein, high-density lipoprotein (HDL), protects against the development of foam cells and atherosclerosis by several potential mechanisms. A major proposed mechanism is reverse cholesterol transport, whereby HDL facilitates the removal of cholesterol from the foam cells and transports this cholesterol out of the vessel wall and back to the liver where it can be removed from the body. In addition, HDL may protect LDL from being oxidized in the vessel wall. Ox—oxidized.

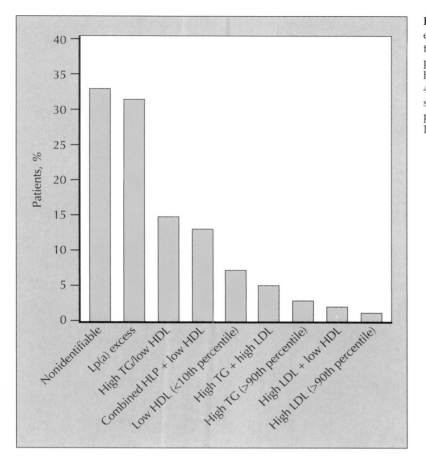

FIGURE 1-16. Frequency of genetic dyslipoproteinemias in patients with established coronary heart disease. An evaluation of patients admitted with the diagnosis of premature myocardial infarction revealed that 67% of patients had an underlying genetic dyslipoproteinemia [16]. A depressed high-density lipoprotein (HDL) cholesterol concentration was present in 42% of these patients. The hypertriglyceridemia-hypoalphalipoproteinemia syndrome (high triglyceride [TG] low HDL) was present in 15% of the probands with established heart disease. HLP—hyperlipoproteinemia; LDL—low-density lipoprotein; Lp(a)–lipoprotein (a).

LOW-DENSITY LIPOPROTEINS

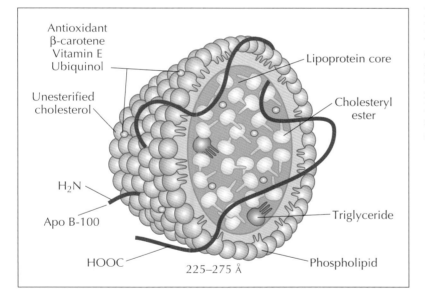

FIGURE 1-17. The structure of a low-density lipoprotein (LDL) particle. LDL is the major cholesterol-carrying plasma lipoprotein. Each particle with a mass exceeding 3,000,000 D has 1500 molecules of cholesterol esters in its core. There is very little triglyceride in the core of normal LDL particles. Considerable amounts of plasma tocopherols, carotenoids, and other lipophilic antioxidants are also present. Other lipophilic molecules, including drugs and proteins, may also be associated with the lipoprotein. Its surface is composed of free cholesterol and phospholipids (predominantly phosphatidylcholine and sphingomyelin) and a single protein, apolipoprotein (apo) B-100.

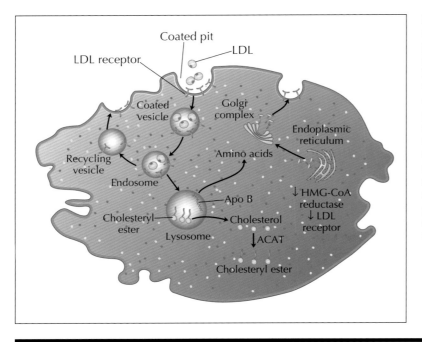

Coated pit
LDL receptor
LDL
Coated vesicle
Golgi complex
Endoplasmic reticulum
Recycling vesicle
Amino acids
Endosome
Apo B
↓ HMG-CoA reductase
↓ LDL receptor
Cholesteryl ester
Cholesterol
Lysosome
↓ACAT
Cholesteryl ester

FIGURE 1-18. Receptor-mediated clearance of low-density lipoprotein (LDL). The LDL receptor is synthesized in the endoplasmic reticulum and processed in the Golgi complex. It is exported to the surface in the mature form to the plasma membrane where it collects in the coated pits. LDL binds to its receptor in the coated pits and is internalized in the coated vesicles. After acidification and uncoating, the resulting endosomes are delivered to the lysosomes for degradation of the lipid and protein components. The receptor dissociates from the LDL and is recycled to the surface. Apo B is hydrolyzed to constituent amino acids and cholesterol esters are degraded to free cholesterol and transported to endoplasmic reticulum. This free cholesterol serves several regulatory functions. It is esterified by acyl coenzyme A:cholesterol acyl transferase (ACAT) for storage as cytoplasmic cholesterol ester droplets. The free cholesterol suppresses activities of the key enzymes of cholesterol biosynthetic pathway (hydroxymethyl glutaryl-coenzyme A [HMG-CoA] synthase and reductase) and suppresses the synthesis of new LDL receptor protein. (*Adapted from* Brown and Goldstein [17].)

MODIFIED LIPOPROTEINS AND SCAVENGER RECEPTOR PATHWAYS

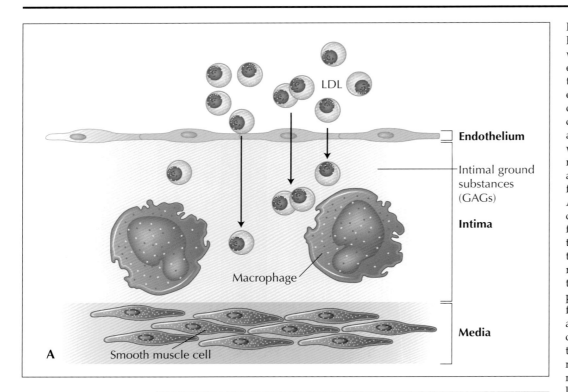

LDL

Endothelium

Intimal ground substances (GAGs)

Intima

Macrophage

Media

A   Smooth muscle cell

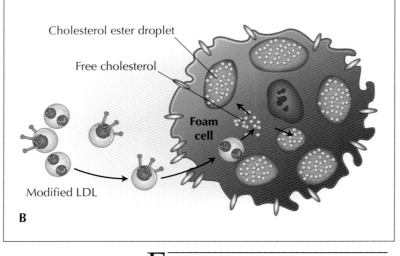

Cholesterol ester droplet

Free cholesterol

Foam cell

Modified LDL

B

FIGURE 1-19. **A,** Infiltration and entrapment of low-density lipoprotein (LDL) in the arterial wall. Circulating LDLs migrate through the endothelial barrier of the arterial wall and penetrate into the intima. A portion of the LDL is entrapped in the subendothelial space as a result of its interaction with extracellular matrix components. These include the proteoglycans and other intimal glycosaminoglycans (GAGs), which have high affinity for apo B. This entrapment increases the residence time of LDL in the artery and renders the LDL susceptible to modifications such as oxidation and aggregation. Aggregates of LDL have been identified in association with matrix components. **B,** Foam cell formation. Foam cells derive their name from their foamy appearance due to lipid accumulation and are the hallmark of early atherosclerotic, fatty streak lesions. The predominant cell type that accumulates lipids is the macrophage, although smooth muscle cell–derived foam cells also occur. Increased chemotactic activity may account for the presence of monocytes or macrophages in the artery. However, the factors that aid in the differentiation of monocytes into differentiated tissue macrophages are yet unknown. Modified lipoproteins are recognized and internalized by the scavenger receptors on the macrophages; there is no feedback regulation of the uptake by this mechanism. The accumulated cellular cholesterol is readily converted to cholesterol ester and stored as large cytoplasmic lipid droplets. Methods have been developed to isolate and study foam cells from the atherosclerotic artery [14]. (*Adapted from* Rosenfeld *et al.* [18].)

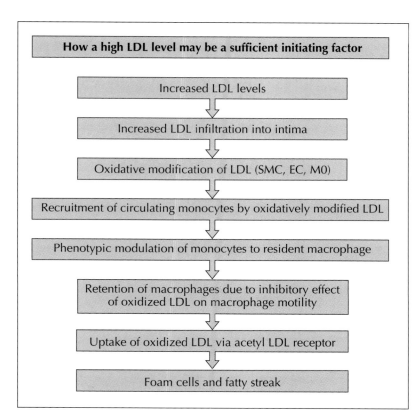

How a high LDL level may be a sufficient initiating factor

Increased LDL levels

↓

Increased LDL infiltration into intima

↓

Oxidative modification of LDL (SMC, EC, M0)

↓

Recruitment of circulating monocytes by oxidatively modified LDL

↓

Phenotypic modulation of monocytes to resident macrophage

↓

Retention of macrophages due to inhibitory effect of oxidized LDL on macrophage motility

↓

Uptake of oxidized LDL via acetyl LDL receptor

↓

Foam cells and fatty streak

FIGURE 1-20. Elevated levels of plasma low-density lipoprotein (LDL) alone may be sufficient to initiate the fatty streak lesion. High levels of plasma LDL may increase the availability of LDL in the intima. Free or matrix-bound LDL may undergo oxidation by cells such as endothelial cells (EC), smooth muscle cells (SMC), or macrophages (M0). The mildly oxidized LDL may increase the chemotactic recruitment of monocytes by inducing the expression of monocyte chemotactic protein-1 (MCP-1) or by generating lysophospholipids (more extensively, oxidized LDL). Monocytes may differentiate into macrophages and components of oxidized LDL may promote retention of macrophages in the artery. Macrophages and oxidized LDL may then interact via scavenger pathways leading to foam cell formation. (*Adapted from* Steinberg [19] and Quinn *et al.* [20].)

SOME PRO-ATHEROGENIC EFFECTS OF OXIDIZED LDL

Oxidized LDL is degraded at a faster rate than native LDL by macrophages leading to lipid accumulation.

Oxidized LDL is chemotactic to monocytes, smooth muscle cells, and T lymphocytes, and induces T-cell activation and monocyte differentiation.

Oxidized LDL inhibits macrophage motility, potentially trapping macrophages in the artery.

Components of oxidized LDL are cytotoxic to cells.

Oxidized LDL inhibits endothelium-dependent relaxation factor.

Minimally oxidized LDL enhances monocyte adhesion to endothelium.

Minimally oxidized LDL induces the expression of monocyte chemotactic protein-1 and granulocyte-macrophage colony stimulating factors.

Oxidized LDL inhibits the migration of endothelial cells.

Oxidized LDL induces the expression of adhesion molecules on the endothelium.

Components of oxidized LDL induces interleukin-1 synthesis and secretion by macrophages.

FIGURE 1-21. Some pro-atherogenic effects of oxidized low-density lipoprotein (LDL). Oxidized LDL used in these studies is not homogeneous and does not represent any specific preparation. The lipoproteins used may vary in their content of oxidized lipids and their decomposition products. Oxidized LDL also has other pro-atherogenic effects on platelet function, on the relaxation of endothelium, and on smooth muscle cells.

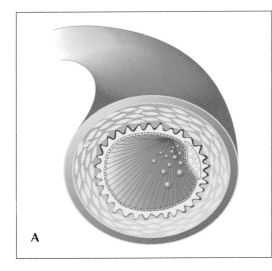

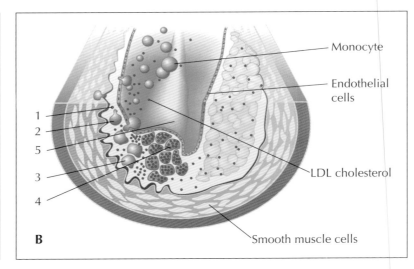

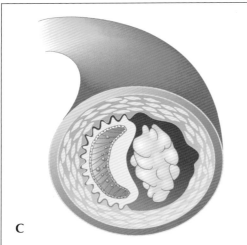

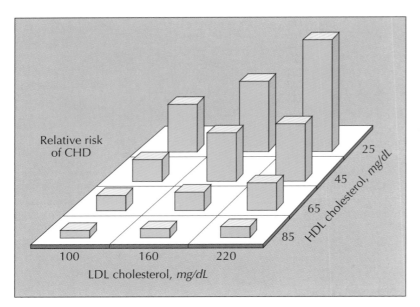

FIGURE 1-22. The atherosclerotic process. **A,** Artery depicting early fatty streak development. **B,** *1,* low-density lipoprotein (LDL) becomes oxidized within the arterial subendothelial space. *2,* Circulating monocytes are recruited to the subendothelial space by chemoattractants including oxidized LDL. *3,* These monocytes undergo differentiation, becoming macrophages, which are scavenger cells that recognize and accumulate oxidized LDL. *4,* The lipid-laden macrophages then become foam cells, which cluster under the endothelial lining to form a bulge into the artery. *5,* This bulge is called a fatty streak and is the first overt sign of atherosclerotic change. **C,** Cross-section of an artery with an atherosclerotic lesion with a narrowed lumen. (*Courtesy of* Merrell Dow Pharmaceuticals Inc., Cincinnati, OH.)

HIGH-DENSITY LIPOPROTEINS

FIGURE 1-23. The Framingham Heart Study: risk of coronary heart disease (CHD) by high-density lipoprotein (HDL) and low-density lipoprotein (LDL) cholesterol. Epidemiologic studies have definitely established that total and LDL cholesterol concentrations are directly correlated with clinical coronary atherosclerosis [21]. The inverse association of HDL cholesterol concentrations with CHD endpoints have also been established in both cross-sectional and prospective epidemiologic studies [22]. In the Framingham Heart Study, the interrelationship between LDL and HDL cholesterol concentrations and the relative risk of developing CHD is particularly striking [23]. For individuals with HDL cholesterol concentrations of 45 mg/dL or less, the risk of CHD increases as the LDL cholesterol concentrations increase. However, patients with elevated HDL cholesterol concentrations appear protected. This protection is striking at 65 mg/dL, and at 85 mg/dL even high concentrations of LDL may increase CHD risk only modestly. Therefore, high concentrations of HDL cholesterol in the blood are associated with a remarkably lower risk for developing vascular disease.

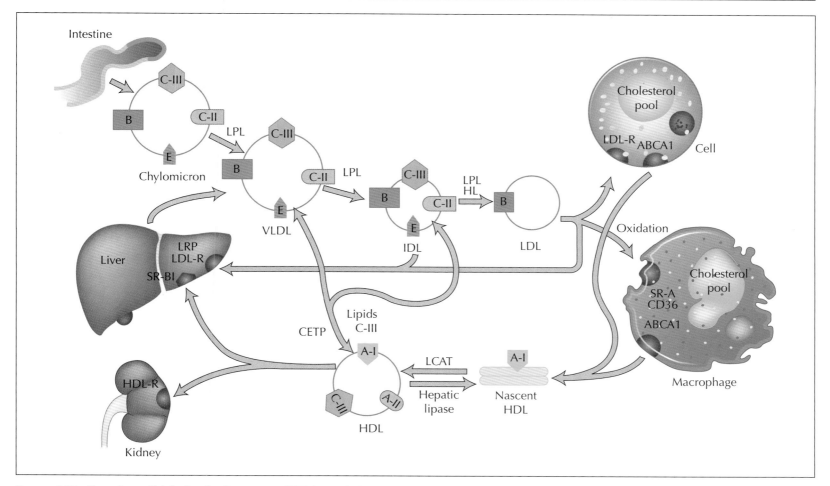

FIGURE 1-24. Overview of high-density lipoprotein (HDL) metabolism and reverse cholesterol transport. Four major pathways are involved in the synthesis of mature HDL. Nascent or pre-HDL, which are composed primarily of apolipoprotein (apo) A-I phospholipid disks, are secreted from the human intestine and liver. Lipids and apolipoprotein constituents of HDL are acquired from the intravascular metabolism and remodeling of both-triglyceride rich chylomicrons and hepatic very low-density lipoprotein (VLDL), which converts nascent HDL to mature HDL. Nascent HDL plays a pivotal role in lipoprotein metabolism and reverse cholesterol transport by facilitating the efflux of excess cholesterol from the membranes of peripheral cells including macrophages by interaction with the ABCA1 transporter [24]. The free cholesterol on nascent HDL is esterified to cholesteryl esters by lecithin cholesterol acyltransferase (LCAT). With the formation of cholesteryl esters, the nascent HDL are converted to spherical lipoproteins with a hydrated density of HDL$_3$. HDL$_3$ are converted to the larger HDL$_2$ by the acquisition of lipids and apolipoproteins (*eg*, apo C-III) released during the stepwise delipidation and remodeling of the triglyceride-rich chylomicrons and VLDL and by the esterification of the choles-

terol removed from peripheral tissues. HDL transports cholesterol back to the liver by two pathways. The first pathway involves a direct delivery of cholesterol to the liver by a newly recognized receptor, SR-BI [24–26], that functions to remove cholesteryl esters selectively from lipoproteins without holoparticle uptake and degradation. Additionally, HDL particles are taken up intact and degraded by receptors primarily in the liver and kidney. In the second pathway, HDL cholesteryl esters are exchanged for triglycerides in the apo B-containing lipoproteins (VLDL, intermediate-density lipoprotein [IDL], low-density lipoprotein [LDL]) by the cholesteryl ester transfer protein (CETP) [27]. A significant fraction of cholesteryl esters present in HDL are transferred back to the liver by the LDL pathway. Thus, cholesterol may be transported back to the liver directly by HDL or following exchange to VLDL-IDL-LDL. It also has been proposed that a variable portion of tissue cholesterol is transported to the liver by HDL particles containing apo E, which may interact with both the hepatic LRP (LDL receptor–related protein) and LDL receptors (LDL-R). HDL-R—high-density lipoprotein receptors; HL—hepatic lipase; LPL—lipoprotein lipase.

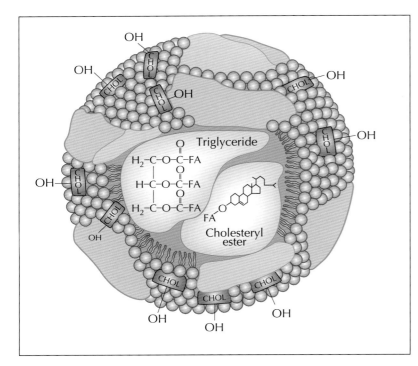

FIGURE 1-25. Schematic model of a plasma high-density lipoprotein particle. The surface of the lipoprotein particle is covered by phospholipids with the polar head groups of the phospholipids interacting with the aqueous environment. The protein components of the lipoprotein, designated apolipoproteins, and cholesterol (CHOL) are intercalated between the polar head groups of the phospholipids. The neutral lipids, cholesteryl esters and triglycerides, fill the core of the lipoprotein particle. Several different apolipoproteins are present on the lipoprotein particle. The apolipoproteins are associated with the lipoprotein particle by protein–protein as well as protein–lipid interactions. The apolipoprotein functions in lipoprotein metabolism as ligands for receptors, cofactors for enzymes, and structural proteins for lipoprotein particle biosynthesis [28].

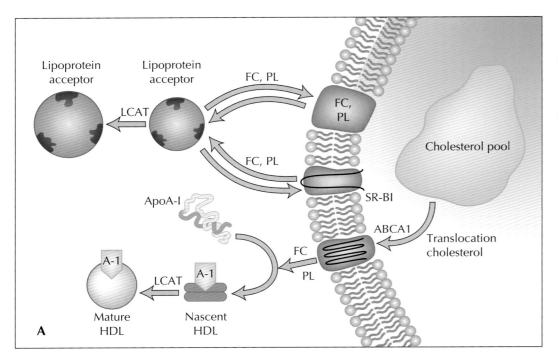

FIGURE 1-26. The ABCA1 transporter. Poorly lipidated apolipoprotein (apo) A1 interacts with the ABCA1 transporter to facilitate the removal of excess cholesterol from peripheral cells. The nascent high-density lipoprotein (HDL) formed following the interaction of apo A1 with the ABCA1 transporter on the cell membrane is converted to mature HDL by the LCAT (**A**). (*continued*)

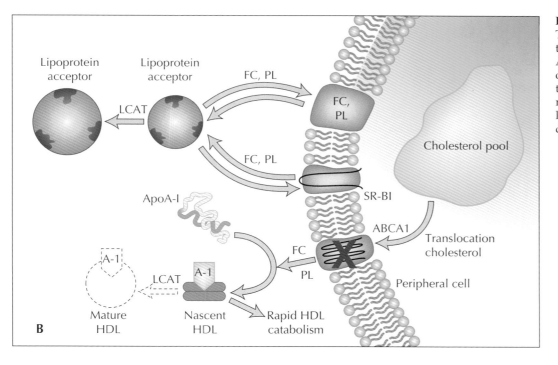

FIGURE 1-26. (*continued*) The genetic defect in Tangier disease (**B**) is a structural mutation in the ABCA1 transporter. The defect in the ABCA1 transporter results in decreased efflux of cholesterol from the cell and reduced lipidation of apo A1. The poorly lipidated HDL is rapidly degraded by the kidney, leading to the low plasma HDL levels characteristic of Tangier disease [29].

TREATMENT OF HYPOALPHALIPOPROTEINEMIA

Beneficial lifestyle changes to increase plasma HDL levels
  Exercise
  Caloric restriction if the patient is not at ideal body weight
  Stop cigarette smoking
Drug treatment of hypoalphalipoproteinemia
  Nicotinic acid
  Fibrates
  Statins
  Bile sequestrants

FIGURE 1-27. Individuals with established coronary heart disease or an increased risk of cardiovascular disease based on family history or other clinical parameters should be considered for diet and lifestyle changes as well as drug treatment when appropriate. In addition, to specifically raise high-density lipoprotein (HDL), the use of agents such as statins to lower low-density lipoprotein cholesterol in a patient with reduced HDL cholesterol is useful. There are no definitive prospective studies to date that have established that raising HDL reduces the risk or decreases the progression of established atherosclerosis in patients with low HDL. Most experts believe that there is enough evidence to warrant drug treatment in those individuals with established disease or with a strong family history of cardiovascular disease cosegregating with low HDL.

TRIGLYCERIDE-RICH LIPOPROTEINS

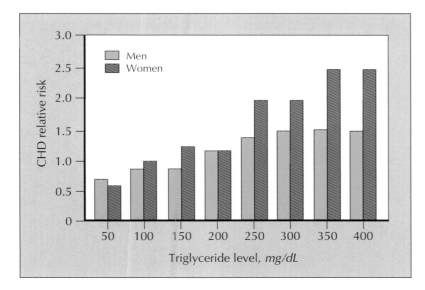

FIGURE 1-28. The incidence of coronary heart disease (CHD)–induced events, such as myocardial infarction and cardiac death, was found to be higher in both men and women with triglyceride levels above the mean for the population. The increase is most obvious as the baseline levels rise from approximately 150 to 350 mg/dL. This relationship of plasma triglycerides to risk of CHD is often stronger in women than in men, as was found in the Framingham Heart Study [23].

RISK FACTORS ASSOCIATED WITH PLASMA TRIGLYCERIDES

Low HDL cholesterol

Low apo A-I

Increased LDL cholesterol

Increased apo B

Small dense LDL

Glucose intolerance

   Insulin resistance/hyperinsulinemia

   Diabetes mellitus

Obesity (abdominal obesity?)

High blood pressure

FIGURE 1-29. Risk factors associated with increased plasma triglycerides include low high-density lipoprotein (HDL) cholesterol, low apolipoprotein A-I (apo A-I), increased low-density lipoprotein (LDL) cholesterol, and small dense LDL particles. In addition, glucose intolerance with insulin resistance and hyperinsulinemia or definite diabetes mellitus is frequently found. Obesity is a common contributing factor to hypertriglyceridemia. The occurrence of intra-abdominal obesity, in particular, appears to be linked to glucose intolerance, high blood pressure, and the lipoprotein abnormalities noted above [30].

RISK OF CHD WITH INCREASING TRIGLYCERIDES

	RELATIVE RISK*	
	MEN	WOMEN
Univariate analysis	1.33	2.02
Adjusted for HDL cholesterol	1.24	1.57

*Risk ratio for CHD in middle-aged persons for each 100 mg/dL rise in serum triglycerides. Data based on meta-analysis of 14 prospective studies [35].

FIGURE 1-30. In recent meta-analyses of several observational studies, the simple measurement of total plasma triglycerides in men has been found to predict an increase in vascular events by 33% for each 100 mg/dL increase in the plasma concentration [31]. A similar rise in plasma triglycerides for women was associated with an increase in risk of coronary heart disease (CHD) by 100%. Men with plasma triglyceride levels of 300 mg/dL would be expected to have 66% more CHD than their counterparts with a plasma triglyceride level of 100 mg/dL. For women, a similar increase in plasma triglycerides would be expected to increase risk of CHD by fourfold.

There is a moderate, but highly significant, inverse relationship between plasma triglyceride and HDL cholesterol concentrations. When the risk associated with a rise in triglycerides from 100 to 300 mg/dL is adjusted for the lower HDL cholesterol, the residual effect is a 47% and 113% increased risk of CHD and in men and women, respectively. Furthermore, individuals with moderately elevated triglycerides (range, 200 to 500 mg/dL) often have higher LDL cholesterol levels; the adjustment for this relationship further reduces the risk that can be assigned specifically to elevations in triglycerides.

The usual daily fluctuations in human plasma levels are much greater for triglycerides than for cholesterol. This variation would significantly weaken any correlation of triglycerides with CHD risk. Few studies have accounted for the true biologic variation in triglycerides and, in fact, virtually all large studies have used single measures for statistical analyses. This may mean that the reported positive relationship between CHD risk and plasma triglycerides may be significantly stronger than current estimates [32].

SYNTHESIS AND METABOLISM OF CHYLOMICRONS AND VLDL

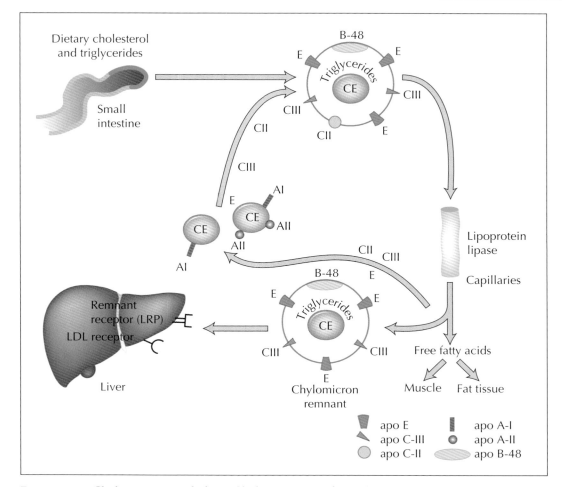

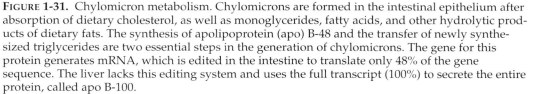

FIGURE 1-31. Chylomicron metabolism. Chylomicrons are formed in the intestinal epithelium after absorption of dietary cholesterol, as well as monoglycerides, fatty acids, and other hydrolytic products of dietary fats. The synthesis of apolipoprotein (apo) B-48 and the transfer of newly synthesized triglycerides are two essential steps in the generation of chylomicrons. The gene for this protein generates mRNA, which is edited in the intestine to translate only 48% of the gene sequence. The liver lacks this editing system and uses the full transcript (100%) to secrete the entire protein, called apo B-100.

Several additional apolipoproteins are transferred from high-density lipoprotein (HDL) to chylomicrons after arrival in the plasma. These include apo C-II, a small (9 kD) protein essential for activity of lipoprotein lipase. Apo C-III is a negatively charged protein of the same size that is believed to 1) stabilize the surface, preventing aggregation of lipid particles, and 2) inhibit uptake by cell surfaces, allowing preferential binding to lipoprotein lipase for hydrolysis at the capillary endothelial cell as mediated by apo C-II. The apo C-II and apo C-III proteins are released during lipase action to return to HDL [33].

A third protein, apo E, is also added to chylomicrons through transfer from HDL. Compared with apo C-II and C-III, a lesser amount of this is released from chylomicrons by lipoprotein lipase. Consequent to this enzyme action, remnant particles are generated that are relatively depleted in triglycerides, apo C-II, and apo C-III but relatively enriched in cholesteryl esters and apo E. A single copy of apo B-48 and many copies of apo E reside on this remnant particle. On circulation through the liver, there are at least two receptors that have high affinity for apo E; these include the LDL receptor and a larger protein referred to as the LDL-receptor related protein (LRP) [34]. Apo B-48 does not have a binding site for either of these receptors.

Uptake in the liver can be regulated by the numbers of apo E and apo C-III molecules. The greater the number of copies of apo E, the higher the affinity of the particle for liver cell surfaces, presumably due to multisite attachment. Increased quantities of apo C-III displace apo E to HDL and reduce the rate of uptake of remnants by the liver.

Hepatic triglyceride lipase is another enzyme on cell surfaces in Disse's spaces. This enzyme may further digest chylomicron remnant triglycerides and phospholipids. It also removes apo E from the surface of these particles [35]. Its role in the clearance of chylomicron remnant lipoprotein is not fully understood.

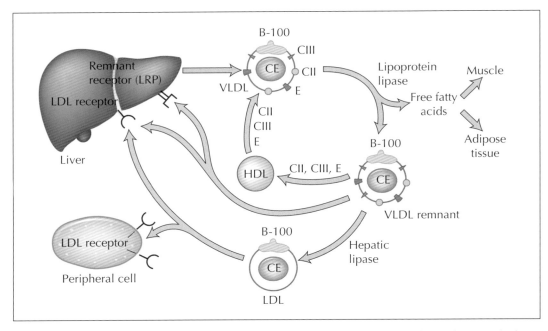

FIGURE 1-32. Metabolism of very low-density lipoproteins (VLDL). Triglyceride synthesis in the liver provides for efficient energy transfer into the plasma as VLDL. The VLDL particle is assembled by adding lipid to a large (550,000 D) protein, apo B-100. This protein is a full transcript of the apo B gene. Several copies of apo C-II, apo C-III, and apo E are also added in the liver cell, although additional copies of these latter proteins are transferred from HDL to the nascent VLDL after their arrival in the plasma. VLDLs follow a process similar to that discussed in Figure 1-31 for chylomicrons involving lipoprotein lipase and the generation of a remnant lipoproteins [33]. Major differences in

the fate of VLDL remnants as compared with chylomicron remnants are possible. VLDL remnants have available an additional binding site for the LDL receptor via apo B-100. However, they are taken up by liver cells less rapidly than are chylomicron remnants. This may be because of their containing fewer apo E molecules per particle—a function of their smaller size and surface area.

The VLDL remnant may alternatively be converted to LDL via the action of hepatic triglyceride lipase, which does not require the presence of apo C-II [36]. The LDL conversion is possible because apo B-100 can adopt a configuration that stabilizes a particle of the size and composition of LDL (apo B-48 does not appear capable of this function). Conversion of VLDL remnants involves removing most of the remaining triglyceride and leaving cholesteryl esters as the major core lipid. In addition, residual apo E, apo C-II, and apo C-III are removed. Most LDL in the plasma of humans appears to be derived from this pathway. Its clearance from the plasma is highly dependent on the LDL receptor because apo B-100 does not bind to the LDL-receptor related protein (LRP). Every cell in the normal human body is capable of expressing LDL receptors. However, most available LDL receptors occur on hepatocytes and, therefore, the liver removes 75% to 80% of LDL. HDL—high-density lipoprotein.

INHERITED SYNDROMES WITH HYPERTRIGLYCERIDEMIA

DYSBETALIPOPROTEINEMIA

Phenotype	Increased concentrations of VLDL and chylomicron remnants
	VLDL cholesterol/triglyceride >0.3 enriched in apo E rich β mobility on electrophoresis
Frequency	1/5000
Inheritance	Polygenic
Probable cause	Apo E defective (E2/E2)
Clinical consequence	Increased production of VLDL
	Increased CHD
	Tubero-eruptive xanthomata
	Palmar xanthomata

FIGURE 1-33. Dysbetalipoproteinemia is an uncommon disorder of remnant clearance caused by the superimposition of at least two common genetic traits. The first is a defective apolipoprotein (apo) E molecule that has very low binding affinity for remnant receptors. There are three common alleles for apo E, two of which (E3 and E4) bind normally [37,38]. A third common allele, E2, results in a defective protein with weak binding affinity. Approximately 15% of the population has at least one defective allele, and approximately 1% is homozygous for this allele. Dysbetalipoproteinemia is usually a recessive trait (ie, requires two defective alleles). Other less common defective E proteins may have no affinity for the receptor and the clinical disorder may

be expressed as a heterozygous defect [38]. Marked elevations in remnants do not usually occur unless there is a concomitant overproduction of very low-density lipoprotein (VLDL) that is separately inherited. The coexistence of two traits, each of which exists in 1% to 2% of the population, gives the observed expression of one in 5000 to one in 10,000 persons.

The clinical diagnosis is suggested by elevations of cholesterol and triglycerides to approximately equivalent levels (250 to 800 mg/dL each). There are tubero-eruptive xanthomata on elbows (see Fig. 1-34), knees, or buttocks in 15% to 30% of patients, and some have planar xanthomata along the palmar creases [39].

The isolation of VLDL can confirm the diagnosis because the remnant particles are relatively rich in cholesterol and apo E, with lesser amounts of apo C-II and apo C-III. Consequently, the cholesterol-to-triglyceride mass ratio for isolated VLDL is greater than 0.3 as compared with a ratio of 0.2 obtained for normal VLDL. In addition, the isolated VLDLs have electrophoretic mobility comparable to β-globulins and LDL rather than normal pre-β mobility.

Atherosclerosis is prevalent in both peripheral arteries and in the coronary arteries of affected persons by midlife.

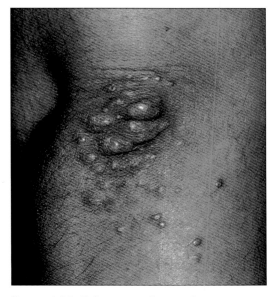

FIGURE 1-34. Tubero-eruptive xanthomata on the elbow of a patient with dysbetalipoproteinemia. (Courtesy of J. Davignon, MD, Montreal, Canada.)

FAMILIAL COMBINED HYPERLIPIDEMIA

Phenotype	Increased VLDL and/or LDL of normal composition; the dominant lipoprotein elevation may present as VLDL *or* LDL
Frequency	1%–2% of population
Inheritance	Autosomal dominant with expression in the third to fourth decade; first-degree relatives may show elevated VLDL and/or LDL
Probable cause	Overproduction of VLDL particles and consequent increased LDL production
Clinical consequences	Increased CHD

FIGURE 1-35. Familial combined hyperlipidemia is one of the most common forms of hypertriglyceridemia [40]. It is usually defined as the existence of elevated triglycerides or elevated LDL cholesterol (exceeding the 95th percentile for age and gender) with one or more first-degree relatives similarly affected. VLDL is normal in composition and has pre-β mobility on electrophoresis. Children usually have high values of triglycerides for their age but may not fully express the disorder until the fourth decade of life [41]. LDL may be only moderately elevated at times, particularly when the triglyceride level exceeds 400 mg/dL.

Overproduction of apo B-100 has been well demonstrated in several kindreds who meet the definition for this disorder [42,43]. The association with coronary heart disease (CHD) in the fifth through seventh decades is well established.

FAMILIAL HYPERTRIGLYCERIDEMIA

Phenotype	Increased VLDL with normal or low LDL; fasting chylomicrons occasionally present
Frequency	1/100
Inheritance	Autosomal dominant
Probable cause	Overproduction of triglycerides without incurred conversion of VLDL to LDL
Clinical consequences	No definite relation to CHD

FIGURE 1-36. Familial hypertriglyceridemia is characterized by increased plasma very low-density lipoprotein (VLDL) triglycerides and, in some cases, with triglycerides above 500 mg/dL, chylomicrons may be present in fasting plasma [42]. The total cholesterol may lie within normal limits because LDL cholesterol and HDL cholesterol are often at or below the lower limits of normal. Hepatic synthesis of triglyceride is increased, although the higher rate of VLDL particle production seen in familial combined hyperlipidemia is not observed [43,44]. The nascent VLDLs are presumed to be larger and relatively more triglyceride-rich than nascent particles.

HDL cholesterol is reduced and small dense LDL and HDL are usually present. The risk of coronary heart disease (CHD) may be only modestly increased, perhaps due to the low LDL cholesterol.

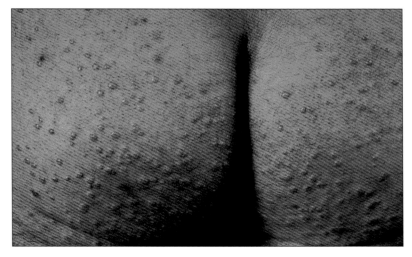

FIGURE 1-37. Eruptive xanthomata on the buttocks of a patient with familial hypertriglyceridemia and hyperchylomicronemic syndrome [45]. (*Courtesy of* J. Davignon, MD, Montreal, Canada.)

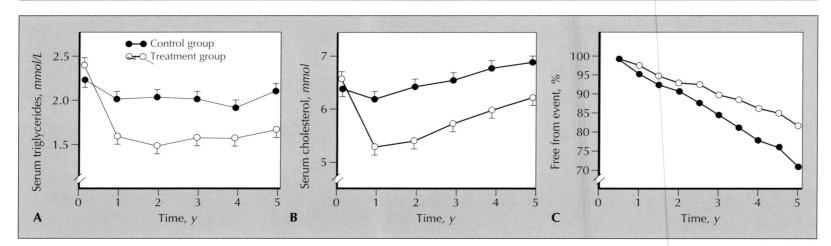

FIGURE 1-38. The Stockholm Ischemic Heart Disease Study was designed to assess plasma lipid reduction as a means of preventing recurrent coronary heart disease (CHD) in those patients who had experienced a myocardial infarction. Five hundred fifty-five men and women age under 79 years of age were assigned randomly to either niacin plus clofibrate or to placebo.

A, The total triglyceride level fell from 2.4 mmol/L (211 mg/dL) to 1.6 mmol/L (140 mg/dL) in the active treatment group. The control group experienced a decline from 2.2 mmol/L (191 mg/dL) to 2.0 mmol/L (176 mg/dL). **B,** The total cholesterol level was reduced from 6.6 mmol/L (254 mg/dL) to 5.2 mmol/L (200 mg/dL) initially; by the end of the study, however, the mean plasma cholesterol had risen to 6.1 mmol/L (235

mg/dL). The control group had a steady rise in cholesterol over the 5 years. **C,** The number of persons suffering a recurrent infarction or cardiovascular death was significantly reduced. At the end of the study, only 71% of the control group had not suffered an event whereas 83% of the treated group were event-free. The total mortality was also significantly reduced because of the marked decline in cardiovascular mortality (36%).

The reduction in CHD events was directly related to triglyceride reduction but had no correlation with the decline in cholesterol. However, low-density lipoprotein cholesterol and high-density lipoprotein (HDL) cholesterol were not measured. Both the drugs used elevated HDL cholesterol significantly, and this probably minimized the change in total plasma cholesterol. (*Adapted from* Carlson and Rosenhamer [46].)

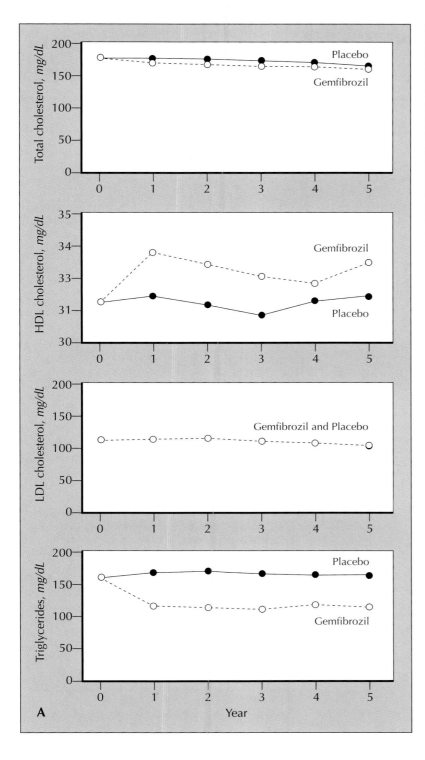

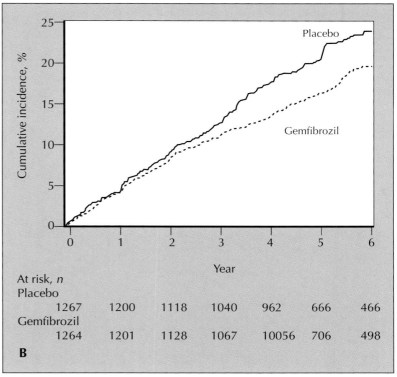

FIGURE 1-39. **A** and **B**, Veterans Affairs Cooperative Studies Program. The High-density Lipoprotein Cholesterol Intervention Trial [VA-HIT] demonstrated that a fibrate (gemfibrozil) can reduce cumulative incidence of coronary death or myocardial infarction without changing low-density lipoprotein (LDL) cholesterol or total plasma cholesterol in patients with low high-density lipoprotein (HDL) cholesterol and pre-existing coronary artery disease [47].

DIETARY TREATMENT

RISK FACTORS

MAJOR CARDIOVASCULAR RISK FACTORS

MODIFIABLE

Lipids and lipoproteins
  Cholesterol*
  Triglycerides*
  LDL*
  HDL*
  Remnant lipoproteins*
  Postprandial lipoproteins*
  Lp(a)
Blood pressure*
Diabetes mellitus*
Cigarette smoking
Central obesity/insulin resistance*

FIXED

Age
Gender
Family history

FIGURE 1-40. The major cardiovascular risk factors can be divided into two main groups: modifiable and fixed. Several lipids and lipoproteins have been demonstrated to be important cardiovascular risk factors, including total cholesterol, low-density lipoprotein (LDL) cholesterol, low levels of high-density lipoprotein (HDL) cholesterol, remnant lipoproteins, postprandial lipoproteins, lipoprotein (a) [Lp(a)], and triglycerides. Other modifiable risk factors include blood pressure, diabetes mellitus, cigarette smoking, and the central obesity/insulin resistance syndrome. Many of these risk factors can be influenced by diet, as designated by the *asterisks*.

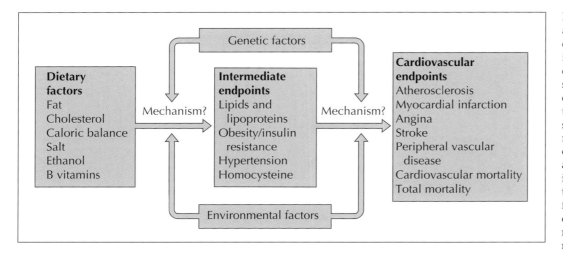

FIGURE 1-41. Ways in which risk factors may affect intermediate and cardiovascular endpoints. Dietary risk factors such as saturated fat, cholesterol, positive caloric balance, salt, and ethanol, and coupled with reduced intake of several B vitamins can affect intermediate endpoints such as lipids, lipoproteins, homocysteine, obesity/insulin resistance, and hypertension. When present in excess, these intermediate markers, or risk factors, can lead to cardiovascular endpoints such as myocardial infarction, angina, peripheral vascular disease, stroke, increased cardiovascular mortality, and increased total mortality. Both genetic and environmental factors may influence the response of intermediate endpoints to dietary factors, although the mechanisms by which genetic and environmental factors contribute remain unclear. Both types of risk factors also may have a direct effect on the response of the arterial wall, independent of these intermediate risk factors, thereby affecting cardiovascular endpoints.

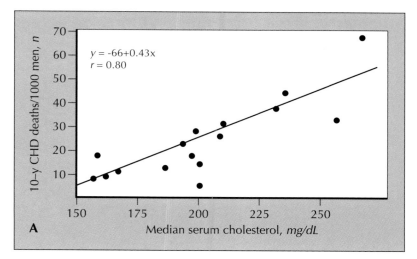

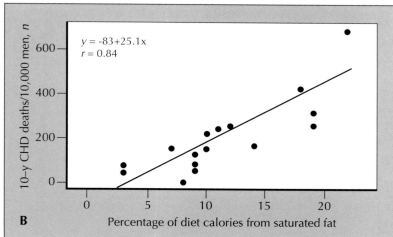

FIGURE 1-42. Comparison of the rates of coronary heart disease (CHD) mortality and serum cholesterol levels in countries consuming different average amounts of dietary fat and cholesterol. In 16 population groups from seven countries (The Seven Countries Study), there was a linear relationship between 10-year CHD mortality rates and median serum cholesterol levels (**A**). A similar relationship was demonstrated between CHD mortality rates and percentage of calories from fat (**B**). For example, in those countries where the consumption of fat constituted about 40% of calories and saturated fat accounted for about 20% of calories such as in Finland, the United States, and the Netherlands, there were higher average serum cholesterol levels and increased mortality from CHD as compared with countries such as Japan and Greece, where saturated fat consumption was less than 10% of calories and serum cholesterol levels were lower. (Part A *adapted from* Keys [48]; part B *adapted from* Keys *et al.* [49].)

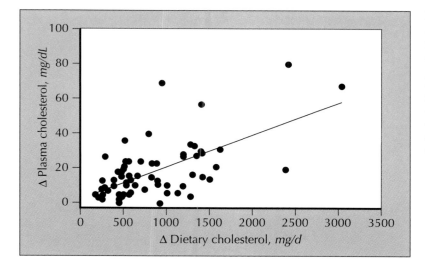

FIGURE 1-43. Relationship between change in dietary cholesterol intake and serum cholesterol levels. The data shown represent 68 clinical studies in 1490 patients summarized by McNamara [50]. There is a positive and significant correlation between the increment in dietary cholesterol intake (in milligrams per day) and the average change in plasma cholesterol levels (in milligrams per deciliter). This change represents an average 1.8 mg/dL change in cholesterol for every 100-mg increment in dietary cholesterol. When the data are normalized per 100 mg/d increment in dietary cholesterol, similar values are obtained, with a mean increase in serum cholesterol of 2.3 mg/dL for every 100 mg/d increase in dietary cholesterol. (*Adapted from* McNamara [50].)

DIETARY INTERVENTION TRIALS ON CORONARY EVENTS

TRIAL*	SUBJECTS IN THE INTERVENTION GROUP	DIETARY INTERVENTION	DIETARY FAT IN THE TREATMENT GROUP, % ENERGY	P:S RATIO IN THE TREATMENT GROUP	DURATION, Y	CHANGE IN SERUM CHOLESTEROL, %†	CHANGE IN CHD, %‡
MRC low-fat diet	123 MI patients, all men	Reduce total fat	22	NR	3	-5	+4
DART	1015 MI patients, all men	Reduce total fat	32	0.8	2	-3.5	-9
Finnish Mental Hospital	676 men	Unsaturated fat → saturated fat	35	1.5	6	-15	-43
Los Angeles Veterans	424 men, most having no evidence of existing heart disease	Unsaturated fat → saturated fat	40	NR	8	-13	-31
Oslo Diet Heart Study	206 MI patients, all men	Unsaturated fat → saturated fat	39	2.4	5	-14	-25
MRC soy oil	199 MI patients, all men	Unsaturated fat → saturated fat	46	2.0	4	-16	-12
Minnesota Coronary Survey	4393 men and 4664 women	Unsaturated fat → saturated fat	38	1.6	4.5	-14	No change
Indian Experiment of Infarct Survival	204 MI patients, primarily men	High fruits, vegetables, nuts, fish, and pulses	24	1.2	1	-9	-40
Lyon Diet Heart Study	302 MI patients, primarily men	Mediterranean diet	31	0.7	2.3	No change	-73

*References for each trial can be found in Hu *et al.* [51].
†Refers to the percentage change in serum cholesterol in the treatment group compared with the change in the control group.
‡Refers to the percentage in coronary event rates in the treatment compared with the control group.

FIGURE 1-44. Dietary intervention trials with clinical endpoints. In general, dietary intervention trials support the benefit of replacing saturated fat with polyunsaturated fat (indicated by the *arrows*).

CHD—coronary heart disease; DART—Diet and Reinfarction Trial; MI—myocardial infarction; MRC—Medical Research Council; NR—not reported. (*Adapted from* Hu *et al.* [51].)

STRATEGIES TO IMPROVE COMPLIANCE

Explain reasons for requiring dietary change
Evaluate baseline (habitual) diet
Set specific dietary goals
  Select nutritious, tasty foods that are low in fat and cholesterol
  Develop diet that matches patient's lifestyle
Offer specific recommendations about dietary change
Provide educational materials
Follow-up regularly
  Reinforcement
  Answer questions
  Address problem areas

FIGURE 1-45. Strategies to improve compliance with a cholesterol-lowering diet. To aid compliance, the patient must understand the reason for recommending dietary change. The patient's baseline (habitual) diet should be assessed to determine what high-fat foods are usually consumed and whether to start with a Step I or Step II diet. It is important to set specific dietary goals for the patient. This includes selection of nutritious and tasty foods that are low in fat and cholesterol and provision of sufficient variety to prevent boredom. It is important to develop a diet that matches the patient's lifestyle, from the standpoints of ethnicity, practicality, and taste preferences. Specific recommendations about dietary change need to be made rather than generalizations. This is best done with the help of a qualified dietitian or nutritionist. Provision of educational materials can be helpful in allowing the patient to study aspects of the diet at leisure. Regular follow-up will enhance compliance. Follow-up will allow a reinforcement of the diet, the opportunity for the patient to ask questions related to specific foods, and to address difficulties with compliance.

FOODS RICH IN MONOUNSATURATED FATTY ACIDS

Olive oil
Canola (rape seed) oil
Peanut oil
Nuts
Avocados

FIGURE 1-46. Sources of monounsaturated fatty acids (oleic acid). The major oils that contain monounsaturated fatty acids are olive oil, rape seed oil (canola oil), and peanut oil. All these oils also contain small amounts of saturated and unsaturated fatty acids. Nuts and avocados are also rich dietary sources of monounsaturated fatty acids.

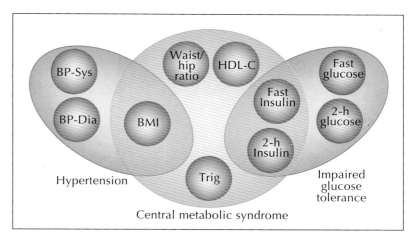

FIGURE 1-48. Risk factors for a metabolic syndrome. Metabolic risk factor clustering was studied in the Framingham offspring. When principal components analysis was used, there appeared to be three distinct domains: one related to hypertension that included measurement of blood pressure measures and body mass index (BMI), a second related to glycemia that included fasting and measurement of postprandial glucose and insulin, and a central core with waist/hip ratio, high-density lipoprotein cholesterol (HDL-C), triglycerides (Trig), fasting and postprandial insulin, and BMI. This approach was undertaken to improve understanding of the insulin resistance syndrome, how factors cluster together, and how coronary heart disease (CHD) risk is increased [52]. BP-Dia—diastolic blood pressure; BP-Sys—systolic blood pressure.

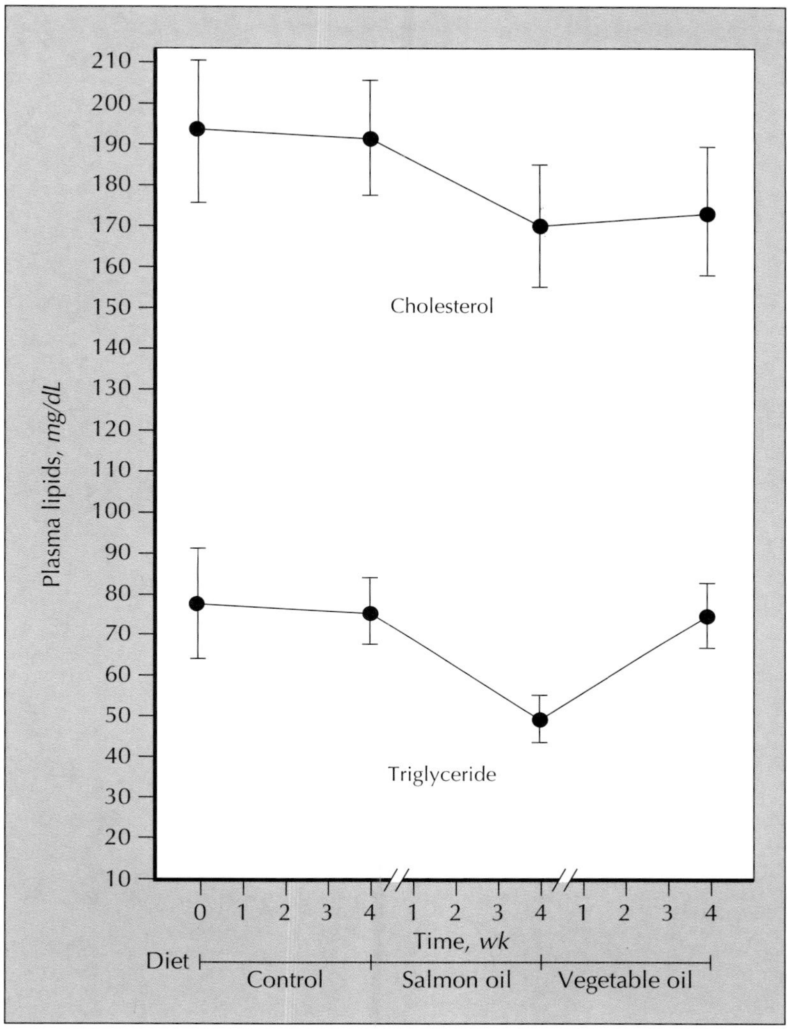

FIGURE 1-47. Effect of fish oils (omega-3 fatty acids) on plasma lipids. In normal subjects, supplements of omega-3 fatty acids primarily lower very low-density lipoprotein (LDL) levels, which leads to a reduction in both triglycerides and cholesterol. However, LDL cholesterol levels do not change (not shown). High-density lipoprotein levels tend to increase, as is commonly seen, when triglyceride levels fall. Several studies in both humans and experimental animals have suggested that omega-3 fatty acids may reduce atherosclerotic artery disease. Several mechanisms may be responsible for this response. Diets rich in fish oils tend to be low in saturated fatty acids. Omega-3 fatty acids may have an antithrombotic effect, both by interfering with platelet aggregation and by modulating prostaglandin and leukotriene metabolism, which in turn may also impact on vascular tone. These fatty acids may thus be antithrombotic, with consequent effects on atherogenesis and thrombosis.

CLINICAL IDENFICATION OF THE METABOLIC SYNDROME

RISK FACTOR	DEFINING LEVEL
Abdominal obesity (waist circumference)	
Men	> 102 cm (> 40 in)
Women	> 88 cm (> 35 in)
Triglycerides	≥ 150 mg/dL
High-density lipoprotein cholesterol	
Men	< 40 mg/dL
Women	< 50 mg/dL
Blood pressure	≥ 130/≥ 85 mm Hg
Fasting glucose	≥ 110 mg/dL

FIGURE 1-49. Metabolic syndrome criteria as proposed by the National Cholesterol Education Program. Core criteria that are being used to help identify persons with insulin resistance and abdominal adiposity (*Adapted from* [53].)

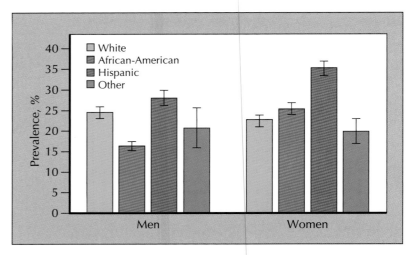

FIGURE 1-50. Age-adjusted prevalence of the metabolic syndrome among 8814 US adults aged at least 20 years, by sex and race or ethnicity. Data are presented as percentage (SE). (*Adapted from* Ford *et al.* [54].)

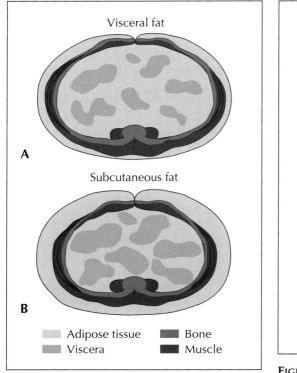

FIGURE 1-51. The concept of intra-abdominal obesity has developed because of observational studies demonstrating a correlation between measures of "central obesity" (waist-hip or waist-thigh ratios) and risk of coronary heart disease [55]. The use of CT of the abdomen allows an improved assessment of central fat illustrating significant independence of visceral as opposed to subcutaneous adipose tissue accumulation [56]. Shown are representative CT scans of two individuals with comparable body mass indices. **A**, Excess visceral fat. **B**, The majority of the fat is present subcutaneously. The blood flow from visceral fat into the portal system and evidence for a relatively enhanced lipolysis with catechol stimuli compared with subcutaneous adipocytes strongly suggests that this type of obesity may have direct metabolic effects, changing glucose and fat metabolism [57].

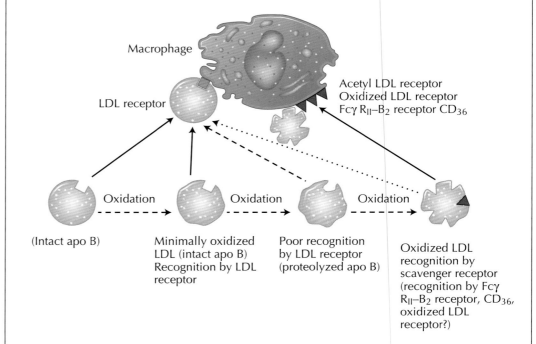

FIGURE 1-52. Low-density lipoprotein (LDL) and scavenger receptor activities as a function of time in culture. LDL and minimally oxidized LDL are recognized by the LDL receptor. Incubation of macrophages with these lipoproteins does not result in lipid accumulation. Further oxidation results in poor recognition by the LDL receptor. More extensively oxidized LDL is recognized by the macrophage scavenger receptors and other uncharacterized receptors. Extensively oxidized LDL may also be recognized by CD_{36}, FcgR11B2, and several other surface proteins. During the differentiation of monocytes in culture, scavenger receptors are induced. The relative contribution of different scavenger receptors in the uptake of oxidized LDL has not been established.

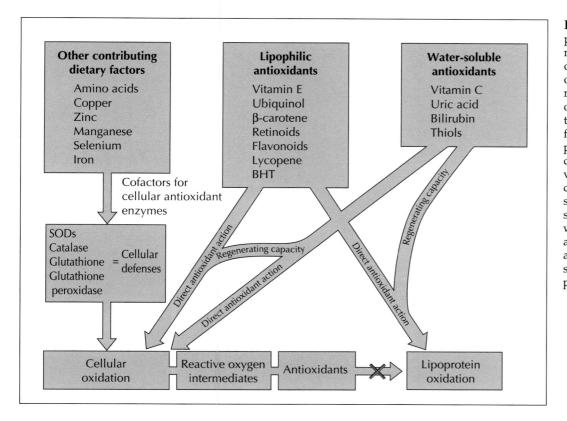

FIGURE 1-53. Potential roles of dietary factors in protection against destructive oxidative mechanisms. Normal cellular oxidative mechanisms occur in the mitochondria or plasma membranes of certain cells and contribute to the oxidative modification of lipoproteins by supplying reactive oxygen intermediates to initiate lipid peroxidation. This illustration demonstrates how dietary factors could contribute to regulating these processes by: 1) acting as chainbreaking antioxidants (*eg*, lipophilic dietary antioxidants such as vitamin E); 2) regenerating the antioxidant capacity of the lipophilic antioxidants (*eg*, water-soluble antioxidants such as vitamin C); or 3) stimulating the normal cellular antioxidant pathways (*eg*, other contributing dietary factors such as copper, zinc, manganese, and selenium, which are cofactors for antioxidant enzymes such as the superoxide dismutases [SODs] and glutathione peroxidase). BHT—butylated hydroxytoluene.

LDL CHOLESTEROL GOALS AND CUTPOINTS FOR TLC AND DRUG THERAPY IN DIFFERENT RISK CATEGORIES

RISK CATEGORY	LDL GOAL, *MG/DL*	LDL LEVEL AT WHICH TO INITIATE TLC, *MG/DL*	LEVEL AT WHICH TO CONSIDER DRUG THERAPY, *MG/DL*
CHD or CHD risk equivalents (10-year risk > 20%)	< 100	≥ 100	≥ 130 (100–129: drug optional)[†]
2 + risk factors (10-year risk ≤ 20%)	< 130	≥ 130	10-year risk 10%–20%: ≥ 130 10-year risk < 10%: ≥ 160
0–1 risk factor*	< 160	≥ 160	≥ 190 (160–189: LDL lowering drug optional)

*Almost all people with 0–1 risk factor have a 10-year risk < 10%; thus, 10-year risk assessment in people with 0–1 risk factor is not necessary.

†Some authorities recommend use of LDL-lowering drugs in this category if an LDL cholesterol level of < 100 mg/dL cannot be achieved by TLC. Others prefer use of drugs that primarily modify triglycerides and high-density lipoprotein, *eg*, nicotinic acid or fibrate. Clinical judgment also may call for deferring drug therapy in this subcategory.

FIGURE 1-54. Low-density lipoprotein (LDL) cholesterol treatment goals set forth in the National Cholesterol Education Program Adult Treatment Panal III guidelines. Include different goals for LDL-cholesterol depending on coronary heart disease (CHD) status of presence of CHD risk factors. TLC—therapeutic lifestyle change. (*Adapted from* [53].)

EFFECT OF DRUGS ON LIPOPROTEIN METABOLISM

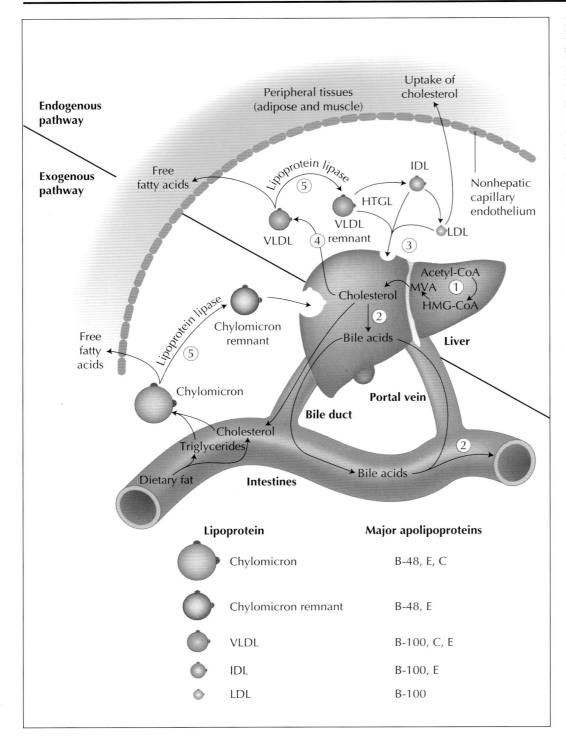

FIGURE 1-55. Overview of lipoprotein metabolism [58]. This illustration depicts the five major sites for drug action that are associated with low-density lipoprotein (LDL) or triglyceride lowering. The major mechanism for lowering LDL involves an increase in LDL receptor numbers (3). Increases in the number of LDL receptors occur when there is a decrease in the cholesterol content of hepatic and other cells. This can occur either by decreasing the rate-limiting enzyme in cholesterol synthesis (hydroxymethyl glutaryl-coenzyme A [HMG-CoA] reductase) (1) or increasing the fecal excretion of bile acids with the resulting decrease in the bile acid pool (2). Enhanced receptor activity (3) increases the removal of LDL plus the precursors of LDL, very low-density lipoprotein (VLDL) remnants, and intermediate-density lipoprotein (IDL). Thus, the formation of LDL can also be decreased. VLDL remnants and IDL also contain triglycerides and thus a modest decrease in triglycerides may be observed. Inhibition of lipoprotein synthesis (4) decreases the synthesis or secretion of VLDL, the major triglyceride-carrying lipoprotein. Secondarily, the formation of VLDL remnants, IDL, and LDL are decreased and both LDL cholesterol and triglyceride levels are reduced. Increased lipoprotein lipase activity (5) facilitates the removal of triglycerides from both chylomicrons and VLDL. These smaller particles may then be removed from the circulation by the remnant receptor. Moreover, the VLDL remnants can proceed to the formation of IDL and LDL, which can be removed by the LDL receptor. Acetyl-CoA—acetyl coenzyme A; HTGL—hepatic triglyceride lipase; MVA—mevalonate.

Lipoprotein	Major apolipoproteins
Chylomicron	B-48, E, C
Chylomicron remnant	B-48, E
VLDL	B-100, C, E
IDL	B-100, E
LDL	B-100

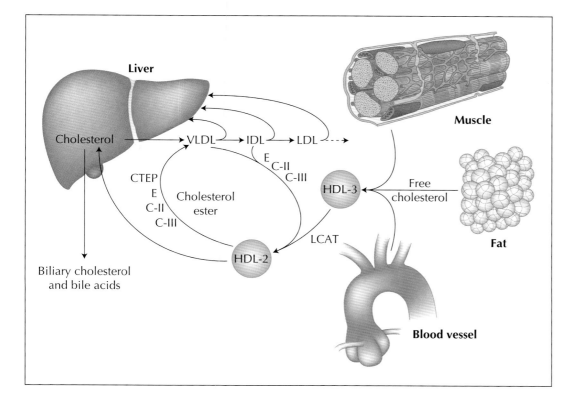

FIGURE 1-56. High-density lipoprotein (HDL) metabolism. The formation and metabolism of HDL are very complex and the mechanism of action of drugs that either increase or decrease HDL have not been well established [59,60]. Apolipoprotein (apo) A-1 is the major protein in HDL, and apo A-1 levels appear to correlate best with changes in HDL levels. Thus, drugs that either increase the synthesis or decrease the catabolism of apo A-1 would be expected to increase HDL levels. However, the origins of the various components of HDL are diffuse and there is an extensive exchange of protein, phospholipid, cholesterol (free and esterified), and triglycerides between HDL and other lipoproteins. Drugs have the potential for influencing HDL levels and function by multiple mechanisms. Because of the complexity and poor understanding, no further discussion of the effects of individual drugs on HDL metabolism is included in this chapter. CETP—cholesteryl ester transfer protein; IDL—intermediate-density lipoprotein; LCAT—lecithin-cholesterol acyltransferase; VLDL—very low-density lipoprotein.

FIGURE 1-57. Relation between coronary heart disease (CHD) events and low-density lipoprotein (LDL) cholesterol in recent lipid trials. The relation between mean LDL cholesterol on therapy and the percent of clinical trial participants developing a CHD event were related and separate slopes were observed for primary prevention trials and secondary prevention studies. Data were derived from a variety of trials [61–66]. Pl—placebo; Rx—treatment.

BILE ACID SEQUESTRANTS

OVERVIEW OF BILE ACID SEQUESTRANTS

Administered as a powder that must be hydrated in an aqueous vehicle

One sequestrant (colestipol) is available in tablet form

Not absorbed from the gastrointestinal tract

Evidence for reduction in risk of coronary heart disease

Evidence of long-term safety

Primary effect is to lower LDL cholesterol levels

Used as single-drug therapy or in combination with other lipid-lowering drugs

Recommended as initial therapy in young adults, women with childbearing potential, or low-risk patients

Acceptance by both patients and health professionals is frequently low because of inconvenience, poor palatability, gastrointestinal complaints, and interference with absorption of other drugs

For active drug in the powder form, efficacy of 5 g of colestipol is equal to 4 g of cholestyramine

FIGURE 1-58. Overview of bile acid sequestrants. Bile acid sequestrants are effective in lowering LDL cholesterol levels but patient acceptance, especially of higher doses, is frequently low. They are ideal drugs for initial therapy in low-risk patients with moderate elevations of LDL cholesterol or in patients in whom long-term safety considerations are of major importance.

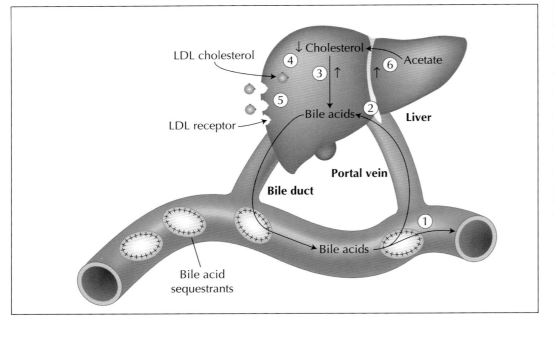

FIGURE 1-59. Mechanism of action of bile acid sequestrants [60,67]. The bile acid sequestrants are highly charged resins that are not absorbed. They form insoluble complexes with bile acids in the gut and increase their fecal excretion (1). There is a decrease in the recirculation and pool of bile acids (2) resulting in a compensatory increase in the conversion of cholesterol to bile acids (3). Hepatic cholesterol content is decreased (4) with an increase in LDL receptor numbers (5) and an increased rate of removal of LDL from the circulation. However, there is also a compensatory increase in cholesterol synthesis (6), which limits the increase in LDL receptors and the decrease in plasma LDL receptors that can be achieved.

STATINS

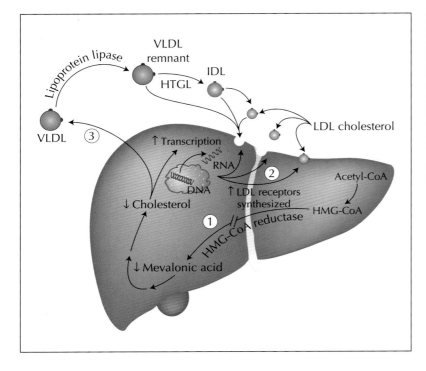

FIGURE 1-60. Mechanism of action of statins [68,69]. The statins inhibit the rate-limiting enzyme, hydroxymethyl glutaryl-coenzyme A (HMG-CoA) reductase, in cholesterol biosynthesis (1). The major organs for cholesterol biosynthesis are the small intestine and liver. The associated decrease in hepatic and cellular cholesterol concentration stimulates the production of low-density lipoprotein (LDL) receptors, which increase the rate of removal of LDL from the plasma (2). There is also increased removal of very low-density lipoprotein (VLDL) remnants and intermediate-density lipoprotein (IDL), which are precursors to LDL formation. In some patients, there may also be a decrease in lipoprotein synthesis (3). The enhanced removal of VLDL remnants and IDL and the inhibition of lipoprotein synthesis may contribute to the modest triglyceride-lowering effect of the statins. Acetyl-CoA—acetyl coenzyme A; HTGL—hepatic triglyceride lipase.

CLINICAL TRIALS WITH STATINS

Clinical endpoint trials

Pravastatin Multinational Study [72]

Scandinavian Simvastatin Survival Study [70]

Most definitive trial to date involving 4444 participants with evidence of CHD who were followed for 5.4 y

Simvastatin administration associated with a 30%–44% reduction in total mortality and major CHD events

West of Scotland Study [71]

Pravastatin treatment reduced CHD events by 32% and mortality by 22%

Cholesterol and Recurrent Events (CARE) Trial [73]

Pravastatin treatment reduced coronary events by 24% in CHD patients with average total cholesterol (209 mg/dL)

Long-term Intervention with Pravastatin in Ischemic Disease (LIPID) Trial [74]

Pravastatin treatment reduced coronary events by 24% in CHD patients

Air Force/Texas Coronary Atherosclerosis Study (AFCAPS/TexCAPS) [75]

Lovastatin reduced fatal and nonfatal myocardial infarction by 40% in normal middle-aged subjects

Heart Protection Study (HPS) [76]

Simvastatin lowered risk of major vascular events 25% in high-risk patients

Prospective Study of Pravastatin in the Elderly at Risk (PROSPER) [77]

Pravastatin lowered low-density lipoprotein cholesterol 34% and reduced risk of a composite cardiovascular disease endpoint in the elderly

Antihypertensive and Lipid-lowering Treatment to Prevent Heart Attack Trial (ALLHAT-LLT) [78]

Pravastatin did not reduce all-cause mortality of CHD when compared with usual care in older participants with well-controlled hypertension and moderately elevated low-density lipoprotein cholesterol

Anglo-Scandinavian cardiac outcomes trial (ASCOT-LLA) [79]

Atorvastatin therapy led to reductions in major cardiovascular events in adults aged 40–79 years

FIGURE 1-61. Clinical endpoint trials with statins. The Scandinavian Simvastatin Survival Study [70] conclusively demonstrated the benefits of low-density lipoprotein cholesterol lowering in patients with coronary heart disease (CHD). The West of Scotland Study [71] has given very similar results in patients who did not have CHD at entry. Recent results are largely confirmatory.

SIDE EFFECTS OF STATINS

INCREASED TRANSAMINASE LEVELS

1%–2% of treated patients develop increases of > 3 × upper-normal limit, especially at higher doses

Rapidly reversible, no evidence of chronic liver disease

MYOPATHY

Diffuse muscle pain and CPK > 10 × upper-normal limit

Primarily seen when higher doses of statins are used in combination with cyclosporine, gemfibrozil, and occasionally erythromycin and niacin

CATARACTS, LENS OPACITIES

No clinical evidence for increased risk

FIGURE 1-62. Side effects of statins [80,81]. The side effect profile of the statins is very favorable, considering their efficacy in lowering LDL cholesterol levels. Initial monitoring of transaminase levels is indicated, but abnormalities are rapidly reversible with a reduction in dosage; discontinuance of drug is rarely required. Myopathy is a clinical diagnosis that is confirmed by marked elevations of creatine phosphokinase (CPK) levels. Early diagnosis and reduction of dose or discontinuance of drug is required to prevent rhabdomyolysis and renal failure. The incidence of all side effects is low. If side effects do occur, use of another statin may be attempted.

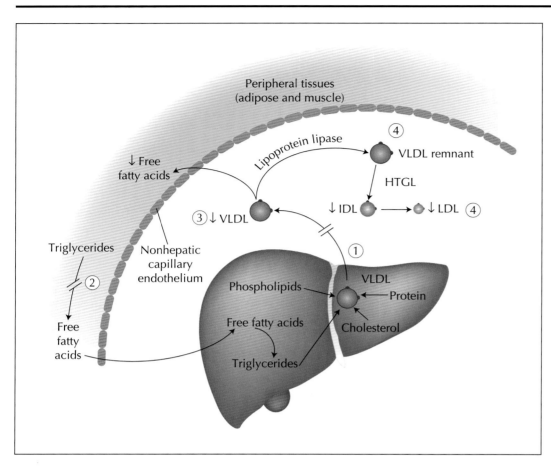

FIGURE 1-63. Mechanism of action of nicotinic acid. Inhibition of lipoprotein synthesis is generally considered to be the major effect of nicotinic acid (1). Inhibition of lipolysis of the stored fat in adipose tissue (2) with the resultant decrease in free fatty acids delivered to the liver could also indirectly decrease lipoprotein synthesis. The clinical significance of this mechanism has not been well documented in humans. Inhibition of lipoprotein synthesis decreases very low-density lipoprotein (VLDL) secretion or synthesis (3), and all subsequent lipoproteins in this pathway (VLDL remnants, intermediate-density lipoprotein [IDL] and LDL) are also decreased (4). Nicotinic acid may also modestly lower lipoprotein (a) levels by unknown mechanism(s). HTGL—hepatic triglyceride lipase.

NICOTINIC ACID PREPARATIONS

<u>NICOTINAMIDE</u>

No lipid-altering effects

<u>NICOTINIC ACID</u>

Crystalline- or immediate-release preparation

Most effective drug for increasing HDL cholesterol

Large doses are required to achieve significant decreases in LDL cholesterol

Sustained or slow-release preparation

Used primarily for lowering LDL cholesterol or if crystalline-release preparation is not tolerated

More effective than crystalline-release preparations for lowering LDL cholesterol, but less effective for raising HDL cholesterol

Risk of severe hepatotoxicity is greater than for crystalline-release preparations

FIGURE 1-64. Nicotinic acid preparations [67,82,83]. Because these preparations are available without a prescription, patients must be instructed to take nicotinic acid or niacin only. The use of slow-release preparations is still controversial and some investigators and clinicians do not recommend their use. HDL—high-density lipoprotein; LDL—low-density lipoprotein.

CLINICAL TRIALS WITH NICOTINIC ACID

CLINICAL EVENTS

Coronary Drug Project [85,86]

Reduction in fatal and nonfatal myocardial infarction in patients with prior myocardial infarction

Reduction in total mortality with follow-up of 15 y

Stockholm Ischemic Heart Study [46]

Reduction of total mortality in unblinded trial with combination therapy, including clofibrate

ANGIOGRAPHIC TRIALS

Reduced rate of progression, increased rate of regression, and suggestion of reduced event rate

Cholesterol Lowering Atherosclerosis Study (CLAS) [87] (nicotinic acid + colestipol)

Familial Atherosclerosis Treatment Study (FATS) [88] (nicotinic acid + colestipol)

FIGURE 1-65. Clinical trials with nicotinic acid. The only major trial with nicotinic acid as single-drug therapy is the Coronary Drug Project [84]. There are no reports of major reported primary prevention trials.

FIBRIC ACIDS

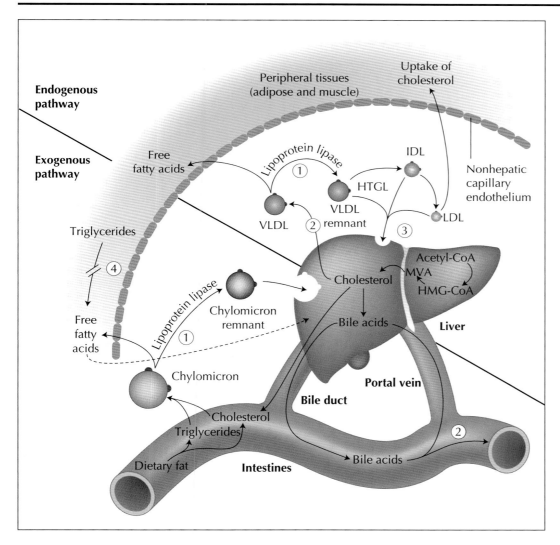

FIGURE 1-66. Mechanism of action of fibric acids [67,86,89]. The mechanism of action of the fibric acids has not been completely established and may also be dependent upon the specific fibric acid used. All fibric acids increase lipoprotein lipase activity (1), which results in decreased very low-density lipoprotein (VLDL) and triglyceride levels. Other reported mechanisms that have been less well documented include decreased lipoprotein synthesis (2), increased LDL receptor activity (3), and decreased lipolysis within adipose tissue (4), which could indirectly decrease lipoprotein synthesis. Acetyl-CoA—acetyl coenzyme A; HMG-CoA—hydroxymethyl glutaryl-coenzyme A; HTGL—hepatic triglyceride lipase; IDL—intermediate-density lipoprotein; MVA—mevalonate.

CLINICAL TRIALS WITH FIBRIC ACIDS

MAJOR PRIMARY PREVENTION TRIALS

WHO Clofibrate Study [90,91]
  Decrease in fatal and nonfatal myocardial infarction
  Increase in non-CHD mortality both during the trial and for entire duration of follow-up
Helsinki Heart Study (gemfibrizol) [92,93]
  34% reduction in fatal and nonfatal myocardial infarction
  Reduction in risk due to both the increase in HDL-C and the decrease in LDL-C
  Increase in non-CHD death rate, especially during post-trial observation

MAJOR SECONDARY PREVENTION TRIALS

Veterans Administration HLD Intervention Trial (gemfibrizol) (VA-HIT) [94]
  Men with coronary disease at baseline and low HDL-C
  Therapy group showed no change in LDL-C during trial and increased HDL-C of 6%
  Decreased hard endpoint cardiovascular disease
Bezafibrate Infarction Prevention Trial (bezafibrate) (BIP) [95]
  Men and women in secondary prevention trial
  No significant benefit shown for CHD risk reduction in treated group

FIGURE 1-67. Clinical trials with fibric acids [90–95]. Major primary prevention trials showed a reduction in coronary heart disease (CHD) events. Clofibrate is no longer used in most countries. HDL-C—high-density lipoprotein cholesterol; LDL-C—low-density lipoprotein cholesterol.

EFFECTS OF ESTROGEN REPLACEMENT ON CHD RISK

Epidemiologic studies indicate that estrogen replacement in postmenopausal women reduced CHD risk
  50% in primary prevention
  80% in secondary intervention
Conjugated estrogens (0.625 mg) or equivalent dose of other estrogen
  LDL-C reduction of 10%–15%
  HDL-C increase of 10%–15%
Clinical trials
  Heart and Estrogen/Progestin Replacement Study (HERS) [97]
    Postmenopausal women with a uterus and clinical evidence of CHD
    Daily administration of 0.625 mg of conjugated equine estrogen and 2.5 mg of medroxyprogesterone acetate for 4+ years
    No significant reduction in fatal and nonfatal MI and increased risk in the first year after initiating therapy
  Women's Health Initiative (WHI) [98]
    Primary prevention
    Daily combined estrogen plus progestin led to 24% greater CHD risk and this arm of trial terminated
    Estrogen only arm of trial still underway
  SERMS
    No clinical trials to date to evaluate potential effect on CHD risk

FIGURE 1-68. Effects of estrogen replacement on coronary heart disease (CHD) risk. Prospective trials with combination therapy of estrogen plus progestin have not shown a reduction in CHD risk [96]. HDL-C—high-density lipoprotein cholesterol; LDL-C—low-density lipoprotein cholesterol; MI —myocardial infarction.

RECOMMENDED COMBINATION THERAPY OF ELEVATED LDL CHOLESTEROL AND NORMAL TRIGLYCERIDES

Statin + bile acid sequestrant
  Both drugs increase LDL cholesterol receptor numbers by differing mechanisms
  Effect is greater than can be achieved by either drug alone; overall effect is additive
    or synergistic
Statin + nicotinic acid
  Statin increases LDL receptor number; niacin inhibits lipoprotein synthesis
  Useful if both LDL cholesterol lowering and HDL cholesterol raising are desired
Bile acid sequestrant + nicotinic acid
  Efficacy in lowering LDL cholesterol is additive
  Documented benefit in vascular disease prevention
  Combination is frequently not tolerated because of frequency of side effects with both drugs
Statin + Ezetimibe
  Efficacy in lowering LDL cholesterol is additive
  Avoids use of high dose statins
  Well tolerated

FIGURE 1-69. Combination therapy for elevated LDL cholesterol levels and normal triglycerides [99]. Statin plus a bile acid sequestrant is an historically effective combination for lowering low-density lipoprotein (LDL) cholesterol. The combination of statin plus nicotinic acid is the ideal combination for both lowering LDL and increasing high-density lipoprotein cholesterol levels.

RECOMMENDED COMBINATION THERAPY OF ELEVATED LDL CHOLESTEROL AND TRIGLYCERIDES

Statin + nicotinic acid
  Effect of two drugs is additive
  Low HDL cholesterol is common, and nicotinic acid increases HDL cholesterol
  Risk of myopathy small
Statin + fibric acid derivative
  If nicotinic acid is not tolerated
  Fibric acid has little effect on LDL cholesterol levels, but decreases triglycerides
    and increases HDL cholesterol
  Risk of myopathy greater
  Useful in non–insulin-dependent diabetes mellitus
Fibric acid + nicotinic acid
  Dose of nicotinic acid that is tolerated is usually insufficient to control LDL cholesterol levels

FIGURE 1-70. Recommended drug combinations for patients with elevations of both low-density lipoprotein (LDL) cholesterol and triglycerides (200 to 400 mg/dL) [99]. HDL—high-density lipoprotein.

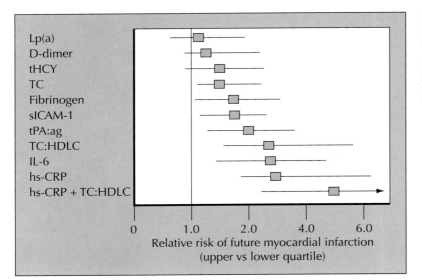

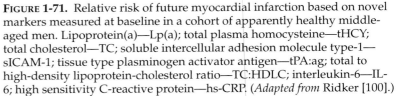

FIGURE 1-71. Relative risk of future myocardial infarction based on novel markers measured at baseline in a cohort of apparently healthy middle-aged men. Lipoprotein(a)—Lp(a); total plasma homocysteine—tHCY; total cholesterol—TC; soluble intercellular adhesion molecule type-1—sICAM-1; tissue type plasminogen activator antigen—tPA:ag; total to high-density lipoprotein-cholesterol ratio—TC:HDLC; interleukin-6—IL-6; high sensitivity C-reactive protein—hs-CRP. (*Adapted from* Ridker [100].)

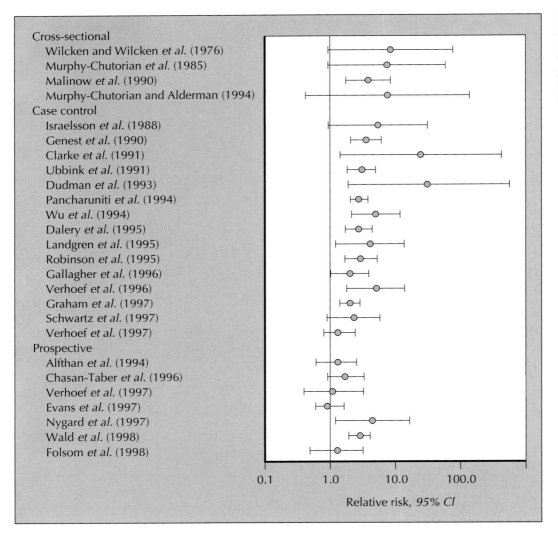

FIGURE 1-72. Fasting homocysteine and coronary artery disease: summary and meta-analysis. This meta-analysis showed that homocysteine levels were highly associated with greater risk for coronary heart disease in a variety of studies. The summary odds ratio for a 5-mol/L difference was approximately 1.60 [101].

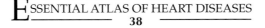

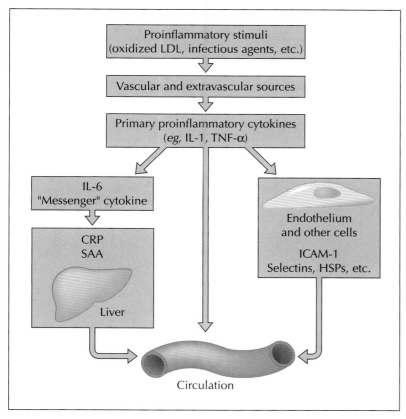

FIGURE 1-73. Cytokine cascade caused by proinflammatory stimuli resulting in circulating levels of inflammatory markers associated with atherothrombosis [102]. CRP—C-reactive protein; HSP—heat shock protein; ICAM-1—intercellular adhesion molecule-1; IL-1—interleukin-1; SAA—serum amyloid A; TNF-α—tumor necrosis factor-α. (*Adapted from* Libby and Ridker [103].)

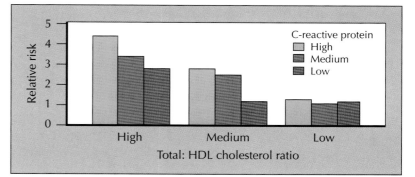

FIGURE 1-74. Relative risk of future myocardial infarction (MI) among healthy men based on total to high-density lipoprotein (HDL)-cholesterol ratio and high sensitivity C-reactive protein (hs-CRP). Plasma levels of hs-CRP appear to add to the predictive value of plasma lipid measurements; this may provide an improved method to determine future risk of MI. (*Adapted from* Ridker *et al.* [104].)

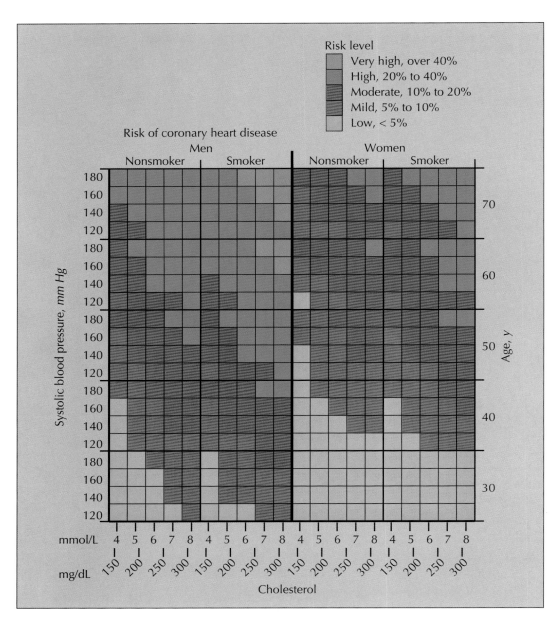

FIGURE 1-75. Coronary risk chart for primary prevention of coronary heart disease (CHD) using cholesterol levels, blood pressure, age, and smoking status. This chart is useful for assessing CHD risk for patients who have not developed symptomatic CHD or other atherosclerotic disease. To estimate a patient's 10-year risk of CHD, locate the appropriate segment for their gender, smoking status, and age. Find the cell nearest to their systolic blood pressure and total cholesterol. The effect of lifetime exposure to risk factors is evident by following the table from bottom to top. High-risk patients are defined as those whose 10-year risk for CHD exceeds 20% or will exceed 20% if projected to age 60. To estimate a patient's relative risk, compare their risk category with that for other people of the same age. CHD risk is higher than indicated in the chart for patients with familial hyperlipidemia, diabetes, familial premature cardiovascular disease, low high-density lipoprotein cholesterol, or triglyceride levels >2.0 mmol/L. (*Adapted from* [105].)

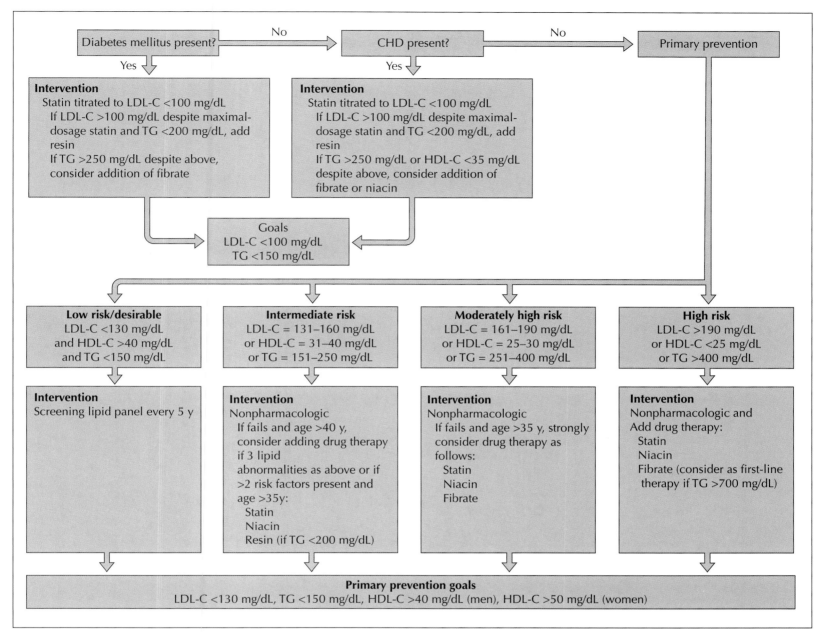

FIGURE 1-76. Algorithm for lipid-lowering therapy based on results from intervention trials. CHD—coronary heart disease; HDL-C—high-density lipoprotein cholesterol; LDL-C—low-density lipoprotein cholesterol; TG—triglycerides. (*Adapted from* Ansell *et al.* [106].)

Category of trial	Trials with data, *n*	Vascular events, *n/n (%)*		Observed-expected	Variance	Odds ratio (CI) Antiplatelet: Control	Odds reduction, % (SE)
		Allocated antiplatelet	Adjusted control				
Aspirin alone, *mg daily*							
500–1500	34	1621/11215 (14.5)	1930/11236 (17.2)	-147.1	707.8		19 (3)
160–325	19	1526/13240 (11.5)	1963/13273 (14.8)	-219.9	742.6		26 (3)
75–150	12	370/3370 (10.9)	517/3406 (15.2)	-72.0	183.8		32 (6)
<75	3	316/1827 (17.3)	354/1828 (19.4)	-18.9	136.5		13 (8)
Any aspirin	65	3829/29 652 (12.9)	4764/29 743 (16.0)	-452.3	1717.0		23 (2)
Other antiplatelet drugs							
Dipyridamole	15	392/2696 (14.5)	458/2734 (16.8)	-30.9	173.0		16 (7)
Sulfinpyrazone	19	315/2411 (13.1)	361/2416 (14.9)	-23.8	140.7		16 (8)
Ticlopidine	42	278/3435 (8.1)	385/3475 (11.0)	-50.5	132.3		32 (7)
Suloctidil	6	47/364 (12.9)	59/367 (16.1)	-5.6	20.5		24 (19)
Picotamide	4	41/1583 (2.6)	66/1602 (4.1)	-12.2	25.8		38 (16)
Sulotroban	4	8/406 (2.0)	14/409 (3.4)	-3.2	5.3		45 (33)
Triflusal	2	10/314 (3.2)	19/309 (6.1)	-4.7	6.7		50 (28)
Other†	9	41/647 (6.3)	73/641 (11.4)	-16.1	25.6		47 (15)
Any other single agent	101	1132/11 856 (9.5)	1435/11 953 (12.0)	-147.0	529.9		24 (4)
Aspirin + another antiplatelet drug							
Asp + dipyridamole	46	1036/9703 (10.7)	1393/9738 (14.3)	-172.6	488.7		30 (4)
Asp + sulfinpyrazone	2	38/283 (13.4)	50/278 (18.0)	-6.5	18.5		30 (20)
Any combination	48	1074/9986 (10.8)	1443/10016 (14.4)	-179.1	507.2		30 (4)
All trials	**188**	**6035/51494 (11.7)**	**7644/51736 (14.8)**	**-715.7**	**2449.6**		**25 (2)**

0.0   0.5   1.0   1.5   2.0

Antiplatelet better   Antiplatelet worse

Treatment effect 2*P* < 0.00001

FIGURE 1-77. Aspirin and prevention of cardiovascular disease. Comprehensive meta-analyses of antiplatelet therapy, considering 287 studies that involved 135,000 patients for prevention of cardiovascular events, have shown that aspirin or other oral therapies are protective in most patients. Even low-dose aspirin (75–150 mg/d) is relatively effective, but in the shorter term a loading dose of at least 150 mg is recommended [107].

REFERENCES

1. Ross R: The pathogenesis of atherosclerosis: a perspective for the 1990s. *Nature* 1993, 362:801–809.

2. Ku DN, Zarins CK, Giddens DP, *et al.*: Pulsatile flow and atherosclerosis in the human carotid bifurcation: positive correlation between plaque localization and low and oscillating shear stress. *Arteriosclerosis* 1985, 5:292–302.

3. Tracy RE, Kissling GE: Age and fibroplasia as preconditions for atheronecrosis in human coronary arteries. *Arch Pathol Lab Med* 1987, 111:957–963.

4. Glagov S, Weisenberg E, Zarins CK, *et al.*: Compensatory enlargement of human atherosclerotic coronary arteries. *N Engl J Med* 1987, 316:1371–1375.

5. Zarins CK, Weisenberg E, Kolettis G, *et al.*: Differential enlargement of artery segments in response to enlarging atherosclerotic plaques. *J Vasc Surg* 1988, 7:386–394.

6. Richardson PD, Davies MS, Born GVR: Influence of plaque configuration and stress distribution on fissuring of coronary atherosclerotic plaques. *Lancet* 1989, 2:941–944.

7. Bini A, Fenoglio JJ Jr, Mesa-Tejada R, *et al.*: Identification and distribution of fibrinogen, fibrin and fibrin(ogen) degradation products in atherosclerosis: use of monoclonal antibodies. *Arteriosclerosis* 1989, 9:109–121.

8. Treasure CB, Alexander RW: The dysfunctional endothelium in heart failure. *J Am Coll Cardiol* 1993, 22:129A–134A.

9. Gokce N, Keaney JF, Jr, Vita JA: Endotheliopathies: clinical manifestations of endothelial dysfunction. In *Thrombosis and Hemorrhage*, edn 2. Edited by Loscalzo J, Schafer AI. Philadelphia: Lippincott Williams & Wilkins; 1998: 901–924.

10. Dobroski DR, Rabbani LE, Loscalzo J: The relationship between thrombosis and atherosclerosis. In *Thrombosis and Hemorrhage*. Edited by Loscalzo J, Schafer AI. Philadelphia: Lippincott Williams & Wilkins; 1998:837–861.

11. Libby P: Molecular bases of the acute coronary syndromes. *Circulation* 1995, 91:2844–2850.

12. Oberman A, Kreisberg RA, Henkin Y, eds: *Principles and Management of Lipid Disorders*. Baltimore: Williams & Wilkins; 1992:87–105.

13. Lindgren FT: The plasma lipoproteins: historical developments and nomenclature. *Ann N Y Acad Sci* 1980, 348:1–15.

14. Segrest JP, Garber DW, Brouillette CG, *et al.*: The amphipathic a helix: a multifunctional structural motif in plasma lipoproteins. *Adv Protein Chem* 1994, 45:303–369.

15. Scanu AM, Fless GM: Lipoprotein (a). Heterogeneity and biological relevance. *J Clin Invest* 1990, 85:1709–1715.

16. Genest JJ Jr, Martin-Munley SS, McNamara JR, *et al.*: Familial lipoprotein disorders in patients with premature coronary artery disease. *Circulation* 1992, 85:2025–2033.

17. Brown MS, Goldstein JL: A receptor-mediated pathway for cholesterol homeostasis. *Science* 1986, 232:34–47.

18. Rosenfeld ME, Khoo JC, Miller E, *et al.*: Macrophage-derived foam cells freshly isolated from rabbit atherosclerotic lesions degrade modified lipoproteins, promote oxidation of low-density lipoproteins, and contain oxidation-specific lipid-protein adducts. *J Clin Invest* 1991, 87:90–99.

19. Steinberg D: Metabolism of lipoproteins and their role in atherogenesis. *Atheroscler Rev* 1988, 18:1–23.

20. Quinn MT, Parthasarathy S, Steinberg D, *et al.*: Oxidatively modified low density lipoproteins: a potential role in recruitment and retention of monocyte/macrophages during atherogenesis: *Proc Natl Acad Sic U S A* 1987, 84:2995–2998.

21. Menotti A, Keys A, Aravanis C, *et al.*: Seven Countries Study. First 20-year mortality data in 12 cohorts of six countries. *Ann Med* 1989, 21:175–179.

22. Keys A: High density lipoprotein cholesterol and longevity. *J Epidemiol Community Health* 1987, 42:60–65.

23. Castelli WP, Garrison RJ, Wilson PWF, *et al.*: Incidence of coronary heart disease and lipoprotein cholesterol levels. The Framingham study. *JAMA* 1986, 256:2835–2838.

24. Acton S, Rigotti A, Landschulz KT *et al.*: Identification of scavenger receptor SR-BI as a high density lipoprotein receptor. *Science* 1996, 271:518–520.

25. Murao K, Terpstra V, Green SR *et al.*: Characterization of CLA-1, a human homologue of rodent scavenger receptor BI, as a receptor for high density lipoprotein and apoptotic thymocytes. *J Biol Chem* 1997, 272:17551–17557.

26. Landschulz KT, Pathak RK, Rigotti A *et al.*: Regulation of scavenger receptor, class B, type I, a high density lipoprotein receptor, in liver and steroidogenic tissues of the rat. *J Clin Invest* 1996, 98:984–995.

27. Tall AR: Metabolic and genetic control of HDL cholesterol levels. *J Intern Med* 1992, 231:661–668.

28. Brewer HB, Jr, Santamarina-Fojo S, Hoeg JM: Molecular biology of the lipoproteins and the apolipoproteins and their role in atherosclerosis. In *Molecular Basis of Cardiology*. Edited by Roberts R. Boston: Blackwell Scientific Publishers; 1992:415–441.

29. Assman G, von Eckardstein A, Brewer HB, Jr.: *The Metabolic and Molecular Basis of Inherited Disease*, edn 8. Edited by Scriver CR, Beaudet AL, Sly WS, et al. New York: McGraw Hill; 2001:2937–2980.

30. Kaplan NM: The deadly quartet: upper-body obesity, glucose intolerance, hypertriglyceridemia, and hypertension. *Arch Intern Med* 1989, 149:1514–1520.

31. Austin MA: Triglycerides, small dense LDL and coronary disease. *Atherosclerosis* 1994, 109:259.

32. NIH Consensus Development Panel on Triglyceride, High-Density Lipoprotein, and Coronary Heart Disease: Triglyceride, high-density lipoprotein, and coronary heart disease. *JAMA* 1993, 269:505–510.

33. Brewer HB Jr, Gregg RE, Hoeg JM, *et al.*: Apolipoproteins and lipoproteins in human plasma: an overview. *Clin Chem* 1988, 34:B4–B8.

34. Beisiegel U, Weber W, Ihrke G, *et al.*: The LDL receptor related protein, LRP, is an apolipoprotein E binding protein. *Nature* 1989, 341:162–164.

35. Rubinstein A, Gibson JC, Paterniti JR: The effect of heparin induced lipolysis on the distribution of apolipoprotein E among lipoprotein subclasses. *J Clin Invest* 1985, 75:710–721.

36. Goldberg IJ, Le N-A, Paterniti JR, *et al.*: Effect of acute inhibition of hepatic triglyceride lipase on very low density lipoprotein metabolism in the cynomolgus monkey. *J Clin Invest* 1982, 70:1184–1192.

37. Zannis VI, Breslow JL: Characterization of a unique human apolipoprotein E variant associated with type III hyperlipoproteinemia. *J Biol Chem* 1980, 255:1759.

38. Rall SC Jr, Weisgraber KH, Innerarity TL, *et al.*: Structural basis for receptor binding heterogeneity of apolipoprotein E from type III hyperlipoproteinemic subjects. *Proc Natl Acad Sci USA* 1982, 79:4696.

39. Fredrickson DS, Morganroth J, Levy RI: Type III hyperlipoproteinemia: an analysis of two contemporary definitions. *Ann Intern Med* 1975, 82:150.

40. Goldstein JL, Schrott HG, Hazzard WR, *et al.*: Hyperlipidemia in coronary artery disease. II. Genetic analysis of lipid levels in 176 families and delineation of a new inherited disorder, combined hyperlipidemia. *J Clin Invest* 1973, 2:1544–1568.

41. Cortner JA, Coates PM, Bennett MJ, *et al.*: Familial combined hyperlipidaemia: use of stable isotopes to demonstrated overproduction of very low-density lipoprotein apolipoprotein B by the liver. *J Inherit Metab Dis* 1991, 14:915–922.

42. Janus CK, Nicoll AM, Turner PR, *et al.*: Kinetic basis of the primary hyperlipidemias: studies of apolipoprotein B turnover in genetically defined subjects. *Eur J Clin Invest* 1980, 10:161–172.

43. Kissebah AH, Alfarsi S, Evans DJ: Low density lipoprotein metabolism in familial combined hyperlipidemia. Mechanisms of the multiple lipoprotein phenotypic expression. *Arteriosclerosis* 1984, 4:614–624.

44. Kesaniemi YA, Vega GL, Grundy SM: Kinetics of apolipoprotein B in normal and hyperlipidemic man: review of current data. In *Lipoprotein in Kinetics and Modeling.* Edited by Berman M, Grundy SM, Howard BV. New York: Academic Press; 1982:181–205.

45. Chait A, Robertson HT, Brunzell JD: Chylomicronemia syndrome in diabetes mellitus. *Diabetes Care* 1981, 4:343–348.

46. Carlson LA, Rosenhamer G: Reduction of mortality in the Stockholm Ischaemic Heart Disease Secondary Prevention Study by combined treatment with clofibrate and nicotinic acid. *Acta Med Scand* 1988, 223:405–418.

47. Rubins HB, Robins SJ, Collins D, *et al.*: Gemfibrozil for the secondary prevention of coronary heart disease in men with low levels of high-density lipoprotein cholesterol. *N Engl J Med* 1999, 341:410–418.

48. Keys A: Coronary heart disease in seven countries. *Circulation* 1970, 41(suppl I):I-1–I-211.

49. Keys A, Menotti A, Karvonen MJ, *et al.*: The diet and 15-year death rate in the seven countries study. *Am J Epidemiol* 1986, 124:903–915.

50. McNamara DJ: Relationship between blood and dietary cholesterol. *Adv Meat Sci* 1990, 6:63–87.

51. Hu FB, Manson JE, Willett WC: Types of dietary fat and risk of coronary heart disease: a critical review. *J Am Coll Nutr* 2001, 20:5–19.

52. Meigs JB, D'Agostino RB, Wilson PWF, *et al.*: Risk variable clustering in the insulin resistance syndrome. *Diabetes* 1997, 46:1594–1600.

53. Executive Summary of the Third Report of the National Cholesterol Education Program (NCEP) Expert Panel on Detection, Evaluation, and Treatment of High Blood Cholesterol in Adults (Adult Treatment Panel III). *JAMA* 2001, 285:2486–2497.

54. Ford ES, Giles WH, Dietz WH: Prevalence of the metabolic syndrome among US adults: findings from the third National Health and Nutrition Examination Survey. *JAMA* 2002, 287:356–359.

55. Bonora E, Zenere M, Branzi P, *et al.*: Influences of body fat and its regional localization on risk factors for atherosclerosis in young men. *Am J Epidemiol* 1992, 135:1272–1278.

56. .Leenan R, van der Kooy K, Seidell JC, *et al.*: Visceral fat accumulation measured by magnetic resonance imaging in relation to serum lipids in obese men and women. *Atherosclerosis* 1992, 94:171–181.

57. Fujioka S, Matsuzawa Y, Tokunaga K, *et al.*: Contribution of intra-abdominal fat accumulation to the impairment of glucose and lipid metabolism in human obesity. *Metabolism* 1987, 36:54–59.

58. Ginsberg HN: Lipoprotein metabolism and its relationship to athero-sclerosis. *Med Clin North Am* 1994, 78:1–20.

59. Shepherd J, Packard CJ: High density lipoprotein metabolism. *Atheroscler Rev* 1993, 24:17–43.

60. Sirtori CR, Manzoni C, Lovati MR: Mechanisms of lipid-lowering agents. *Cardiology* 1991, 78:226–235.

61. Shepherd J, Cobbe SM, Ford I, *et al.*: Prevention of coronary heart disease with pravastatin in men with hypercholesterolemia. West of Scotland Coronary Prevention Study Group. *N Engl J Med* 1995, 333:1301–1307.

62. McKenney JM, Proctor JD, Harris S, *et al.*: A comparison of the efficacy and toxic effects of sustained- vs immediate-release niacin in hypercho-lesterolemic patients. *JAMA* 1994, 271:672–677.

63. The 4S Group: Baseline serum cholesterol and treatment effect in the Scandinavian Simvastatin Survival Study (4S). *Lancet* 1995, 345:1274–1275.

64. Downs JR, Clearfield M, Weis S, *et al.*: Primary prevention of acute coronary events with lovastatin in men and women with average cholesterol levels: results of AFCAPS/TexCAPS. *JAMA* 1998, 279:1615–1622.

65. The Long-Term Intervention with Pravastatin in Ischaemic Disease (LIPID) Study Group: Prevention of cardiovascular events and death with pravastatin in patients with coronary heart disease and a broad range of initial cholesterol levels. *N Engl J Med* 1998, 339:1349–1357.

66. Rubins HB, Robins SJ, Collins D, *et al.*: Gemfibrozil for the secondary prevention of coronary heart disease in men with low levels of high-density lipoprotein cholesterol. Veterans Affairs High-Density Lipoprotein Cholesterol Intervention Trial Study Group. *N Engl J Med* 1999, 341:410–418.

67. Hunninghake DB: Drug treatment of dyslipoproteinemia. *Endocrinol Metab Clin North Am* 1990, 19:345–360.

68. Bilheimer DW, Grundy SM, Brown MS, *et al.*: Mevinolin and colestipol stimulate receptor-mediated clearance of low density lipoprotein from plasma in familiar hypercholesterolemia heterozygoses. *Proc Natl Acad Sci USA* 1983, 80:4124–4128.

69. Blankenhorn DH, Azen SP, Kramsch DM, *et al.*: Coronary angiographic changes with lovastatin therapy. The Monitored Atherosclerosis Regression Study (MARS). *Ann Intern Med* 1993, 19:969–976.

70. Scandinavian Simvastatin Survival Group: Randomized trial of choles-terol lowering 4,444 patients with coronary heart disease: the Scandinavian Simvastatin Survival Study (4S). *Lancet* 1994, 344:1383–1389.

71. Shepherd J, Cobbe SM, Ford I, *et al.*: Prevention of coronary heart disease with pravastatin in men with hypercholesterolemia. *N Engl J Med* 1995, 333:1301–1307.

72. Pravastatin Multinational Study Group for Cardiac Risk Patients: Effects of pravastatin in patients with serum total cholesterol levels from 5.2 to 7.8 mmol/liter (200 to 300 mg/dl) plus two additional atherosclerotic risk factors. *Am J Cardiol* 1993, 72:1031–1037.

73. Sacks FM, Pfeffer MA, Moye LA, *et al.*, for the Cholesterol and Recurrent Events Trial Investigators: The effect of pravastatin on coro-nary events after myocardial infarction in patients with average choles-terol levels. *N Engl J Med* 1996, 335(14):1001–1009.

74. The Long-Term Intervention with Pravastatin in Ischaemic Disease (LIPID) Study Group: Prevention of cardiovascular events and death with pravastatin in patients with coronary heart disease and a broad range of initial cholesterol levels. *N Engl J Med* 1998, 339(19):1349–57.

75. Downs JR, Clearfield M, Weis S, *et al.*, for the Air Force/Texas Coronary Atherosclerosis Research Group: Primary prevention of acute coronary events with lovastatin in men and women with average cholesterol levels: results of AFCAPS/TexCAPS. *JAMA* 1998, 279(20):1615–1622.

76. MRC/BHF Heart Protection Study of cholesterol lowering with simvastatin in 20,536 high-risk individuals: a randomised placebo-controlled trial. *Lancet* 2002, 360:7–22.

77. Shepherd J, Blauw GJ, Murphy MB, *et al.*: Pravastatin in elderly indi-viduals at risk of vascular disease (PROSPER): a randomised controlled trial. *Lancet* 2002, 360:1623–1630.

78. Major outcomes in moderately hypercholesterolemic, hypertensive patients randomized to pravastatin vs usual care: The Antihypertensive and Lipid-Lowering Treatment to Prevent Heart Attack Trial (ALLHAT-LLT). *JAMA* 2002, 288:2998–3007.

79. Sever PS, Dahlof B, Poulter NR, *et al.*: Prevention of coronary and stroke events with atorvastatin in hypertensive patients who have average or lower-than-average cholesterol concentrations, in the Anglo-Scandinavian Cardiac Outcomes Trial - Lipid Lowering Arm (ASCOT-LLA): a multicentre randomised controlled trial. *Lancet* 2003, 361:1149–1158.

80. Bradford R, Sher CL, Chermos AN, *et al.*: Expanded Clinical Evaluation of Lovastatin (EXCEL) Study results: I. Efficacy in modifying plasma lipoproteins and adverse event profile in 8245 patients with moderate hypercholesterolemia. *Arch Intern Med* 1991, 51:43–49.

81. Blum CB: Comparison of properties of four inhibitors of 3-hydroxy-3-methylglutarylcoenzyme A reductase. *Am J Cardiol* 1994, 73(suppl):3D–11D.

82. Illingworth DR, Stein EA, Mitchel YB, *et al.*: Comparative effects of lovastatin and niacin in primary hypercholesterolemia: a prospective trial. *Arch Intern Med* 1994, 154:1586–1595.

83. McKenney JM, Proctor JD, Harris S, *et al.*: A comparison of the efficacy and toxic effects of sustained- vs immediate-release niacin in hyperc-holesterolemic patients. *JAMA* 1994, 271:672–677.

84. Coronary Drug Project Research Group: Clofibrate and niacin in coro-nary heart disease. *JAMA* 1975, 231:360–381.

85. Canner PL, Berge KG, Wenger NK, *et al.*: Fifteen-year mortality in coro-nary drug project patients: long-term benefit with niacin. *J Am Coll Cardiol* 1986, 8:1245–1255.

86. Stewart JM, Packard CJ, Lorimer AR, *et al.*: Effects of bezafibrate on receptor-mediated and receptor-independent low density lipoprotein catabolism in type II hyperlipoproteinaemic subjects. *Atherosclerosis* 1982, 44:355–365.

87. Blankenhorn DH, Nessim SA, Johnson RL, *et al.*: Beneficial effects of combined colestipol-niacin therapy on coronary atherosclerosis and coronary venous bypass grafts. *JAMA* 1987, 257:3233–3240.

88. Brown G, Albers JJ, Fisher LD, *et al.*: Regression of coronary artery disease as a result of intensive lipid-lowering therapy in men with high levels of apolipoprotein B. *N Engl J Med* 1990, 323:1289–1298.

89. Yuan J, Tsai M, Hunninghake DB: Changes in composition and distribution of LDL subspecies in hypertriglyceridemic and hypercholesterolemic patients during gemfibrozil therapy. *Atherosclerosis* 1994, 110:1–11.

90. WHO Monica Project: A co-operative trial in the primary prevention of ischemic heart disease using clofibrate. *Br Heart J* 1978, 40:1069–1118.

91. Committee of Principal Investigators: WHO cooperative trial on primary prevention of ischemic heart disease with clofibrate to lower serum cholesterol: final mortality follow-up. *Lancet* 1984, 2:600–604.

92. Frick MH, Elo O, Haapa K, *et al.*: Helsinki Heart Study: primary-prevention trial with gemfibrozil in middle-aged men with dyslipidemia: safety of treatment, changes in risk factors, and incidence of coronary heart disease. *N Engl J Med* 1987, 317:1237–1245.

93. Huttunen JK, Heinonen OP, Manninen V, *et al.*: The Helsinki Heart Study: an 8.5 year safety and mortality follow-up. *J Intern Med* 1994, 235:31–39.

94. Rubins HB, Robins SJ, Collins D, *et al.*: Gemfibrizol for the secondary prevention of coronary heart disease in men with low levels of high-density lipoprotein cholesterol. Veterans Affairs High-Density Lipoprotein Cholesterol Intervention Trial Study Group. *N Engl J Med* 1999, 341:410–418.

95. Haim M, Benderly M, Brunner D, *et al.*: Elevated serum triglyceride levels and long-term mortality in patients with coronary heart disease: the Benzafibrate Infarction Prevention (BIP) Registry. *Circulation* 1999, 100:475–482.

96. Hulley S, Grady D, Bush T: Randomized trial of estrogen plus progestin for secondary prevention of coronary heart disease in post menopausal women. *JAMA* 1998, 280:605–613.

97. Crouse 3rd JR, Byington RP, Hoen HM, Furberg CD: Reductase inhibitor monotherapy and stroke prevention. *Arch Intern Med* 1997, 157:1305–1310.

98. Manson JE, Hsia J, Johnson KC, *et al.*: Estrogen plus progestin and the risk of coronary heart disease. *N Engl J Med* 2003, 349:523–534.

99. National Cholesterol Education Program: Second report of the National Cholesterol Education Program (NCEP) expert panel on detection, evaluation, and treatment of high blood cholesterol in adults (adult treatment panel II). *Circulation* 1994, 89:1329–1445.

100. Ridker PM: Novel risk factors and markers for coronary disease. *Adv Intern Med* 2000, 45:391–418.

101. Christen WG, Ajani UA, Glynn RJ, Hennekens CH: Blood levels of homocysteine and increased risks of cardiovascular disease: causal or casual? *Arch Intern Med* 2000, 160:422–434.

102. Ridker PM, Genest J, Libby P: In *Heart Disease: A Textbook of Cardiovascular Medicine*, edn 6. Edited by Braunwald E, Zipes DP, Libby P. Philadelphia: WB Saunders; 2001:1010–1039.

103. Libby P, Ridker PM: Novel inflammatory markers of coronary risk: theory versus practice. *Circulation* 1999, 100(11):1148–1150.

104. Ridker PM, Glynn RJ, Hennekens CH: C-reactive protein adds to the predictive value of total and HDL cholesterol in determining risk of first myocardial infarction. *Circulation* 1998, 97(20):2007–2011.

105. Prevention of coronary heart disease in clinical practice. Recommendations of the Second Joint Task Force of European and other Societies on coronary prevention. *Eur Heart J* 1998, 19(10):1434–1503.

106. Ansell BJ, Watson KE, Fogelman AM: An evidence-based assessment of the NCEP Adult Treatment Panel II guidelines. National Cholesterol Education Program. *JAMA* 1999, 282(21):2051–2057.

107. Collaboration AT: Collaborative meta-analysis of randomised trials of antiplatelet therapy for prevention of death, myocardial infarction, and stroke in high risk patients . *BMJ* 2002, 324:71–86.

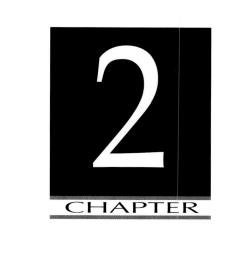

2 CHAPTER

ACUTE MYOCARDIAL INFARCTION AND OTHER ACUTE ISCHEMIC SYNDROMES

Edited by Robert M. Califf

Elliott M. Antman, Paul W. Armstrong, Edwin G. Bovill, Erling Falk, Christopher B. Granger, Judith S. Hochman, David R. Holmes, Jr., Neal S. Kleiman, Anatoly Langer, Colin D. Lee, James E. Muller, Angela Palazzo, Manesh Patel, Prediman K. Shah, Barbara E. Tardiff, Russell P. Tracy, Sergio Waxman, W. Douglas Weaver

OVERVIEW OF THE ACUTE CORONARY SYNDROMES

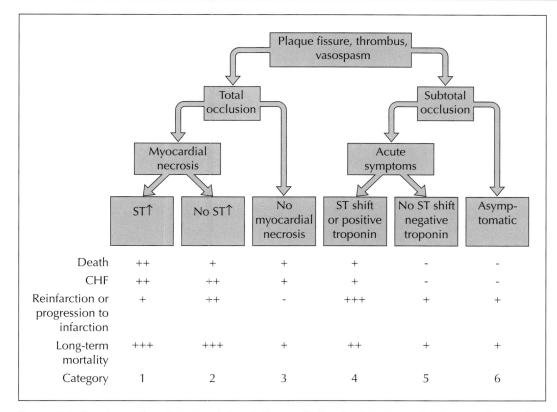

FIGURE 2-1. Spectrum of acute ischemic heart disease. Pathophysiologic mechanisms can be used as a basis for constructing a spectrum of presentations of plaque fissuring that consists of six general categories, each with its own risk profile and potential for effective therapy. A totally occluded vessel with ongoing myocardial necrosis can be present either with or without ST-segment elevation. In general, patients with ST-segment elevation (category 1) are at high risk for death and congestive heart failure (CHF), although the risk in patients without this finding (category 2) appears to be almost as high, perhaps owing to inclusion of the subpopulation with substantial

preexistent myocardial dysfunction. Total occlusion without myocardial necrosis (category 3) generally poses a low risk for any acute events. Subtotally occluded vessels that produce symptoms at rest and ST-segment changes on the electrocardiogram (ECG) or positive troponin in the circulation (category 4) present a high risk for subsequent myocardial infarction, whereas the same morphology without frequent ECG changes or symptoms at rest (category 5) presents a much lower risk. Finally, asymptomatic plaque fissuring that leads to progression of atherosclerosis (category 6) carries no immediate risk, but the long-term outcome will eventually be impaired. The place of sudden death in this spectrum remains unclear.

Interventions to treat or prevent clinical manifestations of acute ischemic heart disease can be considered as layered upon this continuum. Throughout the lifetime of a patient with acute ischemic heart disease, antiplatelet therapy is a mainstay of therapy, and its intensity may be adjusted according to the acuteness and severity of the illness. Antithrombin therapy also plays a major role in most situations in the acute phase, although this issue has recently become more complicated in the chronic phase. Beta blockade also appears to be beneficial across the entire spectrum, and angiotensin converting enzyme inhibitors may be assuming this therapeutic role as well. Nitrates are now relegated to symptom relief only. Standard approaches to secondary prevention are being developed for use as the acute phase of the illness becomes quiescent. All other therapies are known to be beneficial only in selected circumstances.

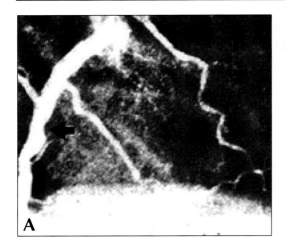

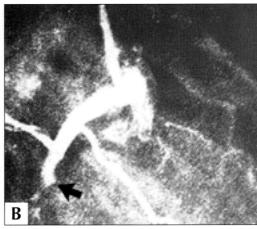

FIGURE 2-2. A, Coronary angiogram of right coronary artery showing only a luminal irregularity at a future infarct site (*arrow*). **B,** A repeat angiogram in the same patient after an inferior infarction 13 days later. The mid-right coronary artery is totally occluded at the site of the previously noted irregularity. The observation that a large number of infarctions are due to the formation of obstructive thrombus at sites of noncritical stenosis [1–4] supports the concept that steps to prevent the triggering of plaque disruption and occlusive thrombus formation could greatly reduce cardiovascular morbidity and mortality. (*From* Little *et al.* [1]; with permission from the American Heart Association, Inc.)

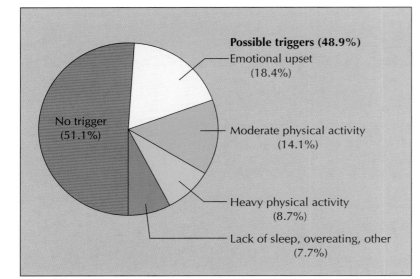

FIGURE 2-3. Possible triggers of myocardial infarction (MI). In the MILIS study [5], 412 of 849 patients (48.5%) with confirmed MI reported one possible trigger. Multiple possible triggers were reported by 109 (13%) patients. The likelihood of reporting possible triggers varied inversely with increasing age, female gender, history of diabetes, and time of onset. No difference in the likelihood of reporting a possible trigger was found for size or type of infarction (Q-wave vs non–Q-wave). The subgroup differences may be accounted for by the possibility that patients whose plaques are more vulnerable to disruption may require a less marked (and thus less easily identifiable) external trigger to cause infarction. Alternatively, in the absence of control data, certain subgroups of patients, such as the elderly, may be less likely to engage in activities that are potential triggers. Sumiyoshi *et al.* [6] have reported similar findings, with 53% of patients reporting that their infarct began during moderate to heavy exercise, emotional stress, or excitement. (*Adapted from* Tofler *et al.* [5].)

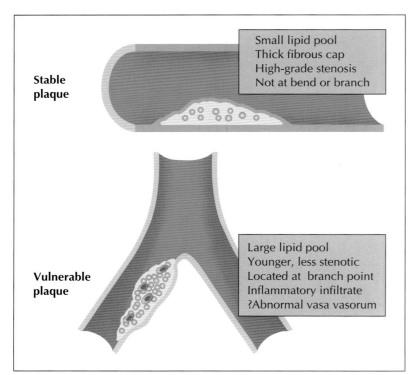

FIGURE 2-4. Specific features of the plaque that are thought to predispose to fissuring or rupture have been elucidated through a series of intricated pathologic studies. The atherosclerotic plaques most likely to lead to acute myocardial infarction are those with a large lipid pool, which is thought to produce instability beneath the fibrous cap and thus to make the plaque more susceptible to shear forces. Most often these vulnerable plaques are not likely stenotic prior to the acute event and are relatively new, without a large amount of fibrotic material. In addition, atherosclerotic plaques located at vessel branch points are more likely to become fissured owing to increased shear forces that create turbulence at the branches. Finally, fissured or disrupted plaques more often show infiltration of macrophages into the fibrous cap. The stimulus to such infiltration remains unclear, but a leading theory is that oxidized low-density lipoprotein (LDL) cholesterol is the culprit; in experimental models, oxidized LDL cholesterol attracts macrophages and other inflammatory cells into tissue and may thus provide a link between antioxidant status and risk for cardiac events. The potential role of infectious agents has been raised in light of these findings, although a direct link to such an agent has not been established. Another line of reasoning supposes that some plaque events are caused by thrombosis or hemorrhage of vasa vasorum, the vessels in the adventitia that supply the vessel wall. As the plaque enlarges, the vasa vasorum may become inadequate or may be compressed by other elements of the plaque.

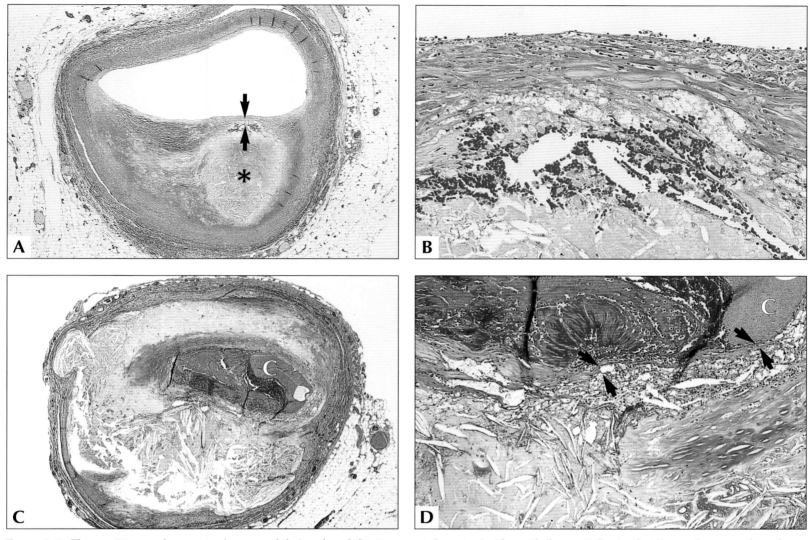

FIGURE 2–5. The consistency of coronary plaques and their vulnerability to rupture differ. The collagen-rich sclerotic plaque component is hard and stable, while the lipid-rich atheromatous component is soft and unstable. **A** and **B,** A thin cap of fibrous tissue (*between arrows*) separates the soft, lipid-rich pool (*asterisk*) from the lumen. Such a thin fibrous cap, infiltrated with macrophage foam cells (clearly seen in *B*), overlying an extracellular lipid pool is mechanically weak and vulnerable to rupture. The presence of erythrocytes just beneath the cap indicates that the cap is ruptured nearby. **C** and **D,** In this case, the thin, foam cell–infiltrated cap (*between arrows* in *D*) has ruptured nearby, and a mural thrombus has evolved at the rupture site where thrombogenic material has been exposed (trichrome stain, showing collagen as blue and thrombus as red). C—contrast medium. (**A** and **B** *from* Falk and Andersen [7]; **C** and **D** *from* Falk [8]; with permission from the American Heart Association, Inc.)

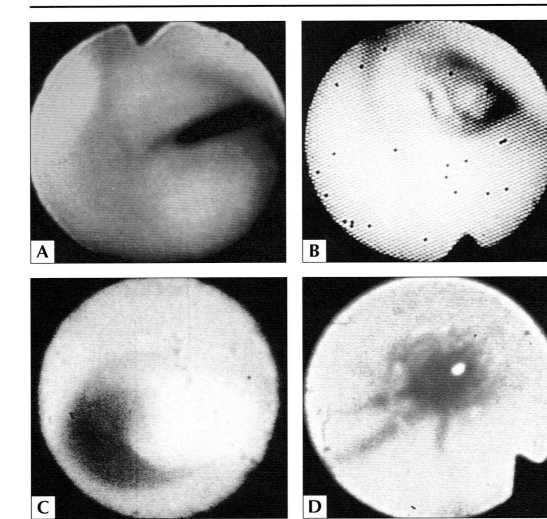

FIGURE 2-6. Intraoperative fiberoptic angioscopic appearance of culprit coronary lesions in patients with various coronary syndromes. **A,** Stable plaque with a smooth intact surface in stable angina. **B,** Culprit plaque with intimal disruption and intralesional hemorrhage in unstable angina. **C,** Nonocclusive crescent-shaped thrombus in the culprit artery in unstable angina. **D,** Occlusive thrombus in the culprit artery in acute myocardial infarction. (*From* Sherman *et al.* [9]; with permission.)

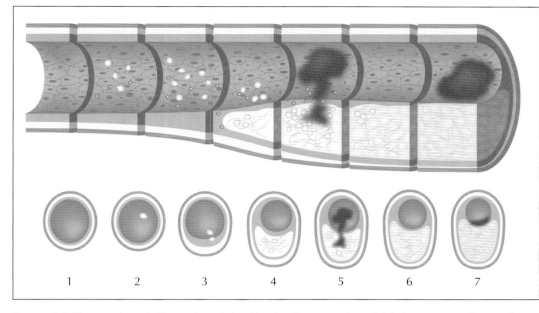

FIGURE 2-7 Progression of atherosclerosis leading to plaque rupture. Initiation, progression, and complication of human coronary atherosclerotic plaque. *Top*, Longitudinal section of artery depicting "timeline" of human atherogenesis from normal artery (1) to atheroma that caused clinical manifestations by thrombosis or stenosis (5, 6, 7). *Bottom*, Cross-sections of artery during various stages of atheroma evolution. 1, Normal artery. Note that in human arteries, the intimal layer is much better developed than in most other species. The intima of human arteries contains resident smooth muscle cells often as early as the first year of life. 2, Lesion initiation occurs when endothelial cells, activated by risk factors such as hyperlipoproteinemia, express adhesion and chemoattractant molecules that recruit inflammatory leukocytes such as monocytes and T lymphocytes. Extracellular lipid begins to accumulate in intima at this stage. 3, Evolution to fibrofatty stage. Monocytes recruited to artery wall become macrophages and express scavenger receptors that bind modified lipoproteins. Macrophages become lipid-laden foam cells by engulfing modified lipoproteins. Leukocytes and resident vascular wall cells can secrete inflammatory cytokines and growth factors that amplify leukocyte recruitment and cause smooth muscle cell migration and proliferation. 4, As lesion progresses, inflammatory mediators cause expression of tissue factor, a potent procoagulant, and of matrix-degrading proteinases that weaken fibrous cap of plaque. 5, If fibrous cap ruptures at point of weakening, coagulation factors in blood can gain access to thrombogenic, tissue factor–containing lipid core, causing thrombosis on nonocclusive atherosclerotic plaque. If balance between prothrombotic and fibrinolytic mechanisms prevailing at that particular region and at that particular time is unfavorable, occlusive thrombosis causing acute coronary syndromes may result. 6, When thrombosis resorbs, products associated with thrombosis such as thrombin and mediators released from degranulating platelets, including platelet-derived growth factor and transforming growth factor-β, can cause healing response, leading to increased collagen accumulation and smooth muscle cell growth. In this manner, the fibrofatty lesion can evolve into advanced fibrous and often calcified plaque, one that may cause significant stenosis, and produce symptoms of stable angina pectoris. 7, In some cases, occlusive thrombi arise not from fracture of fibrous cap but from superficial erosion of endothelial layer. Resulting mural thrombus, again dependent on local prothrombotic and fibrinolytic balance, can cause acute myocardial infarction. Superficial erosions often complicate advanced and stenotic lesions, as shown here. However, superficial erosions do not necessarily occur after fibrous cap rupture, as depicted in this idealized diagram. (*Adapted from* Libby [10].)

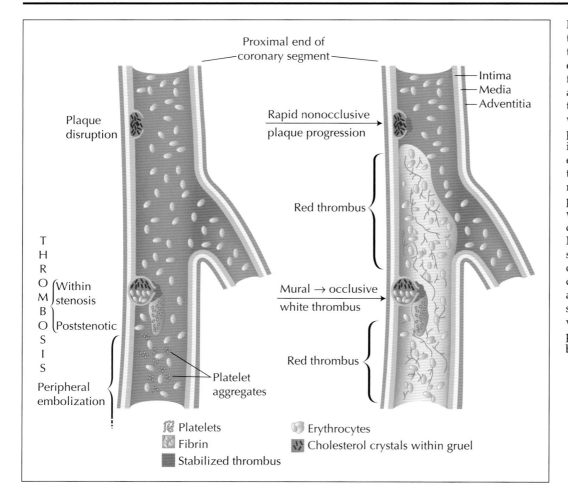

FIGURE 2-8. Pathogenesis of a coronary thrombus. Most coronary thrombi (about three fourths) are initiated by plaque rupture, exposing thrombogenic material to the flowing blood; the atheromatous gruel appears to be highly thrombogenic. The thrombus is platelet-rich and usually gray-white at the rupture site; severe stenosis, if present, promotes thrombosis via shear-induced platelet activation. Fibrin soon enmeshes the platelets, stabilizing the thrombus. Thrombus formation is dynamic: recurrent thrombosis, thrombolysis, and peripheral embolization occur simultaneously, with or without concomitant vasospasm, causing intermittent flow obstruction. Nonoccluding thrombi may extend post-stenotically, and if the platelet-rich thrombus occludes the vessel, the blood proximal and distal to the occlusion may stagnate and co-agulate, giving rise to upstream and/or down-stream propagation of a red, fibrin-dependent, venous-like thrombus. Upstream thrombus propagation does not occlude major side branches. (*Adapted from* Falk [11].)

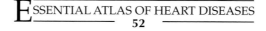

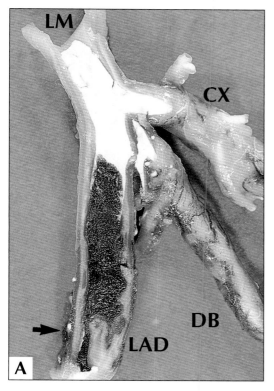

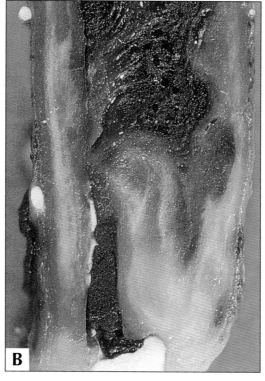

FIGURE 2-9. Secondary to flow reduction, a red stagnation thrombus may propagate upstream. **A** and **B,** The proximal left anterior descending coronary artery (LAD) has been cut open longitudinally. A ruptured plaque with a gray-white occluding thrombus (platelet-rich) can be seen at the *arrow* in *A* (magnified in *B*), and a red thrombus (erythrocyte-rich) is seen propagating upstream up to the first diagonal branch (DB). **C** and **D,** A thrombosed right coronary artery, showing a red thrombus propagating upstream and passing a side branch (SB) without occluding it. The platelet-rich thrombus causing the initial flow reduction is marked (*arrow*). **E** and **F,** Specimen of partly opened, thrombosed right coronary artery and corresponding angiogram showing total occlusion at and just proximal to the acute branch (AB) as well as an extensive filling defect propagating upstream without occluding any major side branches. CX—circumflex branch; LM—left main stem. (**A** *from* Falk [11]; with permission; **D** *from* Falk [12]; with permission.)

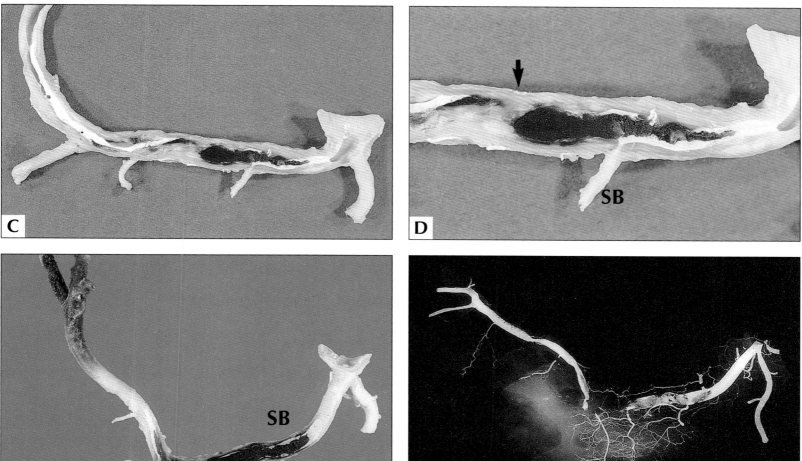

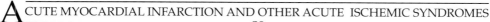

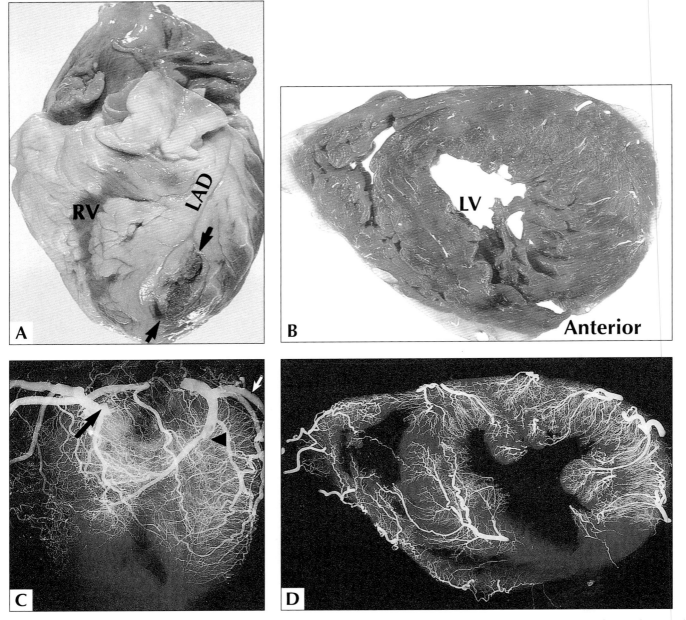

FIGURE 2-10. Rupture of the heart complicates acute myocardial infarction in about 10% of autopsied cases. Typically, it occurs during the first week after a first infarct and is more common in elderly women. The pathoanatomic substrate for postinfarction rupture of the left ventricular free wall or the interventricular septum includes total occlusion of a functional end artery (poor collateral circulation) causing transmural infarction in a perfusion area that was previously healthy (ie, no myocardial fibrosis). Usually, heart weight is normal. **A,** Rupture of the anterior wall of the left ventricle (LV; *between arrows*), parallel to the left anterior descending artery (LAD). **B,** Perforation of the free wall in this 11-hour-old infarct can be seen clearly on the transventricular myocardial slice (short-axis view). Thrombolytic therapy was not given. **C,** Postmortem angiogram of a similar case (28-hour-old infarct) showing LAD occlusion (*arrowhead*). The right coronary (*black arrow*) and left circumflex (*white arrow*) arteries appear almost normal (single-vessel disease). The LAD is occluded just distal to the first septal branch, with no distal collateral filling.

D, Angiographic short-axis view of transventricular myocardial slice reveals no vascular filling in the area normally perfused by the LAD. Note the treelike coronary branching pattern with well-defined perfusion areas, in contrast to the enlarged anastomotic network frequently seen with subendocardial infarction and, in particular, with diffuse subendocardial necrosis. RV—right ventricle.

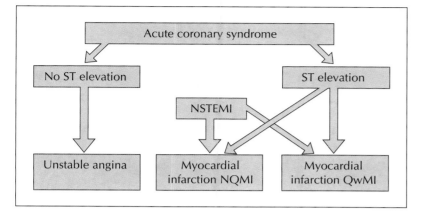

FIGURE 2-11 Nomenclature of acute coronary syndromes. Patients with ischemic discomfort may present with or without ST-segment elevation on the electrocardiogram (ECG). The majority of patients with ST-segment elevation (*thicker arrows*) ultimately develop a Q-wave myocardial infarction (QwMI), whereas a minority (*thinner arrows*) develop a non–Q-wave myocardial infarction (NQMI). Patients who present without ST-segment elevation are experiencing either unstable angina (UA) or a no ST elevation myocardial infarction (NSTEMI). The distinction between these two diagnoses is ultimately made based on the presence or absence of a cardiac marker detected in the blood. Most patients with NSTEMI do not evolve a Q wave on the 12-lead ECG and are subsequently referred to as having sustained NQMI; only a minority of NSTEMI patients develop a Q wave and are later diagnosed as having Q-wave MI. Not shown is Prinzmetal's angina, which presents with transient chest pain and ST-segment elevation but rarely MI. The spectrum of clinical conditions that range from UA to NQMI and QwMI is referred to as acute coronary syndromes. (*Adapted from* Antman and Braunwald [13].)

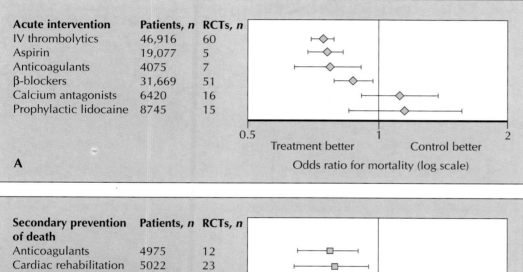

Figure 2-12. Pooled results of randomized controlled trials in *acute* myocardial infarction (MI) [14]. **A,** Meta-analysis of several trials of acute therapy for MI. This graph presents the pooled estimate of the odds of reducing (or increasing) mortality with the test intervention versus control. The 95% confidence intervals (CI) around these point estimates are indicated by the width of the horizontal lines. Therapies that reduce mortality are plotted to the left of the vertical line (Treatment better), while those that increase mortality are plotted to the right (Control better). For example, intravenous (IV) thrombolytic agents were evaluated in 60 trials that collectively enrolled 46,916 patients; the pooled odds ratio for mortality was 0.75 (CI, 0.71 to 0.79), indicating a reduction in the odds of dying by about 25% in those patients who received thrombolytic therapy versus placebo. The pooled data from trials of calcium antagonists and prophylactic lidocaine show a trend toward increased mortality in patients who received active therapy.

B, Meta-analysis of trials of *secondary prevention* of mortality following MI conducted between 1960 and 1990 [14]. Long-term therapy with calcium antagonists shows no significant evidence of benefit, whereas class I antiarrhythmic agents are associated with increased mortality. The other therapies studied were all associated with improvements in survival, although precise dose-ranging information has not been established definitively for important drugs such as warfarin and aspirin. (*Adapted from* Lau *et al.* [14].)

A. POTENTIAL MECHANISMS OF BETA BLOCKADE

Reduce shear force on plaque—plaque and myocardial rupture
Reduce catecholamine effects—arrhythmia, platelet activation
Better endocardial-to-epicardial ratio of myocardial blood flow

FIGURE 2-13. **A,** In addition to reducing myocardial oxygen demand, beta blockade may have a number of other beneficial effects. Blunting of symptomatic surges could prevent lethal arrhythmias as well as rapid fluctuations in shear stress that could promote further plaque fissuring. Epinephrine is also a substantial stimulus to platelet aggregation, so that blunting sympathetic tone could lead to a less thrombogenic environment. Finally, beta blockade redistributes coronary blood flow from the epicardium toward the endocardium, providing a primary anti-ischemic effect. **B,** Vascular mortality during the scheduled treatment period (days 0 to 7) and immediately after (to day 14) among 16,027 patients with suspected acute myocardial infarction enrolled in ISIS-1. (**B** *adapted from* ISIS-1 Collaborative Group [15].)

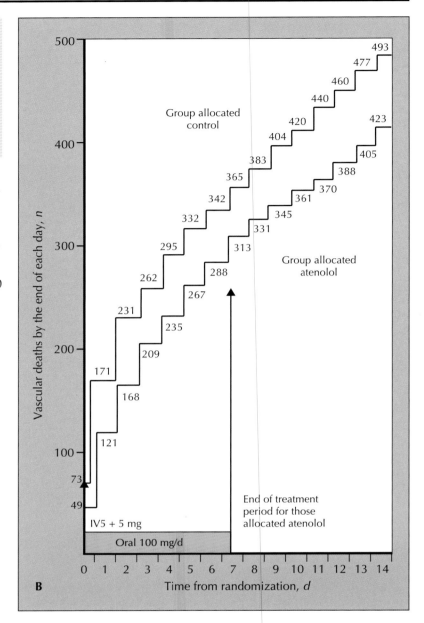

CALCIUM ANTAGONISTS

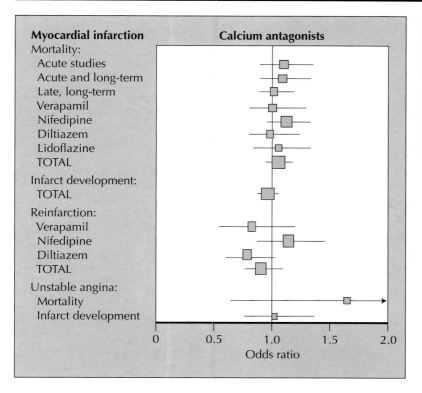

FIGURE 2-14. Results of therapy with calcium antagonists in acute coronary syndromes. This meta-analysis indicates that calcium antagonists have no significant beneficial effect on mortality in patients with acute myocardial infarction (MI) and may even be associated with a trend toward an *increase* in mortality; no evidence of a beneficial effect was detected in patients with unstable angina either. Reinfarction rates tended to be lower in the patients treated with verapamil or diltiazem, but this value did not achieve statistical significance (confidence intervals overlap vertical line). Based on these observations, calcium antagonists cannot be recommended as primary therapy for unstable angina or acute MI. (*Adapted from* Held *et al.* [16].)

NITRATE THERAPY

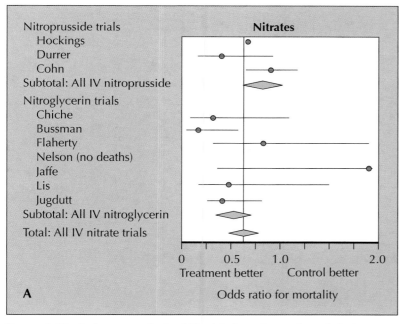

A

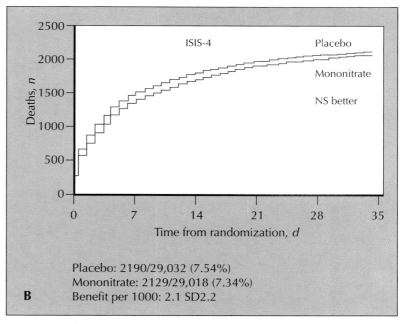

Placebo: 2190/29,032 (7.54%)
Mononitrate: 2129/29,018 (7.34%)
Benefit per 1000: 2.1 SD2.2

B

FIGURE 2-15. A, A meta-analysis of 10 trials from the prethrombolytic era indicated a favorable effect of nitrate-like compounds in the acute phase of myocardial infarction (MI) [17]. **B,** In the current thrombolytic era, when important reductions in mortality can be achieved with reperfusion therapy and aspirin, the relative benefit of nitrates is considerably smaller, although some evidence of a slight reduction in short-term mortality can still be seen in the ISIS-4 [18] and GISSI-3 [19] Trials. IV—intravenous. (**A** *adapted from* Yusuf *et al.* [17]; **B** *adapted from* ISIS-4 Collaborative Group [18].)

ANGIOTENSIN-CONVERTING ENZYME INHIBITION

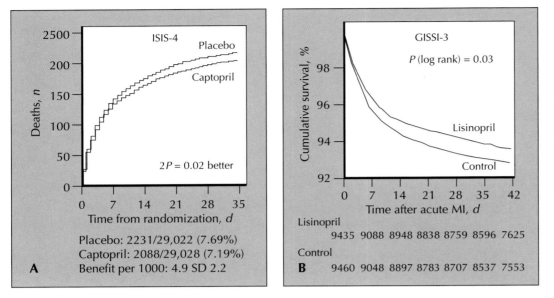

FIGURE 2-16. Results of treatment with angiotensin-converting enzyme (ACE) inhibitors after acute myocardial infarction (MI). Two trials of acute therapy in unselected patients (*ie*, both with and without evidence of left ventricular dysfunction) have shown that ACE inhibitors reduce mortality at 4 to 6 weeks [18,19]. This effect was seen in two different patient populations and with two different ACE inhibitors, captopril (**A**) and lisinopril (**B**), attesting to the consistency and generalizability of the observations. (**A** *adapted from* ISIS-4 Collaborative Group [18]; **B** *adapted from* Gruppo Italiano per lo Studio della Sopravvivenza nell'Infarto Miocardico [19].)

PROPHYLACTIC ANTIARRHYTHMIC DRUG THERAPY

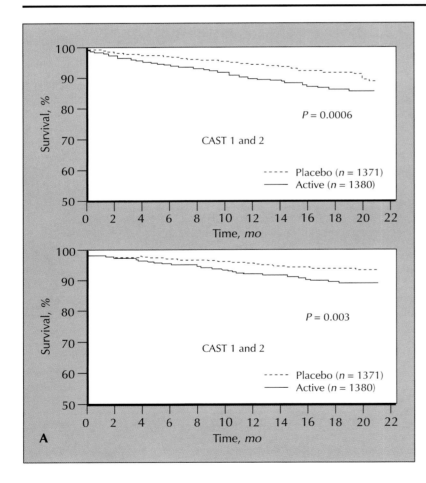

FIGURE 2-17. A, Results of CAST (Cardiac Arrhythmia Suppression Trial) [19]. This trial tested the hypothesis that the use of encainide, flecainide, or moricizine to suppress ventricular arrhythmias detected on Holter monitoring after myocardial infarction (MI) would reduce the long-term risk for cardiac arrest and death. The first phase of the trial (CAST-1), which involved encainide and flecainide (class IC antiarrhythmic agents), was stopped prematurely because these drugs increased mortality; the second phase of the trial (CAST-2), in which moricizine (a class IA agent) was compared with placebo, was also discontinued prematurely due to both an increase in mortality during the titration phase of moricizine dosing and the fact that beneficial effects of moricizine in those patients who survived the titration phase were highly unlikely. Data from both CAST-1 and CAST-2 are combined here and clearly depict the adverse impact on long-term total mortality (*top panel*) and sudden cardiac death (*bottom panel*) with these antiarrhythmic agents versus placebo. (*continued*)

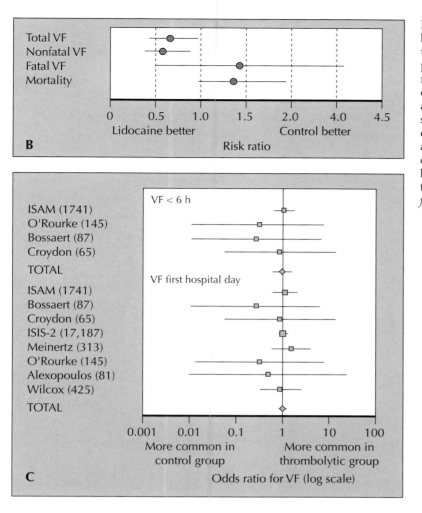

B

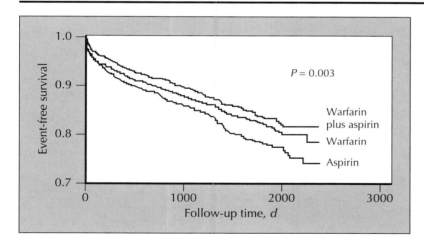

C

Figure 2-17. (*continued*) **B,** Although prophylactic lidocaine was clearly beneficial in reducing the risk for primary ventricular fibrillation (VF) in the absence of congestive heart failure or cardiogenic shock in the prethrombolytic era, its use was associated with a trend toward increased mortality, probably due to fatal bradycardia and asystolic arrest. **C,** Impact of thrombolytic therapy on the development of VF. Despite initial concerns about an increase in VF with reperfusion, the results of this meta-analysis show no difference in the incidence of VF in the first 6 hours or at any time during the first 24 hours in patients treated with a variety of thrombolytic agents compared with those given placebo. Based on this observation, the decision to administer a thrombolytic agent to patients treated in the hospital for acute MI does not appear to increase their risk for VF during the first day of treatment. (**B** *adapted from* MacMahon *et al.* [21]; **C** *adapted from* Solomon *et al.* [22].)

WARFARIN THERAPY

Figure 2-18. Event-free survival curves for the composite endpoint of death, nonfatal reinfarction, and thromboembolic stroke. The *P* value refers to the overall difference among the curves (Tarone-Ware method). A recent trial of 3630 patients in Norway demonstrated a reduction in death in patients treated with warfarin (INR 2.8–4.2) or aspirin plus warfarin (INR 2–2.5) compared with aspirin alone [23].

CLINICAL USE OF ANTITHROMBOTIC THERAPY

ORAL ANTIPLATELET THERAPY

Aspirin	Initial dose of 162–325 mg nonenteric formulation followed by 75–160 mg/d of an enteric or nonenteric formulation
Clopidogrel	75 mg/d, a loading dose of 4 to 8 tablets (300–600 mg) can be used when rapid onset of action is required
Ticlopidine	250 mg twice daily, a loading dose of 500 mg can be used when rapid onset of inhibition is required; monitoring of platelet and white cell counts during treatment is required
Heparins	
Enoxaparin	1 mg/kg subcutaneously every 12 hours; the first dase may be preceded by a 30 mg IV bolus
Heparin (UFH)	Bolus 60–70 units/kg (maximum 5000 units) IV followed by infusion of 12–15 units/kg/h (maximum 1000 u/h) titrated to aPTTT 1.5–2.5 times control
Intravenous antiplatelet therapy	
Abciximab	0.25 mg/kg bolus followed by infusion of 0.125 µg/kg/min (maximum 10 µg/min) for 12 to 24 hours
Eptifibatide	180 µg/kg bolus followed by infusion of 2.0 µg/kg/min for 72 to 96 hours*
Tirofiban	0.4 µg/kg/min for 30 minutes followed by infusion of 0.1 µg/kg/min for 48 to 96 hours*

*Different dose regimens were tested in recent clinical trials before percutaneous interventions.

FIGURE 2-19. Clinical use of antithrombotic therapy. Antithrombotic therapy recommended in the guidelines for unstable angina in non-ST elevation myocardial infarction [24]. The change in heparin dosing is important to note; underdosing of heparin will lead to an increase in thrombotic events while overdosing will lead to an increase in both thrombotic and hemorrhagic events. Care must also be exhibited in combining the glycoprotein (GP) IIb/IIIa inhibitors with heparin or low molecular weight heparin. There is a pharmocodynamic interaction mandating an even lower dose of heparin when a GP IIb/IIIa inhibitor is used; the proper dose of a LVMW when a GP IIb/IIIa inhibitor is under study. UFH—unfractionated heparin.

CLASS I RECOMMENDATIONS FOR ANTITHROMBOTIC THERAPY

POSSIBLE ACS	LIKELY/DEFINITE ACS	DEFINITE ACS WITH CONTINUE ISCHEMIA OR OTHER HIGH-RISK FEATURES* OR PLANNED INTERVENTION
Aspirin	Aspirin + SC LMWH or IV heparin + clopidogiel (if noninvasive strategy planned)	Aspirin + IV heparin + IV GP IIb/IIIa antagonist + clopidogiel (if CABG surgery unlikely)

Clinical data on the combination of LMWH and GP IIb/IIIa antagonist are lacking. Their combined use is not currently recommended.

*High-risk features include diabetes, recent myocardial infarction, and elevated troponin T or I.

FIGURE 2-20. Class I recommendations for antithrombotic therapy. Patients with possible acute coronary syndrome (ACS) should be treated with aspirin. Patients with definite ACS should be treated with aspirin and either low molecular weight heparin (LMWH) or unfractionated heparin. Patients with high-risk features should be treated with aspirin, intravenous (IV) heparin, and an IV glycoprotein (GP) IIb/IIIa antagonist. Aspirin is recommended for possible ACS because of its demonstrated benefit and very low risk of bleeding complications. The addition of the antithrombin regimen is based on less conclusive data, but the global community is convinced of the benefit and the empirical support is substantial. The addition of GP IIb/IIIa inhibitor in high-risk situations is based upon definitive clinical trial results [24]. Based on the results of the CURE trial, clopidogrel should be added in any patient with definite ACS who is unlikely to undergo coronary artery bypass graft (CABG) surgery.

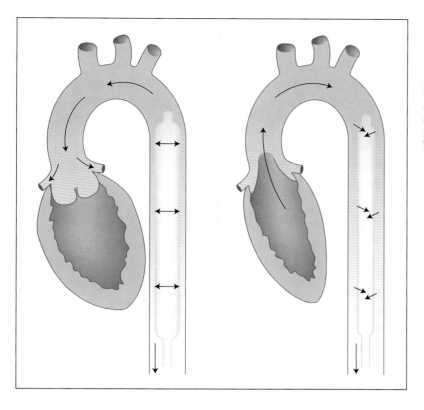

FIGURE 2-21. The major mode of action of the intra-aortic balloon pump (IABP) in unstable angina is improvement of diastolic coronary blood flow. In addition, the mechanical effect of the balloon inflation and deflation decreases afterload substantially, therefore reducing myocardial wall stress. Functioning IABP. During diastole (*left panel*), the balloon is inflated, which increases volume in the aorta, raises diastolic pressure, and increases perfusion of coronary arteries. Just before and during systole (*right panel*), the balloon is deflated, which decreases the volume in the aorta, decreases aortic pressure (afterload), and facilitates ejection by the left ventricle.

OVERVIEW OF MEDICAL MANAGEMENT OF ACUTE CORONARY SYNDROMES

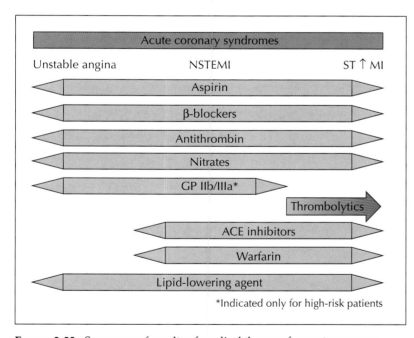

FIGURE 2-22. Summary of results of medical therapy for acute coronary syndromes. Aspirin, beta-blockers, and an antithrombin (*eg*, heparin or the new direct antithrombins), alone and in combination, have been shown to reduce morbidity and mortality across the entire spectrum of acute coronary

syndromes. Although nitrates are useful for relieving recurrent episodes of ischemic-type discomfort, these agents probably provide only a small short-term benefit with regard to reducing mortality in patients with acute myocardial infarction (MI) who receive the other therapies noted above. Of the various forms of medical therapy, intravenous thrombolytic agents offer the most dramatic reductions in mortality for patients with ST-elevation MI. Based on available data, the thrombolytic agents and regimens now available do not appear to benefit patients with unstable angina/NSTEMI. Angiotensin-converting enzyme (ACE) inhibitors have clearly been shown to reduce long-term mortality in patients with left ventricular (LV) dysfunction following MI, and recent data suggest that they reduce short-term mortality (4 to 6 weeks) even when patients are not selected for the presence of LV dysfunction. However, before ACE inhibitors can be recommended on a broad basis for patients with either NSTEMI or ST-elevation MI, even in the absence of LV dysfunction, additional analyses and more long-term follow-up are needed. The benefits of magnesium remain controversial, and decisions regarding the use of class III antiarrhythmic agents such as amiodarone or low-dose warfarin in combination with aspirin should await the findings of ongoing clinical trials.

Lipid-lowering therapy is clearly helpful in reducing risk for recurrent ischemic events and probably will lead to a reduction in mortality, although the latter outcome has not been rigorously established in the current therapeutic era. Recent recommendations from the National Cholesterol Education Program Adult Treatment Panel-2 have proposed a much more aggressive approach to lipid lowering than clinicians have used in the past. A target goal for low-density lipoprotein cholesterol below 100 mg/dL has been recommended for patients with a history of coronary heart disease. NSTEMI—non-ST elevation myocardial infarction.

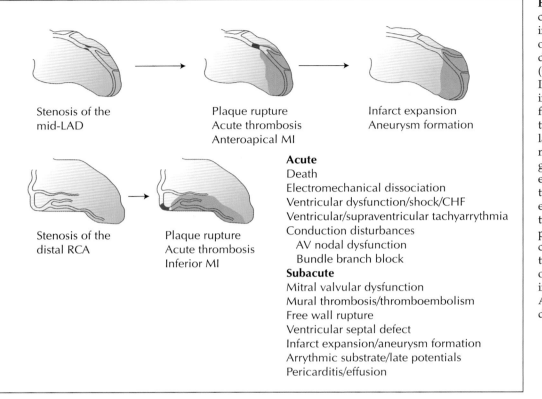

Stenosis of the
mid-LAD

Plaque rupture
Acute thrombosis
Anteroapical MI

Infarct expansion
Aneurysm formation

Stenosis of the
distal RCA

Plaque rupture
Acute thrombosis
Inferior MI

Acute
Death
Electromechanical dissociation
Ventricular dysfunction/shock/CHF
Ventricular/supraventricular tachyarrythmia
Conduction disturbances
  AV nodal dysfunction
  Bundle branch block
Subacute
Mitral valvular dysfunction
Mural thrombosis/thromboembolism
Free wall rupture
Ventricular septal defect
Infarct expansion/aneurysm formation
Arrythmic substrate/late potentials
Pericarditis/effusion

FIGURE 2-23. Myocardial consequences of acute coronary occlusion. Complications of myocardial infarction (MI) are direct consequences of the loss of ventricular myocardium. Acutely, ventricular dysfunction may result in congestive heart failure (CHF) or shock, severely compromising survival. In the subacute period, compromised integrity of infarcted myocardium may lead to rupture of the free wall (usually leading to pericardial tamponade), rupture of the septum (leading to a large intracardiac shunt), or disruption of the mitral apparatus (leading to acute valvular regurgitation). In the convalescent phase, infarct expansion and/or aneurysm formation may lead to unfavorable ventricular mechanics and may exacerbate CHF. Acutely and chronically, noncontractile or dyskinetic myocardial regions predispose to mural thrombosis and thromboembolic complications. Electrical instability predisposing to potentially fatal ventricular arrhythmias may occur in the acute or chronic phase, with the infarct scar serving as arrhythmic substrate. AV—atrioventricular; LAD—left anterior descending artery; RCA—right coronary artery.

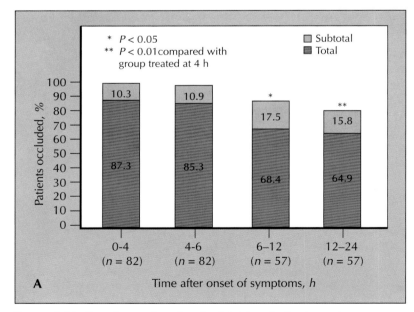

A

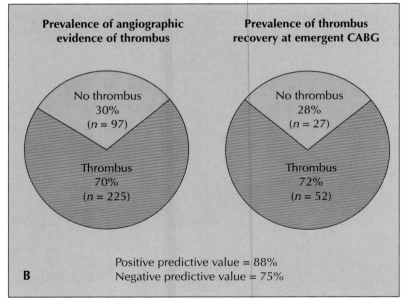

Positive predictive value = 88%
Negative predictive value = 75%

B

FIGURE 2-24. Prevalence of total and subtotal occlusion in acute myocardial infarction (MI). The role of acute thrombotic occlusion in the pathogenesis of MI has guided therapeutic efforts since publication of the landmark study by DeWood *et al.* [25] in 1980. DeWood *et al.* performed coronary angiography on 322 patients (out of 1210 patients admitted with early transmural MI between March 1971 and December 1978) within 24 hours of onset of symptoms. **A,** The prevalence of total and subtotal coronary occlusions was found to be highest in the earliest hours following symptom onset, prompting therapeutic strategies aimed at restoration of coronary blood flow. The numbers inside each bar are percentages of total and subtotal occlusions.

B, The high prevalence of angiographic evidence of thrombus, corroborated by the recovery of thrombus at the time of emergent coronary artery bypass graft surgery (CABG), provides the rationale for the strategy of thrombolytic/antithrombotic approaches to the treatment of acute MI. (*Adapted from* DeWood *et al.* [25].)

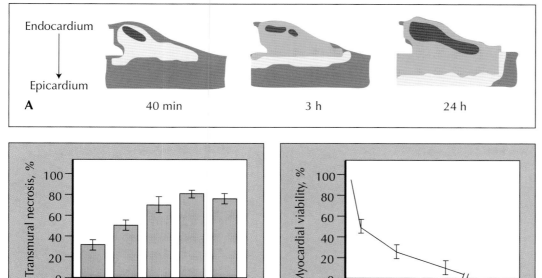

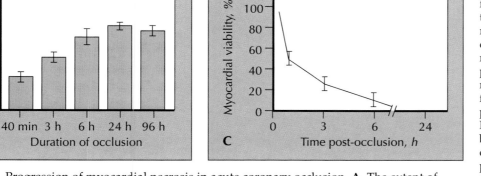

subepicardial region over time. *Yellow area* indicates the anatomic boundary between ischemic circumflex and nonischemic left anterior descending coronary beds. *Orange area* indicates interstitial hemorrhage. *Red area* represents the central core of necrotic muscle devoid of either hemorrhage or inflammatory response, which results from complete cessation of microvascular perfusion.

B, In the dog papillary model, the percentage of sections exhibiting transmural infarction continues to rise over the first 6 hours following coronary occlusion. **C,** Conversely, the amount of viable myocardium diminishes rapidly over the first hour, and continues to decline to small amounts of salvageable myocardium beyond 6 hours (plot shows proportion of viable, potentially salvageable myocardium in a dog papillary model as a function of time after coronary occlusion, plotted as a percentage of 24-hour infarct size). Myocardial loss in acute MI in humans has been found to follow a similar time dependency, forming the basis of the quest for therapeutic strategies emphasizing earlier diagnosis and triage, and the earliest possible restoration of coronary blood flow. *T-bars* indicate ±SEM. (*Adapted from* Reimer *et al.* [26].)

FIGURE 2-25. Progression of myocardial necrosis in acute coronary occlusion. **A,** The extent of myocardial necrosis in acute myocardial infarction (MI) is a time-dependent process, as elucidated by Reimer *et al.* [26] in a dog papillary muscle preparation. Necrosis following coronary occlusion occurs in "wavefront" form, advancing from the endocardial surface outward to the

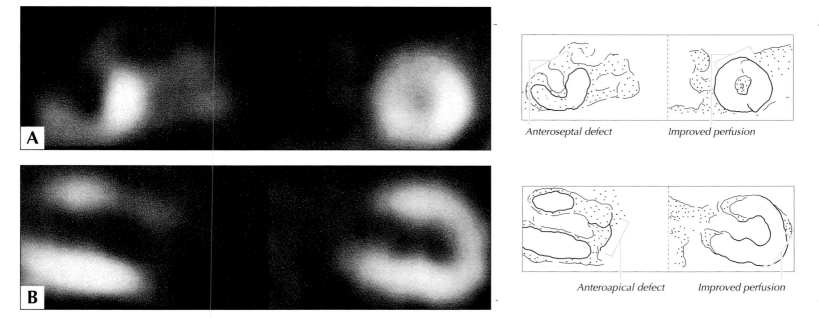

FIGURE 2-26. Radionuclide perfusion imaging: assessment of myocardium at risk and myocardial salvage. Tomographic images of a patient with acute anterior myocardial infarction (MI). **A,** Midventricular short-axis slices. **B,** Vertical long-axis slices. The images in the *left panels* were

acquired following acute MI prior to administration of thrombolytic therapy. Repeat imaging performed 1 week later (*right panels*) revealed resolution of the initial large anterior perfusion defects indicative of successful reperfusion. (*From* Gibbons [27]; with permission.)

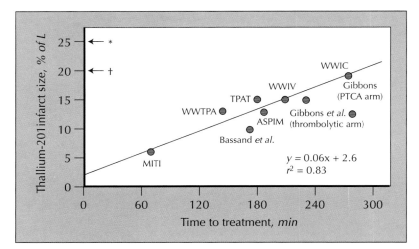

FIGURE 2-27. Effect of time to reperfusion therapy and infarct size. This graph shows infarct size, as determined by radionuclide tomographic

perfusion imaging in trials of thrombolytic therapy and direct angioplasty, plotted against the mean time to initiation of reperfusion therapy. Indicated are the approximate infarct sizes that might be expected in the presence of treated but persistently occluded vessels (*asterisk*), and in patients treated by conservative means (*dagger*) as suggested by the results of the TPAT [28,29] and Western Washington [30,31] trials. A remarkably consistent correlation exists between time to treatment and infarct size across these studies. At approximately 4 to 5 hours, the infarct size might be expected to be similar in treated and untreated groups, thus reperfusion beyond this time is not likely to result in significant myocardial salvage. Of interest, the farthest outlier (not included in regression) is the direct percutaneous transluminal coronary angioplasty (PTCA) group of the study by Gibbons [27]. While the thrombolytic arm of this study [32] appears consistent with other thrombolytic trials, the smaller infarcts experienced by the PTCA group, even at a later time to treatment, may reflect the greater likelihood of *complete reperfusion* with this strategy. The non-zero intersection of the regression line reflects the limitations of both symptom-based infarction diagnosis and reperfusion therapy [33–37]. LV—left ventricle. (*Adapted from* Martin and Kennedy [34].)

CORONARY PATENCY, VENTRICULAR FUNCTION, AND SURVIVAL

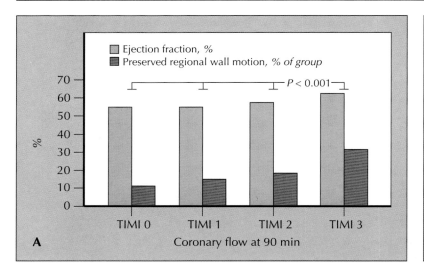

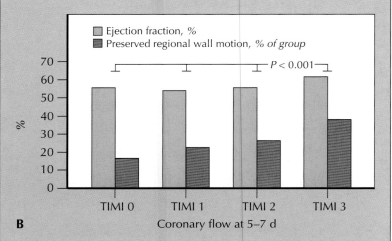

FIGURE 2-28. GUSTO: Coronary patency and ventricular function. The potential for myocardial salvage through restoration of coronary blood flow early in the course of acute myocardial infarction has been demonstrated dramatically by the GUSTO angiographic substudy. In this group of patients treated with various thrombolytic regimens, significant relationships of flow to various measures of ventricular function were observed. In addition to global ejection fraction and the percentage of patients with completely preserved regional wall motion, measures of

end-systolic volume index, wall motion (SD/chord, by left ventriculography), and number of abnormal chords all were significantly better in the group with normal flow (TIMI 3) when compared with no (TIMI 0 to 1) or only partial (TIMI 2) reperfusion. These relationships were observed both acutely (by angiography at 90 minutes post-thrombolytic administration; **A**) and in the convalescent period (5 to 7 days; **B**). (*Adapted from* the GUSTO Angiographic Investigators [38].)

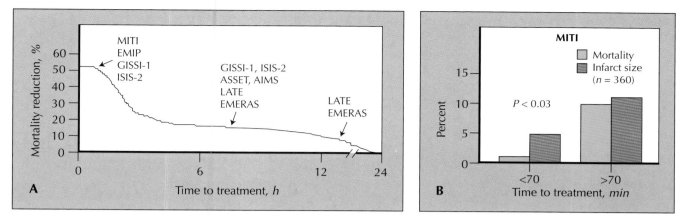

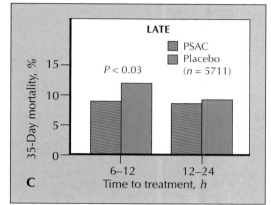

FIGURE 2-29. Mortality reduction and time to initiation of reperfusion therapy. **A,** Mortality reduction through thrombolytic therapy for acute myocardial infarction is clearly a time-dependent phenomenon, reflecting the increased likelihood of successful reperfusion as well as the greater potential for myocardial salvage in the early hours following the onset of symptoms. **B,** The greatest benefit may be achieved in the first 1 to 2 hours. In the MITI trial [33], dramatic decreases in mortality and infarct size were noted in patients treated within 70 minutes (compared with patients treated after 70 minutes). **C,** As demonstrated by the LATE trial [39], modest benefit may still be derived if treatment is initiated as late as 12 hours after the onset of infarction. Therapy initiated between 12 and 24 hours is of uncertain merit; to date, no clinical trials have demonstrated mortality reduction in patients treated with therapy in this time frame. However, individuals with significant coronary collateralization or "stuttering" infarcts may possess significant amounts of viable, vulnerable myocardium, and may be at risk for infarct extension and/or recurrent ischemia during this later time frame. Such situations may warrant revascularization. APSAC—anisoylated plasminogen-streptokinase activator complex. (**A** *adapted from* Lincoff and Topol [40].)

SPECIFIC THROMBOLYTIC AGENTS

CHARACTERISTICS OF MAJOR FIBRINOLYTIC AGENTS

AGENT	STREPTOKINASE	ANISTREPLASE	ALTEPLASE	SARUPLASE	RETEPLASE	TENECTEPLASE	STAPHYLOKINASE
Source	Gp C streptococci	Gp C streptococci; plasminogen; anisoylated	Recombinant, human	Recombinant, human	Recombinant, human deletion mutation	Recombinant, triple substitution mutant	Recombinant *Staphylococcus aureus*
Fibrin specificity	No	No	++	+	+	+++	++++
Half-life, *min*	18–23	70–120	3–4	6–8	18	20	6
Mode of administration	infusion	Single bolus	90-min infusion	infusion	Double bolus	Single bolus	Double bolus
Mode of action	Activator complex	Direct	Direct	Direct	Direct	Direct	Activator complex
Antigenicity	Yes	No	No	No	No	No	Yes
Patency 90 min TIMI-3, %	32	50	54		60	54	68
Estimated hospital cost, in US dollars	280	1700	2200	Not determined	2200	Not determined	Not determined

FIGURE 2-30. Streptokinase remains a commonly used fibrinolytic agent in many parts of the world, especially where there are greater cost restraints. Anistreplase is not commonly used, and saruplase (pro-urokinase) is promising based on patency studies and a trial showing similar clinical outcomes as streptokinase, but it is not approved for acute myocardial infarction in the United States. Alteplase (t-PA) [41], reteplase (rPA) [42], and tenecteplase (TNK-t-PA) [43] all have similar 90-minute coronary artery patency, with reteplase having the advantage of the ease of double-bolus administration, and tenecteplase the ease of single-bolus administration and lower risk of noncerebral bleeding. Staphylokinase, which is even more fibrin specific than tenecteplase, is in development [44]. Angiographic patency rates are derived from different trials and therefore are not directly comparable.

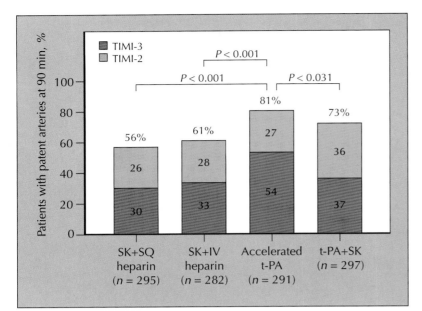

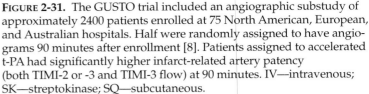

Figure 2-31. The GUSTO trial included an angiographic substudy of approximately 2400 patients enrolled at 75 North American, European, and Australian hospitals. Half were randomly assigned to have angiograms 90 minutes after enrollment [8]. Patients assigned to accelerated t-PA had significantly higher infarct-related artery patency (both TIMI-2 or -3 and TIMI-3 flow) at 90 minutes. IV—intravenous; SK—streptokinase; SQ—subcutaneous.

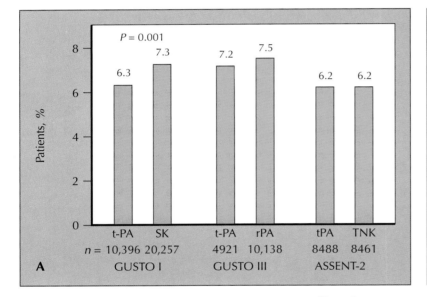

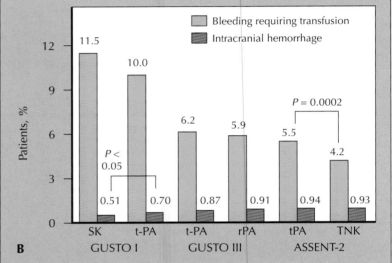

Figure 2-32. A and **B**, Selected clinical trials comparing fibrinolytic agents. Since the ISIS-3 trial [45] that showed that streptokinase (SK), 4-hour t-PA (dutelplase) infusion, and anistreplase resulted in similar mortality when administered with either delayed subcutaneous or no routine heparin, there have been three large trials comparing currently available fibrinolytic agents. All three included patients within 6 hours of symptom onset and with ST segment elevation or left bundle branch block on the qualifying electrocardiogram (ECG). All used 30-day mortality as the primary endpoint. GUSTO I [46] showed a 1.0% absolute survival advantage of accelerated t-PA over streptokinase (95% confidence interval 0.4 to 1.6%). GUSTO III [47] showed a 0.2% excess mortality with reteplase (rPA) compared with alteplase (95% confidence interval -1.1 to 0.6%). ASSENT-2 [48] showed nearly identical mortality with tenecteplase versus alteplase (6.16 vs 6.18%, with the 95% confidence interval of the difference being -0.67 to 0.74). Intracranial hemorrhage was higher with alteplase than streptokinase and was similar for reteplase and tenecteplase versus alteplase. Of concern, the overall rate of intracranial hemorrhage with alteplase has tended to increase since the early 1990s (GUSTO-I) to the late 1990s (ASSENT-2), a finding that cannot be explained by changing patient characteristics such as age. Noncerebral bleeding was higher for those taking streptokinase than alteplase, and higher for those taking alteplase than tenecteplase. Bleeding and transfusion rates are dependent on definitions, country norms, and intervention rates; therefore, comparisons between trials are limited. TNK—tenecteplase.

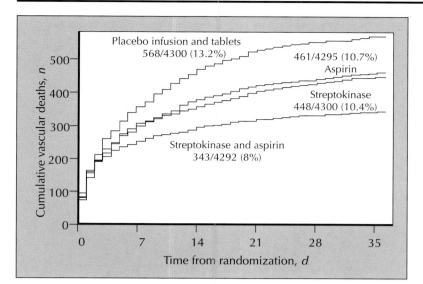

FIGURE 2-33. The ISIS-2 (Second International Study of Infarct Survival [49]) trial confirmed the results of GISSI-1 (Gruppo Italiano per lo Studio della Streptochinasi nell'Infarto Miocardico [50]) by finding a decrease in 5-week mortality from 12.0% with placebo to 9.2% with streptokinase, which indicates a 25% relative reduction. Moreover, aspirin alone resulted in a 23% relative reduction in mortality, and the combination of streptokinase and aspirin resulted in an even more impressive additive effect, with a 42% relative reduction in mortality from 13.2% to 8.0%. (*Adapted from* ISIS-2 Collaborative Group [49].)

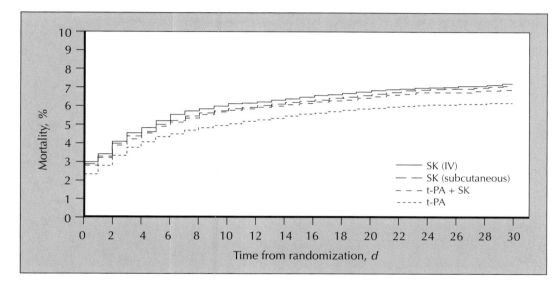

FIGURE 2-34. Accelerated t-PA was associated with the lowest 30-day mortality in the GUSTO trial at 6.30%, compared with 7.25% with streptokinase (SK) with subcutaneous heparin, 7.35% with streptokinase with intravenous (IV) heparin, and 7.0% for the combination of streptokinase and t-PA [51]. The protocol called for combining the streptokinase groups if there was no significant difference between the two in order to get a more reliable estimate of the overall effect of streptokinase. Compared with streptokinase, there was a relative reduction in 30-day mortality of 14% with accelerated t-PA ($P < 0.001$). This corresponds to 10 additional lives saved with accelerated t-PA (compared with streptokinase) per 1000 patients treated, or one of every seven deaths prevented that would have occurred with streptokinase. The survival advantage seems to be explained by the difference in 90-minute patency between the strategies.

COST-EFFECTIVENESS RATIOS FOR T-PA COMPARED WITH SK

GROUP OF PATIENTS	INCREASED LIFE EXPECTANCY WITH T-PA		COST-EFFECTIVENESS RATIO*
	UNDISCOUNTED	DISCOUNTED	
	YEARS OF LIFE SAVED		DOLLARS
Overall	0.14	0.09	32,678
Inferior MI, age ≤ 40 y	0.03	0.01	203,071
Anterior MI, age ≤ 40 y	0.04	0.02	123,609
Inferior MI, age 41–60 y	0.07	0.04	74,816
Anterior MI, age 41–60 y	0.10	0.06	49,877
Inferior MI, age 61–75 y	0.16	0.10	27,873
Anterior MI, age 61–75 y	0.20	0.14	20,601
Inferior MI, age > 75 y	0.26	0.17	16,246
Anterior MI, age > 75 y	0.29	0.21	13,410

*Cost-effectiveness ratios show the cost in dollars per year of life saved (both discounted at 5%); these calculations were based on the assumption that patients treated with t-PA had costs in the first year that were $2845 higher than those for patients treated with SK.

FIGURE 2-35. Cost-effectiveness ratios for tissue-type plasminogen activator (t-PA) compared with streptokinase (SK). Assuming a persistence of the 1.1% 1-year survival advantage of t-PA, an average life expectancy projected from the Duke Cardiovascular Disease Database of 14 years, and an estimated average increased cost of t-PA–treated patients of $2845, the use of t-PA was associated with $33,678 per year of life saved in the overall GUSTO patient population. Young patients with small inferior myocardial infarctions (MIs) had low mortality regardless of thrombolytic assignment, and therefore the cost of each additional year of life was very high. On the other hand, patients at high risk of death, such as the elderly, had a much greater absolute survival advantage and better cost-effectiveness with t-PA [52].

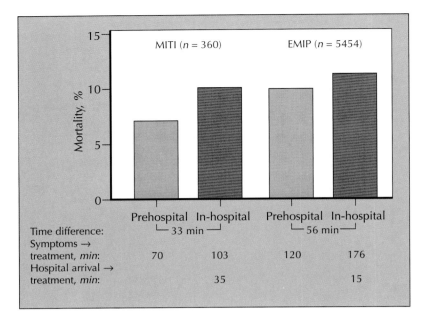

FIGURE 2-36. Both the MITI trial and the European Myocardial Infarction Project (EMIP) [53] randomized patients with acute myocardial infarction to either prehospital or in-hospital initiation of thrombolytic therapy. Both demonstrated a trend toward improved survival with randomization to prehospital treatment, although neither reached statistical significance. This could be explained by the relatively small time differences of 33 and 56 minutes between symptom onset and initiation of thrombolytic therapy in the two trials, respectively. Both also showed that rapid treatment, within 15 to 35 minutes of hospital arrival, is possible, especially if prehospital identification has occurred and electrocardiograms have been obtained.

THROMBOLYTIC THERAPY FOR NON–ST ELEVATION AND UNSTABLE ANGINA

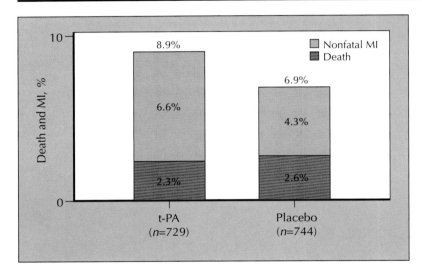

FIGURE 2-37. The TIMI-IIIB trial was the largest trial to investigate whether thrombolytic therapy is beneficial for patients presenting with unstable angina or myocardial infarction (MI) without ST-segment elevation [54]. There were 1473 patients randomized within 24 hours of symptoms to either t-PA or placebo. There was no evidence of benefit from thrombolytic therapy. In fact, there was a slight excess of myocardial (re)infarction among patients treated with t-PA (P=0.4), as well as a trend toward more intracranial hemorrhages. This trial, both alone and when combined with other randomized trials, suggests that patients without ST elevation should not be treated with thrombolytic therapy.

PLATELETS AND THE MECHANISMS OF ARTERIAL THROMBOSIS

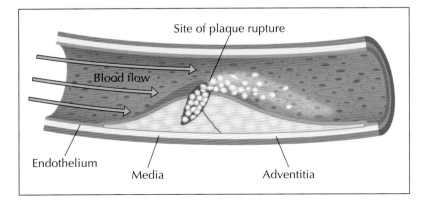

FIGURE 2-38. Diagram of arterial thrombus responsible for acute myocardial infarction. Platelet adhesion and aggregation occur at the site of plaque rupture ("white thrombus"). Activated platelets exert procoagulant effects and the soluble coagulation cascade is activated. Fibrin strands and erythrocytes predominate within the lumen of the vessel and downstream in the "body" and "tail" of the thrombus [55].

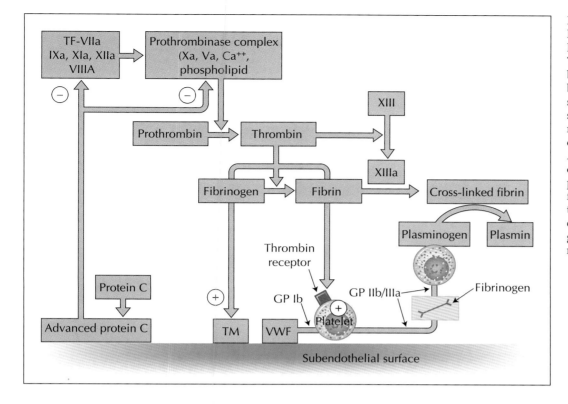

FIGURE 2-39. Investigations over the last decade have shown the interdependence of platelet hemostasis and the coagulation system. Thrombosis is a complex series of interactions between these two systems. The interplay between agonists and inhibitors of these systems maintains the balance between hemostasis and hemorrhage. A fascinating array of new approaches to altering the balance of the coagulation system is becoming available. Agonists and antagonists of each step of the coagulation cascade are now available for preclinical or clinical investigation. The search for the most appropriate balance of inhibition of thrombosis versus production of bleeding will demand substantial empiric evidence. GP—glycoprotein; TF—tissue factor; TM—thrombomodulin; VWF—von Willebrand factor.

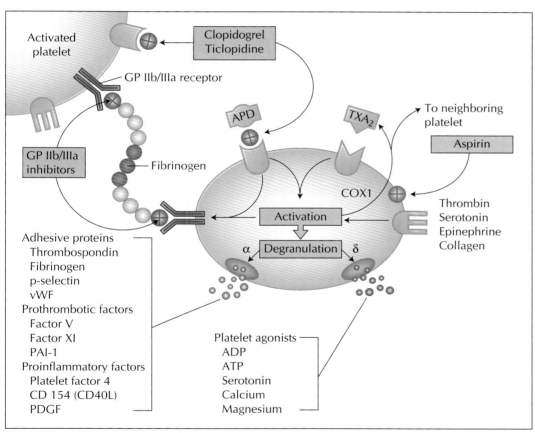

FIGURE 2-40 Platelet aggregation. Platelet activation is an important early step in the pathophysiology of atherothrombosis. Platelet activation involves 1) a shape change in whih the platelet membrane surface area is greatly increased; 2) the secretion of proinflammatory, prothrombotic, adhesive, chemotactic mediators (release reaction), that propagate, amplify, and sustain the atherothrombotic process; and 3) the activation of the glycoprotein (GP) IIb/IIIa receptor from inactive form. Multiple agonists including thromboxane A_2 (TXA_A), ADP, thrombin, serotonin, epinephrine, and collagen can acitvate the platelet and thus contribute toward establishing the environmental conditions necessary for atherothrombosis to occur. Aspirin inhibits the production of TXA_2 by its effect on the enzyme cyclooxygenase (COX) 1. The ADP receptor antagonists clopidogrel and ticlopidine prevent the binding of ADP to its receptor. The effect of combining aspirin and clopidogrel is synergistic in preventing platelet aggregation. Antithrombins such as unfractionated or low-molecular weight heparin, hirudin, or bivalirudin are important in interfering with both thombin-induced platelet activation and coagulation. The GP IIb/IIIa receptor antagonists act at a later step in the process by preventing fibrinogen-mediated cross-linking of platelets, which have already become activated. PAI—plasminogen activator inhibitor; PDGF—platelet-derived growth factor; vWF—von Willibrand factor. (*Adapted from* Mehta and Yusuf [56].)

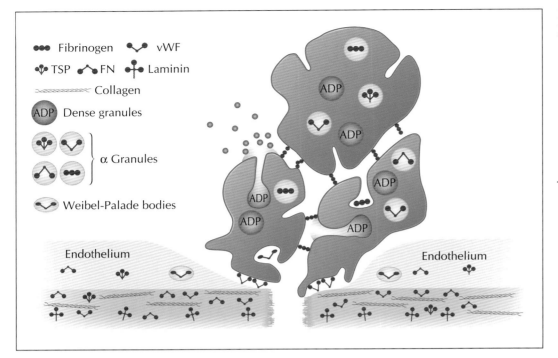

FIGURE 2-41. Platelet aggregation occurs primarily through platelet-platelet cross-linking by fibrinogen. Although the fibrinogen receptor glycoprotein IIb-IIIa is present on the platelet surface at all times, it is able to bind fibrinogen only after the platelet has undergone some level of "activation" and ADP has been provided, from either the platelet itself or other locations such as endothelial cells. Platelets may also be cross-linked through an ADP-dependent mechanism by von Willebrand factor (vWF). FN—fibronectin; TSP—thrombospondin. (*Adapted from* Hawiger [57].)

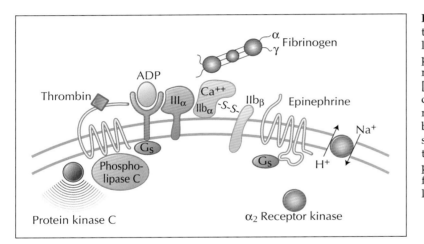

FIGURE 2-42. The three known agonist receptors on human platelets. Once the appropriate ligand has come into place, the role of these receptors is at least in part to activate the glycoprotein IIb-IIIa fibrinogen receptor so that platelet aggregation can take place. Thrombin "receptor" is actually a misnomer, since it is not a receptor at all but rather a substrate for thrombin [58]. This "receptor" and the epinephrine receptor (a true "receptor") are coupled to G proteins (G_s) and phospholipase C. Both receptors are members of a protein superfamily characterized by seven domains believed to be transmembranous. The ADP receptor is not well understood at this time; it is believed to be closely associated with the glycoprotein IIb-IIIa fibrinogen receptor, but the details await discovery. Binding of platelets to other extracellular matrix components such as collagen and fibronectin through specific receptors also results in activation, although less is known about these receptors. (*Adapted from* Hawiger [59].)

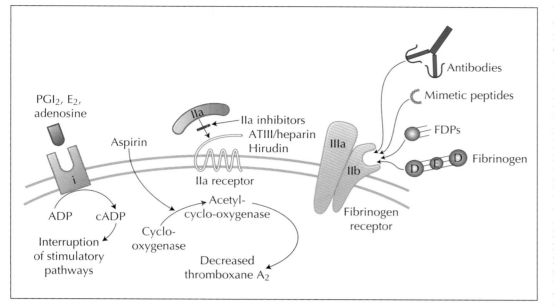

FIGURE 2-43. Four major classes of platelet inhibitors. Inhibitory prostaglandins (PGI₂, PGE₂), along with adenosine, act as inhibitors by binding to specific inhibitory receptors (i), thereby generating cADP, which interrupts the phospholipase A_2 and phospholipase C stimulatory pathways. Aspirin, which is receiving increased attention as a means of preventing coronary heart disease, works by irreversibly acetylating the cyclo-oxygenase enzyme, thereby reducing the concentration of the stimulator thromboxane A_2 [60]. Thrombin (IIa) acts as a platelet agonist by cleaving the thrombin receptor and producing the "tethered ligand." Therefore, any effective thrombin inhibitor will act as a platelet inhibitor. Such inhibitors include heparin, the leech anticoagulant hirudin (and recent genetically engineered modifications of hirudin), and other inhibitors of the thrombin active site. Finally, platelet cross-linking during thrombus formation occurs via the interaction of fibrinogen (and in some cases von Willebrand factor) with the activated glycoprotein IIb-IIIa receptor. Therefore, any compound that can occupy this receptor will act as a platelet inhibitor in the sense that it will inhibit platelet aggregation by competition for the IIb-IIIa receptor. Such compounds include specific anti–IIb-IIIa antibodies; small synthetic peptides that mimic the part of fibrinogen which binds to the receptor; and fibrin(ogen) degradation products (FDPs), which contain the IIb-IIIa binding site from fibrinogen.

ANTIPLATELET THERAPY

ASPIRIN

ANTIPLATELET TRIALISTS' COLLABORATION: REDUCTION IN VASCULAR EVENTS ACHIEVED BY ANTIPLATELET THERAPY FOLLOWING ACUTE MI			
EVENT	REDUCTION, %	STANDARD DEVIATION, %	P VALUE
All vascular events	25	4	< 0.001
Nonfatal infarction	31	5	< 0.001
Nonfatal stroke	42	11	< 0.001
Vascular death	13	5	< 0.005

FIGURE 2-44. In an analysis of 10 trials of antiplatelet agents (predominantly aspirin) for secondary prophylaxis of vascular events following acute myocardial infarction (MI), the Antiplatelet Trialists' Collaboration reported striking reductions in nonfatal MI and nonfatal stroke in patients treated chronically with antiplatelet therapy (n = 18,441). There was also a highly significant reduction in cardiovascular mortality. Interestingly, similar reductions were seen for patients receiving antiplatelet therapy following stroke. There were no differences in effect between varying doses of aspirin or aspirin with or without dipyridamole. Based on these data, it was estimated that if 100 patients underwent treatment with antiplatelet therapy for 2 years following acute MI, two deaths and three nonfatal events would be prevented. Based on a smaller number of patients with unstable angina, one death and two nonfatal events would be prevented [61].

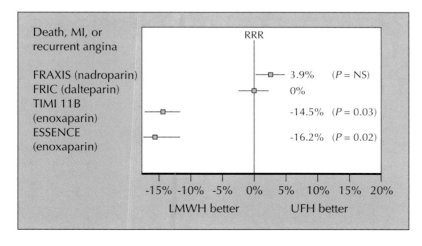

FIGURE 2-45 Meta-analysis of low molecular weight heparin (LMWH) trials in unstable angina/non–ST-segment elevation myocardial infarction. ESSENCE—Efficacy and Safety of Subcutaneous Enoxaparin in Non–Q-wave Coronary Events; FRAXIS—Fraxiparine in Ischemic Syndromes; FRIC—Fragmin in Unstable Coronary Artery Disease; TIMI—Thrombolysis in Myocardial Infarction; UFH—unfractionated heparin.

TRIALS OF ANTITHROMBIN AND ANTIPLATELET THERAPY

TRIALS	n	Active	Placebo		P VALUE
ASA vs placebo					
Lewis, et al. (VA)	1266	5.0	10.1		0.005
Cairns, et al.	555	10.5	14.7		0.137
Théroux, et al.	239	3.3	11.9		0.012
RISC Group	388	7.4	17.6		0.003
All ASA vs placebo	2448	6.4	12.5		0.0005
UFH +ASA vs ASA					
Théroux, et al.	243	1.6	3.3		0.40
RISC Group	399	1.4	3.7		0.140
ATACS Group	214	3.8	8.3		0.170
Gurfinkel, et al.	143	5.7	9.6		0.380
ALL UFH vs ASA	999	2.6	5.5		0.018
LMWH + ASA vs ASA					
Gurfinkel, et al.	141	0.0	9.6		n/a
FRISC Group	1498	1.8	4.8		0.001
All heparin or LMWH vs ASA	2629	2.0	5.3		0.0005
GP IIb/IIIa antagonist + UFH vs UFH					
CAPTURE	1265	4.8	9.0		0.003
PARAGON*	1516	10.6	11.7		0.410
PRISM-PLUS	1570	8.7	11.9		0.034
PRISM†	3232	5.8	7.1		0.110
PURSUIT	9461	3.5	3.7		0.042
All GP IIb/IIIa‡	170444	5.1	6.2		0.0022

PATIENTS WITH EVENT, % DEATH OR MI. Endpoints: 5-day to 2-year; 1-week; 1-week; 30-day. Scale 0.1–1.9. Active Treatment Superior / Active Treatment Inferior.

*Best results group; †GP IIb/IIIa with no heparin; ‡all trials except PRISM compared GP IIb/IIIa with UFH vs UFH.

FIGURE 2-46. Trials of antithrombin and antiplatelet therapy. The aspirin trials in unstable angina all show a benefit; although the number of patients is relatively small, the magnitude of the benefit is great [24].

The trials of unfractionated heparin versus aspirin alone also show a benefit of UFH, but the magnitude of the benefit is difficult to estimate due to the fact that few than 1000 patients have been studied. The small number of patients has created difficulty in the development of new therapies attempting to show equivalence of noninferiority to unfractionated heparin. Definitive equivalence studies require substantial evidence that the active control, standard treatment (in this case, unfractionated heparin) is actually better than no treatment.

The trials of low molecular weight heparin (LMWH) plus aspirin versus aspirin have achieved mixed results. Trials with enoxaparin have shown benefit, while other trials have been neutral. These results have spawned a debate about whether there is heterogeneity in the clinical benefit of

LMWH or whether the apparent differences are due to random chance.

When combining all trials of either LMWH or unfractionated heparin versus aspirin, the magnitude of the benefit is highly significant and very substantial. These results from the combined unfractionated and LMWH trials provide the best support for the Class I recommendation for antithrombin therapy.

It is important to note that all the trials with antithrombin therapy had only a one week endpoint. The small amount of longer term follow-up for unfractionated heparin has shown an erosion of the benefit over time while the result with enoxaparin has been a sustenance of the benefit over time.

The final portion of the figure demonstrates the results of the 4P trials and CAPTURE, all of which used glycoprotein (GP) IIb/IIIa inhibitors in the setting of unstable angina or non-ST elevation myocardial infarction. The overall effect and the result in every trial favor using GP IIb/IIIa inhibitors. ASA—acetylsalicylic acid; UFH—unfractionated heparin.

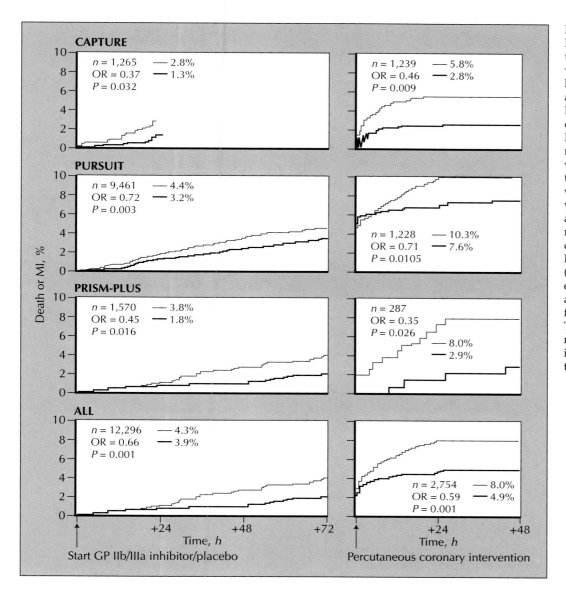

FIGURE 2-47. Results of a complex analysis looking at the CAPTURE trial, the PURSUIT trial, and the PRISM PLUS trial to determine whether glycoprotein (GP) IIb/IIIa inhibitors have an effect under medical treatment as well as in the setting of percutaneous intervention. Because the trials do not include a factorial design with percutaneous intervention and GP IIb/IIIa inhibitor administration, a complex methodology was required in which patients were counted as being medically treated until the time of percutaneous intervention. Patients who died before percutaneous intervention were censored at that point. In this analysis, it is apparent that there is a highly significant 34% reduction in the odds ratio of death or myocardial infarction in patients treated with a GP IIb/IIIa inhibitor undergoing medical treatment (albeit a small absolute benefit due to the low early event rate). This benefit is magnified with an odds ratio demonstrating a 41% reduction from the time of percutaneous intervention. These data form the basis for the Class I recommendation for the use of GP IIb/IIIa inhibitors in patients who are at high risk beginning at the time of diagnosis [24]. OR—odds ratio.

PTCA vs Thrombolysis in the Management of Myocardial Infarction

ADVANTAGES AND DISADVANTAGES OF DIRECT PTCA

ADVANTAGES

Excellent reperfusion rates > 90%

Achieves TIMI-3 flow in > 90% patients

Rare contraindications (*eg*, lack of arterial access, inability to receive heparin, unprotected left main coronary artery stenosis)

Can treat underlying residual stenosis as well as the thrombotic occlusion

Prompt identification of reperfusion

Identification of severity and extent of CAD facilitates triage and enhances therapeutic decision process, *eg*, need for CABG in left main CAD patients

Effective for patients with hemodynamic instability

Facilitates diagnosis in patients with equivocal or indeterminant ECGs

Facilitates access for placement of hemodynamic support devices, *eg*, IABP

DISADVANTAGES

Requires prompt, easy access to catheterization laboratory and trained personnel

Costs of maintenance of 24-h laboratory facilities

Requires placement of large arterial sheaths

Limited controlled scientific data

Specific operator dependence

FIGURE 2-48. Advantages and disadvantages of direct percutaneous transluminal coronary angioplasty (PTCA). Proponents of both PTCA and thrombolytic therapy have been vocal, and valid arguments can be made for either approach. Those favoring direct PTCA have maintained that success rates (usually defined as restoration of antegrade flow in an occluded infarct-related artery and a residual stenosis less than 50%) are far better than those seen with thrombolytic therapy, with improved outcome and the ability to treat larger numbers of patients who did not receive thrombolytic therapy for acute MI. Not only are overall reperfusion rates with direct PTCA superior to those with thrombolytic therapy, but successful PTCA almost always results in TIMI (Thrombolysis in Myocardial Infarction) grade 3 flow, which has been shown to be associated with improved left ventricular (LV) function and improved survival compared with patients in whom only TIMI-2 flow is achieved. In several studies, TIMI-2 flow resulted in outcomes more similar to TIMI-0 flow than TIMI-3 flow. Contraindications to direct PTCA are rare and include the lack of arterial access, the inability to receive heparin, and some specific angiographic subsets such as significant left main coronary artery stenosis or an inability to reach the infarct-related occlusion. An important part of PTCA is the requirement for diagnostic angiography, which allows identification of the extent and severity of the underlying coronary artery disease (CAD).

Patients with severe left main coronary artery stenosis or severe three-vessel disease and decreased LV function may be better served with coronary artery bypass grafting (CABG). Angiography can also substantiate the diagnosis of MI in patients with typical symptoms but indeterminant electrocardiographic (ECG) changes. In these patients, identification of an occlusion with coronary arterial thrombus substantiates the diagnosis. Finally, having the patient in the catheterization laboratory facilitates placement of intra-aortic balloon pumping (IABP) devices.

Major disadvantages of direct PTCA are systems-related. Because salvage of myocardium is enhanced by early reperfusion, the patient must be able to have very prompt access to catheterization laboratories and trained personnel available 24 hours a day if direct PTCA is to be used. Not all patients live in close enough proximity to such hospitals, and not all hospitals are so equipped and trained. This may become more of an issue as hospital closings increase with changing health care delivery systems. The costs of maintaining 24-hour-a-day staffed laboratories are substantial. Another factor is the specific operator-dependence, related to both the experience and the technical expertise of the invasive cardiologist. While somewhat difficult to quantitate, these issues may have a major impact on individual patient outcomes. Dilatation for acute MI can be very difficult, particularly with complex coronary anatomy and hemodynamic instability.

ADVANTAGES AND DISADVANTAGES OF THROMBOLYTIC THERAPY

ADVANTAGES	DISADVANTAGES
Does not require access to catheterization laboratory facilities	Despite widespread availability, thrombolytic therapy is only given in approximately 30%–40% of patients with acute MI; absolute or relative contraindications frequent
Treats the underlying problem of a central occluding thrombus	Not effective for hemodynamic instability
Documented efficacy in large, well-controlled trials	Early reperfusion rates range from 55%–80% depending on agent used
	Achievement of TIMI-3 flow in < 50%–60% of patients
	Reliable assessment of reperfusion often not possible
	Residual stenosis

FIGURE 2-49. Advantages and disadvantages of thrombolytic therapy. Proponents of thrombolytic therapy are equally vocal. One of the most important advantages is that thrombolytic therapy can be given in a variety of settings—primary, secondary, and tertiary hospitals, emergency rooms, and even in the field by trained paramedical personnel. It does not require access to a cardiac catheterization laboratory. This ability to administer the drug in a wider range of settings enhances the chance of giving it early and salvaging substantial myocardium. The other major advantage is that it has been documented to be effective in reducing morbidity and mortality in more than 150,000 patients in well-designed, scientifically controlled trials [25,49,62–66].

There are several disadvantages as well. Even though thrombolytic therapy is widely available, the most recent data indicate that it is given to only 30% to 40% of patients with acute myocardial infarction (MI) in the United States. The frequency of administration in patients with acute MI may be higher in other countries, and it is increasing in this country. It remains the case that a large number of patients presenting with acute MI do not receive thrombolytic therapy either because of relative or absolute contraindications or concerns about risk-benefit issues. Despite the fact that early reperfusion is the goal of therapy, in contrast to direct percutaneous transluminal coronary angioplasty, which is characterized by success rates of more than 90%, lytic therapy results in early reperfusion in only 55% to 80% of patients depending on the agent used [38]. In addition, achievement of TIMI-3 flow is even less frequent, although this may be the most important goal to optimize outcome. As previously mentioned, TIMI-3 flow is associated with substantially better improvement in left ventricular function and survival than TIMI-2 flow [38,67]. Other disadvantages include the fact that reliable assessment of reperfusion noninvasively is often not possible and, finally, that a significant residual stenosis often remains.

CHARACTERISTICS OF TRIALS COMPARING PTCA WITH INTRAVENOUS THROMBOLYSIS

STUDY	PATIENT POPULATION	DURATION OF SYMPTOMS, h	PRIMARY FOLLOW-UP PERIOD	PTCA NO. OF PATIENTS (n = 1290)	TIME TO TREATMENT, MIN	NO. OF PATIENTS (n = 1316)
Zijlstra et al.	≤ 75 y; ST ↑	< 6	Discharge	152	62 †	142
Ribiero et al.	< 75 y; ST ↑	< 6	Discharge	50	238	50
Grinfeld et al.	ST ↑	< 12	30 d	54	63 ‡	58
Zijlstra et al.	ST ↑; low risk	< 6	30 d	45	68 †	50
DeWood	≤ 76 y; ST ↑	< 12	30 d	46	126 †	44
Grines et al.	ST ↑	< 12	Discharge	195	60 ‡	20
Gibbons et al.	< 80 y; ST ↑	< 12	Discharge	47	45 ‡	56
Ribichini et al.	< 80 y; inferior MI; anterior ST ↓	< 6	Discharge	41	40 ‡	42
Garcia et al.	Anterior MI	5	30 d	95	84 †	94
GUSTO IIb	ST ↑; LBBB	< 12	30 d	565	114 ‡	573

* All patients were treated with oral aspirin, except for those in the study by Zijlstra et al., who received intravenous angioplasty.
† From admission.
‡ From randomization.
  LBBB—left bundle branch block; MI—myocardial infarction; ST ↑— ST-segment elevation; ST ↓—ST-segment depression.

FIGURE 2-50. Meta-analysis of ten randomized clinical trials of thrombolytic therapy compared with direct angioplasty. A total of 2606 patients were included in this analysis. Overall, outcome was improved with direct angioplasty; mortality was 4.4% for patients undergoing direct percutaneous transluminal coronary angioplasty (PTCA) and 6.5% in patients receiving thrombolytic therapy. The duration of follow-up reported for some of these trials was confined to the hospital stay and was 30 days for others. For this reason, as well as because of patient selection factors, the observed mortality is lower than that reported in broader epidemiologic studies. Overall, other secondary endpoints such as nonfatal reinfarction and recurrent ischemia were reduced in the primary PTCA groups compared with patients undergoing thrombolysis [68]. These trials were performed before the current era of stent placement and GP IIb/IIIa antagonist therapy, both of which have been associated with improved outcome in primary coronary angioplasty patients. (Adapted from Weaver et al. [68].)

	n (%)		Odds ratio (95% CI)	P
Study	**PTCA**	**Lytic therapy**		
Streptokinase				
Zijlstra *et al.*	5/152 (3.3)	23/149 (15.4)		
Ribeiro *et al.*	5/50 (10.0)	2/50 (4.0)		
Grinfeld *et al.*	6/54 (11.1)	7/58 (12.1)		
Zijlstra *et al.*	1/45 (2.2)	8/50 (16.0)		
Subtotal	17/301 (5.6)	40/307 (13.0)		0.003
t-PA				
DeWood	3/46 (6.5)	2/44 (4.5)		
Grines *et al.*	10/195 (5.1)	24/200 (12.0)		
Gibbons *et al.*	3/47 (6.4)	5/56 (8.9)		
Subtotal	16/288 (5.6)	31/300 (10.3)		0.05
Accelerated t-PA				
Ribichini *et al.*	0/41	1/42 (2.4)		
Garcia *et al.*	7/95 (7.4)	14/94 (14.9)		
GUSTO *et al.*	54/565 (9.6)	70/573 (12.2)		
Subtotal	61/701 (8.7)	85/709 (12.0)		0.05
Total	**94/1290 (7.2)**	**156/1316 (11.9)**		< 0.001

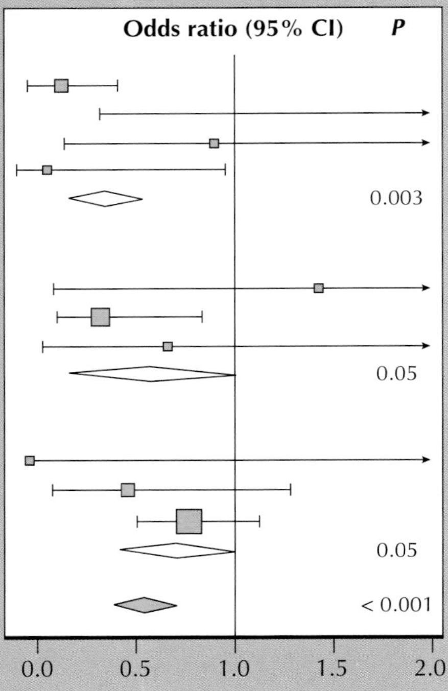

FIGURE 2-51 Meta-analysis of outcomes from percutaneous transluminal coronary angioplasty (PTCA) versus lytic trials in acute myocardial infarction. t-PA—tissue plasminogen activator. (*Adapted from* Weaver *et al.* [68].)

CARDIOGENIC SHOCK

PATHOPHYSIOLOGY OF LEFT VENTRICULAR SHOCK

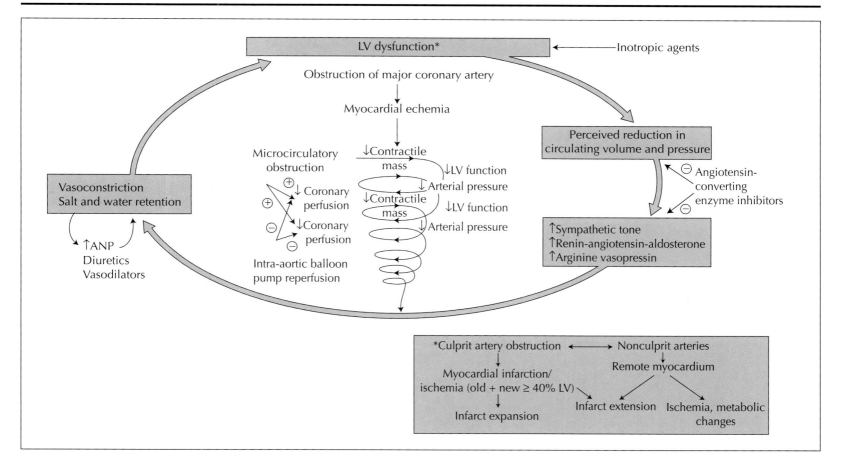

FIGURE 2-52. Cardiogenic shock can develop either early or late after the onset of myocardial infarction. Early cardiogenic shock may be secondary to massive necrosis of the left ventricle (LV), but the combination of more modest necrosis plus widespread ischemia may also be responsible. Cardiogenic shock that develops later reflects more complex pathophysiology. The infarct can extend to areas of myocardium at risk as a result of re-occlusion of a recanalized artery or propagation of the existing thrombus into previously patent branches. In addition, LV dysfunction leads to hypotension and increases in LV end-diastolic pressure (LVEDP), further exacerbating coronary hypoperfusion. This low coronary blood flow compromises not only the jeopardized region but also distant myocardium. This "ischemia at a distance" is particularly profound when multivessel disease is present.

The development of LV dilatation and tachycardia associated with cardiogenic shock markedly increases the metabolic demands of the myocardium at a time when coronary flow reserve is too low to compensate, leading to more global ischemia and further dysfunction. This vicious circle is then perpetuated, as shown in the classic downward spiral of cardiogenic shock presented by Califf and Bengtson [69]. Infarct expansion characterized by thinning and dilatation of the infarct zone as well as acute LV "functional" aneurysm formation can further compromise cardiac output and increase wall stress and metabolic demands. ANP—atrial natriuretic peptide. (*Adapted from* Califf and Bengtson [69].)

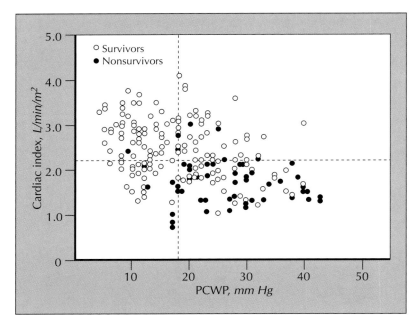

FIGURE 2-53. Cardiac index versus pulmonary capillary wedge pressure (PCWP) in 200 patients after acute myocardial infarction (MI), demonstrating an inverse relationship between mortality and cardiac performance [70]. A PCWP exceeding 18 mm Hg and a cardiac index less than 2.2 L/min/m² represent severe left ventricular (LV) failure (with or

without hypotension) and were associated with the highest mortality. This subset includes patients with classic LV cardiogenic shock. The results of this study by Forrester *et al.* [70] illustrate the importance of optimizing the PCWP to maximize cardiac index.

Based on the American College of Cardiology/American Heart Association (ACC/AHA) Task Force guidelines for the early management of patients with acute MI [71], patients with LV pump failure can be divided into two subsets. Subset 1 includes those with an LV filling pressure above 15 mm Hg, systolic arterial blood pressure above 100 mm Hg, and a cardiac index below 2.5 L/min/m², representing LV failure without classic shock. Subset 2 is defined as an LV filling pressure above 15 mm Hg, arterial pressure below 90 mm Hg, and a cardiac index below 2.5 L/min/m², representing more classic shock. Typically, the cardiac index is lower (*ie*, <2.0 L/min/m²) and PCWP higher (*ie*, >20 mm Hg) when classic cardiogenic shock is the result of LV failure (without hypo-volemia). This distinction has important clinical implications in terms of therapeutic intervention. When systolic arterial blood pressure exceeds 100 mm Hg, treatment options would include afterload reduction with nitroglycerin or nitroprusside, drugs that are usually employed in conjunction with inotropic agents. Agents that combine inotropy and vasodilation, such as dobutamine or milrinone (or amrinone), can be used either alone or in combination.

Subset 2 constitutes the classic cardiogenic shock population. Frank hypotension and hypoperfusion are present. In addition to inotropic and vasopressor support, intra-aortic balloon counterpulsation for afterload reduction, increased coronary blood flow, and augmented systemic diastolic pressure are frequently needed. (*Adapted from* Forrester *et al.* [70].)

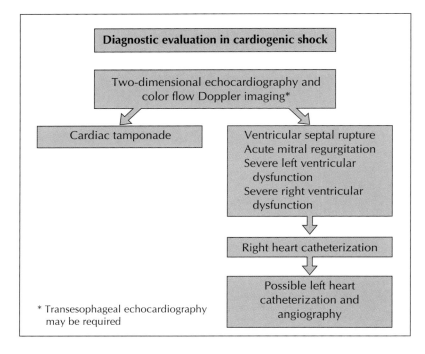

FIGURE 2-54. The diagnostic investigation for patients with cardiogenic shock should include an evaluation of volume status and an assessment of both right and left ventricular function. Swan-Ganz catheterization is used to measure right heart pressures, pulmonary artery pressure, and pulmonary capillary wedge pressure. Oxygen saturation should be measured routinely in the right-sided chambers in all patients with cardiogenic shock to assess whether a left-to-right shunt (*ie*, ventricular septal rupture) is present. Two-dimensional echocardiography and color flow Doppler imaging should be performed in all patients with cardiogenic shock. These tests are invaluable for the bedside assessment of ventricular function and the detection of valvular heart disease, shunts, and tamponade. Left heart catheterization with coronary angio-graphy is indicated when an intervention such as percutaneous transluminal coronary angioplasty or cardiac surgery is contemplated. At times the urgency of the situation (*eg*, acute cardiac tamponade) may preclude such testing prior to the intervention.

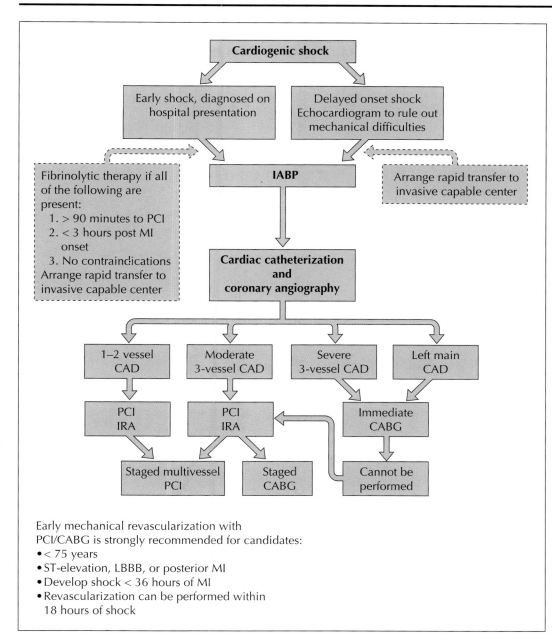

FIGURE 2-55. Recommendations for initial reperfusion therapy when cardiogenic shock complicates acute myocardial infarction (MI). Early mechanical revascularization with percutaneous coronary intervention (PCI) or coronary artery bypass graft (CABG) is strongly recommended for suitable candidates less than 75 years of age and for selected elderly patients. Eight-five percent of shock cases are diagnosed after initial therapy for acute MI, but most patients develop shock within 24 hours. Intra-aortic balloon pump (IABP) is recommended when shock is not quickly reversed with pharmacologic therapy as a stabilizing measure for patients who are candidates for further invasive care. *Dashed lines* indicate that the procedure should be performed in patients with specific indications only. CAD—coronary artery disease; LBBB—left bundle brach block. (*Adapted from* Hochman [72].)

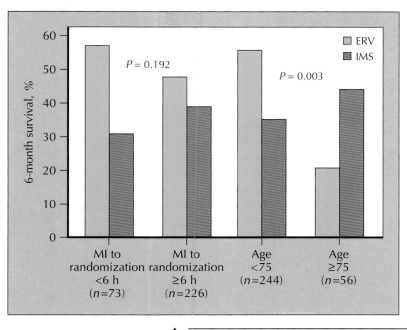

FIGURE 2-56. Six-month survival data from the SHOCK trial [73]. These prospective subgroups were tested for differential treatment effects. The subgroup variable of age (< 75 years vs ≥ 75 years) interacted significantly with treatment effect at 30 days, 6 months, and 12 months ($P = 0.01$, $P = 0.003$, and $P = 0.029$, respectively). There was no significant difference in the treatment effect for those with anterior myocardial infarction (MI) versus those without anterior MI. There was a trend toward survival in the early intervention group with prior MI.

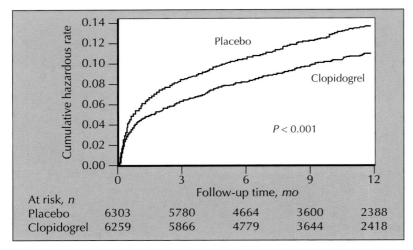

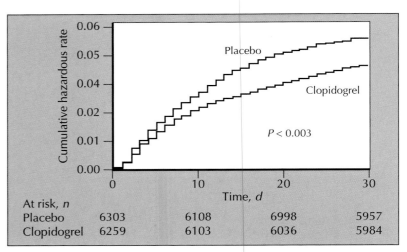

FIGURE 2-57. Clopidogrel in addition to aspirin in patients with acute coronary syndromes without ST-segment elevation (CURE) trial. Hazard rates for the primary outcome of death from cardiovascular causes, nonfatal myocardial infarction, and stroke over the 12 months of follow-up. Results demonstrate a sustained benefit with clopidogrel therapy.

FIGURE 2-58. The cumulative hazard rates for the primary outcome of death from cardiovascular causes, nonfatal myocardial infarction, or stroke in patients with acute coronary syndromes without ST-segment elevation treated with clopidogrel versus placebo. The results demonstrate an early effect of clopidogrel.

MITRAL REGURGITATION, VENTRICULAR SEPTAL DEFECT AND CARDIAC RUPTURE

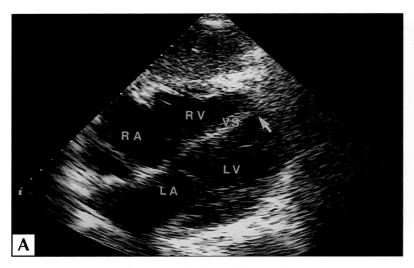

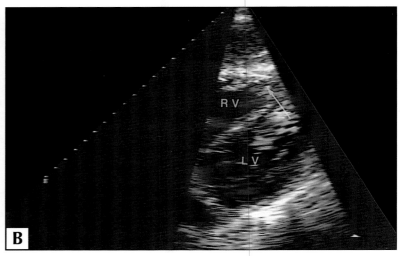

FIGURE 2-59. **A,** Two-dimensional echocardiogram demonstrating ventricular septal (VS) rupture (VSR). The *arrow* indicates the defect in the apical portion of the VS. **B,** Color Doppler flow through the VSR. The *arrow* shows systolic flow from the left ventricle (LV) to the right ventricle (RV) across the VSR. LA—left atrium; RA—right atrium. (*Courtesy of* Alan Mogtader, MD, St. Luke's-Roosevelt Hospital Center and Columbia University, New York, NY.)

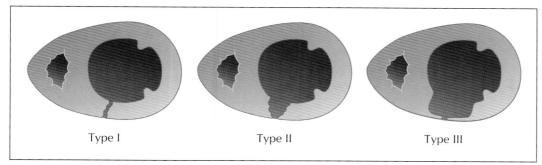

| Type I | Type II | Type III |

FIGURE 2-60. Three pathologic types of cardiac rupture have been described, and the timing of their occurrence after the onset of myocardial infarction (MI) varies greatly [74]. Type I, which appears as a slit through a normal-thickness infarcted ventricular wall, occurs very early after MI, most often within the first day. In this study, the most common location was anterior, and 17 of 29 hearts showed single-vessel coronary artery disease. Subepicardial hemorrhage was sometimes noted. Other authors have noted hemorrhage within the rupture zone [75]. The incidence of rupture on the first day in the ISIS trial was increased in the streptokinase-treated patients (0.5%, compared with 0.3% in the control group) [49]. Perhaps this pathologic type of rupture contributed to the early hazard associated with thrombolysis.

Type II rupture was less frequently seen than type I in this series by Becker and van Mantgem [74]. This type was characterized by localized loss of myocardium with "erosion at the endocardial surface" of the rupture site. The tear is also slitlike, as in type I, with associated hemorrhage in the subepicardium. Most type II ruptures involved posterior infarcts, and seven of 11 of these patients had two-vessel coronary artery disease.

Type III rupture occurred in the setting of marked infarct expansion; thinning and dilation of the infarct zone were also reported by Schuster and Bulkley [76]. Most type III ruptures occurred in anterior infarcts, and six of 10 hearts had single-vessel coronary artery disease. The apparent increase in early cardiac rupture seen with thrombolytic therapy is offset by a decrease in cardiac rupture after the first day, probably due to reduced infarct expansion following thrombolysis [77]. Nonsteroidal anti-inflammatory agents and steroids are known to exacerbate expansion and therefore might increase the risk of rupture. (*Adapted from* Becker and van Mantgem [74].)

REFERENCES

1. Little WC, Constantinescu M, Applegate RJ, *et al.*: Can coronary angiography predict the site of a subsequent myocardial infarction in patients with mild-to-moderate coronary artery disease? *Circulation* 1988, 78:1157–1166.

2. Brown BG, Gallery CA, Badger RS, *et al.*: Incomplete lysis of thrombus in the moderate underlying atherosclerotic lesion during intracoronary infusion of streptokinase for acute myocardial infarction: quantitative angiographic observations. *Circulation* 1986, 73:653–661.

3. Ambrose JA, Tannenbaum MA, Alexopoulos D, *et al.*: Angiographic progression of coronary artery disease and the development of myocardial infarction. *Am J Cardiol* 1988, 12:56–62.

4. Giroud D, Li JM, Urban P, *et al.*: Relationship of site of acute myocardial infarction to the most severe coronary arterial stenosis at prior angiography. *Am J Cardiol* 1992, 69:729–732.

5. Tofler GH, Stone PH, Maclure M, and the MILIS Study Group: Analysis of possible triggers of acute myocardial infarction (the MILIS Study). *Am J Cardiol* 1990, 66:22–27.

6. Sumiyoshi T, Haze K, Saito M, *et al.*: Evaluation of clinical factors involved in onset of myocardial infarction. *Jpn Circ J* 1986, 50:164–173.

7. Falk E, Andersen HR: Pathology of atherosclerotic plaque: stable, unstable, and infarctional. In *Interventional Cardiovascular Medicine: Principles and Practice*. Edited by Roubin GS, Califf RM, O'Neill WW, *et al.* New York: Churchill Livingstone 1994:57–68.

8. Falk E: Why do plaques rupture? *Circulation* 1992, 86(suppl III):30–42.

9. Sherman CT, Litvack F, Grundfest W, *et al.*: Coronary angioscopy in patients with unstable angina pectoris. *N Engl J Med* 1986, 315:913–919.

10. Libby P: Current concepts of the pathogenesis of the acute coronary syndromes. *Circulation* 2001, 104:365–372.

11. Falk E: Coronary thrombosis: pathogenesis and clinical manifestations. *Am J Cardiol* 1991, 68:28B–35B.

12. Falk E: Dynamics in thrombus formation. In Plasminogen activation in fibrinolysis, in tissue remodeling, and in development. *Ann NY Acad Sci* 1992, 667:204–223.

13. Antman EM, Braunwald E: Acute myocardial infarction. In *Heart Disease: A Textbook of Cardiovascular Medicine*. Edited by Braunwald E. Philadelphia: WB Saunders; 1997.

14. Lau J, Antman E, Jimenez-Silva J, *et al.*: Cumulative meta-analysis of therapeutic trials for myocardial infarction. *N Engl J Med* 1992, 327:248–254.

15. ISIS-1 (First International Study of Infarct Survival) Collaborative Group: Randomized trial of intravenous atenolol among 16,027 cases of suspected acute myocardial infarction. ISIS-1. *Lancet* 1986, 2:57–66.

16. Held PH, Yusuf S, Furberg CD: Calcium channel blockers in acute myocardial infarction and unstable angina: an overview. *BMJ* 1989, 299:1187–1192.

17. Yusuf S, Collins R, MacMahon S, *et al.*: Effect of intravenous nitrates on mortality in acute myocardial infarction: an overview of the randomised trials. *Lancet* 1988, i:1088–1092.

18. ISIS-4 (Fourth International Study of Infarct Survival) Collaborative Group: A randomised factorial trial assessing early oral captopril, oral mononitrate, and intravenous magnesium sulphate in 5850 patients with suspected acute myocardial infarction. *Lancet* 1995, 345:669–685.

19. Gruppo Italiano per lo Studio della Sopravvivenza nell'Infarto Miocardico: GISSI-3: effects of lisinopril and transdermal glyceryl trinitrate single and together on 6-week mortality and ventricular function after acute myocardial infarction. *Lancet* 1994, 343:1115–1122.

20. Epstein AE, Hallstrom AP, Rogers WJ, *et al.*, for the CAST Investigators: Mortality following ventricular arrhythmia suppression by encainide, flecainide, and moricizine after myocardial infarction. *JAMA* 1993, 270:2451–2455.

21. MacMahon S, Collins R, Peto R, *et al.*: Effects of prophylactic lidocaine in suspected acute myocardial infarction: an overview of the results from the randomized, controlled trials. *JAMA* 1988, 260:1910–1916.

22. Solomon SD, Ridker PM, Antman EM: Ventricular arrhythmias in trials of thrombolytic therapy for acute myocardial infarction. *Circulation* 1993, 88:2575–2581.

23. Hurlen M, Abdelnoor M, Smith P, *et al.*: Warfarin, aspirin, or both after myocardial infarction. *N Engl J Med* 2002, 347:969–974.

24. Braunwald E, Antman EM, Beasley JW, *et al.*: ACC/AHA guidelines for the management of patients with unstable angina and non-ST-segment elevation myocardial infarction: executive summary and recommendations. A report of the American College of Cardiology/American Heart Association task force on practice guidelines (committee on the management of patients with unstable angina). *Circulation* 2000, 102:1193–1209.

25. DeWood MA, Spores J, Notske R, *et al.*: Prevalence of total coronary occlusion during the early hours of transmural myocardial infarction. *N Engl J Med* 1980, 303:897–902.

26. Reimer KA, Lowe JE, Rasmussen MM, Jennings RB: The wavefront phenomenon of ischemic cell death: 1. Myocardial infarct size vs duration of coronary occlusion in dogs. *Circulation* 1977, 56:786–794.

27. Gibbons RJ: Technetium 99m sestamibi in the assessment of acute myocardial infarction. *Semin Nucl Med* 1991, XXI:213–222.

28. Armstrong PW, Baigrie RS, Daly PA, *et al.*: Tissue plasminogen activator: Toronto (TPAT) placebo-controlled randomized trial in acute myocardial infarction. *J Am Coll Cardiol* 1989, 13:1469–1476.

29. Morgan CD, Roberts RS, Haq A, *et al.*: Coronary patency, infarct size and left ventricular function after thrombolytic therapy for acute myocardial infarction: results from the tissue plasminogen activator: Toronto (TPAT) placebo-controlled trial. TPAT Study Group. *J Am Coll Cardiol* 1991, 17:1451–1457.

30. Kennedy JW, Ritchie JL, Davis KB, et al.: The Western Washington randomized trial of intracoronary streptokinase in acute myocardial infarction. N Engl J Med 1985, 312:1073–1078.

31. Ritchie JL, Cerqueira M, Maynard C, et al.: Ventricular function and infarct size: the Western Washington Intravenous Streptokinase in Myocardial Infarction Trial. J Am Coll Cardiol 1988, 11:689–697.

32. Gibbons RJ, Holmes DR, Reeder GS, et al.: Immediate angioplasty compared with the administration of a thrombolytic agent followed by conservative treatment for myocardial infarction. N Engl J Med 1993, 328:685–691.

33. Weaver WD, Cerqueira M, Hallstrom AP, et al.: Prehospital-initiated vs hospital-initiated thrombolytic therapy: the Myocardial Infarction Triage and Intervention Trial. JAMA 1993, 270:1211–1216.

34. Martin GV, Kennedy JW: Choice of thrombolytic agent. In Management of Acute Myocardial Infarction. Edited by Julian D, Braunwald E. London: WB Saunders; 1994:71–105.

35. Bassand JP, Cassagnes J, Machecourt J, et al.: Comparative effects of APSAC and rt-PA on infarct size and left ventricular function in acute myocardial infarction: a multicenter randomized study. Circulation 1991, 84:1107–1117.

36. Bassand JP, Machecourt J, Cassagnes J, et al.: Multicenter trial of intravenous anisoylated plasminogen streptokinase activator complex (APSAC) in acute myocardial infarction: effects on infarct size and left ventricular function. J Am Coll Cardiol 1990, 13:988–997.

37. Cerqueira MD, Maynard C, Ritchie JL: Radionuclide assessment of infarct size and left ventricular function in clinical trials of thrombolysis. Circulation 1991, 84:I-100–I-108.

38. The GUSTO Angiographic Investigators: The effects of tissue plasminogen activator, streptokinase, or both on coronary-artery patency, ventricular function, and survival after acute myocardial infarction. N Engl J Med 1993, 329:1615–1622.

39. LATE Study Group: Late Assessment of Thrombolytic Efficacy (LATE) study with alteplase 6–24 hours after onset of myocardial infarction. Lancet 1993, 342:759–766.

40. Lincoff AM, Topol EJ: The illusion of reperfusion. Does anyone achieve optimal reperfusion during acute myocardial infarction? Circulation 1993, 87:1792–1805.

41. The GUSTO Angiographic Investigators: The effects of tissue plasminogen activator, streptokinase, or both on coronary artery patency, ventricular function, and survival after acute myocardial infarction. N Engl J Med 1993, 329:1615–1622.

42. Bode C, Smalling RW, Berg G, et al.: Randomized comparision of coronary thrombolysis achieved with double-bolus reteplase (recombinant plasminogen activator) and front-loaded, accelerated alteplase (recombinant tissue plasminogen activator) in patients with acute myocardial infarction. The RAPID II Investigators. Circulation 1996, 94:891–898.

43. Cannon CP, Gibson CM, McCabe CH, et al.: TNK-tissue plasminogen activator compared with front-loaded alteplase in acute myocardial infarction: results of the TIMI 10B trial. Thrombolysis in Myocardial Infarction (TIMI) 10B Investigators. Circulation 1998, 98:2805–2814.

44. Vanderschueren S, Dens J, Kerdsinchai P, et al.: Randomized coronary patency trial of double-bolus recombinant staphylokinase versus front-loaded alteplase in acute myocardial infarction. Am Heart J 1997, 134:213–219.

45. ISIS-3 (Third International Study of Infarct Survival) Collaborative Group: ISIS-3: a randomised comparison of streptokinase vs tissue plasminogen activator vs anistreplase and of aspirin plus hepain vs aspirin alone among 41,299 cases of suspected acute myocardial infarction. Lancet 1992, 339:753–770.

46. The GUSTO Investigators: An international randomized trial comparing four thrombolytic strategies for acute myocardial infarction. N Engl J Med 1993, 329:673–682.

47. The Global Use of Strategies to Open Occluded Infarct Arteries (GUSTO III) Investigators: a comparison of reteplase with alteplase for acute myocardial infarction. N Engl J Med 1997, 337:118–1123.

48. Assessment of the Safety and Efficacy of a New Thrombolytic (ASSENT-2) Investigators: Single-bolus tenecteplase compared with front-loaded alteplase in acute myocardial infarction: the ASSENT-2 double-blind randomised trial. Lancet 1999, 354:716–722.

49. ISIS-2 (Second International Study of Infarct Survival) Collaborative Group: Randomised trial of intravenous streptokinase, oral aspirin, both, or neither among 17,187 cases of suspected acute myocardial infarctions: ISIS-2. Lancet 1988, ii:349–360.

50. Gruppo Italiano per lo Studio della Streptochinasi nell'Infarto Miocardico (GISSI): Effectiveness of intravenous thrombolytic treatment in acute myocardial infarction. Lancet 1986, i:397–402.

51. The GUSTO Investigators: An international randomized trial comparing four thrombolytic strategies for acute myocardial infarction. N Engl J Med 1993, 329:673–682.

52. Mark DB, Hlatky MA, Califf RM, et al.: Cost effectiveness of thrombolytic therapy with tissue plasminogen activator as compared with streptokinase for acute myocardial infarction. N Engl J Med 1995, 332:1418–1424.

53. The European Myocardial Infarction Project Group: Prehospital thrombolytic therapy in patients with suspected acute myocardial infarction. N Engl J Med 1993, 329:383–389.

54. TIMI IIIB Investigators: Effects of tissue plasminogen activator and a comparison of early invasive and conservative strategies in unstable angina and non-Q-wave myocardial infarction: results of the TIMI IIIB Trial. Circulation 1994, 89:1545–1556.

55. Friedman M, Van den Bovenkamp GJ: The pathogenesis of a coronary thrombus. Am J Pathol 1966, 48:19–44.

56. Mehta SR, Yusuf S: Short- and long-term oral antiplatelet therapy in acute coronary syndromes and percutaneous coronary intervention. J Am Coll Cardiol 2003, 41:79S–88S.

57. Hawiger J: Formation and regulation of platelet and fibrin hemostatic plug. Hum Pathol 1987, 18:111–122.

58. Vu T-K, Hung D, Wheaton V, et al.: Molecular cloning of a functional thrombin receptor reveals a novel proteolytic mechanism of receptor activation. Cell 1991, 64:1057–1067.

59. Hawiger J: Repertoire of platelet receptors. Meth Enzymol 1992, 215:131–136.

60. Patrono C: Aspirin as an antiplatelet drug. N Engl J Med 1994, 330:1287–1294.

61. Antiplatelet Trialists' Collaboration: Collaborative overview of randomised trials of antiplatelet therapy—I: prevention of death, myocardial infarction, and stroke by prolonged antiplatelet therapy in various categories of patients. BMJ 1994, 308:81–106.

62. ISAM Study Group: A prospective trial of intravenous streptokinase in acute myocardial infarction (ISAM): mortality, morbidity, and infarct size at 21 days. N Engl J Med 1986, 314:1465–1471.

63. Gruppo Italiano per lo Studio della Streptochinasi nell'Infarto Miocardico (GISSI): Effectiveness of intravenous thrombolytic treatment in acute myocardial infarction. Lancet 1986, 1:397–401.

64. AIMS Trial Study Group: Long-term effects of intravenous antistreplase in acute myocardial infarction: final report of the AIMS study. Lancet 1990, 335:427–431.

65. Wilcox RG, von der Lippe G, Olsson CG, et al., for the ASSET Study Group: Trial of tissue plasminogen activator for mortality reduction in acute myocardial infarction: Anglo-Scandinavian Study of Early Thrombolysis (ASSET). Lancet 1988, 2:525–530.

66. Fibrinolytic Therapy Trialists' (FTT) Collaborative Group: Indications for fibrinolytic therapy in suspected acute myocardial infarction: collaborative overview of mortality and major morbidity results from all randomised trials of more than 1,000 patients. Lancet 1994, 343:311–322.

67. Simes J, Holmes DR, Ross A, et al.: The link between the angiographic substudy and mortality outcomes in a large randomized trial of myocardial infarction: the importance of early and complete infarct artery reperfusion. Circulation 1995, 91:1923–1928.

68. Weaver WD, Simes RJ, Betriu A, et al.: Comparison of primary coronary angioplasty and intravenous thrombolytic therapy for acute myocardial infarction: a quantitative review. JAMA 1997, 278:2093–2098.

69. Califf RA, Bengston JR: Cardiogenic shock. N Engl J Med 1994, 330:1724–1730.

70. Forrester JS, Diamond G, Chatterjee K, et al.: Medical therapy of acute myocardial infarction by application of hemodynamic subsets. N Engl J Med 1976, 295:1356–1362.

71. Gunnar RM (Chairman), on behalf of the ACC/AHA Task Force: ACC/AHA Task Force Report: Guidelines for the early management of patients with acute myocardial infarction. J Am Coll Cardiol 1990, 16:249–292.

72. Hochman JS: Cardiogenic shock complicating acute myocardial infarction: expanding the paradigm. Circulation 2003, 107:2998–3002.

73. Hochman JS, Sleeper L, Webb J, et al.: Effect of early revascularization for cardiogenic shock on one-year mortality: the SHOCK Trial Results [abstract]. Circulation 1999, 100:1939.

74. Becker AE, van Mantgem J-P: Cardiac tamponade: a study of 50 hearts. Eur J Cardiol 1975, 3/4:349–358.

75. Bloor CM: Cardiac Pathology. Philadelphia: JB Lippincott Co; 1978:176–221.

76. Schuster EH, Bulkley BH: Expansion of transmural myocardial infarction: a pathophysiologic factor in cardiac rupture. Circulation 1979, 60:1532–1538.

77. Becker R, Charlesworth A, Wilcox R, et al.: Cardiac rupture associated with thrombolytic therapy: impact of time to treatment in the Last Assessment of Thrombolytic Efficacy (LATE) Study. J Am Coll Cardiol 1995, 25:1063–1068.

CHRONIC ISCHEMIC HEART DISEASE

CHAPTER 3

Edited by George A. Beller

Jonathan Abrams, Barry D. Bertolet, Bernard R. Chaitman,
Delos M. Cosgrove III, Carl J. Pepine, Michael H. Picard,
Eric R. Powers, Michael Ragosta, Malissa J. Wood

PATHOPHYSIOLOGY OF ANGINA

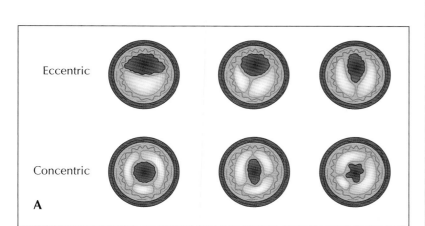

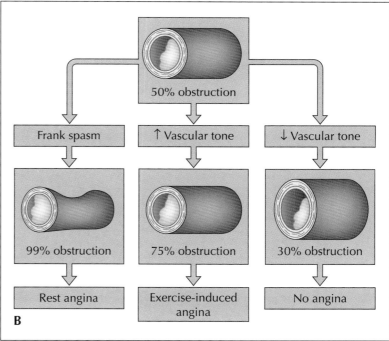

FIGURE 3-1. Coronary stenosis as a cause of angina. It is now recognized that coronary artery obstructions are capable of changing caliber, and constriction or narrowing of a preexisting lesion can be a factor in precipitating angina and myocardial ischemia.

A, If the coronary segment has sufficient smooth muscle (media) that is not involved in the atherosclerotic process, the vessel can dilate or constrict at the site of the stenosis. In general, vasoconstriction is most likely to occur with eccentric or asymmetric lesions, which consist of coronary atherosclerotic plaque in a segment of the vessel wall, with some relatively normal media intact. Concentric stenoses are less likely to constrict further or dilate. In concentric atherosclerosis, the atheroscle-

rotic plaque circumferentially involves the entire area of the vessel. It is believed that at least 25% of an arc or rim of media in the coronary artery must be preserved to allow for stenosis vasomotion.

B, This figure shows how the caliber of eccentric coronary artery stenoses may change, with considerable variation in the degree of stenosis resistance and the propensity to produce angina. Both increased vascular tone (first two examples) and decreased vascular tone (third example) are depicted. This phenomenon has been called dynamic coronary obstruction by some, emphasizing the variability and transitory nature of the actual "obstruction."

Continued on next page

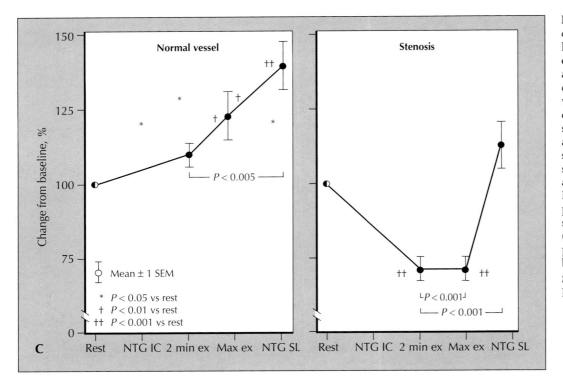

FIGURE 3-1. *(Continued)* **C,** Stenosis constriction can be induced in the cardiac catheterization laboratory by exercise or by the infusion of endothelial-dependent vasodilators, such as acetylcholine or serotonin. In the presence of disordered endothelial function, these substances, which normally cause dilatation, may produce constriction. In this study, patients with severe stable angina exercised (ex) during coronary angiography. At the onset of chest pain, the stenotic site of the culprit coronary artery was smaller (right panel). After nitroglycerin (NTG) administration, the stenosis dilated beyond base-line, thus relieving the chest pain. The normal portion of the coronary artery proximal to the stenosis dilates with exercise and nitroglycerin (left panel). Stenosis constriction could be prevented by the administration of nitroglycerin before exercise. IC—intracoronary; SL—sublingual. (Part B *adapted from* Epstein and Talbot [1]; part C *adapted from* Gage *et al.* [2].)

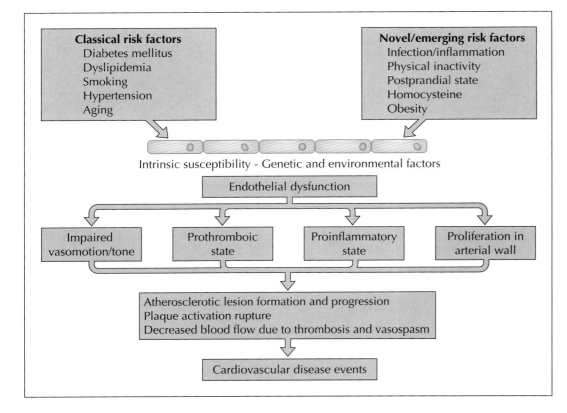

FIGURE 3–2. Endothelial dysfunction leading to a loss of endothelial control of vascular home-ostasis can lead to clinical entities such as stable angina, acute coronary syndromes, peripheral vascular disease symptoms, and stroke. Many of the pharmacologic therapies for patients with coronary heart disease improve endothelial function and reduce risk of future cardiac events. Classic cardiovascular disease risk factors such as diabetes, dyslipidemia, smoking, and hypertension adversely affect endothelial function and contribute to the development and progression of coronary atherosclerosis. Genetic and environmental factors modulate the susceptibility of the endothelium to damage and subsequent dysfunction, which lead to impaired vasomotor tone, a prothrombotic state, a proin-flammatory state, and smooth muscle prolifera-tion or neointimal formation in the arterial wall. The pathophysiologic entities resulting from these states include plaque rupture, intravas-cular thrombosis, vasospasm, and progression of the atherosclerotic process. (*Adapted from* Widlansky *et al.* [3].)

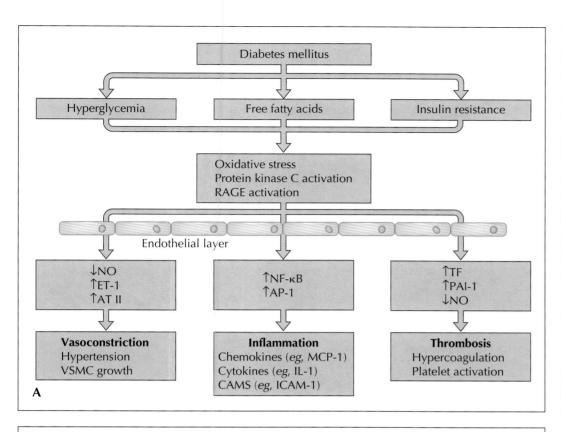

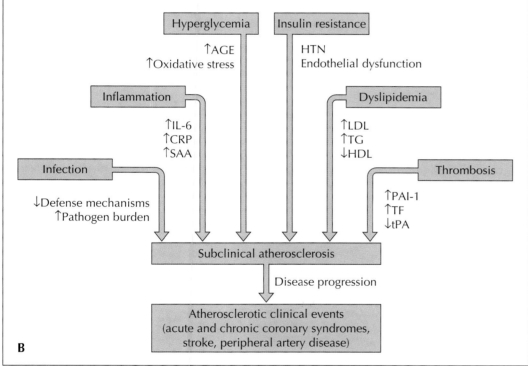

FIGURE 3-3. Type 2 diabetes is a major risk factor for atherosclerotic vascular disease. The epidemic of obesity is leading to a marked increase in number of patients with type 2 diabetes. Patients with diabetes and no coronary heart disease have the same risk for future cardiac death as nondiabetics with prior myocardial infarction. Diabetics have increased mortality and morbidity after myocardial infarction and a worse prognosis with unstable angina. They also have worse outcomes following percutaneous coronary intervention. **A,** Certain metabolic abnormalities that are consequent to diabetes include hyperglycemia, increase in free fatty acids, and insulin resistance. These metabolic abnormalities lead to increased oxidative stress, disturbances in intracellular signal transduction as with activation of protein kinase C, and activation of the receptor for advanced glycation end products (RAGE). This leads to decreased availability of nitric oxide (NO), increased production of endothelin (ET-1), activation of transcription factors such as NF-κB and AP-1.

The metabolic consequences of diabetes also enhance release of prothrombotic factors such as tissue factor (TF) and plasminogen activator inhibitor-1 (PAI-1). Endothelial dysfunction occurs in diabetes consequent to reduced ability of NO-mediated relaxation. Insulin resistance and hyperinsulinemia in diabetics or in patients with the metabolic syndrome are associated with elevated triglycerides, low level of high-density lipoprotein (HDL), increased small dense low-density lipoprotein (LDL), enhanced secretion of LDL, disorders of coagulation, increased vascular resistance, hypertension (HTN), and atherosclerosis progression with inflammation. (*Adapted from* Creager *et al.* [4].)

B, Pathogenetic mechanisms involved in the initiation of subclinical atherosclerosis and disease progression to atherosclerotic events in diabetic patients. Infection, inflammation, hyperglycemia, insulin resistance, dyslipidemia, and thrombosis are all associated with diabetes and contribute to the atherosclerotic process. AGE—advanced glycation end product; CRP—C-reactive protein; IL-6—interleukin-6; PAI-1—plasminogen activator inhibitor-1; SAA—serum amyloid A protein; TPA—tissue-type plasminogen activator. (*Adapted from* Biondi-Zoccai GGL *et al.* [5].)

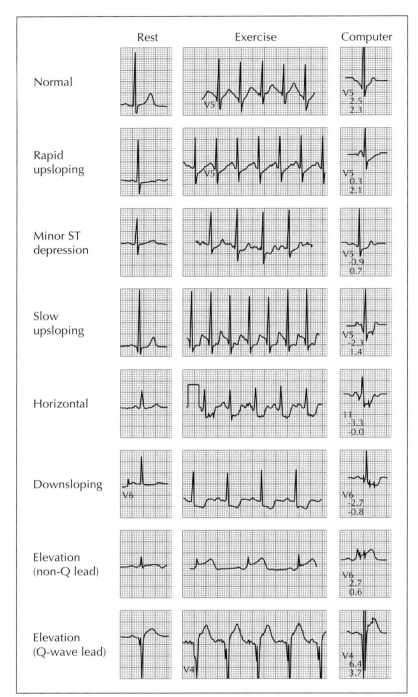

	Rest	Exercise	Computer
Normal			V5 2.5 2.3
Rapid upsloping		V5	V5 0.3 2.1
Minor ST depression			V5 -0.9 0.7
Slow upsloping			V5 -2.3 1.4
Horizontal			11 -3.3 -0.0
Downsloping	V6		V6 -2.7 -0.8
Elevation (non-Q lead)			V6 2.7 0.6
Elevation (Q-wave lead)		V4	V4 6.4 3.7

FIGURE 3-4. Illustration of typical exercise ECG patterns at rest and at peak exertion. The computer-processed incrementally averaged beat corresponds with the raw data taken at the same time during exercise. The patterns represent a gradient of worsening ECG response to myocardial ischemia. In the column of computer-averaged beats, ST-80 displacement (*top number*) indicates the magnitude of ST-segment displacement 80 ms after the J-point relative to the PQ junction or E point. ST-segment slope measurement (*bottom number*) indicates the ST-segment slope at a fixed time after the J-point to the ST-80 measurement. At least three noncomputer averaged complexes with a stable baseline should meet criteria for abnormality before the exercise ECG can be considered abnormal.

The first two tracings illustrate normal and rapid upsloping ST segments; both are normal responses to exercise. Minor ST depression can occur occasionally at submaximal workloads in patients with coronary disease; in the illustration, the ST segment is depressed 0.9 mm (0.09 mV) 80 ms after the J-point. A slow upsloping ST-segment pattern often demonstrates an ischemic response in patients with known coronary disease or those with a high clinical risk before testing. Criteria for slow upsloping ST-segment depression include J-point and ST-80 depression of 1.5 mV/s or greater and an ST segment slope of 0.7 to 1.0 mV/s or greater.

Classic criteria for myocardial ischemia include horizontal ST-segment depression observed when J-point and ST-80 depression are 0.1 mV or greater and the ST-segment slope is within the range of ±0.7 to 1.0 mV/s. Downsloping ST-segment depression occurs when J-point and ST-80 depression are 0.1 mV or greater and ST-segment slope is -0.7 to -1.0 mV/s or greater. ST-segment elevation in a non–Q-wave non-infarct territory lead occurs when J-point and ST-60 are 1.0 mV or greater and represents a severe ischemic response. ST-segment elevation in an infarct territory (Q-wave lead) indicates a severe wall motion abnormality and is usually not an ischemic response.

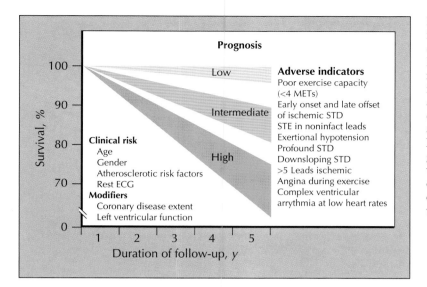

FIGURE 3-5. Actuarial survival curves of patients with normal or mildly impaired left ventricular function who have prognostic low-, intermediate-, and high-risk mortality estimates based on exercise test results. Patients able to exercise to at least seven metabolic equivalents with a normal exercise ECG have an excellent 5-year prognosis for survival, even in the presence of obstructive coronary disease. The presence of several adverse indicators, such as poor exercise capacity and early onset and late offset of myocardial ischemia on the exercise ECG, places the patient into a prognostic high-risk group. Patients in the intermediate category, who have fewer marked adverse indicators than individuals in the higher-risk group, fall into a subgroup for which myocardial perfusion imaging would significantly enhance the prognostic information used to guide the decision for coronary angiography and revascularization. The survival curves shift downward for patients with moderate or severe left ventricular dysfunction. (*Adapted from* Chaitman [6].)

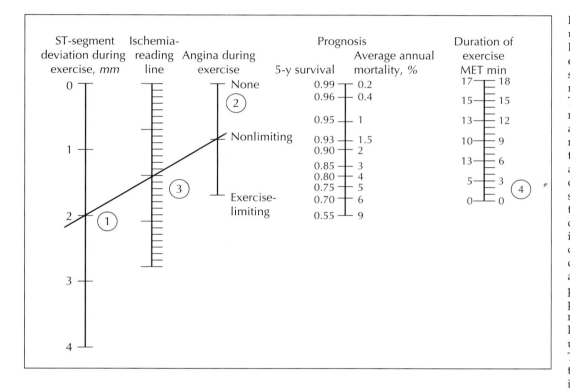

FIGURE 3-6. Nomogram of prognostic relations using the Duke outpatient treadmill score. The Duke treadmill score incorporates duration of exercise (in minutes) - (5 × the maximal ST-segment deviation during or after exercise [in millimeters]) - (4 × the treadmill angina index). Treadmill angina index is 0 for no angina, 1 for nonlimiting angina, and 2 for exercise-limiting angina. Of 613 outpatients with suspected coronary disease referred for exercise testing, two of three had a treadmill score of 5 or more with an associated 4-year survival rate of 99%. Only 4% of outpatients had scores less than 10, with a 4-year survival rate of 79%. The nomogram can be used to assess ambulatory outpatients referred for exercise testing. The observed amount of exercise-induced ST-segment deviation (minus resting changes) is marked on the line for ST-segment deviation during exercise (1). Next, the degree of angina during exercise is plotted (2), and the two points are connected with a straight edge. The point of intersection on the ischemia reading line is noted (3). Next, the number of metabolic equivalents (or minutes of exercise if the Bruce method is used) is marked on the exercise duration line (4). The mark on the ischemia reading line and duration of exercise line are connected, and the point of intersection on the prognosis line determines the 5-year survival rate and average annual mortality for patients with the selected specific variables. The 5-year prognosis is estimated at 78% for this case of exercise-induced 2-mm ST depression, nonlimiting exercise-induced angina, and peak exercise workload of five metabolic equivalents. (*Adapted from* Mark *et al.* [7].)

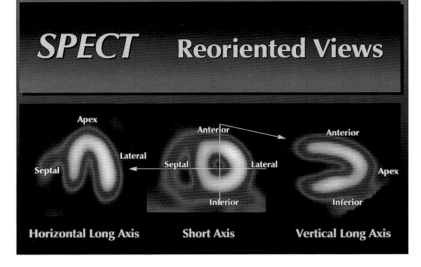

FIGURE 3-7. Single-photon emission computed tomography (SPECT) radionuclide imaging with either thallium-201 or one of the technetium-99m–labeled imaging agents such as technetium-99m–sestamibi or technetium-99m–tetrofosmin provides supplementary diagnostic and prognostic value to treadmill exercise testing or pharmacologic stress imaging. The major tomographic views are the horizontal long-axis, short-axis, and vertical long-axis slices. Defects in the anterior wall, apex, and interventricular septum most commonly are associated with a significant stenosis of the left anterior descending coronary artery. Defects extending throughout the postero-lateral wall are usually attributed to stenoses in the left circumflex coronary artery. Defects in the inferior wall which extend to the infero-lateral and infero-septal regions are most often attributed to stenoses in the right coronary artery.

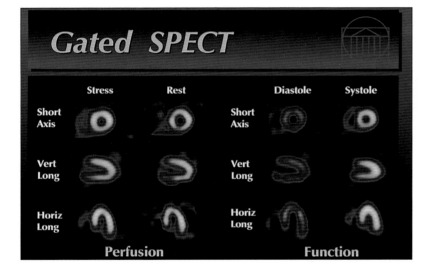

FIGURE 3-8. Single-photon emission computed tomographic (SPECT) imaging most often is performed using electrocardiographic-gated imaging in order to evaluate regional wall motion or regional systolic thickening. Stress and rest images are compared for determination of significant perfusion abnormalities. End-diastolic and end-systolic images are employed to evaluate abnormal regional myocardial dysfunction either secondary to myocardial scar, post-ischemic stunning, or myocardial hibernation. When color images are used, the increasing intensity of the color (*eg*, from red to orange) represents the degree of systolic thickening from end-diastole to end-systole. These images are from a normal individual.

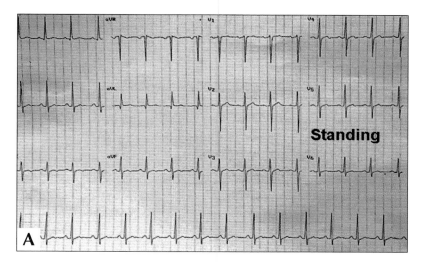

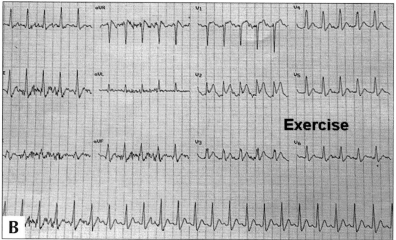

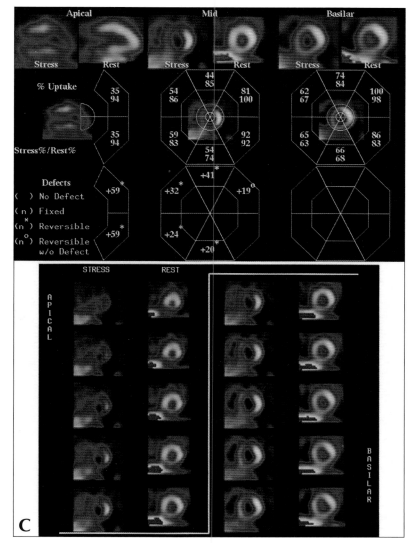

FIGURE 3-9. Myocardial perfusion imaging with radionuclide imaging agents provides supplementary diagnostic and prognostic value to exercise or pharmacologic stress testing in patients presenting with chest pain. High-risk patients are those with extensive areas of inducible ischemia. **A**, The standing resting electrocardiogram in a patient referred for exercise myocardial perfusion imaging. **B**, The exercise electrocardiogram at peak stress showing new ST-segment elevation in leads V_1 and V_2 with upsloping ST-segment depression in the infero-lateral leads. **C**, Stress and rest short-axis technetium-99m tomograms from the same patient showing an extensive defect on the poststress images involving the anterior wall, septum, and inferior wall. The defect also involves the apex. Transient ischemic left ventricular (LV) cavity dilation is observed in this imaging study. It is a high-risk finding where the LV cavity is larger on the stress than the resting scan and reflects stress-induced subendocardial ischemia. The resting images show significant reversibility in the entire defect region.

Continued on next page

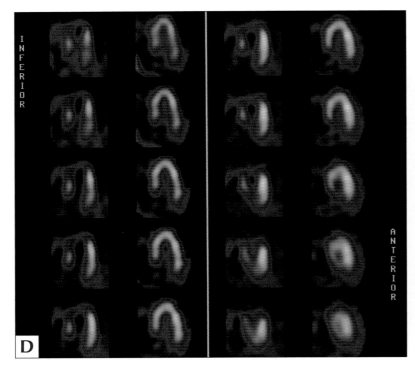

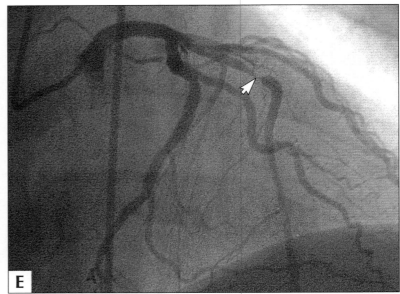

FIGURE 3-9. *(Continued)* **D**, Stress and rest horizontal long-axis tomograms from the same patient showing a significant reversible defect involving the apex and intraventricular septum. **E**, The coronary angiogram from the same patient showing a very high-grade stenosis in the left anterior descending coronary (LAD) artery *(arrow)*.

This patient is representative of a high-risk noninvasive stress perfusion imaging finding with an inducible transmural ischemia on the exercise electrocardiogram and an extensive stress-induced hypoperfusion involving the entire LAD risk area. Coronary angiography confirmed the presence of a severe stenosis in the LAD, which was successfully stented.

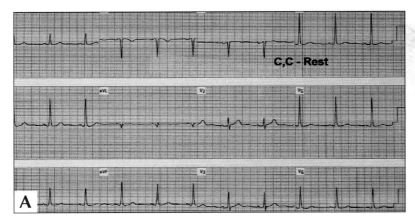

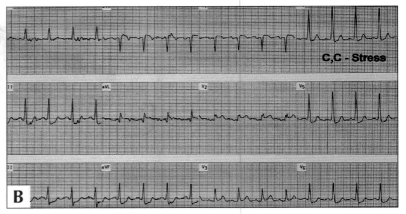

FIGURE 3-10. **A**, Resting electrocardiogram in a patient referred for exercise myocardial perfusion imaging. **B**, The exercise electrocardiogram at peak exercise stress showing significant slow upsloping ST-segment depression in multiple leads with 1.0 to 2.0 mm of ST-segment elevation in V_1 and V_2.

Continued on next page

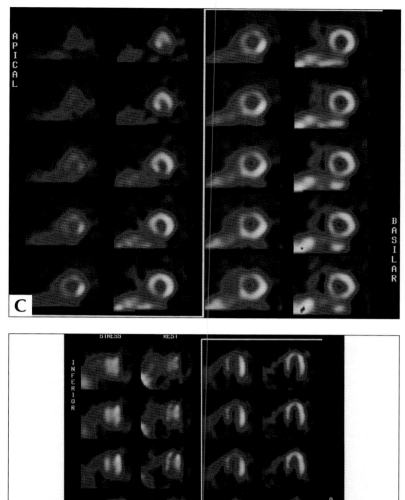

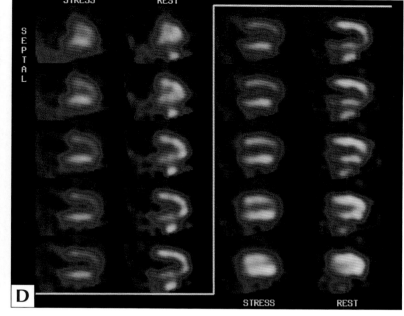

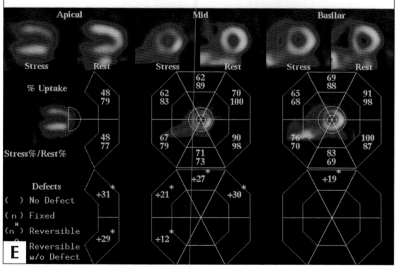

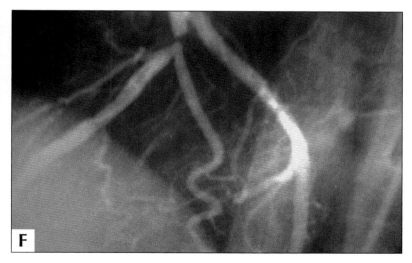

FIGURE 3-10. *(Continued)* **C,** Stress and rest short-axis tomograms showing an extensive anterior defect extending to the intraventricular septum and apex. The resting study shows total reversibility of this defect. **D,** Stress and rest vertical long-axis tomograms showing defect reversibility in the anterior wall and apex. **E,** Horizontal long-axis images in the same patient showing reversible defects involving the apex and intraventricular septum. **F,** Left anterior oblique projection of a coronary angiogram from the same patient showing a high-grade proximal left anterior descending coronary artery stenosis. This patient is similar to the one depicted in Figure 3-9 except that transient left ventricular cavity dilation is not observed.

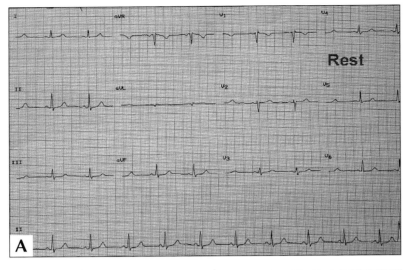

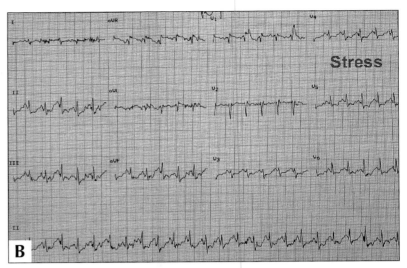

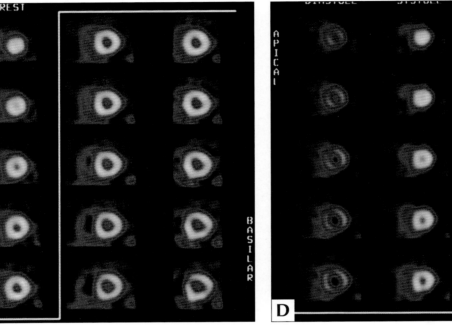

FIGURE 3-11. Stress perfusion imaging is useful in differentiating true from false positive ST-segment responses on exercise treadmill testing. This is an example of a patient with a false-positive electrocardiogram stress test response, who had a normal gated single-photon emission computed tomography (SPECT) perfusion scan. A, Resting electrocardiogram showing no abnormalities. B, The exercise electrocardiogram at peak stress showing ST-segment depression in multiple leads and most prominent in leads V_4–V_6. For most complexes, the ST depression is

approximately 1 mm. C, Stress and rest short-axis tomographic images showing uniform technetium-99m–sestamibi uptake in all myocardial segments. The resting study is also within normal limits. D, End-diastolic and end-systolic short-axis images showing uniform systolic thickening of all myocardial segments.

This patient was told that the ST-segment response was false-positive for ischemia and that no coronary artery disease was present.

SURVIVAL CURVE FOR DIABETIC MEN VERSUS WOMEN RELATIVE TO EXTENT OF ISCHEMIA

	DEATH/MI		
	0-VESSEL ISCHEMIA	1-VESSEL ISCHEMIA	≥ 2-VESSEL ISCHEMIA
Diabetic men	86	77	79
Diabetic women	96	72	60

FIGURE 3-12. Stress perfusion imaging is particularly useful in patients with diabetes who present with chest pain and possible coronary artery disease. The greater the extent of myocardial ischemia (MI), the greater the subsequent cardiac event rate. In this multicenter trial, diabetic women who had ischemia in two or more coronary territories (*eg*, left anterior descending and left circumflex supply regions) had only a 60% survival free of death or infarction during a 3-year follow-up. Diabetic men have a 79% event-free survival. In contrast, diabetic women with normal scans (0-vessel ischemia) had a substantially better event-free survival than diabetic men with no inducible ischemia (96% vs 86%). (*$P < 0.05$). (*Adapted from* Giri *et al.* [8].)

PROGNOSTIC VALUE OF MYOCARDIAL PERFUSION IMAGING

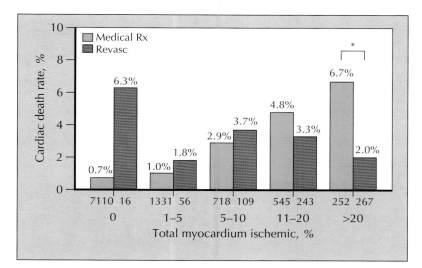

FIGURE 3-13. Stress myocardial perfusion single-photon emission computed tomography (SPECT) can be employed for determining which patients with no prior coronary artery disease may have a better outcome with revascularization compared with medical therapy. In this study, a total of 10,627 consecutive patients who underwent exercise or adenosine myocardial perfusion imaging were followed for an average of 1.9 ± 0.6 years. To adjust for nonrandomization of treatment, a propensity score was developed using logistic regression to model the decision to refer to revascularization. As shown, the observed cardiac death rates over the follow-up period in patients undergoing revascularization (revasc), versus medical therapy (medical Rx), were related to the amount of inducible ischemia. The increase in cardiac death frequency was a function of the amount of ischemia where patients who had more than 11% of the total myocardium rendered ischemic showed a more favorable survival with revascularization compared with medical therapy. However, the difference in outcome between revascularized patients and patients treated medically was only seen when more than 20% of the total myocardium was judged to be ischemic. Note also that with medical therapy, the greater the extent of ischemia, the worse the outcome. Patients with no ischemia ($n = 7110$) had only a 0.7% annual cardiac death rate with medical therapy. Patients with more than 20% of the myocardium rendered ischemic had a 6.7% annual cardiac death rate. (*$P < 0.0001$.) (*Adapted from* Hachamovitch *et al.* 9].)

ECHOCARDIOGRAPHY

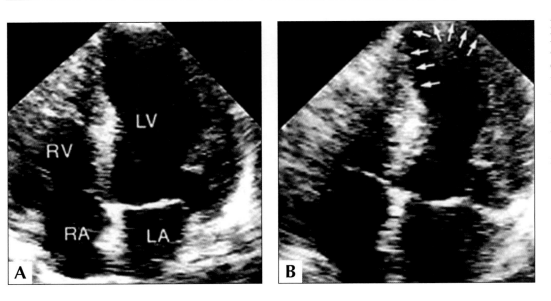

FIGURE 3-14. Wall motion abnormality is the hallmark of coronary artery disease on echocardiography. This abnormality is one of the earliest signs of myocardial ischemia or infarction. **A,** Two-dimensional echocardiographic apical four-chamber view at end-diastole. **B,** Two-dimensional echocardiographic apical four-chamber view at end-systole. The right ventricle (RV) and the septal and lateral walls at the base of the left ventricle (LV) demonstrate normal inward motion from diastole through systole; however, the distal septum and apex demonstrate akinesis (arrows in B). The wall motion abnormality demonstrated in this frame was caused by ischemia from a lesion in the mid-left anterior descending artery. LA—left atrium; RA—right atrium.

NATURAL HISTORY OF WALL MOTION ABNORMALITIES

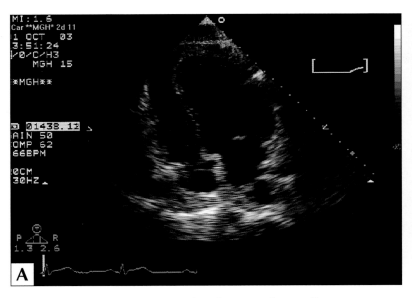

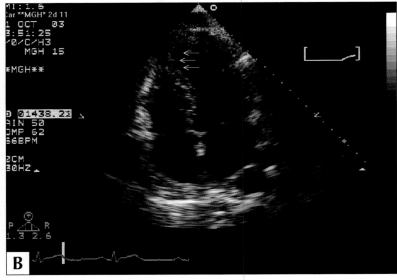

FIGURE 3-15. Example of a regional wall motion abnormality on two-dimensional echocardiography. The hallmark of myocardial ischemia and infarction on echocardiography is regional dysfunction. **A,** Apical four-chamber view in diastole. **B,** Same view in systole demonstrating akinesis of the distal septum due to prior infarction (*arrows*). As shown in this example, the hallmark of myocardial ischemia and infarction is the regional wall motion abnormality. The wall motion abnormality occurs almost immediately upon occlusion of the coronary artery. In patients with significant coronary artery disease, the left ventricular wall motion may be normal at rest and then regional wall motion abnormalities are induced with exercise. The presence of a resting wall motion abnormality is also of value in detecting ischemia and infarction in a patient with symptoms but an uninterpretable electrocardiogram such as left bundle branch block.

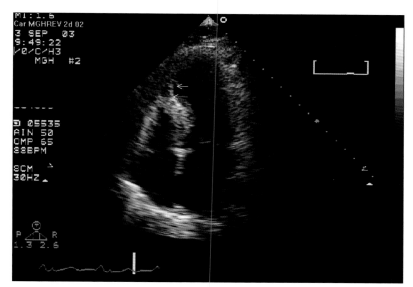

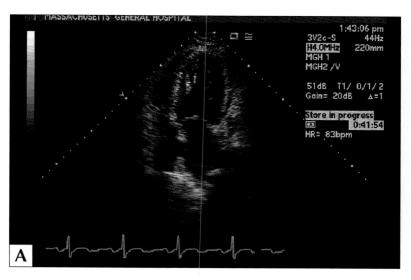

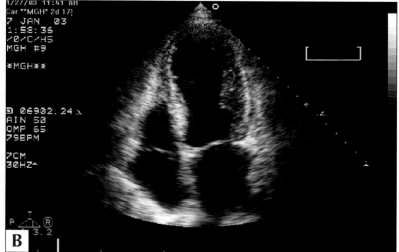

FIGURE 3-16. Left ventricular (LV) aneurysm detected by echocardiography. An aneurysm of the LV apex (*arrows*) was due to chronic persistent total occlusion of the mid-left anterior descending coronary artery. This aneurysm is seen in this apical four-chamber view. A true aneurysm of the left ventricle can be a sequelae of myocardial infarction and a chronically occluded coronary artery. The true aneurysm is noted on echocardiography by its wide neck and distortion of the normal ventricular contour in both diastole and systole. The wall of the true aneurysm is composed of these myocardial elements. Thrombus formation within the aneurysm is an additional complication of this distortion of ventricular shape and function.

FIGURE 3-17. Infarct expansion occurring following acute myocardial infarction that contributes to the left ventricular (LV) remodeling process can be detected by echocardiography. **A,** Example of a normal left ventricular shape at end-systole and an apical four-chamber view. **B,** End-systolic shape alterations 2 months after anterior myocardial infarction. The LV cavity is dilated, and the LV apex is remodeling with hypertrophy of normal segments. Infarct expansion is noted by enlargement of infarcted portions of the ventricle, a decrease in global LV function and hypertrophy of non-infarcted segments. This process is an attempt to compensate for the decrease in function that accompanies large infarctions. Infarct expansion is responsible for much of the congestive heart failure and ventricular arrhythmias noted late after myocardial infarction. Pharmacologic therapy, especially with angiotensin-converting enzyme inhibitors, can attenuate this process. Early interventions to limit infarct size, including early revascularization by catheter ("primary" angioplasty or stenting) also reduces the incidence of infarct expansion.

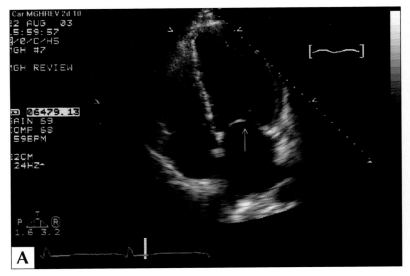

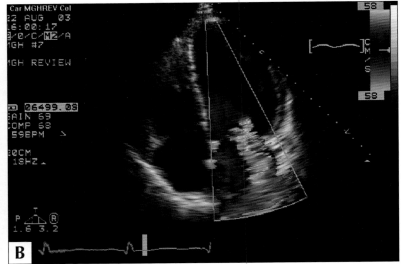

FIGURE 3-18. Mitral regurgitation can occur as a complication of chronic coronary artery disease. Mitral regurgitation after myocardial infarction is commonly due to left ventricular dilation and resultant displacement of the papillary muscles away for the valvular apparatus. This results in an apical tenting of the mitral valve (the "incomplete mitral leaflet closure pattern"). Increasing severity of mitral regurgitation after infarction is a marker of decreased long-term event-free survival. **A,** In this chronically ischemic heart, the left ventricle is dilated resulting in apical tenting of the mitral valve (*arrow*), also known as "incomplete mitral leaflet closure pattern." It is due to displacement of the papillary muscles away from the mitral valve annulus. **B,** Color Doppler demonstrating severe mitral regurgitation.

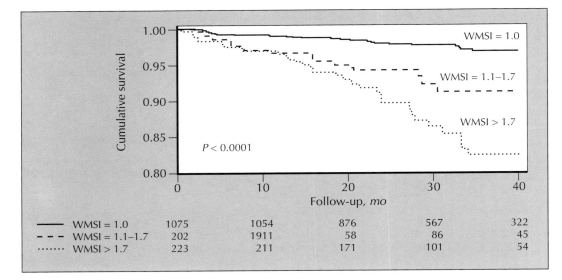

FIGURE 3-19. Stress echocardiography is a valuable technique for detecting coronary artery disease and determining prognosis. These curves represent groups of patients stratified by a wall motion score index (WMSI), which is a measure of regional function at peak stress. Patients with a normal WMSI (*upper curve*) have an excellent prognosis, whereas patients with a WMSI greater than 1.7 have a significantly worse event-free survival. (*Adapted from* Yao *et al.* [10].)

—— WMSI = 1.0	1075	1054	876	567	322
- - - WMSI = 1.1–1.7	202	1911	58	86	45
······ WMSI > 1.7	223	211	171	101	54

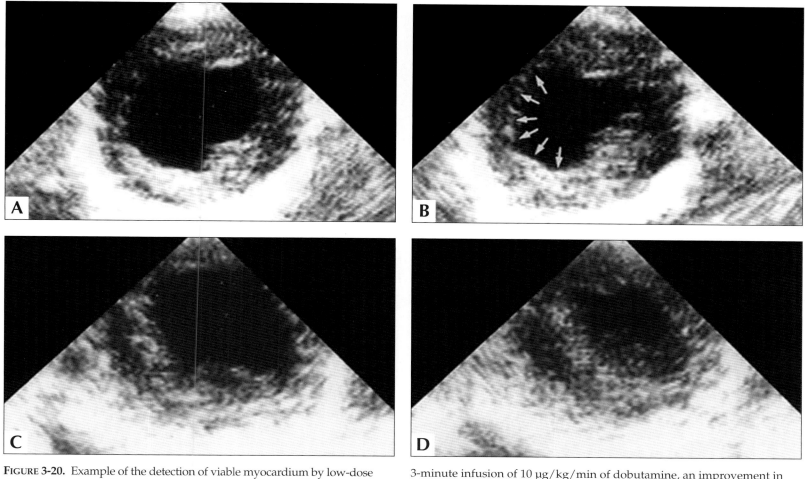

FIGURE 3-20. Example of the detection of viable myocardium by low-dose dobutamine echocardiography in an experimental model of ischemic but viable myocardium. **A,** Short-axis end-diastolic image of the left ventricular apex at rest. **B,** Accompanying end-systolic image. A wall motion abnormality is present (*arrows* in *B*) involving 50% of the circumference and results from reduction of flow in the mid-left anterior descending artery. **C** and **D,** With a 3-minute infusion of 10 μg/kg/min of dobutamine, an improvement in wall motion is noted in the segments that formerly exhibited abnormal wall motion. *C* is of the apex at end-diastole, and *D* is at end-systole. Following restoration of normal flow in the left anterior descending artery, wall motion in the apex returned to normal.

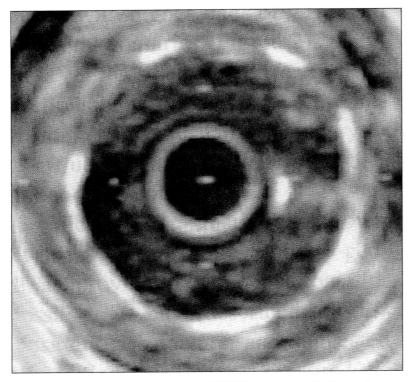

FIGURE 3-21. Intravascular ultrasound (IVUS) can be applied in conjunction with coronary stenting to assure that the stent is well deployed against all of the coronary artery walls. This is an example of an intravascular ultrasound image of a stented right coronary artery. (*From* Jang *et al*. 11]; with permission.)

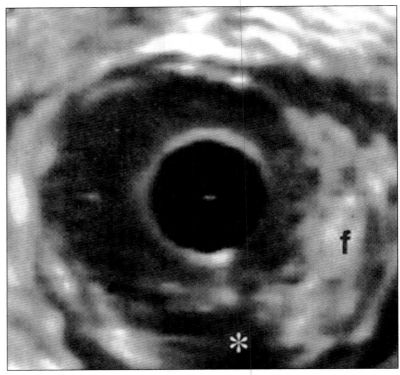

FIGURE 3-22. Intravascular ultrasound (IVUS) has value in determining the type of tissue responsible for certain coronary lesions. This degree of detail is not available on angiography and may assist in determining the appropriate type of intervention. For example, in this image, a fibrous plaque (f) is identified. The full circumferential extent of plaque is partially obscured by a shadow artifact created by the guidewire (*). (From Jang *et al*. [12]; with permission.)

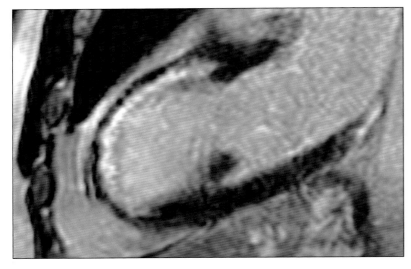

FIGURE 3-23. Contrast-enhanced cardiac magnetic resonance imaging is gaining increasing popularity for the detection and quantification of the extent of a transmural myocardial scar. This figure is a two-chamber long-axis mid-diastolic image from a patient 1 week after a reperfused anterior myocardial infarction. The images were obtained with an inversion recovery fast gradient echo technique (turboFLASH) 20 minutes after the infusion of 0.1 mL/kg of Gd-DTPA. In this image type, signal from normal myocardium is nulled and appears dark and infarcted myocardium appears quite bright with an increase in signal of up to 500% of that of normal myocardium. In this particular example, the infarct is a subendocardial anterior infarction that subtends 50% of the transmural extent of the anterior wall from the base to the apex. Studies have shown that the transmural extent of acute infarction correlates with functional recovery months after the infarct.

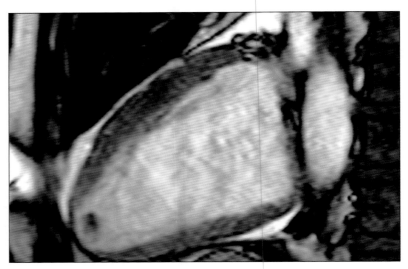

FIGURE 3-24. Shown is an end-diastolic two-chamber long-axis image from a steady state free precession cine image set obtained in a patient with multivessel coronary artery disease prior to coronary artery bypass graft surgery. The contrast to noise between the myocardium and blood pool is excellent using this technique. The apex appears quite thin relative to the anterior wall and inferior wall. Within the blood pool in the apex is an oblong shape that appears to be as dark as the myocardium and represents an *apical mural thrombus*. Cine imaging after contrast has been shown to be more sensitive for left ventricular thrombus than either cine imaging alone or echocardiography in such patients.

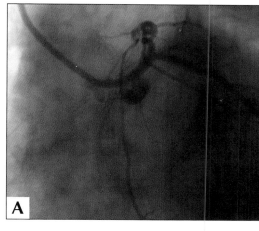

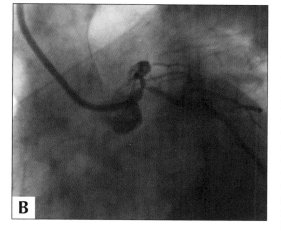

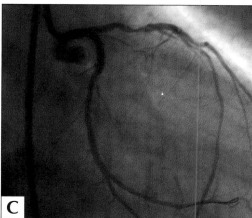

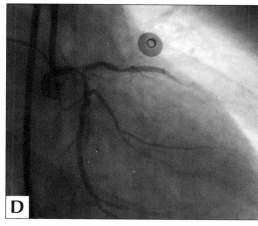

FIGURE 3-25. Coronary stenting in a high-risk patient. The arteriographic frames are from a 58-year-old woman with newly diagnosed pancreatic cancer who presented with severe chest pain unresponsive to full medical therapy. Catheterization and then percutaneous coronary intervention (PCI) was offered for palliation of her unrelenting chest pain. **A,** Right anterior oblique (RAO) caudal view demonstrating a severe lesion involving the left main coronary and proximal left anterior descending (LAD) and circumflex arteries. **B,** Left anterior oblique (LAO) caudal view demonstrating the same abnormalities. **C,** RAO caudal view at conclusion of PCI. A stent was placed in the LAD followed by placement of a long stent, treating both the circumflex artery and the left main. **D,** LAO caudal view at the conclusion of the PCI procedure.

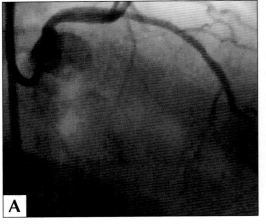

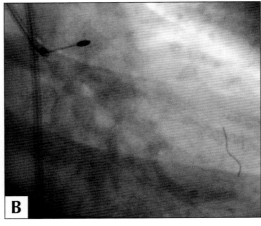

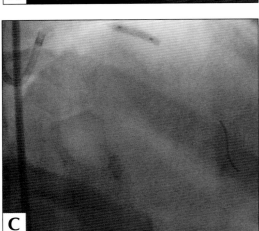

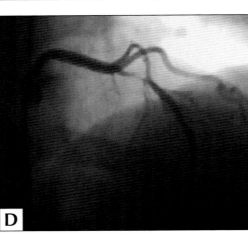

FIGURE 3-26. In-stent restenosis treated with rotational atherectomy followed by balloon angioplasty. These coronary arteriographic frames are from a 54-year-old man who presented with severe exertional chest pain. For a similar problem, he had undergone left anterior descending (LAD) coronary artery stenting 5 months previously. He was treated with rotational atherectomy followed by balloon angioplasty. This approach to in-stent restenosis has largely been replaced by brachytherapy. **A**, Right anterior oblique (RAO) cranial view demonstrating a tight LAD in-stent restenosis. **B**, RAO cranial view showing wire across lesion in distal LAD and atherectomy burr in LAD proximal to stenosis. **C**, Same view showing balloon inflation following rotational atherectomy. **D**, Same view at conclusion of procedure, demonstrating good angiographic result.

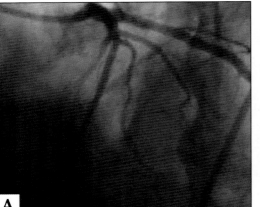

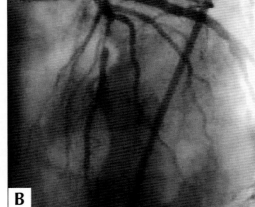

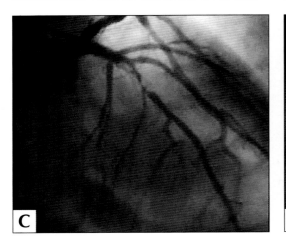

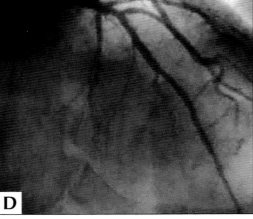

FIGURE 3-27. Example of pre- and poststenting of a tight left anterior descending (LAD) coronary artery stenosis in a 61-year-old man who presented with an acute coronary syndrome. **A**, Right anterior oblique (RAO) cranial view demonstrating a tight stenosis in the LAD. **B**, Left anterior oblique (LAO) cranial view demonstrating tight stenosis. **C**, RAO cranial view following placement of a single stent. **D**, LAO cranial view following stent placement.

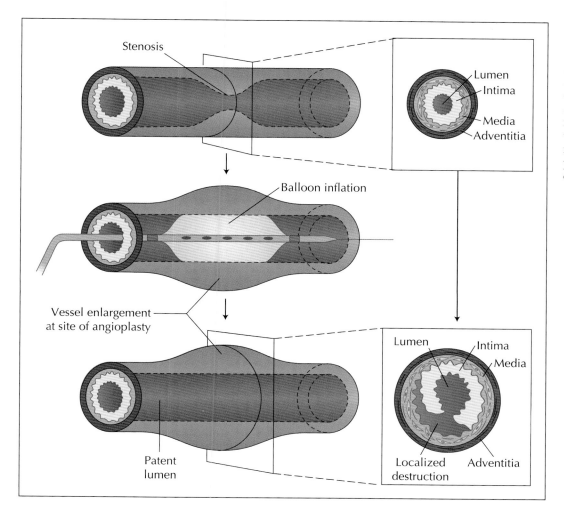

Stenosis

Lumen
Intima
Media
Adventitia

Balloon inflation

Vessel enlargement
at site of angioplasty

Lumen
Intima
Media
Adventitia

Patent
lumen

Localized
destruction

FIGURE 3-28. The mechanism of percutaneous transluminal coronary angioplasty (PTCA). Balloon PTCA enlarges the vessel lumen by stretching the entire vessel, creating a localized aneurysm. Immediately after the balloon is deflated, elastic recoil occurs and re-narrows the artery by 20% to 30%; however, the artery remains larger than it was before initial dilatation. In the process of stretching the artery, the inelastic components of the arterial wall are torn, particularly if the artery is narrowed in a concentric fashion.

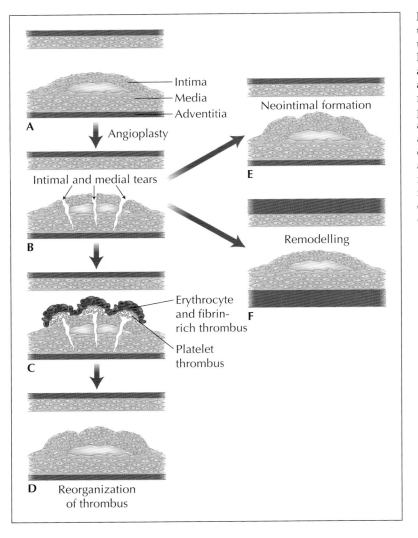

FIGURE 3-29. Restenosis occurs in a significant number of patients who undergo balloon angioplasty and to a lesser extent in those who have undergone intracoronary stenting. Over-distension of an atherosclerotic lesion causes endothelial damage, fracture of the internal elastic lamina, and medial dissection. The figure shows possible outcomes following angioplasty and the mechanisms responsible for restenosis. **A,** Schematic representation of the diseased vessel before intervention. **B,** After angioplasty, dissection of both the intima and the media is shown, which is then associated with enlargement of the dilated segment. As shown in **C,** angioplasty may be complicated by acute thrombosis. In **D,** the thrombus can become organized. Neointima formation (**E**) can result from migration and proliferation of medial and intimal vascular smooth muscle cells resulting from the injury. Restenosis may also be caused by negative remodeling (**F**). In this situation, the adventitia is shown to have expanded, with increased collagen formation resulting in the overall decrease in lumen diameter. (Adapted from Bennett and O'Sullivan [13].)

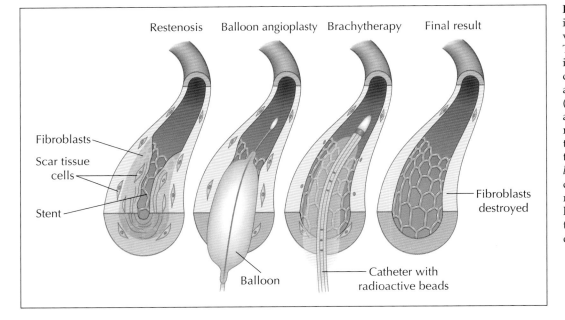

FIGURE 3-30. Brachytherapy in which radiation is delivered to a coronary lesion has proven valuable for treatment of in-stent restenosis. The diagram shows the steps in performing intracoronary brachytherapy, beginning with a depiction of in-stent restenosis (*left*). Balloon agioplasty of the stenotic segment is performed (*second from left*). The balloon is then removed and replaced with a catheter that contains the radioactive source. The radioactive source is then left in place for a calculated length of time to give an appropriate radiation dose (*third from left*). The catheter is then removed. At *right* is a depiction of the final result with the in-stent restenosis being successfully dilated and fibroblasts and other cells that might cause a proliferative response to the treatment having been destroyed by the brachytherapy.

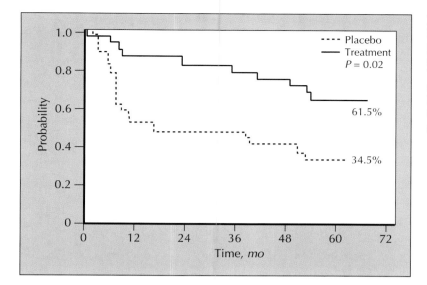

FIGURE 3-31. Five-year follow-up data for patients receiving either brachytherapy with an iridium-192 gamma-emitting source versus placebo. Plotted against time is the probability of being free from death, myocardial infarction, or repeated revascularization of the target lesion. The curves begin to separate at approximately 3 months, and the difference between the curves persists throughout follow-up. Thus, brachytherapy with a gamma source was found to be superior in long-term follow-up to placebo treatment in this group of patients with in-stent stenosis. (*Adapted from* Grise *et al.* [14].)

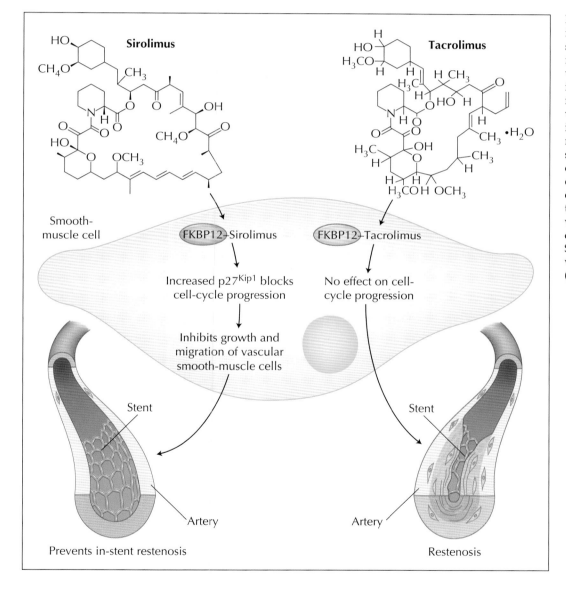

FIGURE 3-32. Drug-eluting stents have emerged in the field of interventional cardiology and show great promise in reducing the incidence of restenosis after a percutaneous coronary intervention. Sirolimus (rapamycin), an inhibitor of in-stent restenosis of the coronary arteries, has made a significant impact in the field of interventional cardiology. Sirolimus is a potent inhibitor of the proliferation of vascular smooth muscle cells. Sirolimus and the related immunosuppressant tacrolimus both bind to the same cystolic receptor FKBP12, but their actions are different. FKBP12-sirolimus inhibits the growth of vascular smooth cells, whereas FKBP12-tacrolimus does not (*arrows*). The mechanism by which sirolimus inhibits cells growth involves cell-cycle arrest at the transition G_1 to S. Sirolimus prevents in-stent restenosis (*lower left*), whereas tacrolimus does not (*lower right*). (*Adapted from* Marks [15].)

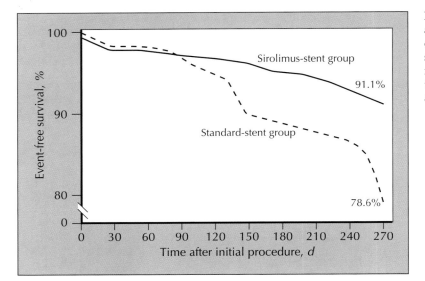

FIGURE 3-33. Actuarial rate of survival free from target-vessel failure among patients who received either a sirolimus-eluting stent or a standard stent. Event-free survival was significantly higher in the sirolimus-stent group than in the standard stent group ($P < 0.001$). This study was a randomized, double-blind trial comprising 1508 patients at 53 centers in the United States who had a newly diagnosed lesion in a native coronary artery. (*Adapted from* Moses *et al.* [16].)

MEDICAL THERAPY

AGGRESSIVE RISK FACTOR MODIFICATION

RISK FACTOR	SPECIFIC THERAPY
Dyslipidemia Increased LDL cholesterol, decreased HDL cholesterol, increased triglyceride and low HDL combination (typically associated with insulin resistance, obesity, or diabetes)	Dietary modification, weight loss, hypolipidemic agents
Cigarette smoking	Smoking cessation programs, behavioral therapy, nicotine patches
Hypertension	Weight loss, low sodium intake, pharmacologic therapy
Diabetes	Diet, oral agents, insulin
Estrogen deficiency	

FIGURE 3-34. Coronary risk factors. Identification and vigorous intervention in coronary risk is an underestimated and under-utilized aspect of the medical approach to angina pectoris. The risk factors listed should be modified aggressively with lifestyle or hygienic changes, behavior modification, or pharmacologic therapy. The new National Cholesterol Education Programs Guidelines and many experts favor aggressive risk factor modification for high-risk individuals with established vascular disease (*eg*, patients with angina pectoris). HDL—high-density lipoprotein; LDL—low-density lipoprotein.

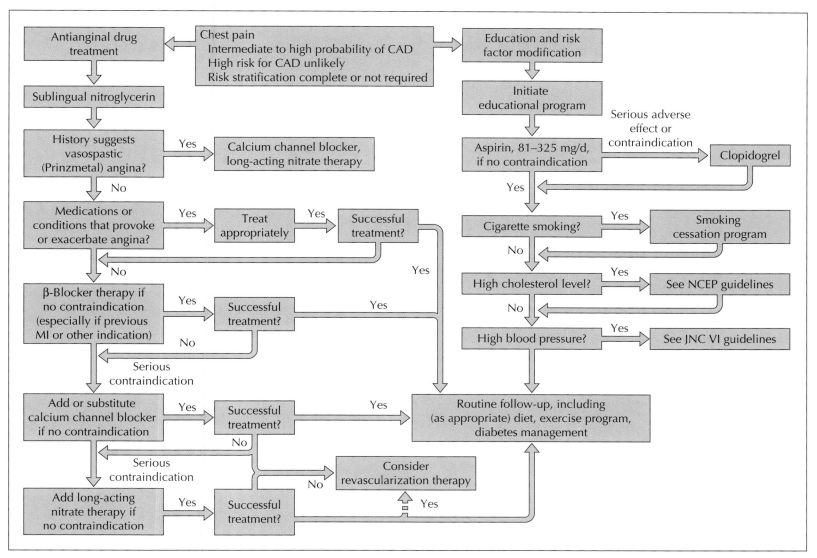

FIGURE 3-35. Guidelines for the management of patients with chronic stable angina are shown in this diagram. Patients with intermediate to high probability of coronary artery disease (CAD) for whom referral to early invasive strategies is not required are given antianginal treatment (*left*) as well as education and risk factor modification (*right*). The essentials of antianginal pharmacologic therapy include beta-blockers, calcium antagonists, and nitrates. Beta-blockers are particularly indicated in patients with previous myocardial infarction (MI). Contraindications to beta-blockers are severe bradycardia, advanced atrial ventricular block, sick sinus syndrome with bradyarrhythmias, asthma, and perhaps severe depression or severe peripheral vascular disease. Patients intolerant of beta-blockers can be treated with a heart rate–lowering calcium channel blocker. Long-acting nitrates are also highly effective in reducing episodes

as angina and nitroglycerin consumption. Aspirin is a mainstay of treatment for patients with antianginal therapy as are cholesterol-lowering drugs in conjunction with diet, smoking cessation, and vigorous blood pressure control (< 140/90 mm Hg). Patients with stable angina need to be engaged in an exercise program and, if diabetes exists, tight control of blood sugar is required. Invasive treatment with either a view toward percutaneous coronary intervention or coronary bypass surgery is recommended for patients with refractory symptoms, those with high-risk noninvasive findings consistent with extensive ischemia, and patients with left main disease or proximal three-vessel disease or two-vessel disease including a high-grade stenosis of the proximal left anterior descending coronary artery. (*Adapted from* Fihn *et al.* [17].)

RECOMMENDATIONS FOR PHARMACOTHERAPY TO PREVENT MI AND DEATH IN ASYMPTOMATIC PATIENTS

Class I

Aspirin in the absence of contraindications in patients with prior MI (level of evidence: A)

Beta-blockers as initial therapy in the absence of contraindications in patients with prior MI (level of evidence: B)

Lipid-lowering therapy in patients with documented CAD and LDL cholesterol greater than 130 mg/dL, with a target LDL of less than 100 mg/dL (level of evidence: A)

ACE inhibitor in patients with CAD* who also have diabetes and/or left ventricular systolic dysfunction (level of evidence: A)

Class IIa

Aspirin in the absence of contraindications in patients without prior MI (level of evidence: B)

Beta-blockers as initial therapy in the absence of contraindications in patients without prior MI (level of evidence: C)

Lipid-lowering therapy in patients with documented CAD and LDL cholesterol 100 to 129 mg/dL, with a target LDL of 100 mg/dL (level of evidence: C)

ACE inhibitor in all patients with CAD* or other vascular disease (level of evidence: B)

*Significant CAD by angiography or previous MI.

FIGURE 3-36. American College of Cardiology/American Heart Association 2002 guideline update for the management of patients with chronic stable angina. Shown are the recommendations for pharmacotherapy to prevent myocardial infarction (MI) and death in asymptomatic stable coronary artery disease (CAD) patients. Class I indications, implying that these treatment regimens should be implemented if no contraindications exist, include aspirin and beta-blockers in patients with prior MI, lipid-lowering therapy into a target low-density lipoprotein (LDL) of < 100 mg/dL, and an angiotensin-converting enzyme (ACE) inhibitor in patients who have diabetes and/or left ventricular dysfunction. The evidence is very strong for such treatment modalities. Class IIa indications include aspirin and beta-blockers in patients without prior MI and when there are no contraindications, and ACE inhibitor therapy in all patients with CAD defined by coronary angiography or by history of a previous MI. (*Adapted from* Gibbons *et al.* [18].)

ANTI-ISCHEMIC MECHANISMS OF MEDICAL THERAPY IN STABLE ANGINA

ACTION	DRUG CLASS		
	NITROGLYCERIN OR NITRATES	β-BLOCKERS	CALCIUM ANTAGONISTS
Decreased myocardial demand	++	+++	+ to ++
Increased coronary blood supply	+++	0 to +	++ to +++
Prevent coronary spasm or vasoconstriction	++	0 to -	++ to +++
Coronary stenosis enlargement	++	0 to +	+ to ++
Left ventricular function	Improves	- to 0	- to 0
Other	Reverse disordered endothelial function; antiplatelet action	Electrical stabilization; antiarrhythmic; antihypertensive	Antihypertensive

0—no effects; - —negative effects or may worsen; +—minor effects; ++—moderate effects; +++—major effects.

FIGURE 3-37. Anti-ischemic mechanisms of medical therapy in stable angina. It is traditionally believed that all classes of drugs act predominantly through lowering myocardial oxygen consumption, thereby lessening cardiac energy demands. The β-blockers are the most potent in this regard. The nitrates and calcium antagonists increase coronary blood flow and thus are used in the presence of coronary artery vasoconstriction.

Coronary atherosclerotic stenosis constriction is believed to be an important cause of angina in some patients. Data regarding drugs other than nitrates in preventing or reversing stenosis constriction are limited. The nitrates are the favored drugs for patients with angina and left ventricular dysfunction or congestive heart failure. The β-blockers and calcium antagonists are ideal for angina occurring in the presence of hypertension.

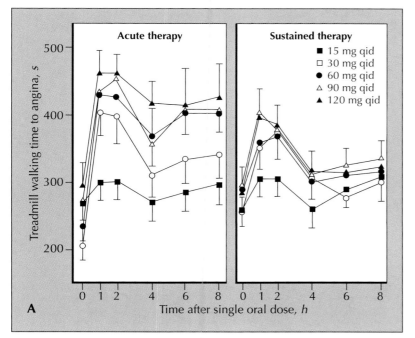

A

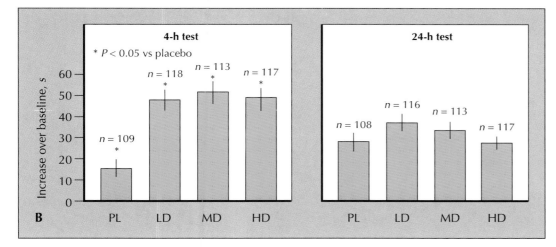

B

FIGURE 3-38. Nitrate tolerance. These two studies of nitrate tolerance in patients with angina are typical of numerous clinical trials in the literature. **A,** The first study was a pivotal investigation documenting the appearance of tolerance with various doses of oral isosorbide dinitrate. In this placebo-controlled, double-blind study, dosing with 15 mg of isosorbide four times daily (qid) for 1 to 2 weeks resulted in decreased duration of nitrate efficacy as well as a loss of the dose-response relationship. **B,** Results of a more recent 2-month trial with continuous administration of nitroglycerin by means of a patch at various doses. A complete loss of nitrate anti-ischemic effect occurred after the first dose on the first day. This effect was demonstrated for all doses studied. Very large doses were employed in many of the patient groups [19]. HD—high-dose group; LD—low-dose group; MD—medium-dose group; PL—placebo group. (Part A *adapted from* Thadani *et al.* [20]; part B *adapted from* Steering Committee, Transdermal Nitroglycerin Cooperative Study [21].)

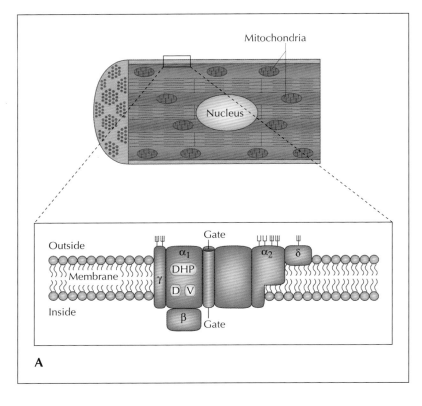

A

<u>DETERMINANTS OF MYOCARDIAL OXYGEN CONSUMPTION</u>

Heart rate–slowing calcium blockers (verapamil, diltiazem)

Decreased blood pressure (all)

<u>CORONARY BLOOD FLOW</u>

Increased coronary epicardial diameter

Prevention of exercise-induced coronary stenosis (diltiazem)

Prevention or reversal of coronary vasoconstriction or spasm

Increased collateral blood flow

FIGURE 3-39. Mechanisms of action of calcium antagonists. **A,** Intracellular aspects of calcium blockade in cardiac and vascular smooth muscle cells. There are several binding sites for the various calcium antagonists in the cell membrane. **B,** Changes in heart rate, blood pressure, and coronary blood flow with administration of calcium antagonists [22,23]. D—diltiazem; DHP—dihydropyridine; V—verapamil; α_1—α_1 receptor; α_2—α_2 receptor.

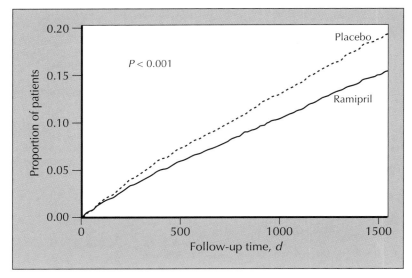

FIGURE 3-40. The Heart Outcomes Prevention Evaluation (HOPE) randomized trial sought to determine whether the angiotensin-converting enzyme inhibitor, ramipril, could significantly reduce rates of death, myocardial infarction, and stroke in patients at high risk for cardiovascular events but who did not have left ventricular dysfunction or heart failure. Treatment with ramipril reduces the rate of death from cardiovascular causes (6.1% vs 8.1% in the placebo group; relative risk, 0.74; $P < 0.001$), myocardial infarction (9.9% vs 12.3%; relative risk, 0.80; $P < 0.001$), and stroke (3.4% vs 4.9%; relative risk, 0.68; $P < 0.001$). Also, death from any cause, revascularization procedures, cardiac arrest, heart failure, and complications related to diabetes were all reduced in the ramipril patients compared with placebo-treated patients. Shown are the Kaplan-Meier estimates of the composite outcome of myocardial infarction, stroke, or death from cardiovascular causes in the ramipril group and the placebo group. (*Adapted from* The Heart Outcomes Prevention Evaluation Study Investigators [24].)

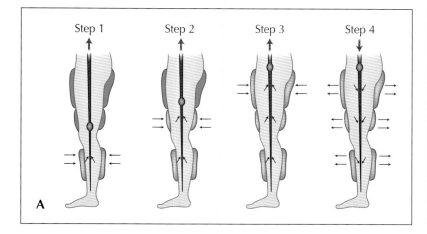

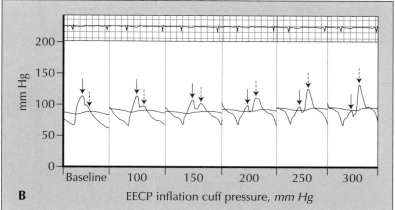

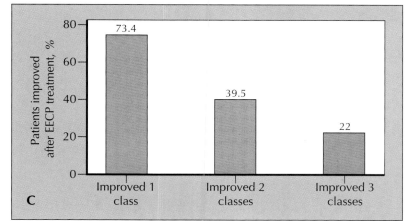

FIGURE 3–41. Enhanced external counterpulsation (EECP) is an effective treatment for patients with coronary artery disease and angina refractory to conventional medical therapy and where revascularization is not an option. **A,** EECP involves the use of three paired inflatable cuffs wrapped around the patient's lower extremities. The cuffs are sequentially inflated during diastole; the calves followed by lower thighs and followed by upper thighs and buttocks. The pressure is released at the onset of systole. The sequential cuff compression enhances venous return and significantly augments diastolic pressure. (*Adapted from* Sinvhal *et al.* [25].)

B, Intracoronary phasic and mean pressure tracings at baseline and at increasing cuff inflation pressure in the EECP device. With increasing inflation pressure, the diastolic (*dashed arrows*) and mean pressures increase, whereas the systolic pressure (*solid arrows*) decreases. Note that the diastolic augmentation is significant at an EECP inflation cuff pressure of 250 mm Hg. (*Adapted from* Michaels *et al.* [26].)

C, An analysis of the potential benefits of EECP has been conducted in a registry cohort of 2289 consecutive patients enrolled in the EECP consortium. Patients were assessed using the Canadian Cardiovascular Society angina classification system (Class 1–4). The figure shows improvement in angina class for patients enrolled in the consortium. Shown is that 73.4% of enrolled patients improved by at least one angina class. (*Adapted from* Lawson *et al.* [27].)

CORONARY ARTERY BYPASS SURGERY

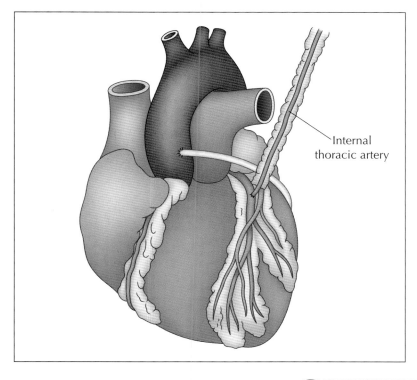

FIGURE 3-42. Prior to the advent of coronary angiography, Vineberg harvested the internal thoracic artery (ITA) to draw it into ischemic myocardium in an attempt to revascularize the area. In 1970, Green created a directed anastomosis of the ITA to the coronary tree using this conduit. Use of the ITA gave surgeons a second type of conduit for revascularization. These early efforts employed a surgical microscope. Loop simplified the technique by describing a method for direct anastomosis that eliminated the need for high-power optical magnification [28].

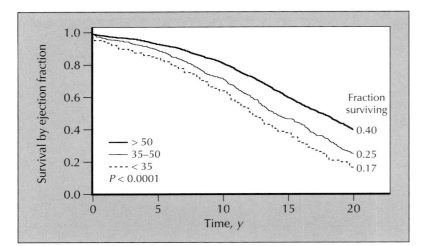

FIGURE 3-43. Twenty-year survival free from myocardial infarction and repeat coronary bypass graft (CABG) surgery stratified by preoperative ejection fraction. Note that patients with an ejection fraction of less than 35% had the worst prognosis. In this study, multivariate correlates of late mortality were age, female sex, hypertension, angina class, prior CABG, ejection fraction, number of diseased vessels, and weight. (*Adapted from* Weintraub *et al.* [29].)

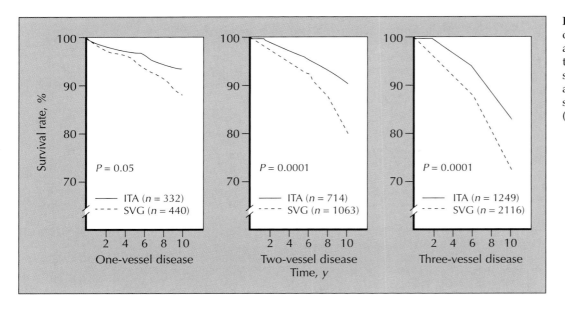

FIGURE 3-44. The relative importance of the type of conduit, regardless of the extent of disease, is apparent through study of disease affecting one, two, or three vessels. All groups demonstrated statistically significant improved survival when an internal thoracic artery (ITA) as opposed to a saphenous vein graft (SVG) was used [30]. (*Adapted from* Loop *et al.* [30].)

COMPARISON OF TREATMENT MODALITIES

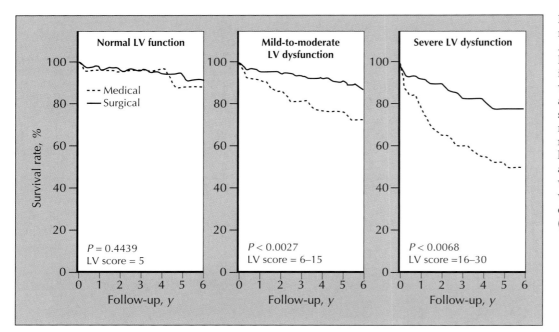

FIGURE 3-45. The effect of surgery versus medical therapy among patients in the Coronary Artery Surgery Study with moderate and severe left ventricular (LV) function compared with individuals with normal LV dysfunction. The LV wall motion score is assessed from the 30° right anterior oblique view in which the cardiac silhouette is divided into five segments, and wall motion in each segment is graded from 1 to 6 (1, normal; 2, moderate hypokinesis; 3, severe hypokinesis; 4, akinesis; 5, dyskinesis). A truly aneurysmal segment is assigned a score of 6. The wall motion score was obtained by adding values for each segment, with a combined score of 5 indicative of normal ventricular function. (*Adapted from* Mock *et al.* [31].)

REFERENCES

1. Epstein S, Talbot T: Dynamic coronary tone in precipitation, exacerbation and relief of angina pectoris. *Am J Cardiol* 1981, 48:797–803.

2. Gage JE, Hess OM, Murakami T, *et al.*: Vasoconstriction of stenotic coronary arteries during dynamic exercise in patients with classic angina pectoris: reversibility by nitroglycerin. *Circulation* 1986, 73:865–876.

3. Widlansky ME, Gokce N, Keaney JF Jr, Vita JA: The clinical implications of endothelial dysfunction. *J Am Coll Cardiol* 2003, 42:1149–1160.

4. Creager MA, Lüscher TF, Consentino F, Beckman JA: Diabetes and vascular disease. Pathophysiology, clinical consequences, and medical therapy: part I. *Circulation* 2003, 108:1527–1532.

5. Biondi-Zoccai GGL, Abbate A, Liuzzo G, Biasucci LM: Atherothrombosis, inflammation, and diabetes. *J Am Coll Cardiol* 2003, 41:1071–1077.

6. Chaitman BR: Exercise stress testing. In *Heart Disease*, edn 6. Edited by Braunwald E, Zipes D, Libby P. Philadelphia:WB Saunders; 2001:129–159.

7. Mark DB, Shaw L, Harrell FE, *et al.*: Prognostic value of a treadmill exercise score in outpatients with suspected coronary artery disease. *N Engl J Med* 1991, 325:849–853.

8. Giri S, Shaw LJ, Murthy DR, *et al.*: Impact of diabetes on the risk stratification using stress single-photon emission computed tomography myocardial perfusion imaging in patients with symptoms suggestive of coronary artery disease. *Circulation* 2002, 105:32–40.

9. Hachamovitch R, Hayes SW, Friedman JD, *et al.*: Comparison of the short-term survival benefit associated with revascularization compared with medical therapy in patients with no prior coronary artery disease undergoing stress myocardial perfusion single photon emission computed tomography. *Circulation* 2003, 107:2900–2906.

10. Yao S-S, Qureshi E, Sherrid MV, Chaudhry FA: Practical applications in stress echocardiography. Risk stratification and prognosis in patients with known or suspected ischemic heart disease. *J Am Coll Cardiol* 2003, 42:1084–1090.

11. Jang I-K, Tearney G, Bouma B: Visualization of tissue prolapse between coronary stent struts by optical coherence tomography. Comparison with intravascular ultrasound. *Circulation* 2001, 104:2574.

12. Jang I-K, Bouma BE, Kang D-H, *et al.*: Visualization of coronary atherosclerotic plaques in patients using optical coherence tomography: comparison with intravascular ultrasound. *J Am Coll Cardiol* 2002, 39:604–609.

13. Bennett MR, O'Sullivan M: Mechanisms of angioplasty and stent restenosis: implications for design of rational therapy. *Pharmacol Ther* 2001, 91:149–166.

14. Grise MA, Massullo V, Jani S, *et al.*: Five-year clinical follow-up after intracoronary radiation. Results of a randomized clinical trial. *Circulation* 2002, 105:2737–2740.

15. Marks AR: Sirolimus for the prevention of in-stent restenosis in a coronary artery. *N Engl J Med* 2003, 349:1307–1309.

16. Moses JW, Leon MB, Popma JJ, *et al.*: Sirolimus-eluting stents versus standard stents in patients with stenosis in a native coronary artery. *N Engl J Med* 2003, 349:1315–1323.

17. Fihn SD, Williams SV, Daley J, Gibbons RJ: Guidelines for the management of patients with chronic stable angina: treatment. *Ann Intern Med* 2001, 135:616–632.

18. Gibbons RJ, Abrams J, Chatterjee K, *et al.*: ACC/AHA 2002 guideline update for the management of patients with chronic stable angina–summary article: a report of the American College of Cardiology/American Heart Association Task Force on Practice Guidelines (Committee on the Management of Patients with Chronic Stable Angina). *J Am Coll Cardiol* 2003, 41:159–168.

19. Parker JD, Parker JO: Nitrate therapy for stabel angina pectoris. *N Engl J Med* 1998, 338:520–531.

20. Thadani U, Fung H-L, Darke AC, *et al.*: Oral isosorbide dinitrate in angina pectoris: comparison of duration of action and dose response relationship during acute and sustained therapy. *Am J Cardiol* 1982, 49:411–419.

21. Steering Committee, Transdermal Nitroglycerin Cooperative Study: Acute and chronic antianginal efficacy of continuous twenty-four-hour application of transdermal nitroglycerin. *Am J Cardiol* 1991, 68:1263–1273.

22. Abernathy DR, Schwartz JB: Calcium antagonist drugs. *N Engl J Med* 1999, 341:1447–1457.

23. Opie LH: Calcium channel antagonists in the treatment of coronary artery disease: fundamental pharmacological properties relevant to clinical use. *Prog Cardiovasc Dis* 1996, 38:273–290.

24. The Heart Outcomes Prevention Evaluation Study Investigators: Effects of an angiotensin-converting enzyme inhibitor, ramipril, on cardiovascular events in high-risk patients. *N Engl J Med* 2000, 342:145–153.

25. Sinvhal RM, Gowda RM, Khan IA: Enhanced external counterpulsation for refractory angina. *Heart* 2003, 89:830–833.

26. Michaels AD, Accad M, Ports TA, Grossman W: Left ventricular systolic unloading and augmentation of intracoronary pressure and Doppler flow during enhanced counterpulsation. *Circulation* 2002, 106:1237–1242.

27. Lawson WE, Hui JC, Lang G: Treatment benefit in the enhanced external counterpulsation consortium. *Cardiology* 2000, 94:31–35.

28. Green GE, Spencer FC, Tice DA, *et al.*: Arterial and venous microsurgical bypass grafts for coronary artery disease. *J Thorac Cardiovasc Surg* 1970, 60:491–501.

29. Weintraub WS, Clements SD Jr, Crisco LV-T, *et al.*: Twenty-year survival after coronary artery surgery. An institutional perspective from Emory University. *Circulation* 2003, 107:1271–1277.

30. Loop FD, Lytle BW, Cosgrove DM, *et al.*: Influence of the internal mammary artery graft on 10-year survival and other cardiac events. *N Engl J Med* 1986, 314:1–6.

31. Mock MB, Fisher LD, Holmes DR Jr, *et al.*: Comparison of effects of medical and surgical therapy on survival in severe angina pectoris and two-vessel coronary artery disease with and without left ventricular dysfunction: a Coronary Artery Surgery Study Registry study. *Am J Cardiol* 1988, 61:1198–1203.

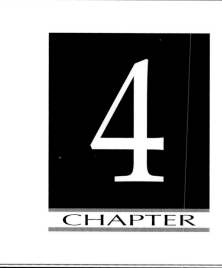

HEART FAILURE

Edited by Wilson S. Colucci

*Robert J. Cody, Jay N. Cohn, Mark A. Creager, Jorge A. Cusco,
Joshua M. Hare, Arnold M. Katz, Ralph A. Kelly, Carl V. Leier,
Marc A. Pfeffer, Thomas S. Rector, Thomas W. Smith, Mark R. Starling,
Lynne Warner Stevenson, Cynthia M. Thaik, James B. Young*

NORMAL CONTRACTION

CONTRACTILE PROTEIN INTERACTIONS

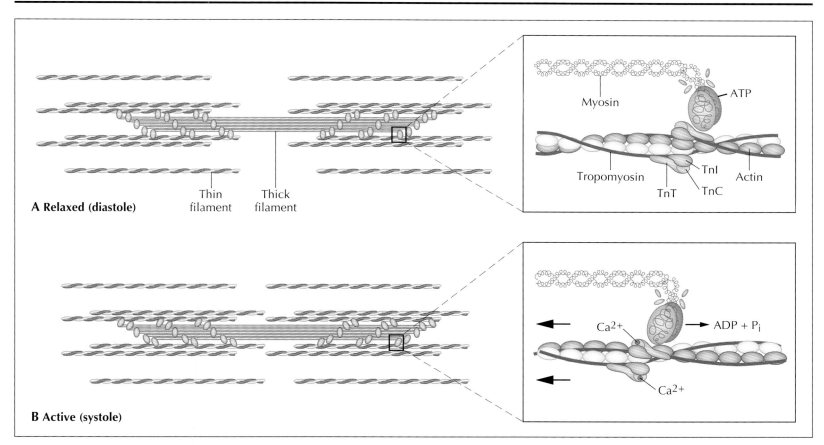

FIGURE 4-1. Cardiac contraction is brought about by interactions between actin in the thin filament and myosin cross-bridges that project from the thick filament. **A**, In relaxed muscle, where troponin C (TnC) is not bound to calcium, the "relaxed" conformation of the troponin complexes and tropomyosin prevents actin in the thin filament from interacting with the myosin cross-bridges. As a result, actin is unable to convert the chemical energy of the ATP bound to the myosin cross-bridges into mechanical work.

B, In active muscle, Ca^{2+} bound to TnC has shifted the troponin complexes and tropomyosin to an "active" conformation that enables actin to interact with the myosin cross-bridges. Release of chemical energy when actin stimulates hydrolysis of myosin-bound ATP enables the cross-bridges to "row" the thin filaments toward the center of the sarcomere. TnI—troponin I; TnT—troponin T.

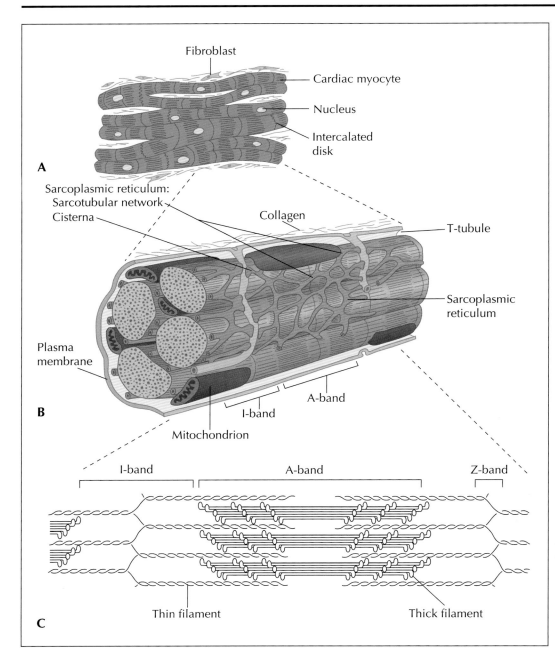

A

B

C

Fibroblast

Cardiac myocyte

Nucleus

Intercalated disk

Sarcoplasmic reticulum:
Sarcotubular network
Cisterna

Collagen

T-tubule

Sarcoplasmic reticulum

Plasma membrane

A-band

I-band

Mitochondrion

I-band

A-band

Z-band

Thin filament

Thick filament

FIGURE 4-2. Structure of the heart. The heart is composed of both myocytes and nonmyoctes. **A,** Nonmyocytes include connective tissue cells (mainly fibroblasts), vascular smooth muscle cells, and endothelial cells. Whereas large cardiac myocytes make up most of the heart's mass, the majority of the cells of the heart (approximately 70%) are smaller nonmyocytes. The large, branched cardiac myocytes, which are enmeshed in a collagen network, are separated longitudinally by intercalated discs, which represent specialized cell-cell junctions. The intercalated discs provide strong mechanical connections between adjacent cells and contain gap junctions that provide low-resistance pathways for electrical conduction.

B, Cardiac myocytes that are specialized for contraction contain myofilaments whose organization in a regular array of thick and thin filaments gives rise to the characteristic striated appearance. Also prominent within these cells are two membrane structures: energy-producing mitochondria and the sarcoplasmic reticulum, which regulates cytosolic Ca^{2+} concentration. The latter is an intracellular membrane system that contains the calcium channels that initiate systole by delivering activator calcium to the myofilaments, and calcium pumps that, by removing calcium from the cytosol, dissociate this activator cation from its binding sites on the thin filament.

Myofilaments contain about 70% of the protein of the cardiac myocytes, and most of the membrane surface is found in the mitochondria. Other important membranes include the plasma membrane, which is continuous with the transverse tubular membranes (t-tubules) that extend toward the center of the cell and carry depolarizing currents into the myocardial cell. **C,** Each sarcomere, which is delimited by two Z-bands, contains one A-band and two half I-bands. The A-bands are made up of thick, myosin-containing filaments into which thin filaments interdigitate from the adjacent two half I-bands. The latter are made up of actin and the regulatory proteins, tropomyosin and the troponin complex. Bisecting each Z-band is a lattice of axial and cross-connecting filaments that includes the overlapping ends of thin filaments from adjacent sarcomeres. (Part B *adapted from* Katz [1].)

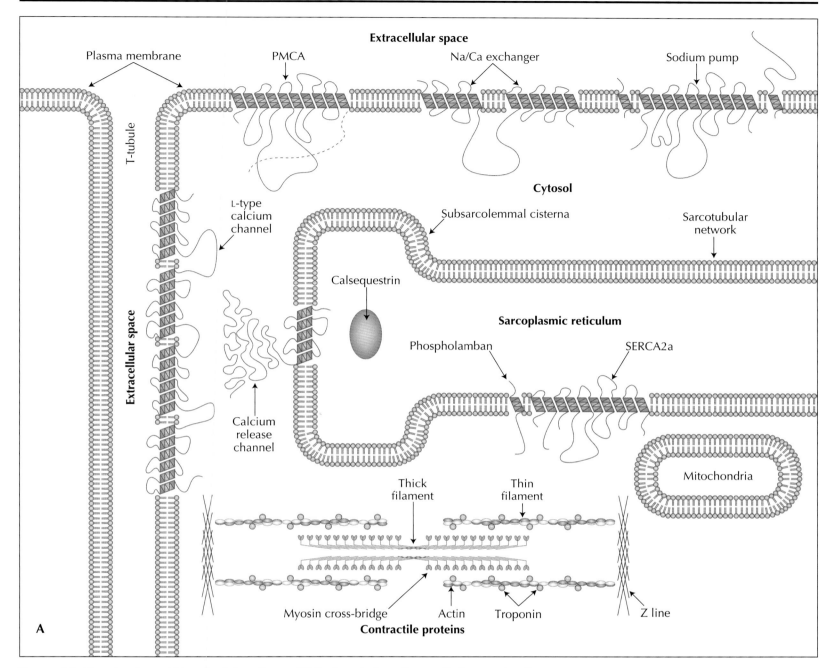

FIGURE 4-3. Key structures (**A**) and calcium fluxes (**B**) that control cardiac excitation-contraction coupling and relaxation. Calcium "pools" are in bold capital letters (**A**).

Continued on next page

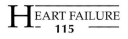

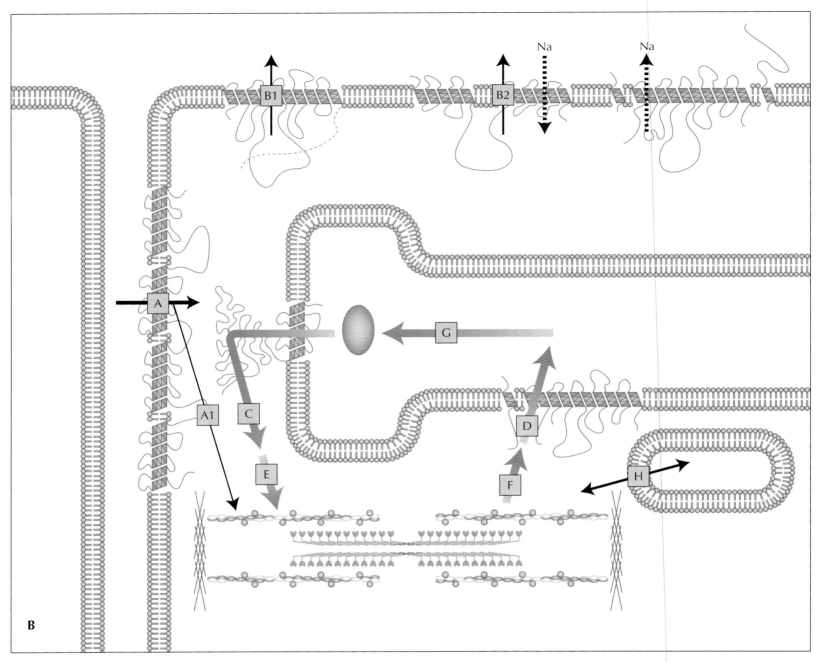

FIGURE 4-3. *(Continued)* In **B**, the thickness of the arrows indicates the magnitude of the calcium fluxes, while their vertical orientations describe their "energetics": *down arrows* represent passive calcium fluxes; *up arrows* represent energy-dependent active calcium transport. Most of the calcium that enters the cell from the extracellular fluid via ʟ-type calcium channels (*arrow A*) triggers calcium release from the sarcoplasmic reticulum; only a small portion directly activates the contractile proteins (*arrow A1*). Calcium is actively transported back into the extracellular fluid by the plasma membrane calcium pump ATPase (PMCA; *arrow B1*), and the Na/Ca exchanger (*arrow B2*). The sodium that enters the cell in exchange for calcium (dashed line) is pumped out of the cytosol by the sodium pump. Two calcium fluxes are regulated by the sarcoplasmic reticulum: calcium efflux from the subsarcolemmal cisternae via calcium release channels (*arrow C*) and calcium uptake into the sarcotubular network by the sarco(endo)plasmic reticulum calcium pump ATPase (*arrow D*). Calcium diffuses within the sacroplasmic reticulum from the sarcotubular network to the subsarcolemmal cisternae (*arrow G*), in which it is stored in a complex with calsequestrin and other calcium-binding proteins. Calcium binding to (*arrow E*) and dissociation from (*arrow F*) high-affinity calcium-binding sites of troponin C activate and inhibit the interactions of the contractile proteins. Calcium movements into and out of mitochondria (*arrow H*) buffer cytostolic calcium concentration. The extracellular calcium cycle is show at arrows A, B1, and B2, whereas the intracellular cycle involves arrows C, E, F, D, and G. (*Adapted from* Katz [3].)

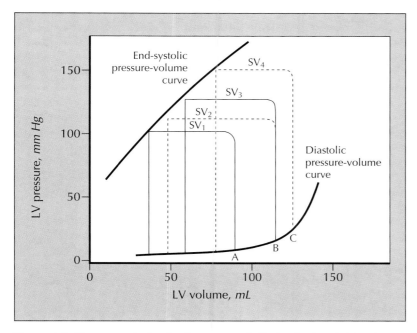

infusions without volume loading, stroke volume (SV) was progressively reduced. This relationship between left ventricular (LV) stroke volume and either end-diastolic pressure or volume was shifted upward and to the right when an angiotensin II infusion was combined with volume loading. The LV appeared to operate on a single diastolic and end-systolic pressure-volume relationship, suggesting no change in LV diastolic chamber elastance or contractility.

An attempt to graphically depict this relationship in an intact circulation that is allowed to freely adapt to alterations in LV pressure and volume is shown here, assuming a single diastolic and end-systolic pressure-volume relationship. Starting at point A and following the solid line at a constant contractile state, SV_1 is generated. With volume loading alone, movement up the diastolic pressure-volume curve to point B occurs and the dashed line is followed generating SV_2, which is greater than SV_1, indicating the presence of preload reserve. Similarly, with pressure loading there is an increase in end-diastolic volume and pressure to point B along the diastolic pressure-volume curve; the solid line is followed generating SV_3, which is equal to SV_1. Therefore, despite an increase in LV pressure, stroke volume is maintained owing to preload reserve. In contrast, with a further increase in LV pressure, stroke volume is decreased, as shown by SV_4, due to an afterload mismatch. Preload reserve is exhausted at point C on the diastolic pressure-volume curve and is therefore insufficient to compensate for the increase in afterload. This is consistent with the observations of Lee *et al.* [5] in conscious animals, indicating that preload reserve is substantial in the normal heart and that it can compensate for increases in afterload on a beat-to-beat basis without changes in the passive diastolic pressure-volume relation or contractility as long as venous return is adequate.

FIGURE 4-4. The concept of preload reserve and afterload mismatch has been proposed by Ross [4]. As illustrated in studies in normal conscious dogs by Lee *et al.* [5], this concept provides a possible explanation for the descending limb of the Starling curve. During acute angiotensin II

SYSTOLIC AND DIASTOLIC FAILURE

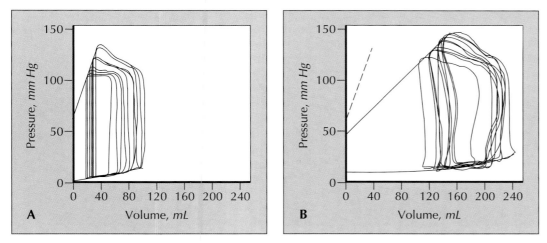

cardiovascular performance. Pressure-volume diagrams can be used to characterize systolic dysfunction, altered diastolic compli-ance, and the influence of loading conditions on cardiac function.

A, A series of pressure-volume loops obtained from a patient with normal cardiac function. Each loop represents a cardiac cycle sampled during inflation of a balloon in the inferior vena cava to alter loading conditions. The slope of the end-systolic pressure-volume loop relationship (ESPVR, *solid line*) reflects end-systolic ventricular elastance, a relatively load-independent index of contractility. **B,** In dilated cardiomy-opathy ventricular volumes are higher, and the ESPVR slope is reduced compared with normal (*dashed line*). Ventricular enlargement is a final common pathway in the heart with systolic impairment. (*continued*)

FIGURE 4-5. Systolic and diastolic heart failure. Abnormalities of ventricular function during systole, diastole, or both, may produce congestive heart failure. Furthermore, the interaction of the heart with the circulation (*ie*, the loading conditions placed on the heart) is an important determinant of overall

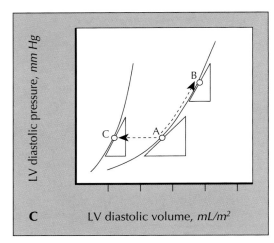

C

FIGURE 4-5. (*continued*) **C,** Diastolic dysfunction also may produce heart failure, either primarily or in conjunction with systolic failure. Myocardial ischemia, fibrosis, myocyte hypertrophy, elevated afterload, and pericardial constriction all may contribute to diastolic dysfunction [6]. The end-diastolic pressure-volume relationship (EDPVR) can be used to assess the passive properties of the ventricular chamber. The *operative volume stiffness* of the ventricle is defined as dP/dV (the slope of a tangent to the EDPVR), and the *compliance* of the ventricle is defined as the reciprocal of stiffness (*ie*, dV/dP). Alterations in diastolic function may occur because of increases in stiffness due to rises in chamber preload (A toward B) or actual shifts in the EDPVR (A toward C). Leftward shifts in the EDPVR can occur acutely with ischemia or chronically with fibrosis and hypertrophy. With such shifts, the EDPVR is steeper, and increments in volume produce an exaggerated rise in pressure. LV—left ventricular. (Parts A and B *courtesy of* David Kass, Baltimore, MD; part C *adapted from* Gaasch et al. [7].)

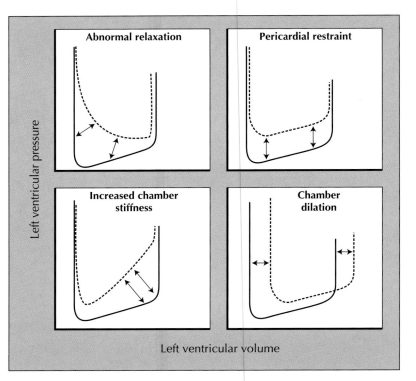

FIGURE 4-6. Diastolic dysfunction reflected in the pressure-volume relation. This figure illustrates the mechanisms that cause diastolic dysfunction. Only the bottom half of the pressure-volume loop is depicted. *Solid lines* represent normal subjects; *dashed lines* represent patients with diastolic dysfunction. (*Adapted from* Zile [8].)

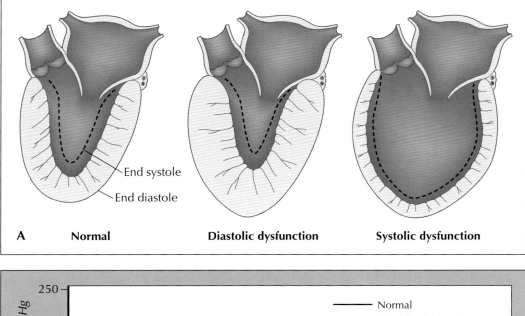

A   **Normal**   **Diastolic dysfunction**   **Systolic dysfunction**

FIGURE 4-7. Heart failure resulting from systolic and diastolic dysfunction.

A, The extremes of ventricular remodeling that lead to distinctly different abnormal hemodynamic profiles and therapeutic interventions. The extreme example of systolic dysfunction shown is typically the result of a dilated cardiomyopathy and is characterized by large ventricular chamber dimensions, high end-diastolic pressures, and a low ejection fraction. The opposite extreme is also illustrated, in which a thickened ventricular wall caused, for example, by chronic, poorly controlled hypertension, results in decreased ventricular distensibility and high diastolic filling pressures but a normal ejection fraction.

B, The hemodynamic profiles, illustrated as the relationship between ventricular pressure and volume throughout a representative cardiac cycle, for the three hearts shown in *panel A*.

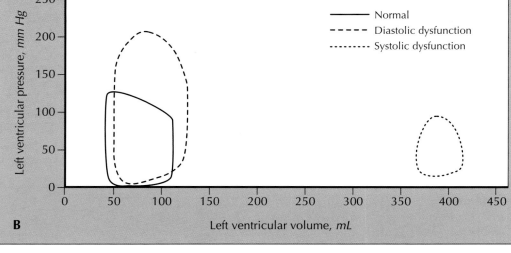

B

	Normal	Acute load	Compensatory hypertrophy	Cardiac failure
LV systolic pressure	N	+	+	+
LV radius	N	+	+	+
LV wall thickness	N	N	+	+
LV diastolic volume	N	+	±	++
Systolic wall stress	N	+	N	+
Diastolic wall stress	N	+	N	+

FIGURE 4-8. Hemodynamic overload is the most common stimulus for myocardial hypertrophy and remodeling. A frequent cause of hemodynamic overload is an increase (+) in left ventricular (LV) systolic pressure, as may occur in patients with hypertension or aortic stenosis. The normal (N) relationship between LV wall thickness (h) and chamber radius (r) is shown (*first panel*). An acute increase in systolic pressure causes an increase in systolic wall stress, which can be approximated by the equation $P \times r/h$, where P is LV systolic pressure. Diastolic wall stress is also increased when there is chamber dilatation or when diastolic pressure is elevated (*second panel*). If sufficient compensatory hypertrophy occurs, the increase in ventricular wall thickness may normalize the systolic and diastolic wall stresses (*third panel*). However, if additional chamber dilatation occurs or the increase in wall thickness is insufficient, systolic and diastolic wall stresses remain abnormally elevated. In this situation, further chamber dilatation may occur in association with hemodynamic failure (*fourth panel*). (*Adapted from* Swynghedauw *et al.* [6].)

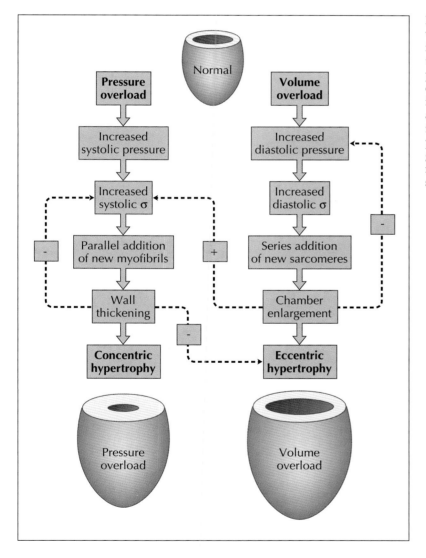

FIGURE 4-9. Patterns of ventricular hypertrophy. Specific patterns of ventricular remodeling occur in response to the imposed augmentation in workload. A pattern of hypertrophic growth characterized as concentric, in which increased mass is out of proportion to chamber volume, is particularly effective in reducing systolic wall stress (σ) under conditions of heightened pressure load. In contrast, in volume overload conditions, in which the major stimulus is diastolic loading, a predominant finding is an increase in the cavity size or volume. Although there can be extensive increases in mass, the relationship between mass and volume is either preserved or, in severe cases, reduced. The fundamental response is generated by cellular hypertrophy. However, the configuration of the new contractile tissue is specific and is related to the type of mechanical stimulus. (*Adapted from* Grossman *et al.* [9].)

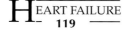

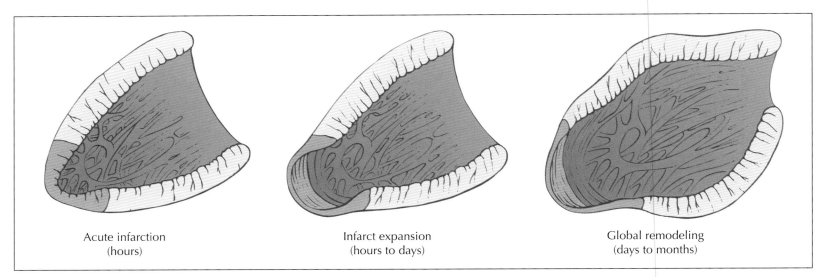

Acute infarction
(hours)

Infarct expansion
(hours to days)

Global remodeling
(days to months)

FIGURE 4-10. Left ventricular remodeling after myocardial infarction (MI). During the critical initial hours after MI when acute ischemia progresses to true necrosis, regional systolic dysfunction is already present. However, in this particularly crucial period measures to restore the balance between O_2 demand and delivery can lead to salvage of contractile tissue. Once cell death has occurred, and particularly if there is a transmural infarction involving the ventricular apex, there is a high likelihood that this will lead to infarct expansion. The distorted ventricle undergoes further remodeling as a consequence of heightened wall stress on the remaining viable myocardium, which leads to further cavity enlargement and shape distortion. The latter insidious process is associated with a greater likelihood of cardiovascular morbidity and mortality.

MOLECULAR AND CELLULAR MECHANISMS OF MYOCARDIAL REMODELING

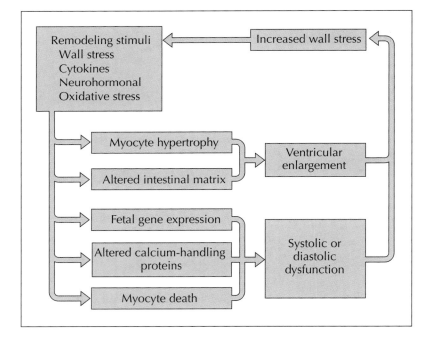

FIGURE 4-11. Remodeling stimuli. Chronic hemodynamic stimuli such as pressure and volume overload lead to ventricular remodeling through increases in myocardial wall stress, cytokines, signaling peptides, neuroendocrine signals, and perhaps, oxidative stress. The myocardium responds with adaptive as well as maladaptive changes. Re-expression of fetal contractile proteins and calcium handling proteins may contribute to impaired contraction and relaxation. Myocytes unable to adapt might be triggered to undergo programmed cell death (apoptosis). The net result of these changes is further impairment in pump function and increased wall stress, thus completing a vicious cycle that leads to further progression of the myocardial dysfunction.

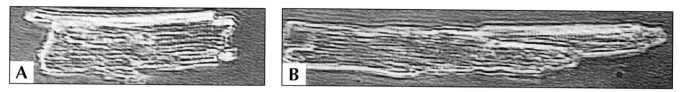

FIGURE 4-12. Isolated cardiac myocytes obtained from mice showing cellular hypertrophy. **A,** Myocyte from the left ventricle of the normal mouse heart. **B,** Hypertrophied myocyte from the left ventricle of a mouse 6 months after myocardial infarction, viewed at the same magnification as in A. In the myocyte from the failing heart, there has been a series of sarcomeres, which are otherwise organized into a normal pattern. The resulting myocyte elongation, a form of hypertrophy, likely contributes to ventricular dilatation that occurs during myocardial remodeling.

CALCIUM HANDLING IN HEART FAILURE

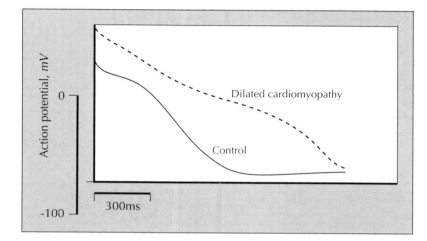

FIGURE 4-13. There is evidence that calcium handling is deranged in the myocardium of patients with end-stage heart failure.

The action potentials in single human cardiac myocytes obtained from patients with normal ventricular function (control) or dilated cardiomyopathy. The action potential is substantially prolonged in the cell from the patient with dilated cardiomyopathy. In failing myocardium there is elevation of the basal concentration of intracellular calcium and attenuation of the peak rise with depolarization. These functional abnormalities are associated with alterations in the mRNA levels for proteins involved in myocyte excitation-contraction coupling, suggesting that at least some of the functional abnormalities in failing myocardium are caused by alterations in gene expression. (*Adapted from* Beuckelmann *et al.* [10].)

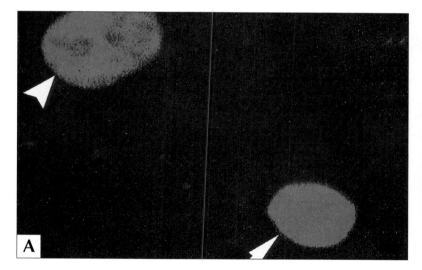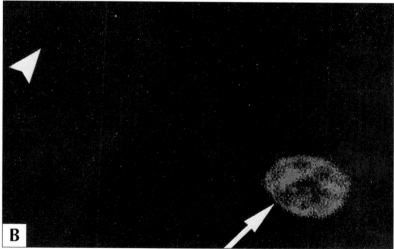

FIGURE 4-14. Loss of myocytes in heart failure. The slow loss of myocytes may contribute to the progressive decline in systolic function in heart failure. All cells have the ability to undergo programmed cell death, or apoptosis, in the presence of stimuli that activate the necessary signaling cascades. Cardiac apoptosis appears to play an important role in embryonic life as the heart "remodels" during development. Thus, apoptosis may be part of a fetal gene program. Apoptosis also occurs as a defense mechanism to rid an organ of infected or damaged cells without activation of inflammatory systems as would occur with necrosis. Olivetti *et al.* [11] demonstrated that apoptosis occurs in myocardium obtained from patients with heart failure by staining for fragmented DNA, a hallmark of the apoptotic process. **A,** Confocal microscopy of myocardial nuclei stained with propridium iodide. **B,** DNA fragments labeled with deoxyuridine triphosphate (Tunel) in apoptotic nucleus (*arrow*) but not normal nucleus (*arrowhead*).

Continued on next page

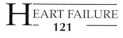

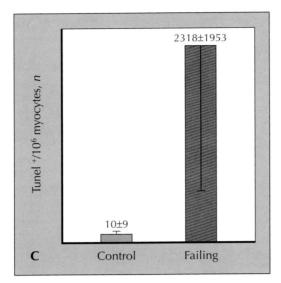

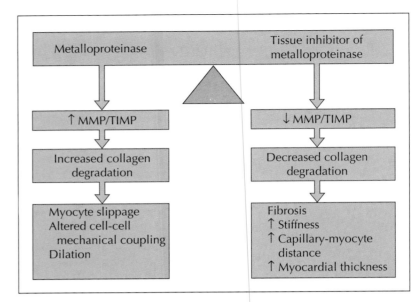

FIGURE 4-14. *(Continued)* **C,** Counting of stained cells shows a large number of apoptotic cells (Tunel+) in failing, but not normal, myocardium. (Parts A and B *from* Olivetti *et al.* [11]; with permission. Part C *adapted from* Olivetti *et al.* [11].)

FIGURE 4-15. The balance between metalloproteinase (MMP) and tissue inhibitors of metalloproteinase (TIMP) activity. This balance determines the rate of matrix degradation and turnover. Increased MMP activity theoretically favors myocyte slippage, with reduced myocyte-to-myocyte mechanical coupling and dilation. Increased TIMP activity results in a net decrease in MMP activity and therefore theoretically favors matrix deposition. This perhaps leads to interstitial fibrosis, which may lead to increased stiffness and impaired supply of nutrients to myocytes because of an increased capillary-to-myocyte distance.

NEUROHUMORAL ADJUSTMENTS

THE ADRENERGIC NERVOUS SYSTEM

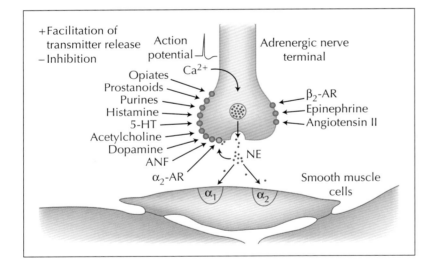

FIGURE 4-16. Sympathetic nerve terminal. Sympathetic nerve activity can be measured directly by measuring the electrical activity in the peripheral nerves and indirectly by measuring the plasma norepinephrine (NE) concentration. Plasma NE is derived from sympathetic nerves, but the amount that reaches the circulation depends on several processes. Plasma NE can be increased by increased nerve release, decreased local uptake, or reduced systemic clearance. Neurotransmitter release at the sympathetic neuroeffector junction is also modulated locally by a variety of hormones and other substances that act on specific receptors located on the presynaptic nerve ending. Several α_2-receptor agonists, including NE itself (via α_2-adrenergic receptors [α_2-AR]), opioids, prostanoids, purines, histamine, 5-hydroxytryptamine (5-HT), atrial natriuretic factor (ANF), dopamine, and acetylcholine, *inhibit* NE release. In contrast, epinephrine (via β_2-adrenergic receptors [β_2-AR]) and angiotensin II *increase* NE release from the neuroeffector junction. (*Adapted from* Vanhoutte and Luscher [12].)

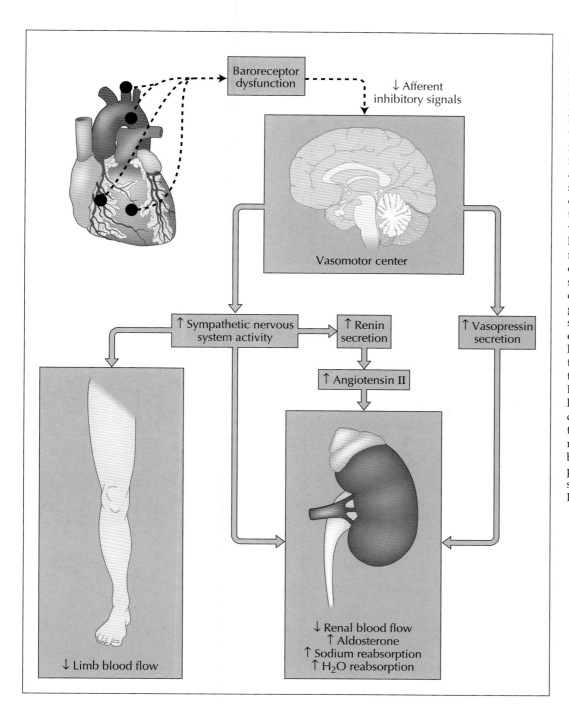

Baroreceptor
dysfunction

↓ Afferent
inhibitory signals

Vasomotor center

↑ Sympathetic nervous
system activity

↑ Renin
secretion

↑ Vasopressin
secretion

↑ Angiotensin II

↓ Renal blood flow
↑ Aldosterone
↑ Sodium reabsorption
↑ H₂O reabsorption

↓ Limb blood flow

FIGURE 4-17. Baroreceptor dysfunction may account for increased sympathetic and reduced parasympathetic nervous system activity in most patients with congestive heart failure. Normally, autonomic balance is regulated by afferent input from multiple peripheral receptors, including baroreceptors in the heart, lungs, and great vessels, chemoreceptors in the carotid bodies, metaboreceptors in skeletal muscle, sensory receptors in skin, a variety of visceral receptors, and from signals originating in the central nervous system. Of these, the baroreceptors are the principal modulators of sympathetic and parasympathetic activity during changes in intravascular volume or pressure. Mechanoreceptors in the heart and pulmonary vasculature (cardiopulmonary baroreceptors) and in the aortic arch and carotid sinus (arterial baroreceptors) respond to stretch by relaying afferent neural signals to the central system via branches of the vagus and glossopharyngeal nerves. These signals *inhibit* sympathetic and *augment* parasympathetic efferent activity. In plasma volume depletion or hypotension, decreased receptor stretch reduces the afferent stimuli, thus decreasing parasympathetic activity and increasing sympathetic activity. Because baroreceptor function is impaired in heart failure, inhibitory input from arterial and cardiopulmonary baroreceptors is decreased, thereby leading to excessive sympathetic and reduced parasympathetic activity. Abnormal baroreceptor function may also facilitate vasopressin release from the neurohypophysis and stimulate renal release of renin. (*Adapted from* Paganelli *et al.* [13].)

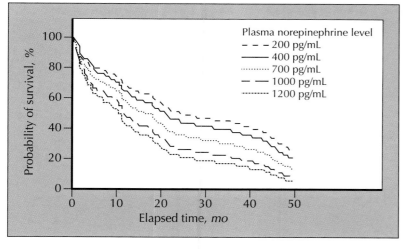

Plasma norepinephrine level
- - - 200 pg/mL
——— 400 pg/mL
········· 700 pg/mL
— — 1000 pg/mL
------- 1200 pg/mL

FIGURE 4-18. Activation of adrenergic nervous system activity, as reflected by elevated plasma norepinephrine levels, has been associated with a poor prognosis in patients with congestive heart failure. Cohn *et al.* [14] measured supine plasma norepinephrine levels in 106 patients with moderate to severe congestive heart failure. A multivariate analysis found that resting plasma norepinephrine levels were a significant independent predictor of mortality among these patients ($P < 0.002$). In addition, the norepinephrine level was higher in patients who died from progressive heart failure (1014 ± 699 pg/mL) than in those who died suddenly (619 ± 238 pg/mL). The figure illustrates predicted survival curves for groups of patients with different baseline plasma norepinephrine levels. (*Adapted from* Cohn *et al.* [14].)

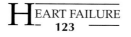

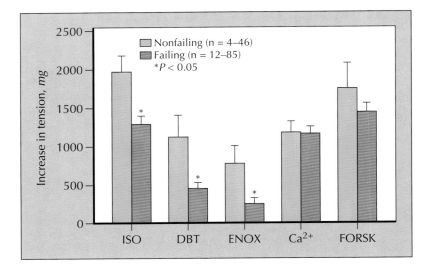

FIGURE 4-19. A characteristic physiologic abnormality in patients with heart failure is a reduction in the inotropic and chronotropic responses to exercise and other types of sympathetic stimulation. The responsiveness of trabeculae from normal hearts and hearts with end-stage failure was examined by determining the development of contractile tension in response to several agonists. By this approach, it was shown that although the contractile response to calcium (Ca^{2+}) is preserved in failing myocardium, the contractile responses to the β-adrenergic agonists isoproterenol (ISO) and dobutamine (DBT) are significantly reduced, as is the response to enoximone (ENOX), a phosphodiesterase inhibitor that is dependent on the availability of cAMP. In contrast, forskolin (FORSK), a substance that directly activates adenylate cyclase, thereby bypassing the β-adrenergic receptor, elicited a normal response in failing myocardium. These observations suggest that, in heart failure, reduced adrenergic responsiveness of the myocardium is relatively specific for the β-adrenergic receptor pathway. (*Adapted from* Bristow [15].)

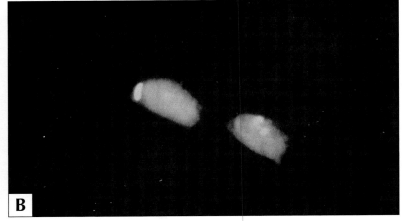

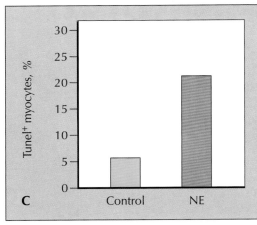

FIGURE 4-20. Apoptosis in cardiac myocytes. Neurohormonal systems, including the sympathetic nervous system, have been implicated in the induction of apoptosis. Communal *et al.* [16] have shown that norepinephrine (NE) can stimulate apoptosis in isolated rat ventricular myocytes as demonstrated here by an increase in the number of cells staining positive for fragmented DNA using the Tunel method. **A**, Control myocytes. **B**, Apoptotic myocytes after 24 hours' treatment with 10 μm NE. **C**, The percent of apoptotic cells increases approximately fourfold. This effect is mediated by β-adrenergic receptors since it is blocked by the β-adrenergic antagonist propranolol but not the α-adrenergic antagonist prazosin. These observations suggest that increased sympathetic tone could contribute to progressive myocyte loss and provide a possible mechanism by which β-adrenergic antagonists might exert beneficial effects in patients with heart failure. DUTP—deoxyuridine triphosphate. (Parts A and B *from* Communal *et al.* [16]; with permission. Part C *adapted from* Communal *et al.* [16].)

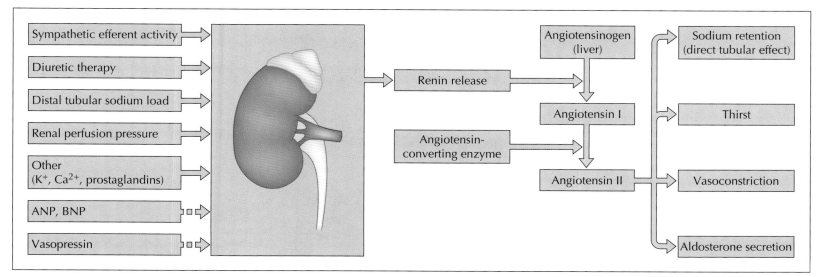

FIGURE 4-21. The renin-angiotensin system is activated in patients with congestive heart failure. The major site of release of circulating renin is the juxtaglomerular apparatus of the kidney, where multiple stimuli may contribute to renal release of renin into the systemic circulation, including increased renal sympathetic efferent activity, decreased distal tubular sodium delivery, reduced renal perfusion pressure, and diuretic therapy. Atrial natriuretic factor and vasopressin (*dashed arrows*) may inhibit the release of renin. Renin enzymatically cleaves angiotensinogen, a tetrapeptide produced in the liver, to form the inactive decapeptide angiotensin I. Angiotensin I is converted to the octapeptide angiotensin II by the angiotensin-converting enzyme. Angiotensin II is a potent vasoconstrictor; it promotes sodium reabsorption by increasing aldosterone secretion and by a direct effect on the tubules, and it stimulates water intake by acting on the thirst center. Angiotensin II causes vasoconstriction directly and may also facilitate the release of norepinephrine by acting on sympathetic nerve endings. ANP—A-type natriuretic peptide; BNP—B-type natriuretic peptide. (*Adapted from* Paganelli *et al.* [13].)

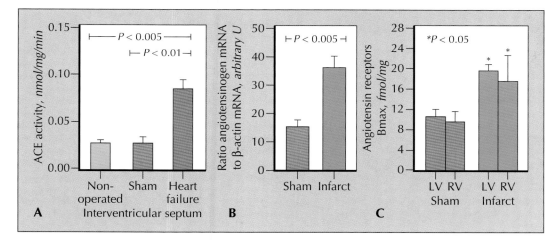

FIGURE 4-22. There is an upregulation of several components of the renin-angiotensin system (RAS) in the noninfarcted myocardium of rats after myocardial infarction. There are significant increases in ACE activity (**A**), the level of angiotensinogen mRNA (**B**), and the density of angiotensin-II receptors (**C**). The increase in angiotensin-II receptor density suggests that, in addition to increased activity of the tissue RAS, the responsiveness of the tissue to angiotensin may be increased. LV—left ventricle; RV—right ventricle. (*Adapted from* Hirsch *et al.* [17]; Lindpainter *et al.* [18]; Meggs *et al.* [19].)

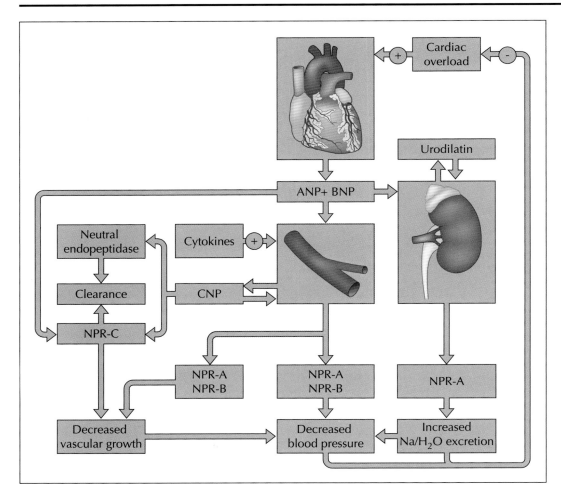

FIGURE 4-23. The natriuretic peptide family. The natriuretic peptides include atrial natriuretic peptide (ANP), brain natriuretic peptide (BNP), C-type natriuretic peptide (CNP), and urodilatin. ANP is derived from a prohormone composed of 126 amino acids, and it is secreted primarily from cardiac atria. The prohormone is cleaved to an N-terminal fragment (ANP1-98) and a C-terminal fragment (ANP99-126). BNP, identified initially in the brain, is secreted from atria and ventricles, particularly the latter. CNP has been identified primarily in the brain, but also is present in vascular endothelial cells. Urodilatin, or ANP95-126, is found in urine. Stretch receptors in the atria and ventricles detect changes in cardiac chamber volume related to increased cardiac filling pressures, resulting in release of ANP and BNP, but not CNP. The natriuretic peptides are mediated by natriuretic peptide receptors (NPRs), designated NPR-A, NPR-B, and NPR-C. NPR-A and NPR-B are particulate guanylate cyclases, activation of which increase levels of 3',5'-cyclic guanosinemonophosphate. NPRs have been localized in vascular smooth muscle, endothelium, platelets, the adrenal glomerulosa, and the kidney. ANP and BNP increase urine volume and sodium excretion, decrease vascular resistance, and inhibit release of renin and secretion of aldosterone and vasopressin. CNP reduces vascular resistance, but, despite its name, does not have natriuretic properties. (*Adapted from Wilkins et al.* [20].)

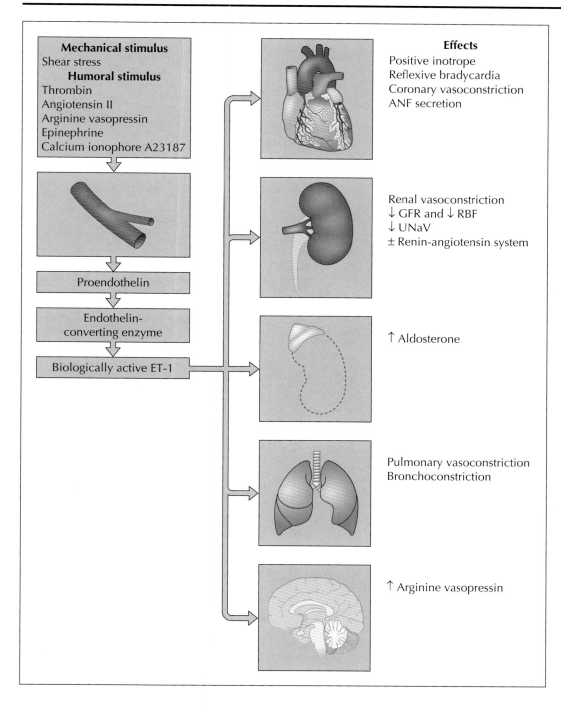

FIGURE 4-24. Summary of the stimuli for endothelin secretion and effects of endothelin in several organs. Mechanical (shear stress) and humoral (thrombin, angiotensin II, vasopressin, epinephrine, calcium ionophore A23187) stimuli may cause the release of endothelin-1 (ET-1). Endothelin increases circulating levels of atrial natriuretic factor (ANF), vasopressin, and aldosterone. It also modulates renin release. Endothelin has a positive inotropic effect and produces coronary and systemic vasoconstriction. These responses produce an increase in blood pressure that is associated with a reflex decrease in heart rate. ET-1 constricts human pulmonary resistance vessels and has a potent bronchoconstrictor effect. Furthermore, ET-1 causes renal vasoconstriction, leading to a reduction in renal blood flow (RBF) and glomerular filtration rate (GFR) and a decrease in urinary sodium excretion (UNaV). (*Adapted from* Underwood et al. [21].)

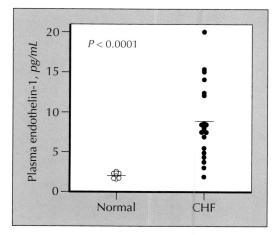

FIGURE 4-25. Cody *et al.* [22] measured immunoreactive circulating endothelin-1 in 12 normal control subjects and in 20 patients with congestive heart failure (CHF). Plasma endothelin-1 was 3.7 ± 0.6 pg/mL in the control group and 9.1 ± 4.1 pg/mL in the CHF group. Increased endothelin synthesis by angiotensin I and vasopressin stimulation and decreased endothelin clearance may contribute to the increased plasma endothelin levels in CHF. Of note, there was a strong positive correlation between endothelin levels and the severity of reactive pulmonary hypertension. (*Adapted from* Cody et al. [22].)

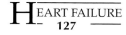

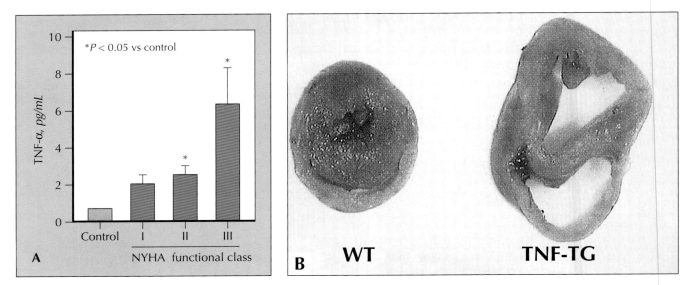

FIGURE 4-26. Proinflammatory cytokines such as tumor necrosis factor-α (TNF-α), interleukin-1β, (IL-1β), and interleukin-6 (IL-6) may play an important pathyphysiologic role in the progression of myocardial failure. The circulating levels of TNF-α and IL-6 were analyzed in randomly selected plasma samples from 63 patients in functional classes I to III enrolled in the neurohormonal substudies of the SOLVD trial. Compared with age-matched controls, patients with left ventricular dysfunction had elevated TNF-α levels (**A**) in direct proportion to functional class. Interestingly, this decrease in LV function was completely reversed 30 days after the infusion was stopped. When Bryant *et al.* [23] caused overexpression of TNF-α in transgenic mice, there was ventricular dilation and impaired survival of mice that was related to the intensity of TNF-α expression (**B**). TG—transgenic; WT—wild type. (Part A *adapted from* Torre-Amione *et al.* [24]; part B *from* Bryant *et al.* [23]; with permission.)

CLINICAL FEATURES

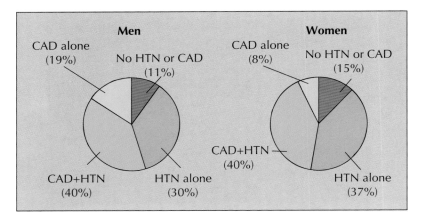

FIGURE 4-27. The epidemiology of congestive heart failure in the United States. The Framingham Heart Study, which followed a cohort of 9405 Americans over a 40-year period, has provided valuable information regarding the etiologic basis of congestive heart failure in the United States [23]. Of 331 men and 321 women who developed heart failure, the majority had coronary artery disease (CAD) with or without hypertension (HTN), and approximately one third had HTN alone. At present, idiopathic dilated cardiomyopathy has replaced HTN as the second most important etiologic factor in the development of heart failure. CAD continues to be the most common risk factor for the development of heart failure in the United States. (*Adapted from* Ho *et al.* [25].)

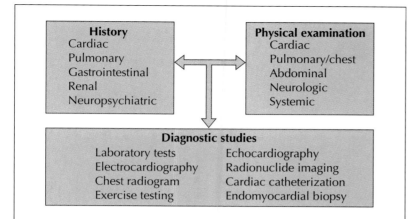

History
Cardiac
Pulmonary
Gastrointestinal
Renal
Neuropsychiatric

Physical examination
Cardiac
Pulmonary/chest
Abdominal
Neurologic
Systemic

Diagnostic studies

Laboratory tests
Electrocardiography
Chest radiogram
Exercise testing

Echocardiography
Radionuclide imaging
Cardiac catheterization
Endomyocardial biopsy

FIGURE 4-28. Approach to the problem of assessing heart failure. To adequately assess patients with heart failure, historical information, data from the physical examination, and diagnostic study information should be obtained and integrated. It should be emphasized that although information from all three categories may be used in the evaluation, not every test needs to be, or should be, performed. In most patients, an electrocardiogram, a chest radiograph, and an echocardiogram are performed. Additional diagnostic studies should be tailored to the patient. Echocardiography could include M-mode, two-dimensional, and Doppler studies. Radionuclide examination might consist of perfusion, performance, or positron-emission tomographic studies. Cardiac catheterization could include angiography, hemodynamics, or endomyocardial biopsy in certain circumstances. Computed tomography and magnetic resonance imaging are sometimes useful, as is determination of maximal exercise oxygen consumption. Information obtained from the history and physical examination should dictate the need for and type of ancillary testing.

FRAMINGHAM CRITERIA FOR DIAGNOSIS OF CONGESTIVE HEART FAILURE

MAJOR CRITERIA

Paroxysmal nocturnal dyspnea
Neck vein distention
Rales
Cardiomegaly
Acute pulmonary edema
S_3 gallop
Increased venous pressure (>16 cm H_2O)
Positive hepatojugular reflux

MINOR CRITERIA

Extremity edema
Night cough
Dyspnea on exertion
Hepatomegaly
Pleural effusion
Vital capacity reduced by one third from normal
Tachycardia (≥120 bpm)

MAJOR OR MINOR

Weight loss ≥ 4.5 kg over 5 days' treatment

FIGURE 4-29. A constellation of symptoms and abnormal physical findings should be used in making the diagnosis of congestive heart failure. The Framingham Study, for example, suggested that several specific clinical criteria be combined and weighted. To establish a clinical diagnosis of congestive heart failure by this method, at least one major and two minor criteria are required [26–28].

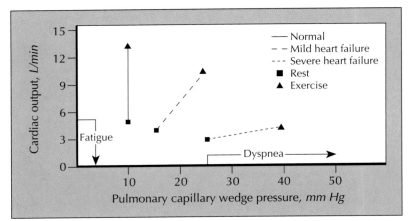

FIGURE 4-30. Symptoms of heart failure are related to pathophysiology. Exercise testing is important in patients with heart failure because it may unmask significant symptomatology. In patients with significant systolic ventricular dysfunction, the cardiac output fails to increase normally under the physiologic stress of exertion, and the pulmonary pressures become disproportionately elevated.

SYSTOLIC VS DIASTOLIC DYSFUNCTION IN HEART FAILURE

A

PARAMETERS	SYSTOLIC	DIASTOLIC
History		
Coronary heart disease	++++	+
Hypertension	++	++++
Diabetes	+++	+
Valvular heart disease	++++	-
Paroxysmal dyspnea	++	+++
Physical examination		
Cardiomegaly	+++	+
Soft heart sounds	++++	+
S$_3$ gallop	+++	+
S$_4$ gallop	+	+++
Hypertension	++	++++
Mitral regurgitation	+++	+
Rales	++	++
Edema	+++	+
Jugular venous distention	+++	+

B

PARAMETERS	SYSTOLIC	DIASTOLIC
Chest roentgenogram		
Cardiomegaly	+++	+
Pulmonary congestion	+++	+++
Electrocardiograms		
Low voltage	+++	-
Left ventricular hypertrophy	++	++++
Q waves	+++	+
Echocardiograms		
Low ejection fraction	++++	-
Left ventricular dilation	+++	-
Left ventricular hypertrophy	++	++++

remember that the clinical features of heart failure may be similar whether left ventricular systolic function is normal or is substantively depressed [30]. The pathophysiology of heart failure with normal systolic ventricular function is different, however, from that noted in patients with depressed left ventricular ejection fraction [31,32]. Furthermore, certain aspects of the history and physical examination (*panel A*), along with clinical measurements (*panel B*), help to distinguish diastolic problems from those more often associated with systolic failure. Patients with hypertensive heart disease, for example, particularly severe left ventricular hypertrophy, often experience heart failure because of diastolic dysfunction. *Plus signs* indicate "suggestive" (the number reflects relative weight). *Minus signs* indicate " not very suggestive."

FIGURE 4-31. A and **B**, Although it is common, congestive heart failure in which diastolic dysfunction is preponderant (vs systolic dysfunction) may be difficult to diagnose [29]. It is important to

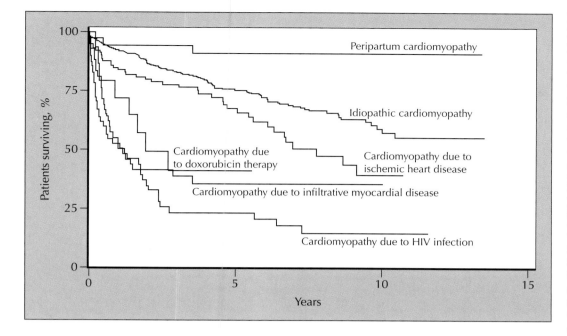

FIGURE 4-32. Survival according to the underlying cause of heart failure. A total of 1230 patients referred to Johns Hopkins Hospital for assessment of unexplained cardiomyopathy underwent a comprehensive diagnostic evaluation including endocardial biopsy, enabling identification of underlying etiology in 50% of cases [33]. Patients with peripartum cariomyopathy had the best prognosis, whereas patients with an ischemic etiology did worse than those with idiopathic cardiomyopathy, consistent with the results of previous studies [34]. This study is limited by the referral nature of the study population, resulting in under-representation of patients with common causes of heart failure. Further, the poor outcome seen among patients with doxorubicin cardiotoxicity, infiltrative myocardial disease, and HIV infection may relate more to the underlying disease process than to cardiac involvement. Nevertheless, this study provides important information on survival, and demonstrates the prognostic value of identifying the underlying cause of cardiomyopathy.

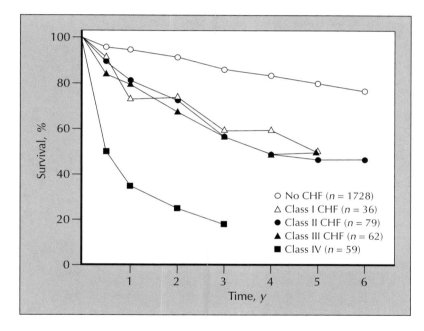

FIGURE 4-33. Survival among patients with different degrees of heart failure symptoms compared with similar patients without congestive heart failure (CHF) [35]. Classification of heart failure was based on the worst clinical condition 6 weeks before cardiac catheterization at Duke University Medical Center (1969 to 1981). All patients had coronary artery disease that was managed medically. These data demonstrate the effect, per se, of heart failure on mortality. The difference in survival between groups with a recent history of CHF and patients without overt heart failure was 27% after 3 years of follow-up. Patients who were symptomatic with any physical activity (class IV) had a very poor prognosis. (*Adapted from* Califf *et al.* [35].)

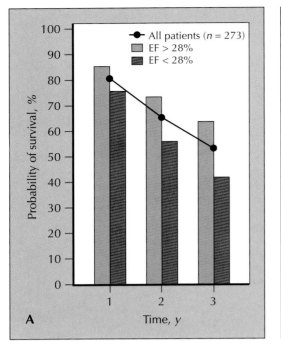

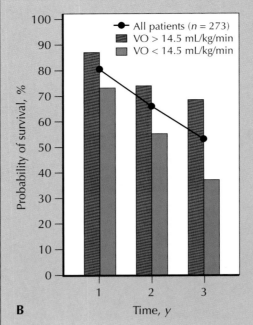

FIGURE 4-34. Examples of the prognostic information available from measurement of the left ventricular ejection fraction (EF; **A**) and peak oxygen consumption (VO$_2$; **B**) in the Vasodilator Heart Failure Trial (V-HeFT I). These data from the placebo group (patients treated with digoxin and diuretic) [36] indicate that the probability of survival over 3 years in different risk strata can differ by 20% to 30%. Strata were defined arbitrarily by the median values in this sample and may not represent the most discriminating cutpoints for these prognostic variables.

MANAGEMENT OF HEART FAILURE

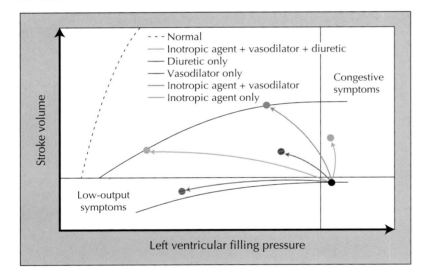

FIGURE 4-35. Physiologic response to pharmacologic intervention in heart failure. These curves represent the Frank-Starling relationship between left ventricular end-diastolic filling pressure and stroke volume for a normal heart and for the patient with heart failure symptoms resulting from predominant systolic dysfunction before and after treatment with digoxin or diuretics, alone or in combination with a vasodilator. Note that only positive inotropic agents, such as digoxin, and vasodilators shift the patient's hemodynamic profile upward and leftward to a more favorable ventricular function curve, resulting in an improvement in cardiac output despite a reduction in ventricular filling pressure. Diuretics reduce heart failure symptoms by lowering ventricular filling pressures, but they may cause a reduction in cardiac output in patients who have decompensated heart failure and marginal systolic reserve.

DIURETICS

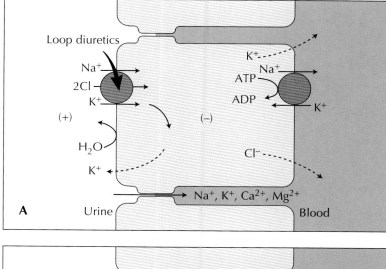

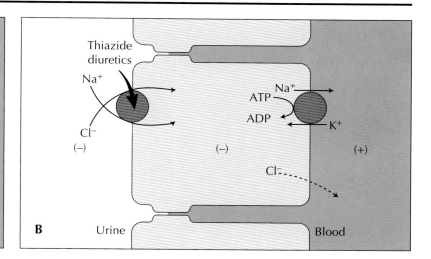

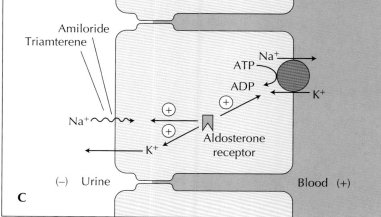

FIGURE 4-36. Loop diuretics in heart failure. **A,** The introduction in the 1960s of diuretics that act within the loop of Henle, so-called "high-ceiling" or "loop" diuretics, dramatically affected the ability of clinicians to improve symptoms of congestive heart failure with minimum toxicity and predictable efficacy compared with other drugs available at that time. These diuretics act on a specific transport protein, the $Na^+K^+/2Cl^-$ cotransporter, located on the apical membrane of renal epithelial cells in the ascending limb of Henle's loop. Ions transported into the cell are then transferred out of the cell by Na^+K^+-ATPase (the "sodium pump") on the basolateral membranes of these cells. Loop diuretics also decrease the absorption of Ca^{2+} and Mg^{2+} in this portion of the nephron, cations whose absorption is indirectly linked to NaCl uptake. Thus, hypocalcemia and hypomagnesia, as well as hypokalemia and volume depletion, may result from prolonged use of these drugs.

Loop diuretics also reduce the tonicity of the medullary interstitium by preventing the normal uptake of solute in the absence of water in the thick ascending limb of Henle's loop. This limits the kidney's ability to concentrate the urine and may contribute to the development of hyponatremia. The loop diuretics are clearly the most useful diuretics as single

agents for patients with decompensated congestive failure, in large part because of the magnitude of the natriuresis that can be achieved over a short period, which can reach as high as 20% of the filtered load of sodium. Typically, the fraction of NaCl filtered at the glomerulus and reabsorbed in the ascending limb of the loop of Henle declines from about 20% to 13% with a loop diuretic, resulting in a 1% to 2% increase in the fractional excretion of sodium over 24 hours [37].

B, Thiazide diuretics. In general, the thiazide diuretics are not useful as single drugs for the therapy of volume retention in heart failure patients, largely because their site of action in the distal convoluted tubule permits rapid adjustment of water and solute absorption in other more proximal nephron segments. Interestingly, the target renal tubular protein of the thiazide class of diuretics, the electroneutral Na^+Cl^- cotransporter, has recently been cloned and sequenced. This is the last of the known diuretic-responsive renal epithelial cell transport proteins to be identified. Many other tissues also express this transport protein, which may have important implications for understanding the effectiveness of these drugs in the treatment of hypertension as well as their less desirable metabolic effects on lipid and glucose metabolism. Unlike loop diuretics, thiazides enhance calcium reabsorption but not that of magnesim, although magnesium wasting is much more pronounced with loop diuretics [37].

C, Potassium-sparing diuretics. The potassium-sparing diuretics fall into two categories: agents such as amiloride and triamterene, which reduce Na^+ conductance through an apical membrane sodium channel; and aldosterone antagonists, which, by inhibiting the actions of aldosterone at its intracellular receptor in renal epithelial cells of the distal collecting duct, reduce Na^+ uptake from the tubular lumen and decrease K^+ secretion by several mechanisms. Aldosterone antagonists also limit the kidney's ability to acidify the urine by inhibiting the action of aldosterone on a renal tubular proton pump. Although none of these diuretics is effective as a single agent in the treatment of heart failure, they play a useful role in diminishing renal K^+ wasting. When combined with loop or thiazide diuretics, the aldosterone antagonists also prevent Mg^{2+} depletion. Because ACE inhibitors increase the serum K^+ concentration, an effect that may be magnified by β-blockers and NSAIDs, potassium-sparing diuretics should be prescribed cautiously for patients who are already receiving vasodilators of this class [37].

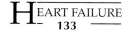

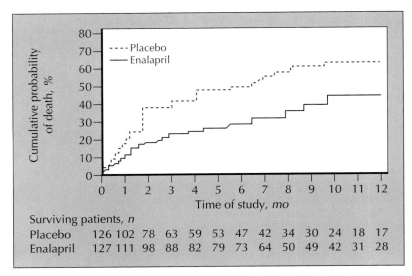

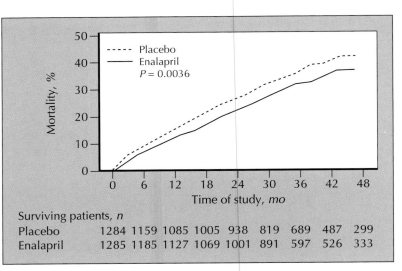

FIGURE 4-37. The CONSENSUS (Cooperative North Scandinavian Enalapril Survival Study) trial, the first mortality study of an ACE inhibitor in patients with congestive heart failure, demonstrated that an ACE inhibitor improved mortality compared with placebo. A lesser-known aspect of the study was that the mean age of the patients at randomization was 70 years. In addition, the majority of patients were elderly and belonged to New York Heart Association functional class IV despite digoxin and diuretic therapy. Approximately 25% of the patients in this trial were also receiving other vasodilators, such as nitrates, before randomization. Early diagnosis of the placebo and enalapril treatment groups prompted early termination of the study. The mean dose of enalapril was just under 20 mg/d. Careful dose titration obviated the excess hypotension observed in early stages of the study. (*Adapted from* CONSENSUS Trial Study Group [38].)

FIGURE 4-38. The SOLVD (Studies of Left Ventricular Dysfunction) treatment subgroup demonstrated mortality benefit in moderate heart failure. The treatment subgroup included patients who already had symptomatic congestive heart failure and were randomized to either placebo or enalapril therapy. Criteria for randomization were a baseline ejection fraction of 35% or less and symptomatic heart failure. The majority of patients in this study had functional class II congestive heart failure. Enalapril was associated with a significant reduction in mortality compared with placebo in these patients. This mortality benefit was primarily the result of reducing mortality due to congestive heart failure. Mortality due to presumed arrhythmic death was not significantly different from placebo. (*Adapted from* the SOLVD Investigators [39].)

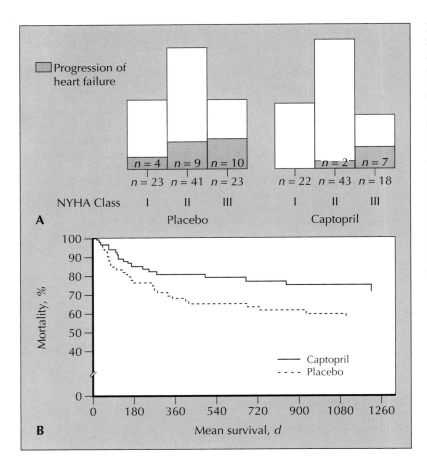

FIGURE 4-39. The Munich Mild Heart Failure Study prospectively determined whether an ACE inhibitor would alter the natural outcome in heart failure by reducing the progression to severe heart failure from milder heart failure. **A,** Patients were randomized to placebo or captopril, and subclassified according to New York Heart Association (NYHA) functional class I, II, or III. The majority of patients in this study were either asymptomatic (NYHA functional class I) or mildly symptomatic (NYHA functional class II), although patients with more severe heart failure (NYHA functional class III) contributed to both treatment groups. In the placebo group, 23 of 87 patients demonstrated progression of heart failure. In the captopril group, only nine of 83 patients demonstrated progression of heart failure. **B,** The mean survival time until the development of progressive heart failure was 223 days longer in the captopril group compared with placebo. Patients treated with the ACE inhibitor could anticipate a greater interval without progression of their heart failure symptoms once the ACE inhibitor had been initiated, compared with the placebo. However, total mortality in the study for the two treatment groups was virtually identical. Twenty-two of the 83 patients receiving captopril died, compared with 22 of the 87 patients receiving placebo. (*Adapted from* Kleber *et al.* [40].)

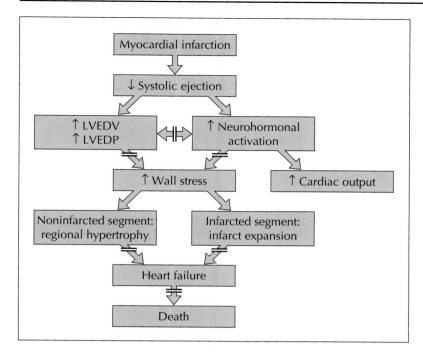

FIGURE 4-40. Although the pathophysiology of infarct healing is complex, there are several potential mechanisms by which an ACE inhibitor may favorably improve left ventricular remodeling. Shown with *intersecting bars* are sites at which an ACE inhibitor may interrupt an adverse consequence of myocardial infarction that would contribute to heart failure or death. LVEDP—left ventricular end-diastolic pressure; LVEDV—left ventricular end-diastolic volume. (*Adapted from* McKay *et al.* [41].)

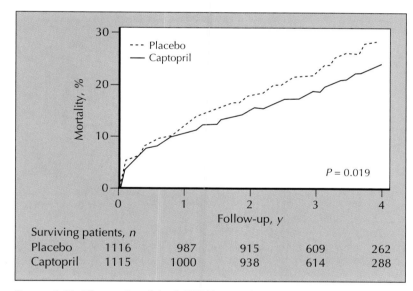

FIGURE 4-41. The results of the SAVE (Survival and Ventricular Enlargement) study demonstrated that an ACE inhibitor given to the high-risk anterior myocardial infarction subgroup was associated with a 19% reduction in all-cause mortality. There was no effect of captopril compared with placebo on short-term mortality during the first year of follow-up. After 1 year of follow-up, mortality reduction was evident in the captopril group. This suggested that the reduction may be due to a decrease in deaths related to the development of heart failure. (*Adapted from* Pfeffer *et al.* [42].)

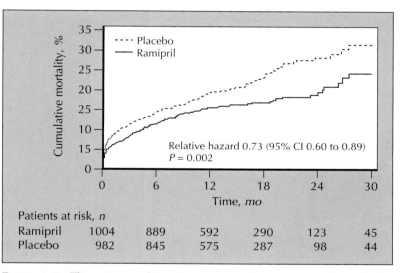

FIGURE 4-42. The outcome of the all-cause mortality primary endpoint in the AIRE (Acute Infarction Ramipril Evaluation) trial, based on intention to treat. It is instructive to compare this figure with the results of the SAVE (Survival and Ventricular Enlargement) trial in Figure 4-38. In AIRE there is an early divergence of survival benefit for ramipril, which is not apparent in SAVE. Many believe that this reflects the greater clinical severity of heart failure in AIRE, whereas patients in SAVE had asymptomatic left ventricular dysfunction. In fact, clinical evidence of heart failure excluded patients from SAVE. In AIRE, this early survival benefit persisted throughout follow-up, as the survival curves continue to diverge. This suggests that, in contrast to SAVE, early survival benefit results from reduction of mortality related to heart failure, which continues through follow-up. CI—confidence interval. (*Adapted from* AIRE Study Investigators [43].)

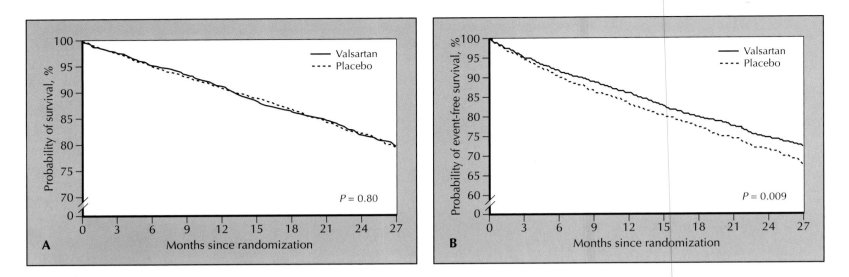

C. EFFECT OF ANGIOTENSIN I RECEPTOR BLOCKADE ON MORBIDITY AND MORTALITY IN ADDITION TO STANDARD HEART FAILURE MEDICATIONS (PRIMARY AND SECONDARY ENDPOINTS)

VARIABLE	PLACEBO	VALSARTAN	RR (CI)	P VALUE
Patients, n	2499	2511		
All-cause mortality, n(%)	484 (19.4%)	495 (19.7%)	1.02 (0.90–1.15)	0.80
Mortality + hospitalization + sudden death + inotrope need, n (%)	801 (32.1%)	723 (28.8%)	0.87 (0.79–0.96)	0.009
Heart failure hospitalizations, n (%)	455 (18.2%)	246 (13.8%)	0.73 (0.63–0.83)	0.001

FIGURE 4-43. The effects of angiotensin receptor blockade on morbidity and mortality in the Valsartan in Heart Failure Trial (Val-HeFT) study [44]. This randomized, double-blind, placebo-controlled trial studied the clinical effect of the addition of valsartan to standard heart failure care that included angiotensin-converting enzyme (ACE) inhibitor therapy. This study enrolled 5010 patients and included two primary endpoints: all-cause mortality, and the composite endpoint of mortality hospialization, and the need for intravenous inotropes for greater than 4 hours. The patient population studied was largely New York Heart Association class II and III. The majority received an ACE inhibitor (93%), some received a β-blocker (35%), and only 5% received spironolactone. The addition of valsartan to standard heart failure care resulted in no improvement in all-cause mortality (A). However, the risk of reaching the composite endpoint was reduced by 13% with valsartan (B). The vast majority of the benefit found in this composite endpoint was through reduction in heart failure hospitalizations. Hospitalizations were reduced by 27.5% with the addition of valsartan, with a highly significant P value of 0.001 (C). (*Adapted from* Cohn *et al.* [44].)

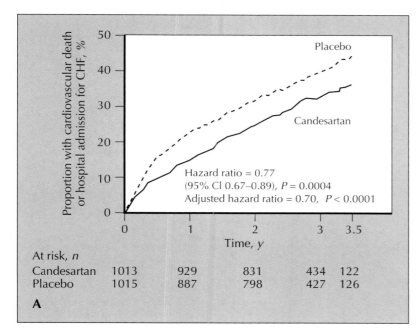

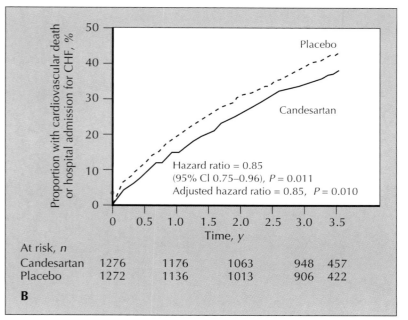

FIGURE 4-44. A and B, Kaplan-Meier cumulative event curves for primary outcome. There are theoretic reasons why an angiotensin receptor antagonist (ARB) may be more or less effective than an ACE inhibitor in patients with heart failure. The CHARM (Candesartan in Heart failure Assessment of Reduction in Mortality and morbidity) Trial program provided important information about the effects of ARBs when used as an alternative to or in combination with ACE inhibitors in patients with systolic heart failure, and as therapy for patients with diastolic heart failure [45]. **A**, In the CHARM-Alternative Trial [46], candesartan or placebo was given to 2028 patients who were intolerant of ACE inhibitors. Candesartan resulted in a 30% reduction in the primary endpoint of death or hospitalization for heart failure (*P* < 0.0001). **B**, In the CHARM-Added Trial [47], candesartan or placebo was given to 2028 patients who were receiving ACE inhibitors. Candesartan resulted in a 15% decrease in primary endpoint of death or hospitalization for heart failure (*P* < 0.011). Of note, this added benefit tended to be greater in patients who were receiving a beta blocker in addition to the ACE inhibitor. In patients with preserved systolic function [48], candesartan decreased the primary endpoint of death or hospitalization for heart failure by 14% (*P* = 0.051), and reduced the composite endpoint, which included nonfatal myocardial infarction and nonfatal stroke by 14% (*P* < 0.037).

POSTINFARCTION LEFT VENTRICULAR DYSFUNCTION

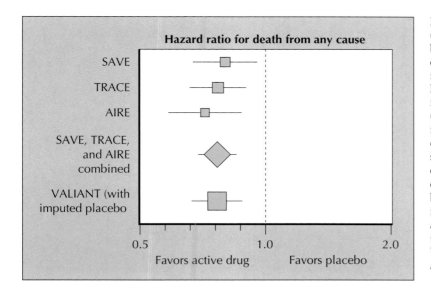

FIGURE 4-45. The Valsartan in Acute Myocardial Infarction Trial (VALIANT) trial [49] compared the effects of the angiotensin-receptor blocker valsartan, the angiotensin-converting enzyme (ACE) inhibitor captopril, and the combination of the two on mortality in patients with myocardial infarction complicated by left ventricular systolic dysfunction, heart failure, or both. Patients receiving conventional therapy were randomly assigned to valsartan (4909 patients), valsartan plus captopril (4885 patients), or captopril (4909 patients) 0.5 to 10 days after myocardial infarction. During a median follow-up of 2 years, mortality and the composite endpoint of fatal and nonfatal cardiovascular events were similar in the three groups, leading to the conclusion that valsartan is as effective as captopril in patients who are at high risk for cardiovascular events after myocardial infarction. The combination was no more effective, but was associated with an increased the rate of adverse events. As the figure illustrates, in VALIANT the hazard ratio for death with valsartan alone versus an imputed placebo group is essentially identical to that for the three prior survival trials with ACE inhibitors (SAVE [Survival and Ventricular Enlargement trial], TRACE [Trandolapril Cardiac Evaluation], and AIRE [Acute Infarction Ramipril Efficacy trial]) combined.

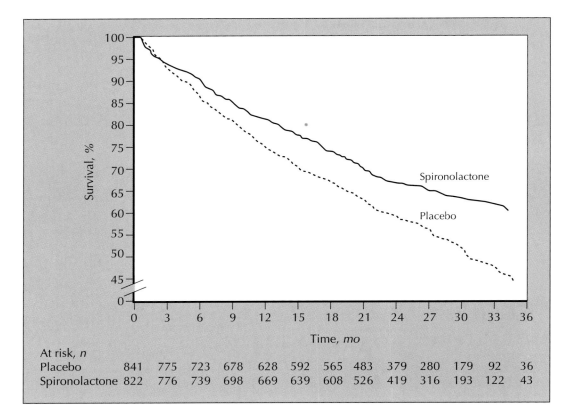

FIGURE 4-46. Effect of spironolactone on survival in patients with severe heart failure. Patients with severe heart failure have been shown to have elevated levels of aldosterone compared with that of normal subjects. Treatment with angiotensin-converting enzyme (ACE) inhibitors reduces aldosterone release by limiting the production of angiotensin II. Because of non–ACE-dependent produc-

tion of angiotensin II (serine protease pathways), aldosterone levels have been shown to rise over time in patients treated with recommended doses of ACE inhibitor. Aldosterone has direct effects on the kidney, leading to sodium retention and reduction in serum potassium concentration. Additionally, animal models of heart failure have shown that aldosterone may be responsible for myocardial fibrosis and myocyte hypertrophy seen with chronic heart failure. The Randomized Aldactone Evaluation Study (RALES) was performed in 1663 patients with ejection fraction of 35% or lower and New York Heat Association (NYHA) IV symptoms, or patients with NYHA III symptoms who had experience NYHA IV symptoms within the past 6 months. Patients were randomly assigned to receive 25 to 50 mg of spironolactone daily versus placebo, delivered in a double-blind fashion. The survival plot demonstrates the effect of spironolactone on all-cause mortality, with a reduction of 30% compared with placebo. This reduction in the risk of death among patients in the spironolactone group was attributed to a lower risk of death from progressive heart failure and sudden death from cardiac causes. The frequency of hospitalization for worsening heart failure was 35% lower in the spironolactone group than in the placebo group. Patients receiving spironolactone treatment should have close monitoring of the serum potassium level, particularly in the first month of therapy [50].

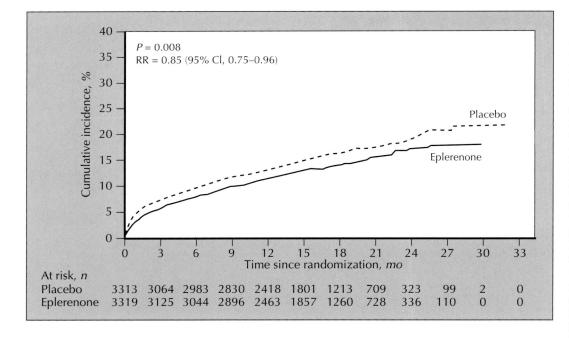

FIGURE 4-47. Kaplan-Meier estimates of the rate of death from any cause. The role of mineralocorticoid receptor blockade was tested further in the Eplerenone Post-acute Myocardial Infarction Heart Failure Efficacy and Survival (EPHESUS) Study. In this trial, 6632 patients who had left ventricular dysfunction and heart failure in the setting of an acute myocardial infarction were randomized to eplerenone (25 mg per day, titrated to a maximum of 50 mg per day) or placebo in addition to standard care. The primary endpoints were 1) all-cause death and 2) cardiovascular death or hospitalization for heart failure, acute myocardial infarction, stroke, or ventricular arrhythmia. Treatment with eplerenone initiated 3 to 14 days after infarction reduced all-cause mortality by 15%. In addition, cardiovascular death or hospitalization for heart failure, acute myocardial infarction, stroke, or ventricular arrhythmia was reduced by 13%. There eplerenone was associated with an increase in the rate of serious hyperkalemia (5.5% vs 3.9% in placebo; $P = 0.002$), and a decrease in the rate of serious hyperkalemia (8.4% vs 13.1% in placebo; $P = 0.001$) [51].

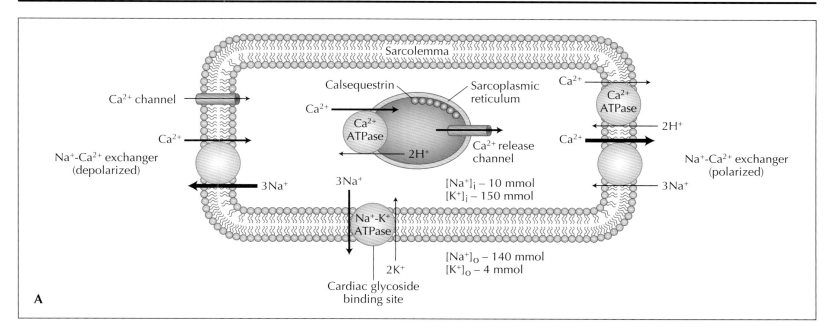

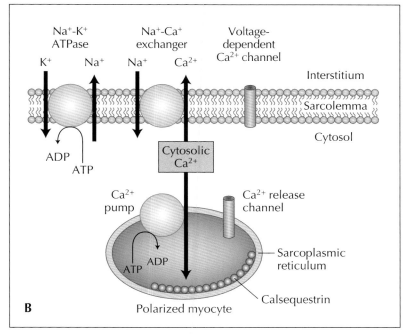

FIGURE 4-48. Sodium pump inhibition by cardiac glycosides. The present understanding of the mechanism by which the cardiac glycosides induce a positive inotropic effect in cardiac muscle is based on the specificity of these drugs for Na^+K^+-ATPase (or the "sodium pump"), a cell membrane protein responsible for the active (*ie*, ATP-consuming) transport of the monovalent cations Na^+ and K^+.

A, Both Na^+ and Ca^{2+} ions enter cardiac muscle cells during each cycle of depolarization, contraction, and repolarization. Ca^{2+} is also released from internal stores in an intracellular compartment called the sarcoplasmic reticulum (SR), where it is bound to the protein calsequestrin. During cellular repolarization, Na^+ is actively extruded by Na^+K^+-ATPase, while Ca^{2+} is

either pumped back into the SR by a Ca^{2+}-ATPase or is removed from the cell by a cell membrane transport protein that exchanges Na^+ for Ca^{2+}. This Na^+ for Ca^{2+} exchanger transports three Na^+ ions in for every Ca^{2+} ion out when the cell is polarized, using the favorable chemical and electrical potential of Na^+ to drive the exchange reaction. **B,** The direction and magnitude of Na^+ and Ca^{2+} transport during diastole (polarized myocyte).

C, The direction and magnitude of Na^+ and Ca^{2+} transport during systole (depolarized myocyte). Note that the exchanger may briefly run in reverse during cell depolarization when the electrical gradient across the plasma membrane is transiently reversed. The capacity of the exchanger to extrude Ca^{2+} from the cell depends critically on the intracellular Na^+ concentrations.

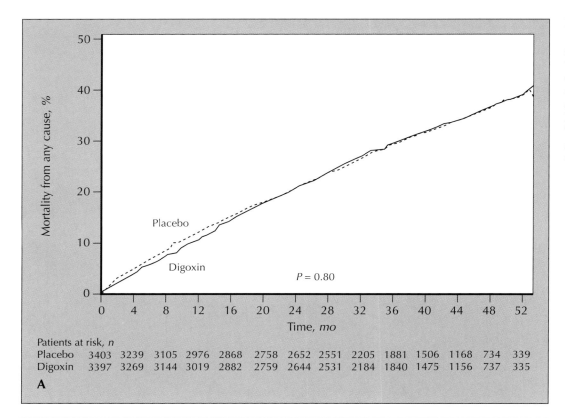

Patients at risk, n

Placebo	3403	3239	3105	2976	2868	2758	2652	2551	2205	1881	1506	1168	734	339
Digoxin	3397	3269	3144	3019	2882	2759	2644	2531	2184	1840	1475	1156	737	335

A

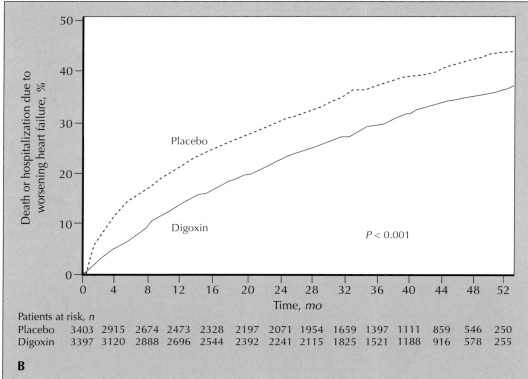

Patients at risk, n

Placebo	3403	2915	2674	2473	2328	2197	2071	1954	1659	1397	1111	859	546	250
Digoxin	3397	3120	2888	2696	2544	2392	2241	2115	1825	1521	1188	916	578	255

B

FIGURE 4-49. The Digitalis Investigation Group (DIG) trial evaluated the effects of digoxin on survival in 6800 patients. The average follow-up was 37 months. Digoxin did not increase or decrease overall mortality (A). However, digoxin-treated patients had a reduction in the overall rate of hospitalization and also the rate of hospitalization for worsening heart failure (B). There was no increased risk of ventricular arrhythmias in the digoxin-treated group. (*Adapted from* Digitalis Investigation Report [52].)

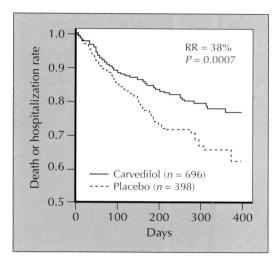

FIGURE 4-50. United States Carvedilol Heart Failure Trials Program: effect on major clinical events. In 1997, the US Food and Drug Administration approved carvedilol, a nonselective β-adrenergic antagonist with α_1-adrenergic receptor blocking and antioxidant properties, as adjunctive therapy for patients with mild to moderate heart failure. This decision was based in large part on the results of the US Carvedilol Heart Failure Trials Program, which randomized 1094 patients with chronic heart failure and a left ventricular ejection fraction of 35% or less to placebo or carvedilol in addition to conventional therapy with digoxin, diuretics, and an agiotensin-converting enzyme inhibitor. Patients were assigned to one of four treatment protocols based on exercise capacity as assessed by a 6-minute walk test. After a mean follow-up of 7 months, carvedilol resulted in a 27% reduction in the risk of cardiovascular hospitalization ($P = 0.036$) and a 38% reduction in the combined endpoint of death or cardiovascular hospitalization. (*Adapted from* Packer *et al.* [53].)

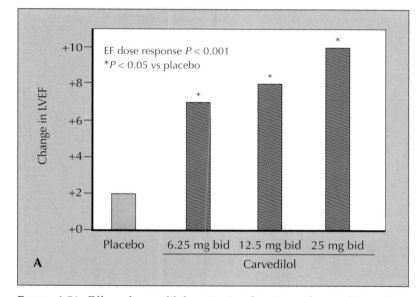

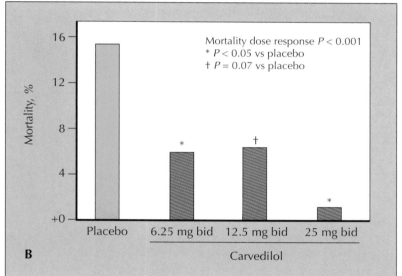

FIGURE 4-51. Effect of carvedilol on ejection fraction and mortality in the Multicenter Oral Carvedilol Heart Failure Assessment (MOCHA) trial. The MOCHA trial, a component of the US Carvedilol Heart Failure Trials Program, tested whether the effects of carvedilol were dose-related. Patients ($n = 345$) with mild to moderate heart failure were randomly assigned to treatment with placebo or carvedilol in one of three target doses: 6.25 mg twice a day (low-dose group), 12.5 mg twice a day (medium-dose group), or 25 mg twice a day (high-dose group). Although carvedilol had no effect on the primary endpoint of submaximal exercise, there were significant dose-related improvements in left ventricular function (**A**) and all-cause mortality (**B**). In this study, carvedilol also lowered the hospitalization rate by approximately 60%. bid—twice a day. (*Adapted from* Bristow *et al.* [54].)

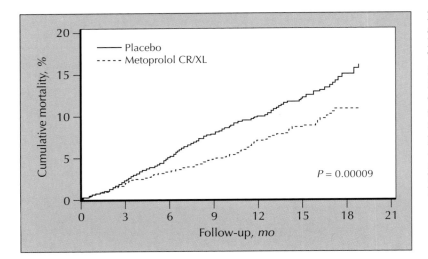

FIGURE 4-52. Effect of metoprolol on all-cause mortality, sudden death, and death due to worsening heart failure in the Metoprolol CR/XL Randomized Intervention Trial in Congestive Heart Failure (MERIT-HF) Trial. In this trial 3991 patients with New York Heart Association (NYHA) functional class II, III, or IV heart failure and a left ventricular ejection fraction below 40% were randomized to treatment with metoprolol controlled release/extended release (CR/XL) or placebo, in addition to optimal standard therapy. Metoprolol CR/XL was begun in a dose of 12.5 mg per day (NYHA III and IV patients) or 25 mg per day (NYHA class II patients), and titrated to a target dose of 200 mg per day over 8 weeks. After a mean follow-up of 1 year, metoprolol CR/XL decreased all-cause mortality by 34% ($P = 0.00009$). The risk of sudden death was decreased by 41% and the risk of death due to worsening heart failure was reduced by 49%. (*Adapted from* MERIT-HF Study Group [55].)

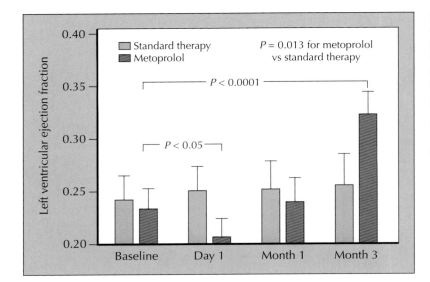

FIGURE 4-53. Time course of the effect of beta-adrenergic blockade on left ventricular ejection fraction in patients with heart failure. Twenty-six patients with dilated cardiomyopathy and a reduced ejection fraction were treated with standard therapy or metoprolol and followed by serial echocardiograms for 18 months. In standard therapy patients there was no change in ejection fraction over time. In patients treated with metoprolol, ejection fraction initially declined at 1 day, returned to baseline at 1 month, and increased markedly above baseline at 3 months. At 18 months, there were decreases in left ventricular mass and sphericity. These observations demonstrate that beta-blockade causes a time-dependent reversal of pathologic remodeling. (*Adapted from* Hall *et al.* [56].)

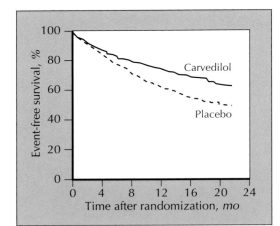

FIGURE 4-54. The Carvedilol Prospective Randomized Cumulative Survival (COPERNICUS) Study examined the effect of carvedilol in 2289 patients with severe heart failure as defined by symptoms of heart failure at rest or with minimal exertion, and an ejection fraction < 25% [57]. Over an average follow-up of 10.4 months, patients treated with carvedilol had a 31% decrease ($P < 0.00004$) in the risk of death or hospitalization for heart failure. In addition, carvedilol-treated patients were more likely to feel improved and less likely to have an adverse event.

STEPS IN CLINICAL AND HEMODYNAMIC STABILIZATION OF ACUTE HEART FAILURE

1. Administer oxygen ($\uparrow$ F$_i$O$_2$)

2. When accompanied by fluid volume overload or a "congestive" component

    Sublingual nitroglycerin

    Intravenous furosemide

    Consider morphine sulfate

    Consider additional preload-afterload reduction

3. Evaluate early for

    Readily reversible causes of acute heart failure (eg, cardiac dysrhythmias, pericardial tamponade). If present initiate appropriate intervention

    Myocardial ischemia-infarction. If present, promptly initiate appropriate interventions (eg, thrombolytic therapy)

4. If patient is refractory to above therapies, hypotensive, or in cardiogenic shock

    Consider fluid or intravenous inotropic and/or vasopressor agents

    Consider catheterization (pulmonary and systemic arterial)

    Obtain echocardiogram to assist in diagnosis, evaluation, and reparability of the culprit lesion or condition

    Consider need for mechanical circulatory assistance (intra-aortic balloon counterpulsation)

5. Proceed to definitive diagnostic and interventional procedures

FIGURE 4-55. The major steps in the initial management of acute heart failure are presented [58–77]. The interventions are arranged in the general order of application and according to the general types of acute heart failure encountered.

1) When possible, it is informative to obtain arterial blood for gas analysis before oxygen administration.

2) Sublingual nitroglycerin can be administered at a dose of 1 tablet (1 or 2 sprays) every 5 minutes three or four times until intravenous nitroglycerin or nitroprusside can take effect. Furosemide is usually administered in a dose range of 20 to 80 mg intravenously. Preload-afterload reduction beyond sublingual nitroglycerin is best achieved by intravenous administration of nitroglycerin or nitroprusside.

3) The medical history and electrocardiogram are obtained early in the evaluation of the patient with acute heart failure to determine whether myocardial ischemia-infarction is the underlying cause for the acute event and whether the patient is a candidate for acute intervention (eg, thrombolytic therapy, coronary angioplasty).

4) Dobutamine, dopamine, and norepinephrine represent the principal inotropic and/or vasopressor agents used in this clinical setting.

5) Once the patient's condition is stabilized, diagnostic and interventional procedures can be performed.

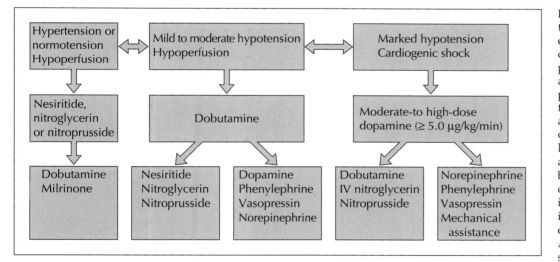

FIGURE 4-56. A practical working diagram of the cardiovascular support drugs commonly employed in the initial short-term management of acute or severe heart failure. It is assumed that patients who require these support drugs have adequate to high left ventricular diastolic filling pressures ($\geq$ 18 mm Hg) or clinical evidence of fluid volume overload. Systemic hypoperfusion and hypotension in a patient without evidence of volume overload or with filling pressures of less than 18 mm Hg should be approached with a fluid volume challenge as the first step. On the basis of the clinical presentation and the state of systemic perfusion and blood pressure, the initial drug of choice is selected and its dosage is increased until clinical or hemodynamic endpoints are achieved or adverse effects appear. At this point, inadequate improvement of clinical status usually requires either the addition of a second agent as combination therapy or mechanical assistance. IV—intravenous.

PRINCIPAL PRELOAD- AND AFTERLOAD-REDUCING DRUGS FOR ACUTE OR SEVERE HEART FAILURE

DRUG	DOSING	POTENTIAL ADVANTAGE	POTENTIAL DISADVANTAGES
Nitroglycerin	Sublingual: 1 tablet (or 1–2 sprays) × 3–4 at 5-min intervals Intravenous: 0.4 µg/kg/min initially; increase as needed	Favorable effect on coronary vasculature and in myocardial ischemia-infarction	Tolerance during prolonged infusion Fluid retention Inadequate afterload reduction in catastrophic cardiovascular disorders (eg, acute valvular insufficiency, ventricular rupture)
Nitroprusside	Intravenous: 0.2 µg/kg/min initially; increase as needed	Relatively powerful afterload reduction	Less favorable effect on coronary vasculature and myocardial ischemia; administration must be closely monitored to avoid marked hypotension; thiocyanate or cyanide toxicity during high-dose or prolonged infusions, particularly in patients with renal failure

FIGURE 4-57. Nitroglycerin and nitroprusside are the primary vasodilators employed to reduce excessive preload and afterload in acute or severe heart failure. Nitroglycerin is used most often, particularly in conditions caused by occlusive atherosclerotic coronary artery disease. Nitroprusside is the drug of choice when more aggressive afterload and preload reduction are needed; examples include catastrophic cardiovascular events (eg, acute, severe mitral or aortic regurgitation), hypertensive emergencies (eg, aortic dissection, pulmonary edema), and inadequate response to nitroglycerin.

PHARMACOLOGIC PROPERTIES AND THERAPEUTIC CONSIDERATIONS IN USING INOTROPIC-VASOPRESSOR AGENTS

PHARMACOLOGIC FEATURES	DOBUTAMINE	DOPAMINE LOW DOSE	DOPAMINE HIGH DOSE	NOREPINEPHRINE
Receptor agonism				
α	+	+	+++	++++
β_1	++++	+	++	+
β_2	++	0	0	0
Dopaminergic	0	+++	++	0
Systemic vascular resistance	↓↓	↓	↑↑	↑↑↑↑
Stroke volume and cardiac output	↑↑↑↑	↑	↑↑	↑
Ability to increase systemic blood pressure	→ to ↑	→	↑↑↑	↑↑↑↑
Ventricular filling pressure	↓↓	↓ to →	→ to ↑↑	→ to ↑↑
Chronotropic	→ to ↑↑	→	→ to ↑↑↑	→ to ↑
Myocardial oxygen demand/supply	→ to ↑	→	→ to ↑↑	→ to ↑↑

FIGURE 4-58. Principal pharmacologic properties and therapeutic considerations in the use of the major inotropic/vasopressor agents in acute or severe heart failure.

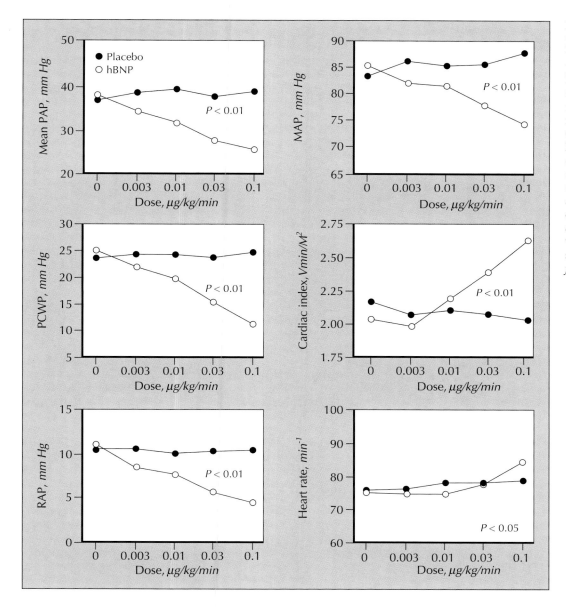

Figure 4-59. Synthetic human brain natriuretic peptide (hBNP) is undergoing clinical investigation as a vasodilator and natriuretic agent in patients with heart failure. In one phase II study, 20 patients with functional class II to IV heart failure and a mean ejection fraction of 20% were randomized in a double-blind crossover trial to receive 90-minute infusions of hBNP (0.003, 0.01, 0.03, and 0.1 µg/kg/min) or placebo. hBNP (*open circles*) caused dose-related decreases in mean pulmonary artery pressure (PAP), pulmonary capillary wedge pressure (PCWP), right atrial pressure (RAP), and mean arterial pressure (MAP). It caused an increase in cardiac index compared with placebo (*closed circles*) and a slight reduction in heart rate. Urine volume and sodium excretion also increased significantly during hBNP infusion. (*Adapted from* Marcus *et al.* [78].)

SELECTION OF CANDIDATES

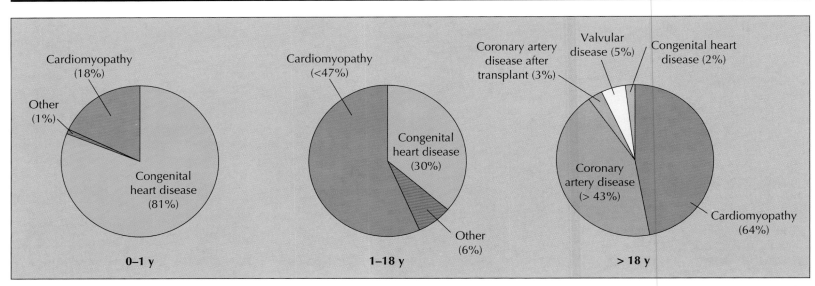

FIGURE 4-60. The primary diagnoses that lead to cardiac transplantation are indicated for candidates in three age groups, based on data that have been collected since 1981 by the Inter-national Registry for the Society of Heart and Lung Transplantation [77]. Congenital heart disease is the leading cause for infants, in whom viral cardiomyopathy is the second most common cause. Cardiomyopathy is the most common cause for older children. In adults, the relative proportion of cardiomyopathy is decreasing as more older patients with coronary artery disease are being considered for transplantation. Valvular heart disease and congenital heart disease in adults are less common indications. Retransplantation in previous transplant recipients, for which the indication is usually acceler-ated graft vasculopathy, accounts for at least 3% of hearts transplanted.

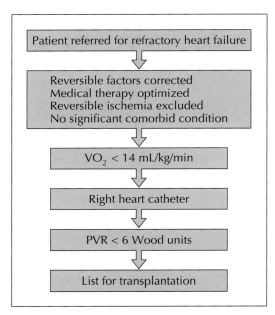

FIGURE 4-61. Proposed algorithm for cardiac transplantation recipient selection. All referred candidates should be New York Heart Association Class III or IV after optimization of medical therapy [79]. PVR—pulmonary vascular resistance.

INDICATIONS FOR SELECTION OF HEART TRANSPLANT RECIPIENTS

ACCEPTED INDICATIONS

Peak VO$_2$ ≤10 mL/kg/min
Severe ischemia limiting routine activity
Recent symptomatic ventricular arrhythmia

PROBABLE INDICATIONS

Peak VO$_2$ <14 mL/kg/min with major daily limitation
Recurrent unstable ischemia
Instability of fluid balance, renal function

INADEQUATE INDICATIONS

EF >20%
History of class III or IV symptoms
Previous ventricular arrhythmia
Peak VO$_2$ >15 mL/kg without other indications

Formal reevaluation recommended at 3–6 mo

FIGURE 4-62. Guidelines for recipient selection as summarized in the 24th Bethesda Conference [80]. The report emphasizes that "patients should not be considered to have refractory hemodynamic decompensation until therapy with intravenous followed by oral vasodilator and diuretic agents has been pursued using continuous hemodynamic monitoring to approach hemodynamic goals. Once reversible factors of decompensation and the adequacy of medical therapy have been thoroughly addressed, exercise capacity should be assessed by direct measurement of peak oxygen consumption."

Although absolute numbers for peak oxygen consumption (VO$_2$) are suggested as criteria, these should be considered in the context of the patient's age, gender, and evidence for achievement of an anaerobic threshold. The indication of symptomatic ischemia requires objective evidence of ischemia and full consideration of revascularization by means of angioplasty or bypass surgery, even if the ejection fraction (EF) is low. Instability of fluid balance and renal function is an indication only if it persists despite good patient compliance with salt restriction and a flexible regimen of diuretics guided by daily weights.

Low EF and a history of previous severe heart failure symptoms are not in themselves adequate indications for transplantation, because many patients with these descriptors can be maintained at a good functional level while receiving optimal medical therapy. Candidacy for cardiac transplantation should be considered a dynamic state from which a patient can be removed and to which he or she can be returned according to changes in condition. Reevaluation within 3 to 6 months from initial listing should include clinical assessment and repeat exercise testing if the patient appears clinically stable.

CONTRAINDICATIONS TO CARDIAC TRANSPLANTATION

Older age (usual limit 60–65 y)

Active infection

Severe diabetes mellitus with other end-organ disease

Pulmonary function < 60%* predicted,
  or chronic bronchitis

Serum creatinine > 2 mg/dL or clearance < 40 mL/min*

Bilirubin > 2.5 mg/dL, transaminases 2 × normal*

PAS > 60 mm Hg, TPG > 15 mm Hg*

High risk of life-threatening noncompliance

FIGURE 4-63. Specific contraindications to cardiac transplantation [80]. These vary slightly among programs, particularly with regard to age. Older patients have been shown in large studies to have a slightly higher mortality during extended follow-up [81–83]. Relative or borderline contraindications are usually weighed more heavily in the older potential candidate. Chronically elevated filling pressures lead to pulmonary hypertension and compromised pulmonary and hepatic function. Renal function is usually impaired to some degree in cardiac transplant candidates. Several days of intravenous therapy to optimize hemodynamics are frequently required to determine whether pulmonary hypertension and organ dysfunction (*asterisks*) are intrinsic or are secondary to hemodynamic compromise (and therefore presumably reversible). The patient and family are considered together as a unit that requires extensive psychological and social work evaluation regarding the potential for good outcome. Noncompliance remains a major cause of late mortality. PAS—pulmonary artery systolic pressure. TPG—transpulmonary gradient: mean pulmonary artery pressure minus capillary wedge pressure.

ASSESSMENT OF DONOR FOR HEART TRANSPLANTATION

Brain death
Age
  Up to 60 y
  Angiography performed
    after age 40–50 y
Cardiac function
  History of risk factors
  Recent insult
    Cause of death
    Anoxia
    Prolonged CPR
  Echocardiographic function
  Need for pressor support

Potential infection
  Acute infection
  Risk factors for AIDS
  Hepatitis
  CMV status
Compatibility with recipient
  Blood type
  Circulating antibodies
  Size

FIGURE 4-64. Considerations in the evaluation of a donor for heart transplantation [84]. Definitions of brain death vary among states. Age restrictions are being liberalized to expand the pool of donor hearts. A history of hypertension or smoking is a greater cause for concern in the older heart,

particularly in male donors. Angiography is frequently performed in the older hearts to determine the presence of coronary artery disease, for which hearts may be rejected; or, in cases of urgent candidate need, bypasses can sometimes be performed at the time of implantation. In the setting of brain injury and death, left ventricular function may be abnormal either globally or regionally, attributable to catecholamine surges and other endocrine derangement, and does not always recover. Cardiac abnormalities may be more often reversible in younger patients and in those with intracranial hemorrhage as opposed to head trauma.

Many potential donors require moderate support with dopamine or dobutamine, usually not exceeding 5 to 10 µg/kg/min, but the need for higher doses may indicate more severe cardiac injury, assuming that fluid replacement has been monitored adequately in the setting of the central diabetes insipidus that often occurs. Hearts from donors with active infection, such as bacteremia or pneumonia, may occasionally be accepted for a critically ill recipient. Risk factors for acquired immunodeficiency syndrome (AIDS) are usually contraindications. Hepatitis B infection is also a contraindication, but decisions regarding hepatitis C infection are still controversial. Evidence of previous cytomegalovirus (CMV) infection is common in both donors and recipients, who may be matched in the future for CMV status. Blood types between donor and recipient are matched as for transfusions. Except in rare cases of multiple sensitization, a donor heart is not given to a recipient with specific preformed antibodies against lymphocytes from that donor. Size matching remains controversial, usually within 20% body weight, depending on the urgency, relative heights of donor and recipient, and recipient cardiomegaly. CPR—cardiopulmonary resuscitation.

FIGURE 4-65. Recipient heart explantation in preparation for bicaval anastomoses rather than biatrial anastomoses, which have frequently been employed. The atrial septum and right atrium are resected with the ventricles of the diseased heart, leaving only a small cuff at the origin of the venae cavae. The left atrium is further resected, leaving a cuff of tissue around the ostia of the pulmonary veins. (*Adapted from* Kapoor and Laks [85].)

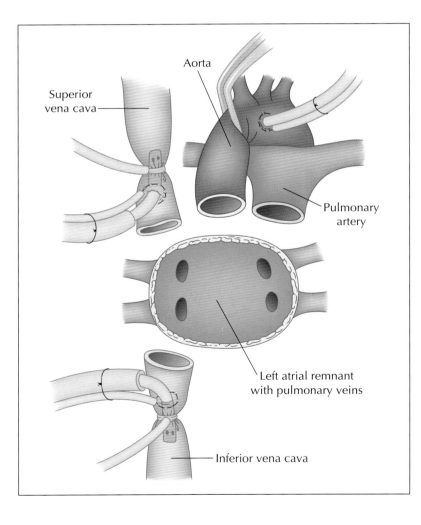

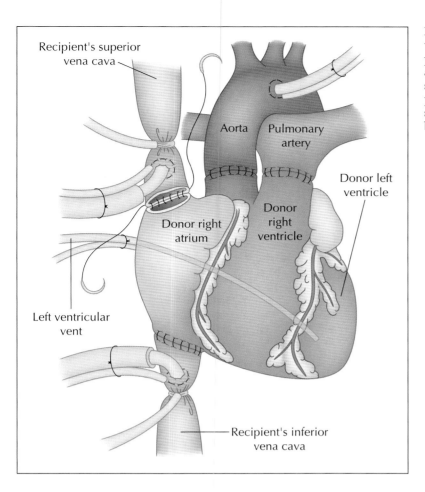

Recipient's superior vena cava

Aorta

Pulmonary artery

Donor left ventricle

Donor right atrium

Donor right ventricle

Left ventricular vent

Recipient's inferior vena cava

FIGURE 4-66. The left atrial anastomosis is completed and a left ventricular vent is inserted through the suture line. After the recipient and donor pulmonary artery anastomosis is completed except for the anterior part, the aortic anastomosis is completed. The heart is de-aired and modified reperfusion is instituted. During reperfusion the inferior vena caval anastomosis is performed. The heart is then de-aired and the cross-clamp is released. The superior vena caval anastomosis is then completed while the heart is beating. (*Adapted from* Kapoor and Laks [85].)

MANAGEMENT OF THE TRANSPLANT PATIENT

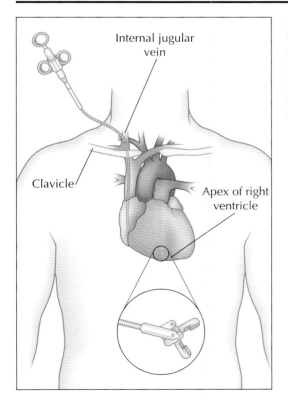

Internal jugular vein

Clavicle

Apex of right ventricle

FIGURE 4-67. Bioptome and access route for right ventricular endomyocardial biopsies from the superior vena cava. Improvements in disposable bioptomes, the instruments used to obtain biopsy specimens, now yield sample quality comparable to that of other bioptomes that require sterilization and sharpening. The majority of biopsies are performed through the right internal jugular approach, but scarring, thrombosis, and other technical problems sometimes necessitate the use of the left internal jugular, subclavian, or femoral veins. With repeated biopsies, some tissue specimens reveal only fibrosis from old biopsy sites. Three to four pieces containing at least 50% myocytes are required for 90% to 95% confidence in the interpretation [86].

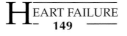

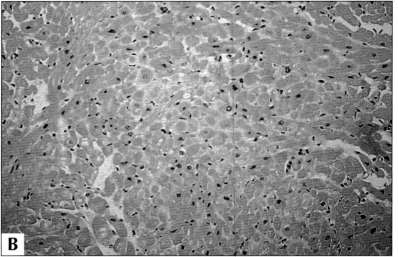

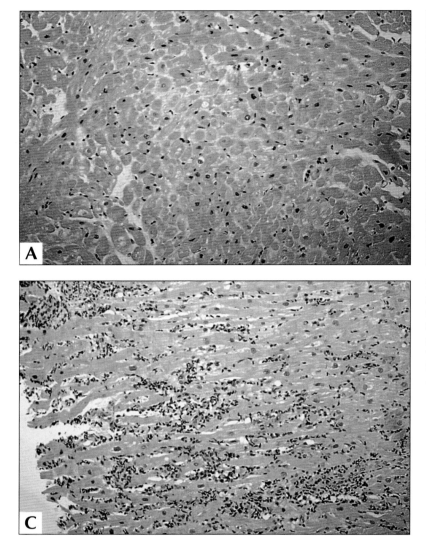

FIGURE 4-68. A–C, Right ventricular endomyocardial biopsy specimens stained with hematoxylin and eosin, demonstrating normal myocardium (A), mild rejection with focal lymphocyte infiltrate without evidence of myocyte necrosis (grade 1) (B), and moderate rejection demonstrating more intensive lymphocytic infiltration with evidence of myocyte vacuolization and loss (grade 3) (C). The refinements of grading relate to the extent of involvement in different areas and samples. (*Courtesy of* Jon A. Kobashigawa, Los Angeles, CA.)

SAMPLE REGIMEN OF MEDICATIONS AFTER TRANSPLANTATION

Cyclosporine	Clotrimazole troches
Azathioprine	Trimethoprim-sulfamethoxazole
Prednisone	HMG-CoA reductase inhibitor
Diltiazem or ACE inhibitor	Aspirin
Furosemide	Calcium carbonate
H_2-receptor blocker	Vitamin D

FIGURE 4-69. Typical regimen of medications for 4 months after cardiac transplantation. In addition to immunosuppressive medications, approximately 75% of patients require drug therapy for hypertension, often with diltiazem, which decreases the metabolism and cost of cyclosporine and may decrease coronary artery disease, and/or an ACE inhibitor. A loop diuretic is required to control fluid retention in most patients during the first 6 months and is less commonly required thereafter. Ranitidine or cimetidine is commonly given to decrease gastrointestinal side effects of prednisone. Clotrimazole troches are used to decrease mucosal candidiasis during the first 3 months. Trimethoprim-sulfamethoxazole may be given twice weekly to decrease the incidence of *Pneumocystis carinii* pneumonia during the first 6 months. Both prophylactic antibiotics may be resumed briefly after subsequent therapy for rejection. There is increasing interest in lowering cholesterol in transplant recipients, who respond well to HMG-CoA reductase inhibitors but require lower doses and careful monitoring to avoid rhabdomyolysis [87]. Aspirin is often used to decrease platelet aggregation as a potential factor in the vasculopathy. Calcium and vitamin D are recommended in postmenopausal women and other patients with decreased bone density, which can result from cyclosporine and corticosteroid use. HMG-CoA—hepatic hydromethylglutaryl coenzyme A; H_2—histamine$_2$.

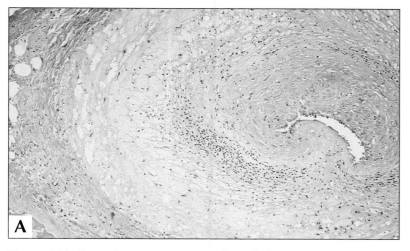

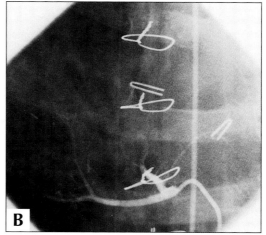

FIGURE 4-70. Transplantation coronary allograft disease (TCAD). The major cause of late death after cardiac transplantation is the development of TCAD, a unique, accelerated form of coronary artery disease. By 1 year posttransplant, about 30% of patients demonstrate some TCAD, and the incidence and severity continue to increase with time [88]. The pathogenesis of TCAD is thought to begin with immunologic and nonimmunologic injury to the arterial endothelium, with resultant loss of endothelial integrity [89]. Microthrombi, cellular proliferation, and plasma lipids accumulate at the site of the injured intima. **A,** This leads to further cellular proliferation and finally profound myointimal hyperplasia leding to diffuse coronary artery lumen narrowing. **B,** Selective left coronary angiography from a patient with severe TCAD, which shows diffuse tapering of the left anterior descending and circumflex arteries as well as pruning of all the secondary vessels. Immunologic mechanisms resulting in endothelial injury include both cellular and humoral factors [90]. Nonimmunologic risk factors also contribute to the development of cardiac allograft vasculopathy. Recipient age and gender, donor age and gender, obesity, hyperlipidemia, and donor ischemic time may impact on the development of vasculopathy [91]. An association has also been found between the presence of active cytomegalovirus infection and the development of vasculopathy [92]. Given the diffuse, concentric nature of this disease, percutaneous transluminal coronary angioplasty and coronary artery bypass grafting are not useful strategies for management. Unfortunately, patients with TCAD have a fivefold greater risk of cardiac events such as myocardial infarction, severe refractory heart failure, and sudden death. Presently retransplantation is the only treatment for severe TCAD; however survival after repeat transplantation is significantly reduced. Consequently, preventative strategies have assumed clinical importance. Hyperlipidemia management with HMG Co-A (3-hydroxy-3-methylglutaryl-coenzyme A) reductase inhibitors and routine aspirin use are two such approaches.

SURVIVAL

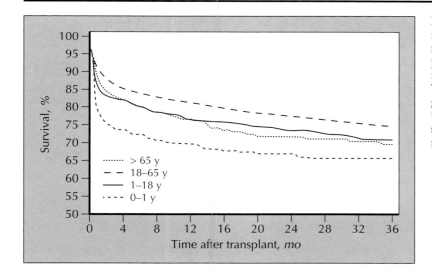

FIGURE 4-71. Actuarial survival according to recipient age, calculated from 15,000 heart transplant recipients in the Registry from the International Society of Heart and Lung Transplantation [81]. Neonatal transplants are associated with a poorer survival, as are those performed in recipients over 65 years of age. Five-year survival for adults is now 68%. The first-year survival in the Registry may continue to improve as a greater proportion of patients followed have received cyclosporine from the time of transplantation. There will be less improvement in later survival, largely limited by transplant vasculopathy, which has *not* been noticeably decreased in the cyclosporine era [82]. (*Adapted from* Kaye [81].)

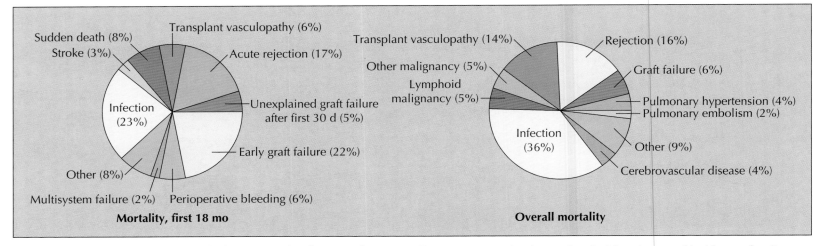

Mortality, first 18 mo

- Sudden death (8%)
- Stroke (3%)
- Transplant vasculopathy (6%)
- Acute rejection (17%)
- Infection (23%)
- Unexplained graft failure after first 30 d (5%)
- Early graft failure (22%)
- Other (8%)
- Multisystem failure (2%)
- Perioperative bleeding (6%)

Overall mortality

- Transplant vasculopathy (14%)
- Other malignancy (5%)
- Lymphoid malignancy (5%)
- Infection (36%)
- Rejection (16%)
- Graft failure (6%)
- Pulmonary hypertension (4%)
- Pulmonary embolism (2%)
- Other (9%)
- Cerebrovascular disease (4%)

FIGURE 4-72. Causes of death during the first 18 months after transplantation and overall. The data for the first 18 months are derived from the Cardiac Transplant Research Database and include 911 patients who underwent transplantation between January 1990 and June 1991 [93]. Early graft failure can be caused by hyperacute or early rejection, acute right heart failure, poor donor selection, or poor preservation of the donor heart. The causes of overall mortality reflect the Stanford experience with 310 patients who underwent transplantation with cyclosporine since 1980 [82].

Immunosuppression is associated with an increased incidence of malignancy, particularly lymphoproliferative disorders, of which the majority in transplant recipients are B-cell lymphomas with a predilection for extranodal sites [94]. Death from transplant vasculopathy accounts for an increasing proportion of late mortality as the frequency of death from acute rejection and infection declines. Sudden cardiac death, which accounts for 5% to 10% of mortality, is usually attributed to rejection in the first year after transplantation and to transplant vasculopathy in the subsequent years.

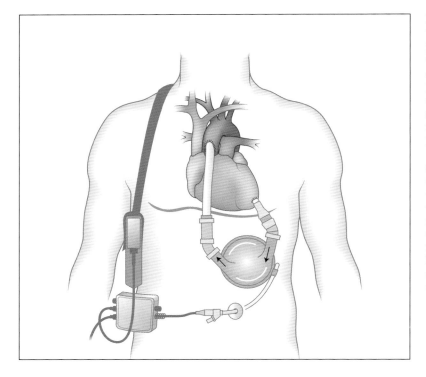

FIGURE 4-73. This electrical-powered device is still undergoing clinical trials. This device requires an external power source. Two external portable batteries linked via the external drive lines provide 6 to 8 hours of power and thus render patients free to engage in a variety of indoor and outdoor activities while awake. Overnight, the patients are linked to a power base station. The Novacor system (not shown) is the other most commonly used left ventricular assist device (LVAD) bridge. The Novacor system does not contain a textured surface. Despite anticoagulation, the incidence of embolic cardiovascular accidents remains high with the present Novacor system.

At the Columbia-Presbyterian Medical Center in New York, the TCI system has been used in 111 patients as a bridge to transplantation. A total of 72 patients (65%) successfully proceeded to transplantation, 27 patients (24%) died while on LVAD support, 5 patients (4.5%) were explanted, and the remainder are awaiting cardiac transplantation. Causes of mortality following LVAD insertion include infection, right heart failure, bleeding complications, and embolic events. With refinement of selection criteria for suitable device candidates, mortality continues to decrease. Moreover, because of the rapidly evolving technology, the possibility for completely implantable devices appears promising in the not-too-distant future. (*Adapted from* Rose and Goldstein [95].)

REFERENCES

1. Katz AM: Congestive heart failure: role of altered myocardial cellular control. *N Engl J Med* 1975, 293:1184–1191.

2. Katz AM: *Physiology of the Heart*, edn 2. New York: Raven Press; 1992.

3. Katz AM: *Physiology of the Heart*, edn 3. Philadelphia: Lippincott Williams & Wilkins; 2001.

4. Ross J: Afterload mismatch and preload reserve: a conceptual framework for the analysis of ventricular function. *Prog Cardiovasc Dis* 1976, 18:255–264.

5. Lee JD, Tajimi T, Ptritti J, *et al.*: Preload reserve and mechanisms of afterload mismatch in normal conscious dog. *Am J Physiol* 1986, 250:H464–H473.

6. Swynghedauw B, Moalic JM, Delcayre C: The origins of cardiac hypertrophy. In *Research in Cardiac Hypertrophy and Failure*. Edited by Swynghedauw B. London: INSERM/John Libbey Eurotext; 1990:23–50.

7. Gaasch WH, Levine HJ, Quinones NM, *et al.*: Left ventricular compliance: mechanisms and clinical implications. *Am J Cardiol* 1976, 38:645–653.

8. Zile MR: Diastolic dysfunction: detection, consequences, and treatment: II. Diagnosis and treatment of diastolic dysfunction. *Mod Concepts Cardiovasc Dis* 1990, 59:1.

9. Grossman W, Carabello BA, Gunther S, *et al.*: Ventricular wall stress and the development of cardiac hypertrophy and failure. In *Perspectives in Cardiovascular Research. Myocardial Hypertrophy and Failure*, vol 7. Edited by Alpert NR. New York: Raven Press; 1993:1–15.

10. Beuckelmann DJ, Nabauer M, Erdmann E: Intracellular calcium handling in isolated ventricular myocytes from patients with terminal heart failure. *Circulation* 1992, 85:1046–1055.

11. Olivetti G, Abbi R, Quaini F, *et al.*: Apoptosis in the failing human heart. *N Engl J Med* 1997, 336:1131–1141.

12. Vanhoutte PM, Luscher TF: Peripheral mechanisms in cardiovascular regulation: transmitters, receptors and the endothelium. In *Handbook of Hypertension*, vol 8. Edited by Tarazi RC, Zanchetti A. Amsterdam: Elsevier Science Publishers; 1986:96–123.

13. Paganelli WC, Creager MA, Dzau VJ: Cardiac regulation of renal function. In *The International Textbook of Cardiology*. Edited by Cheng TO. New York: Pergammon Press; 1986:1010–1020.

14. Cohn JN, Levine B, Olivari MT, *et al.*: Plasma norepinephrine as a guide to prognosis in patients with chronic congestive heart failure. *N Engl J Med* 1984, 311:819–823.

15. Bristow MR: Changes in myocardial and vascular receptors in heart failure. *J Am Coll Cardiol* 1993, 22:61A–71A.

16. Communal C, Singh K, Pimentel DR, Colucci WS: Norepinephrine stimulates apoptosis in adult rat ventricular myocytes by activation of the β-adrenergic pathway. *Circ Res* 1998

17. Hirsch AT, Talsness CE, Schunkert H, *et al.*: Tissue-specific activation of cardiac angiotensin-converting enzyme in experimental heart failure. *Circ Res* 1991, 69:475–482.

18. Lindpainter K, Lu W, Niedermajer N, *et al.*: Selective activation of cardiac angiotensinogen gene expression in post-infarction ventricular remodeling in the rat. *J Mol Cell Cardiol* 1993, 25:133–143.

19. Meggs LG, Coupet J, Huang H, *et al.*: Regulation of angiotensin II receptors on ventricular myocytes after myocardial infarction in rats. *Circ Res* 1993, 72:1149–1162.

20. Wilkins MR, Redondo J, Brown LA: The natriuretic-peptide family. *Lancet* 1997, 349:1307–1310.

21. Underwood RD, Chan DP, Burnett JC: Endothelin: an endothelium derived vasoconstrictor peptide and its role in congestive heart failure. *Heart Failure* 1991, 7:50–58.

22. Cody RJ, Haas GJ, Binkley PF, *et al.*: Plasma endothelin correlates with the extent of the pulmonary hypertension in patients with chronic congestive heart failure. *Circulation* 1992, 85:504–509.

23. Bryant D, Becker L, Richardson J, *et al.*: Cardiac failure in transgenic mice with myocardial expression of tumor necrosis factor-α. *Circulation* 1998, 97:1375–1381.

24. Torre-Amione G, Kapadia S, Benedict C, *et al.*: Proinflammatory cytokine levels in patients with depressed left ventricular ejection fraction: a report from the Studies of Left Ventricular Dysfunction (SOLVD). *J Am Coll Cardiol* 1996, 27:1201–1206.

25. Ho KKL, Pinsky JL, Kannel WB, *et al.*: The epidemiology of heart failure: the Framingham Study. *J Am Coll Cardiol* 1993, 22(suppl A):6A–13A.

26. Kannel WB, Belanger AJ: Epidemiology of heart failure. *Am Heart J* 1991, 121:951–957.

27. McKee PA, Castelli WP, McNamara PM, *et al.*: The natural history of congestive heart failure: the Framingham Study. *N Engl J Med* 1971, 285:1441–1446.

28. Ho KKL, Anderson KM, Kannell WB, *et al.*: Survival after the onset of congestive heart failure in Framingham Heart Study subjects. *Circulation* 1993, 88:107–115.

29. Kessler KM: Heart failure with normal systolic function: update of prevalence, differential diagnosis, prognosis, and therapy [editorial]. *Arch Intern Med* 1988, 148:2109–2111.

30. Goldsmith SR, Dick C: Differentiating systolic from diastolic heart failure: pathophysiologic and therapeutic considerations. *Am J Med* 1993, 95:645–655.

31. Kitzman DW, Higginbotham MB, Cobb FR, *et al.*: Exercise intolerance in patients with heart failure and preserved left ventricular systolic function: failure of the Frank-Starling mechanism. *J Am Coll Cardiol* 1991, 17:1065–1072.

32. Litwin SE, Grossman W: Diastolic dysfunction as a cause of heart failure. *J Am Coll Cardiol* 1993, 22(suppl A):49A–55A.

33. Felker GM, Thompson RE, Hare JM, *et al.*: Underlying causes and long-term survival in patients with initially unexplained cardiomyopathy. *N Engl J Med* 2000, 342:1077–1084.

34. Bart BA, Shaw LK, McCants CB, Jr., *et al.*: Clinical determinants of mortality in patients with angiographically diagnosed ischemic or nonischemic cardiomyopathy. *J Am Coll Cardiol* 1997, 30:1002–1008.

35. Califf RM, Bounous P, Harrell FE, *et al.*: The prognosis in the presence of coronary artery disease. In *Congestive Heart Failure: Current Research and Clinical Applications*. Edited by Braunwald E, Mock B, Watson JT. New York: Grune & Stratton; 1982:31–40.

36. Cohn JN, Johnson GR, Shabetai R, *et al.*: Ejection fraction, peak exercise oxygen consumption, cardiothoracic ratio, ventricular arrhythmias, and plasma norepinephrine as determinants of prognosis in heart failure. *Circulation* 1993, 87(suppl VI):5–16.

37. Kelly RA, Smith TW: Treatement of stable heart failure: digitalis and diuretics. In *Atlas of Heart Diseases: Hypertension: Mechanisms and Therapy*. Edited by Braunwald E, Colucci WS. Philadelphia; Current Medicine; 1995:10.1–10.16.

38. CONSENSUS Trial Study Group: Effects of enalapril on mortality in severe congestive heart failure. *N Engl J Med* 1987, 316:1429–1435.

39. The SOLVD Investigators: Effect of enalapril on survival in patients with reduced left ventricular ejection fractions and congestive heart failure. *N Engl J Med* 1991, 325:293–302.

40. Kleber FX, Niemoller L, Doering W: Impact of converting enzyme inhibition on progression of chronic CHF: results of the Munich Mild CHF Trial. *Br Heart J* 1992, 67:289–296.

41. McKay RG, Pfeffer MA, Pasternal RC, *et al.*: Left ventricular remodeling after myocardial infarction: a corollary to infarct expansion. *Circulation* 1986, 74:693–702.

42. Pfeffer MA, Braunwald E, Moy LA, *et al.* on behalf of the SAVE Investigators: Effect of captopril on mortality and morbidity in patients with left ventricular dysfunction after myocardial infarction: results of the Survival and Ventricular Enlargement Trial. *N Engl J Med* 1992, 327:669–677.

43. Acute Infarction Ramipril Efficacy (AIRE) Study Investigators: Effect of ramipril on mortality and morbidity of survivors of acute myocardial infarction with clinical evidence of CHF. *Lancet* 1993, 342:821–827.

44. Cohn J, Tognoni G, Valsartan Heart Failure Trial Investigators: A randomized trial of the angiotensin receptor blocker valsartan in chronic heart failure. *N Engl J Med* 2001, 345:1667–1675.

45. Pfeffer MA, Swedberg K, Granger CB, *et al.*: Effects of candesartan on mortality and morbidity in patients with chronic heart failure: the CHARM-Overall programme. *Lancet* 2003, 362:759–766.

46. Granger CB, McMurray JJ, Yusuf S, *et al.*: Effects of candesartan in patients with chronic heart failure and reduced left-ventricular systolic function intolerant to angiotensin-converting enzyme inhibitors: the CHARM-Alternative trial. *Lancet* 2003, 362:772–776.

47. McMurray JJ, Ostergren J, Swedberg K, *et al.*: Effects of candesartan in patients with chronic heart failure and reduced left-ventricular systolic function taking angiotensin-converting enzyme inhibitors: the CHARM-Added trial. *Lancet* 2003, 362:767–771.

48. Yusuf S, Pfeffer MA, Swedberg K, *et al.*: Effects of candesartan in patients with chronic heart failure and preserved left-ventricular ejection fraction: the CHARM-Preserved trial. *Lancet* 2003, 362:777–781.

49. Pfeffer MA, McMurray JJ, Velazquez EJ, *et al.*, Valsartan in Acute Myocardial Infarction Trial Investigators: Valsartan, captopril, or both in myocardial infarction complicated by heart failure, left ventricular dysfunction, or both. *N Engl J Med* 2003, 349:1893–1906.

50. Pitt B, Zannad F, Remme WJ, *et al.*: The effect of spironolactone on morbidity and mortality in patients with severe heart failure randomized aldactone evaluation study investigators. *N Engl J Med* 1999, 341:709–717.

51. Pitt B, Remme W, Zannad F, *et al.*: Eplerenone, a selective aldosterone blocker, in patients with left ventricular dysfunction after myocardial infarction. *N Engl J Med* 2003, 348:1309–1321.

52. Digitalis Investigation Group: The effect of digoxin on mortality and morbidity in patients with heart failure. The Digitalis Investigation Group (DIG) Trial. *N Engl J Med* 1997, 336:525–533.

53. Packer M, Bristow MR, Cohn JN, *et al.*: The effect of carvedilol on morbidity and mortality in patients with chronic heart failure. US Carvedilol Heart Failure Study Group. *N Engl J Med* 1996, 334:1349–1355.

54. Bristow MR, Gilbert EM, Abraham WT, *et al.*: Cavedilol produces dose-related improvements in left ventricular function and survival in subjects with chronic heart failure. MOCHA Investigators. *Circulation* 1996, 94:2807–2816.

55. MERIT-HF Study Group: Effect of metoprolol CR/XL in chronic heart failure: Metoprolol CR/XL Randomized Intervention Trial in Congestive Heart Failure. *Lanet* 1999; 353:1471–1472.

56. Hall SA, Cigarroa CG, Marcoux L, *et al.*: Time course of improvement in left ventricular function, mass, and geometry in patients with congestive heart failure treated with beta-adrenergic blockade. *J Am Coll Cardiol* 1995; 25:1154–1161.

57. Packer M, Coats AJ, Fowler MB, *et al.*: Effect of carvedilol on survival in severe chronic heart failure. *N Engl J Med* 2001, 344:1651–1658.

58. Leier CV, Bambach D, Thompson MJ, *et al.*: Central and regional hemodynamic effects of intravenous isosorbide dinitrate, nitroglycerin, and nitroprusside in patients with congestive heart failure. *Am J Cardiol* 1981, 48:1115–1123.

59. Franciosa JA, Guiha NH, Limas CL, *et al.*: Improved left ventricular function during nitroprusside infusion in acute myocardial infarction. *Lancet* 1972, 1:650–654.

60. Miller RR, Vismara LA, Zelis R, *et al.*: Clinical use of sodium nitroprusside in chronic ischemic heart disease. *Circulation* 1975, 51:328–336.

61. Leier CV: Acute inotropic support: intravenously administered positive inotropic drugs. In *Cardiotonic Drugs*, edn 2. Edited by Leier CV. New York: Marcel Dekker; 1991:63–106.

62. Francis GS, Sharma B, Hodges M: Comparative hemodynamic effects of dopamine and dobutamine in patients with acute cardiogenic circulatory collapse. *Am Heart J* 1982, 103:995–1000.

63. Leier CV, Heban PT, Huss P, *et al.*: Comparative systemic and regional hemodynamic effects of dopamine and dobutamine in patients with heart failure. *Circulation* 1978, 58:466–475.

64. Loeb HS, Winslow EBJ, Rahimtoola SH, *et al.*: Acute hemodynamic effects of dopamine in patients with shock. *Circulation* 1971, 44:163–173.

65. Holzer J, Karliner JS, O'Rourke RA, *et al.*: Effectiveness of dopamine in patients with cardiogenic shock. *Am J Cardiol* 1973, 32:79–84.

66. Beregovich J, Bianchi C, Rubler S, *et al.*: Dose-related hemodynamic and renal effects of dopamine in congestive heart failure. *Am Heart J* 1974, 87:550–557.

67. Forrester JS, Diamond G, Chatterjee K, *et al.*: Medical therapy of acute myocardial infarction by application of hemodynamic subsets. *N Engl J Med* 1976, 295:1356–1362, 1404–1413.

68. Scheidt S, Ascheim R, Killip T III: Shock after acute myocardial infarction: a clinical and hemodynamic profile. *Am J Cardiol* 1970, 26:556–564.

69. Alonso DR, Scheidt S, Post M, *et al.*: Pathophysiology of cardiogenic shock: quantification of myocardial necrosis, clinical, pathologic and electrocardiographic correlations. *Circulation* 1973, 48:558–596.

70. Gutovitz AL, Sobel BE, Roberts R: Progressive nature of myocardial injury in selected patients with cardiogenic shock. *Am J Cardiol* 1978, 41:469–475.

71. Hands ME, Rutherford JD, Muller JE, *et al.*: The in-hospital development of cardiogenic shock after myocardial infarction: incidence, predictors of occurrence, outcome and prognostic factors. *J Am Coll Cardiol* 1989, 14:40–46.

72. Goldberg RJ, Gore JM, Alpert JS, *et al.*: Cardiogenic shock after acute myocardial infarction. *N Engl J Med* 1991, 325:1117–1122.

73. Sander CA, Buckley MJ, Leinbach RC, *et al.*: Mechanical circulatory assistance: current status and experience with combining circulatory assistance, emergency coronary angiography, and acute myocardial revascularization. *Circulation* 1972, 45:1291–1313.

74. Bardet J, Masquet C, Kahn J-C, *et al.*: Clinical and hemodynamic results of intra-aortic balloon counterpulsation and surgery for cardiogenic shock. *Am Heart J* 1977, 93:280–288.

75. Johnson SA, Scanlon PJ, Loeb HS, *et al.*: Treatment of cardiogenic shock in myocardial infarction by intra-aortic balloon counter-pulsation and surgery. *Am J Med* 1977, 62:687–692.

76. O'Rourke MF, Sammel N, Chang VP: Arterial counterpulsation in severe refractory heart failure complicating acute myocardial infarction. *Br Heart J* 1979, 41:308–316.

77. DeWood MA, Notski RN, Hensely GR, *et al.*: Intra-aortic balloon counter-pulsation with and without reperfusion for myocardial infarction shock. *Circulation* 1980, 61:1105–1112.

78. Marcus LS, Hart D, Packer M, *et al.*: Hemodynamic and renal excretory effects of human brain natriuretic peptide infusion in patients with congestive heart failure: a double-blind, placebo-controlled, randomized crossover trial. *Circulation* 1996, 94:3184–3189.

79. Costanzo MR: Selection and treatment of candidates for heart transplantation: a statement for health professionald from the Committee on Heart Failure and Cardiac Transplantation of the Council on Clinical Cardiology, American Heart Association. *Circulation* 1995, 92:3593–3612.

80. Mudge GH, Goldstein S, Addonizio LJ, *et al.*: Bethesda Conference on Transplantation Task Force 3: recipient guidelines/prioritization. *J Am Coll Cardiol* 1993; 22:21–31.

81. Kaye MP: Registry of the International Society for Heart and Lung Transplantation: Tenth Official Report—1003. *J Heart Lung Transplant* 1993, 12:541–548.

82. Grattan MT, Moreno-Cabral CE, Starnes VA, *et al.*: Eight-year results of cyclosporine-treated patients with cardiac transplants. *J Thorac Cardiovasc Surg* 1990, 99:500–509.

83. Sharples LD, Caine N, Mullins P, *et al.*: Risk factor analysis for the major hazards following heart transplantation: rejection, infection, and coronary occlusive disease. *Transplantation* 1991, 52:244–252.

84. Baldwin JC, Anderson JL, Boucek MM, *et al.*: Bethesda Conference on Transplantation Task Force 2: donor guidelines. *J Am Coll Cardiol* 1993, 22:14–20.

85. Kapoor AS, Laks H: *Atlas of Heart-Lung Transplantation*. New York: McGraw-Hill; 1994.

86. Billingham ME, Cary NRB, Hammond ME, *et al.*: A working formulation for the standardization of nomenclature in the diagnosis of heart and lung rejection: Heart Rejection Study Group. *J Heart Transplant* 1990, 9:587–593.

87. Kobashigawa JA, Murphy FL, Stevenson LW, *et al.*: Low-dose lovastatin safely lowers cholesterol after cardiac transplantation. *Circulation* 1990, 82:IV-281–IV-283.

88. Michler RE, McLaughlin MJ, Chen JM, *et al.*: Clinical experience with cardiac retransplantation. *J Thorac Cardiovasc Surg* 1993, 106:622–629.

89. Ventura HO, Mehra MR, Smart FW, Stapleton DD: Cardiac allograft vasculopathy: current concepts. *Am Heart J* 1995, 129:791–798.

90. Costanzo-Nordin MR: Cardiac allograft vasculopathy: relationship with acute cellular rejection and histocompatibility. *J Heart Lung Transplant* 1992, 11(suppl):90–104.

91. Johnson MR: Transplant coronary artery disease: nonimmunologic risk factors. *J Heart Lung Transplant* 1992, 11(suppl)124–132.

92. McDonald K, Rector TS, Braunlin EA, *et al.*: Association of coronary artery disease in transplant recipients with cytomegalovirus infection. *Am J Cardiol* 1989, 64:359–362.

93. Bourge RC, Naftel DC, Costanzo-Nordin MR, *et al.*: Pre-transplantation risk factors for death after heart transplantation: a multi-institutional study. *J Heart Lung Transplant* 1993, 12:549–562.

94. Penn I: Cancers after cyclosporine therapy. *Transplant Proc* 1988, 30:276–279.

95. Rose EA, Goldstein DJ: Wearable long-term mechanical support for patients with end-stage heart disease: a tenable goal. *Ann Thorac Surg* 1996, 61:399–402.

CARDIOMYOPATHY, MYOCARDITIS, AND PERICARDIAL DISEASE

Edited by Kenneth L. Baughman

CHAPTER 5

Aftab A. Ansari, Noble Fowler, James J. Glazier, Ahvie Herskowitz, Yuzo Hirota, Ralph H. Hruban, Edward K. Kasper, Allan D. Kitching, Joseph K. Perloff, Harry Rakowski, E. Douglas Wigle

Cardiomyopathies are among the most common causes of both systolic and diastolic heart failure. The most common forms of cardiomyopathy are hypertrophic, dilated, and restricted.

HYPERTROPHIC CARDIOMYOPATHY

Hypertrophic cardiomyopathy (HCM) is characterized by left ventricular hypertrophy without apparent cause. Asymmetric hypertrophy and myocardial disarray are important pathologic features.

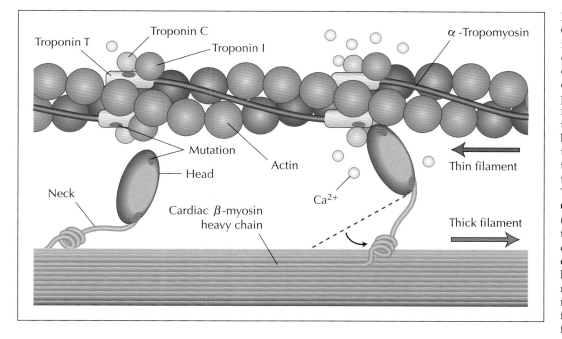

FIGURE 5-1. Components of the myofiber. Cardiac muscle is composed of myosin (thick filament) and actin (thin filament) layers as depicted in this illustration. Cardiac contraction occurs when calcium binds the troponin complex (subunits I, C, and T) and α-tropomyosin and releases the inhibition of the myosin-actin interactions maintained by troponin I. ATPase activity and binding of actin by the globular myosin head causes a conformational change that bends the neck (lever arm) of the thick filament, resulting in sliding of the thick filament in relation to the thin filament. This movement results in cardiac contraction. Genetic alterations in the sarcomeric proteins (including cardiac [beta] myosin heavy chain, troponin T, troponin I, α-tropomyosin, and cardiac myosin binding protein C) may cause an enhancement of contractile function resulting in hypertrophic cardiomyopathy. Alternatively, mutations in the myosin or actin components may cause reduced production of contractile force by the sarcomere resulting in a genetic form of dilated cardiomyopathy [1].

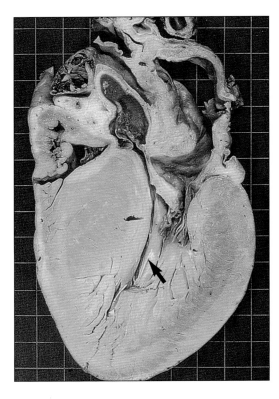

FIGURE 5-2. Asymmetric septal hypertrophy. Longitudinal section of the heart of a 32-year-old woman with subaortic obstructive hypertrophic cardiomyopathy who died suddenly while on propranolol therapy. Hemodynamic investigation confirmed subaortic obstruction as well as mitral regurgitation. The regurgitation was partially due to an abnormal mitral valve (insertion of an anomalous papillary muscle (*arrow*) onto the ventricular surface of the anterior mitral leaflet). Note the asymmetric hypertrophy with a grossly thickened ventricular septum. A narrowed outflow tract between the upper septum and the anterior mitral leaflet, which is thickened and fibrosed from repeated contact with the septum, can also be seen. There was microscopic evidence of extensive myocardial fiber disarray involving the septum and free wall of the left ventricle [2]. (*Courtesy of* L. Horlick.)

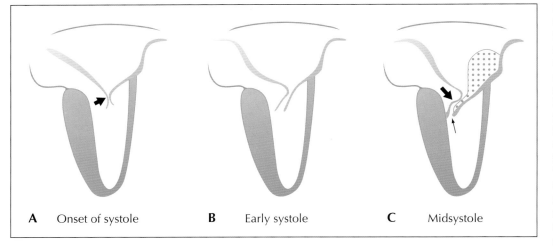

FIGURE 5-3. Myocardial fiber disarray. Microscopic section of the ventricular septum of a 28-year-old patient with hypertrophic cardiomyopathy who died while jogging. This section shows a typical area of myocardial fiber disarray. The muscle cells are short and plump, and the nuclei are large and hyperchromatic. Note the extensive amount of loose intercellular connective tissue that may become transformed into diffuse myocardial fibrosis late in the disease (magnification, × 100). (*From* Wigle *et al.* [2]; with permission.)

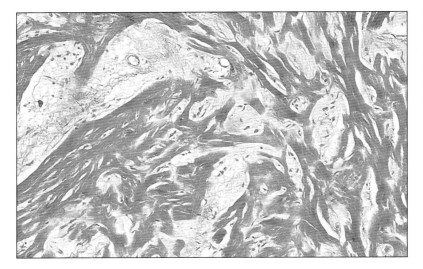

| A | Onset of systole | B | Early systole | C | Midsystole |

FIGURE 5-4. Functional anatomy of mitral leaflet systolic anterior motion and mitral regurgitation in subaortic obstructive hypertrophic cardiomyopathy. Drawing of a transesophageal echocardiogram (frontal long-axis plane) demonstrating the anterior and superior motion of the anterior mitral leaflet to produce mitral leaflet–septal contact and failure of leaflet coaptation in midsystole. **A,** At the onset of systole, the coaptation point (*arrow*) is in the body of the anterior and posterior leaflets rather than at the tip of the leaflets, as in normal subjects [3,4]. The portion of the leaflets beyond the coaptation point is referred to as the residual length of the leaflet [3,4]. During early systole (**B**) and midsystole (**C**) there is anterior and superior movement of the residual length of the anterior mitral leaflet (*thick arrow* in C), with septal contact and failure of leaflet coaptation (*thin arrow* in C) with consequent mitral regurgitation directed posteriorly into the left atrium (*dotted area*). (*Adapted from* Grigg *et al.* [4].)

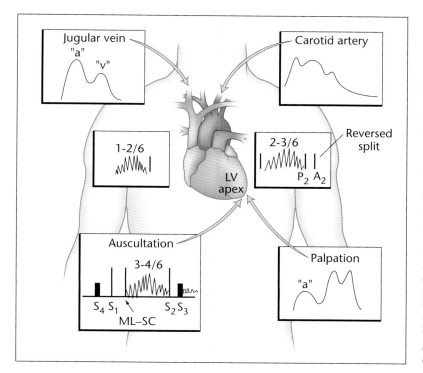

FIGURE 5-5. Physical examination in subaortic obstructive hypertrophic cardiomyopathy (HCM). There are seven physical signs in subaortic obstructive HCM that are not found in nonobstructive HCM. On palpation, a spike-and-dome arterial pulse can often be felt in the carotid artery or in a peripheral pulse. On palpation of the left ventricular (LV) apex, there may be a triple apex beat caused by a palpable left atrial gallop and a double systolic impulse—one impulse comes before the onset of obstruction and the other after. On auscultation, at or just medial to the LV apex, there is a late onset, diamond-shaped systolic murmur of grade 3 to 4/6 in intensity. This murmur is caused by both the subaortic obstruction and the concomitant mitral regurgitation, causing the murmur to radiate to both the left sternal border and to the axilla. Because of the mitral regurgitation, there is often a short diastolic inflow murmur after the third heart sound. Rarely, a mitral leaflet– septal contact (ML–SC) sound may be heard preceding the systolic murmur at the apex. Finally, if there is severe subaortic obstruction, reversed splitting of the second heart sound may occur. In nonobstructive HCM, there is often a third or fourth heart sound at the apex, depending on the type of diastolic dysfunction. If the fourth heart sound is palpable, there will be a double apex beat, which is quite different in timing and significance from the double *systolic* apex beat that occurs in subaortic obstructive HCM. In nonobstructive HCM, there is either no apical systolic murmur or at most a grade 1 to 2/6 murmur of mitral regurgitation. In any type of HCM, a grade 1 to 3/6 systolic ejection murmur at or below the pulmonary area may be heard. This murmur may reflect obstruction to right ventricular (RV) outflow. Examining the jugular venous pulse frequently reveals a prominent a-wave that rises on inspiration, depending on the degree of RV diastolic dysfunction. Rarely, this is accompanied by an RV fourth heart sound.

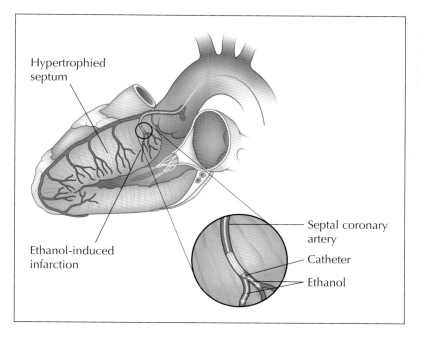

FIGURE 5-6. Alcohol septal ablation. A catheter is inserted into the left anterior descending artery and directed into the septal branch that supplies blood to the hypertrophied portion of the septum. The septal artery catheter balloon is inflated preventing backwash of alcohol into the remainder of the coronary tree. Through a distal port on the balloon-tipped catheter, ethanol is injected into the septal artery resulting in a controlled myocardial infarction [5].

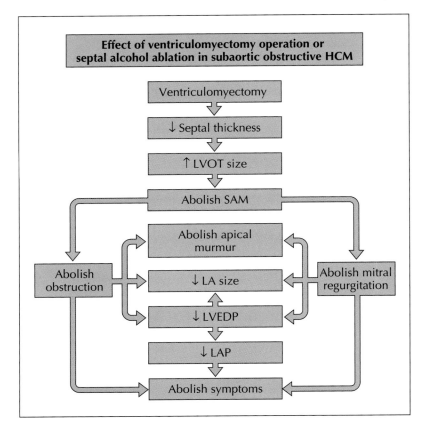

Effect of ventriculomyectomy operation or septal alcohol ablation in subaortic obstructive HCM

Ventriculomyectomy

↓ Septal thickness

↑ LVOT size

Abolish SAM

Abolish apical murmur

Abolish obstruction

↓ LA size

Abolish mitral regurgitation

↓ LVEDP

↓ LAP

Abolish symptoms

FIGURE 5-7. Management of obstructive hypertrophic cardiomyopathy (HCM) that does not respond to medical therapy. When patients with obstructive HCM are unresponsive to medical therapy, or are dissatisfied by the disease-imposed limitations or the side effects of medication, atrioventricular sequential pacemaker therapy, alcohol septal ablation, or surgery may be considered. Ventricular pacing from the right ventricular apex may cause a rightward septal shift and alleviation of the subaortic obstruction with resultant symptomatic improvement in some patients. This form of therapy is not, however, effective in all patients. The obstruction in some patients is not completely relieved, and up to 25% of patients require atrioventricular nodal ablation to achieve ventricular capture [6,7]. Ventriculomy-ectomy surgery, on the other hand, has been performed for over 30 years, and a number of centers have had extensive experience (and good to excellent results) [8–11]. The mechanisms of benefit of this procedure are illustrated. Myectomy thins the ventricular septum and widens the left ventricular outflow tract (LVOT), which abolishes mitral leaflet systolic anterior motion (SAM). This in turn abolishes the obstruction and mitral regurgitation. These effects eliminate the apical murmur and decrease the left ventricular end-diastolic pressure (LVEDP) as well as left atrial pressure (LAP) and size. Symptoms are dramatically relieved by these mechanisms. Myectomy is also indicated in recurrent atrial fibrillation to decrease left atrial size and restore normal sinus rhythm. The procedure should be performed in patients with obstructive HCM with unexplained syncope or cardiac arrest.

Alcohol ablation attempts to reduce the subaortic gradient by creation of myocardial dysfunction. Alcohol is injected into the septal branch or branches of the left anterior descending artery that supply the hypertrophied septum. If successful, the myocardial infarction decreases septal contraction and reduces the outflow gradient.

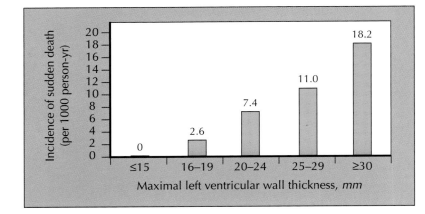

FIGURE 5-8. Patients with asymmetric septal hypertrophy die of progressive heart failure or sudden cardiac death. The risk of sudden death appears to correlate with the maximal left ventricular wall thickness. Severe hypertrophy may be present in young patients with mild or no symptoms [12]. (*Adapted from* Spirito *et al.* [12].)

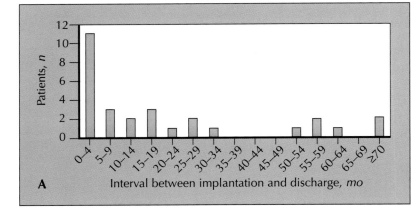

A

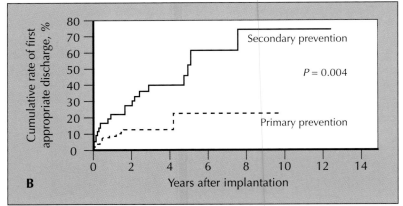

B

FIGURE 5-9. Implantable cardiovertor/defibrillators appear to prevent sudden cardiac death in some patients with hypertrophic cardiomyopathy. In patients who had defibrillators placed after sudden cardiac death or sustained ventricular tachycardia (secondary prevention), 11%

received an appropriate AICD discharge per year. However, in patients where placement was used as primary prevention, 5% received appropriate discharges per year (**A**). Occasionally, the interval between implantation and discharge is long (**B**) [13]. (*Adapted from* Maron *et al.* [13].)

IDIOPATHIC DILATED CARDIOMYOPATHY

According to the World Health Organization, idiopathic dilated cardiomyopathy is characterized by dilatation of the left, right, or both ventricles with impaired systolic function and is of unknown cause.

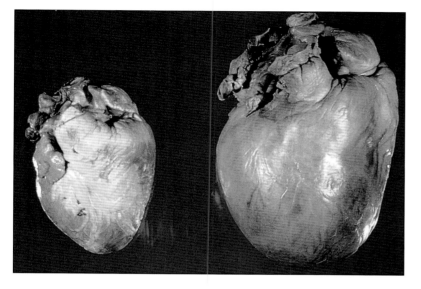

FIGURE 5-10. Gross pathology. In contrast to the normal heart (*left*), the heart in idiopathic dilated cardiomyopathy (*right*) is characterized by biventricular hypertrophy and four-chamber enlargement. The weight is often 25% to 50% above normal. Enlargement of the heart can be seen easily on chest radiography or cardiac echocardiography.

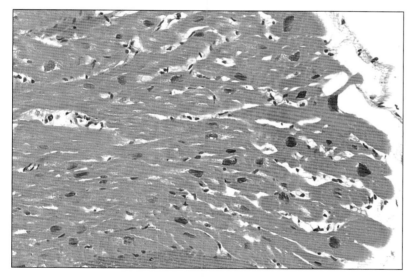

FIGURE 5-11. Endomyocardial biopsy from a patient with idiopathic cardiomyopathy. Large, irregularly shaped hyperchromatic nuclei are present, consistent with myocyte hypertrophy. The interstitium is cellular, but this should not be confused with myocarditis. These features, although nonspecific, support the diagnosis of idiopathic dilated cardiomyopathy. A completely normal endomyocardial biopsy does not support a diagnosis of idiopathic dilated cardiomyopathy and should suggest a focal cause, such as sarcoidosis, which requires further investigation [14].

SPECIFIC HEART-MUSCLE DISEASES

Heredofamilial
  Familial cardiomyopathy
  Muscular dystrophies
Infectious
  Bacterial
  Viral
  Human immunodeficiency virus
  Other
Metabolic
  Endocrine
  Nutritional
  Storage diseases
Myocarditis
Neoplastic
Peripartum
Systemic
  Infiltrative
  Connective tissue disease

Sensitivities and toxic reactions
  Ethanol
  Anthracycline
  Cocaine
  Cobalt
  Catecholamines
  Corticosteroids
  Lithium
  Radiation
  Heavy metal
  Scorpion sting
Other
  Uremia
  Anemia
  Leukemia
  Obesity

FIGURE 5-12. Specific causes of dilated cardiomyopathy. These are also called secondary cardiomyopathies or specific heart-muscle diseases. Almost any disease process can involve cardiac muscle, as can be seen from this list. Multiple factors may actually play a causative role in any single patient. (*Adapted from* Abelmann [15].)

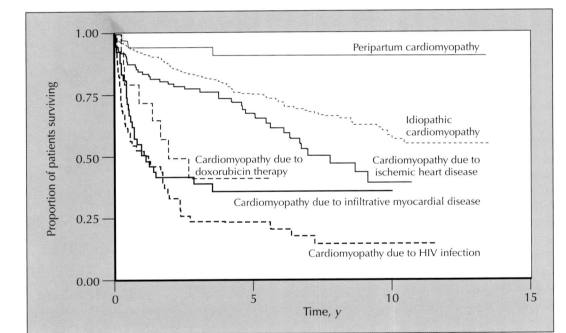

FIGURE 5-13. Although the prognosis in patients with heart failure is poor, it is dramatically influenced by the etiology of the left ventricular compromise [18]. (*Adapted from* Felker *et al.* [16].)

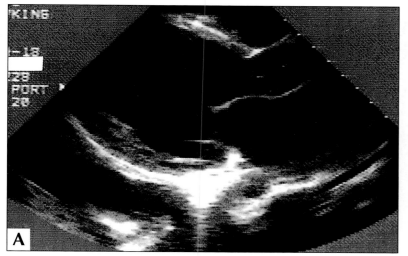

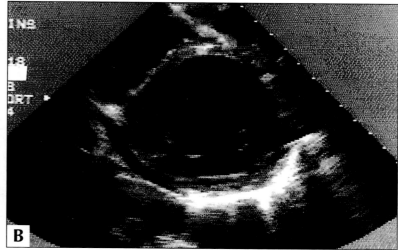

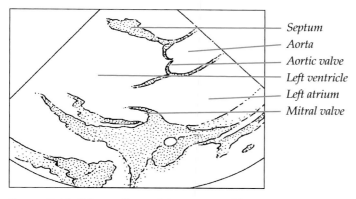

Septum
Aorta
Aortic valve
Left ventricle
Left atrium
Mitral valve

Left ventricular wall
Papillary muscle

FIGURE 5-14. Echocardiographic parasternal long-axis (**A**) and short-axis (**B**) views in a 26-year-old patient with idiopathic dilated cardiomyopathy. The chambers are dilated and the walls are thin. Mitral and tricuspid regurgitation are common. The presence of a segmental wall motion abnormality does not necessarily imply the presence of coronary artery disease. In a study of 50 patients with dilated cardiomyopathy, 64% had segmental wall motion abnormalities and a better prognosis compared with those who had diffuse wall motion abnormalities [17].

SPECIFIC HEART MUSCLE DISEASE

LYME DISEASE

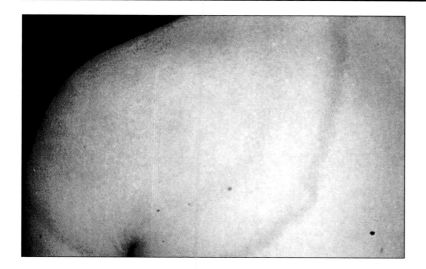

FIGURE 5-15. Erythema chronicum migrans (ECM). Lyme disease is usually contracted during the summer and is heralded by the appearance of a pathognomonic skin lesion, ECM. The appearance of ECM is generally annular, with a sharply demarcated outer border, and it is erythematous or bluish, warm to the touch, flat, and minimally tender or nontender. This unique cutaneous lesion is the best clinical marker of Lyme disease. ECM is followed in weeks to months by joint, neurologic, or cardiac involvement. However, in perhaps one third of cases, the skin lesion is absent or missed and patients present with symptoms of disseminated disease. (*From* Fitzpatrick *et al.* [18]; with permission.)

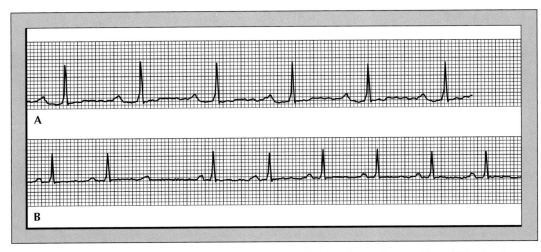

A

B

FIGURE 5-16. Development of first- and second-degree heart block in Lyme disease. About 10% of patients with Lyme disease develop evidence of transient cardiac involvement. The most common cardiac manifestation is variable degrees of atrioventricular (AV) block [19,20]. First-degree heart block (**A**) may progress to second-degree (**B**) or complete heart block over hours. According to some authorities, the risk for progression to complete heart block is much higher when the P-R interval exceeds 0.3 seconds. Syncope from complete heart block is common with cardiac involvement, as there is often associated depression of ventricular escape rhythm. McAlister *et al.* [19], in reviewing 52 reported cases of Lyme carditis, noted that 45 (87%) of these patients had documented AV block; 28 experienced either complete or high-grade AV block and were almost always symptomatic. When AV block of unknown origin develops suddenly, Lyme carditis should be considered, especially in younger patients who live in an area in which the vector is endemic [19,20].

ANTIBIOTIC TREATMENT REGIMENS FOR LYME DISEASE

EARLY INFECTION (LOCAL OR DISSEMINATED)

Adults: doxycycline 100 mg orally twice daily for 14–21 days, amoxicillin 500 mg orally three times daily for 14–21 days; alternatives in case of doxycycline or amoxicillin allergy, cefuroxime axetil 500 mg orally twice daily for 14–21 days, erythromycin 250 mg orally four times a day for 14–21 days

Adults: ceftriaxone 2 g intravenously once a day for 14–28 days, cefotaxime 2 g intravenously every 8 hours for 14–28 days, penicillin G sodium 20 million U intravenously in six divided doses every 4 hours for 14–28 days; alternative in case of ceftriaxone or penicillin allergy, doxycycline 100 mg orally three times a day for 30 days, but this regimen may be ineffective for late neuroborreliosis; facial palsy alone: oral regimens may be adequate

FIGURE 5-17. Antibiotic treatment regimens for Lyme disease [21].

CARDIAC SARCOIDOSIS

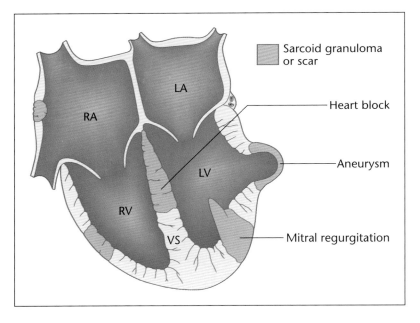

Sarcoid granuloma or scar

Heart block

Aneurysm

Mitral regurgitation

FIGURE 5-18. Distribution and consequences of sarcoid granulomas in sarcoid heart disease. In an autopsy series of 26 patients reported by Roberts *et al.* [22], cardiac granulomas were observed grossly in 25 hearts. Sarcoid granulomas were present in the left ventricular (LV) free wall of all 25 patients, in the right ventricular (RV) septum in 19, in the RV wall in 12, in the right atrial (RA) wall in three patients, and in the left atrial (LA) wall in two. Involvement of the cephalad portion of the muscular ventricular septum was associated with complete heart block. Important consequences of the involvement of the LV wall were aneurysm formation and mitral regurgitation. VS—ventricular septum. (*Adapted from* Roberts *et al.* [22].)

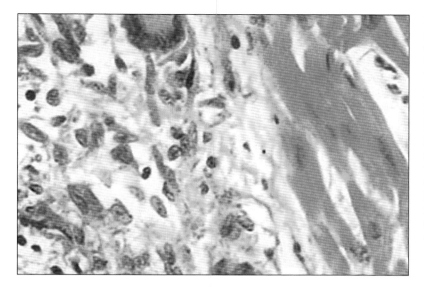

FIGURE 5-19. Endomyocardial biopsy sample demonstrating a sarcoid granuloma. Endomyocardial biopsy is the only technique that allows definitive diagnosis of myocardial sarcoidosis during life [23,24]. The depicted histologic specimen, obtained from the left ventricle, shows a typical noncaseating granuloma, that is characteristic of sarcoidosis (magnification, × 250). In some series, demonstration of sarcoid granulomas on endomyocardial biopsy is possible in only a small percentage of patients with probable myocardial sarcoidosis. This seeming discrepancy may relate to the patchy, diffuse nature of granulomatous involvement. Support for this concept is provided by the observations of Sekiguchi *et al*. [25], who simulated endomyocardial biopsy at different sites in both the left and right ventricles of the autopsied hearts of seven patients with fatal myocardial sarcoidosis. All seven hearts exhibited gross sarcoid involvement. Despite this, the sensitivity of biopsy was only 60% in the right ventricle and 47% in the left ventricle. Therefore, nonspecific biopsy findings do not exclude the diagnosis of myocardial sarcoidosis in clinically suspected cases. (*From* Uretsky [24]; with permission.)

CARDIAC AMYLOIDOSIS

CLINICAL PRESENTATIONS OF CARDIAC AMYLOIDOSIS

Restrictive cardiomyopathy
Jugular venous distention
Narrow pulse pressure
Protodiastolic gallop
Hepatomegaly
Peripheral edema

Congestive heart failure due to systolic dysfunction
Orthostatic hypotension
Abnormalities of cardiac impulse formation and conduction (resulting in arrhythmias and conduction disturbances)

FIGURE 5-20. In amyloidosis associated with an immunocyte dyscrasia (primary amyloidosis), pathologic evidence of cardiac involvement is virtually the rule. However, clinically apparent heart disease is present in only one third to one half of patients [26,27]. The most common clinical presentation of cardiac amyloidosis is that of a restrictive cardiomyopathy, in which right-sided findings dominate the clinical picture [27]. A second common presentation is congestive heart failure due to systolic dysfunction. Much less commonly, patients may present with orthostatic hypotension or with symptoms caused by abnormalities of cardiac impulse formation and conduction.

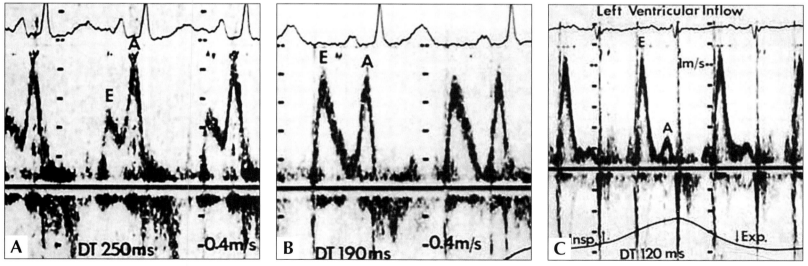

FIGURE 5-21. The spectrum of abnormal Doppler echocardiographic patterns in cardiac amyloidosis. Echocardiography is of considerable value in the diagnosis of infiltrative amyloid heart disease [28]. Typical features on two-dimensional echocardiography include a granular appearance of the myocardium and increased thickness of the myocardial walls. A number of studies have clearly shown that diastolic dysfunction in cardiac amyloidosis exhibits a spectrum of abnormalities that can be followed up serially by Doppler echocardiography. In earlier stages of amyloid heart disease, abnormal relaxation is the Doppler pattern seen (A). The E wave is of lower magnitude than the a-wave and the deceleration time is prolonged. As the disease progresses, a pseudonormalization Doppler pattern may emerge (B: the same patient as in *panel A*, taken 6 months later). Eventually, a restrictive pattern (C) emerges. As shown in this example (pulsed-wave Doppler recording of a left ventricular inflow profile), there is increased E/A ratio (3.7) and short deceleration time (120 ms). (*Adapted from* Klein *et al*. [28].)

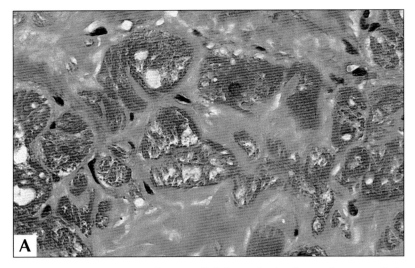

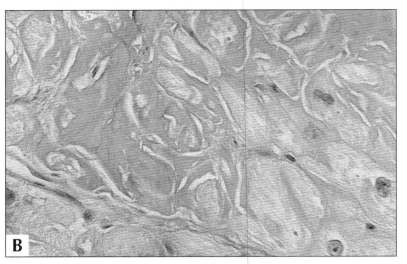

FIGURE 5-22. Appearance of myocardial tissue obtained at endomyocardial biopsy in cardiac amyloidosis. Endomyocardial biopsy may provide a definitive diagnosis in cardiac amyloidosis [27]. The depicted images are those of myocardium obtained at endomyocardial biopsy in a 53-year-old woman with rapidly progressive heart failure, in whom neither cardiac amyloidosis nor a blood dyscrasia was suspected prior to biopsy. **A,** Hematoxylin and eosin staining shows pink eosinophilic deposits of amyloid. **B,** Sulfated Alcian blue staining demonstrates apple green staining of the deposits. (*Courtesy of* Vijaya Reddy, Maywood, IL.)

RESTRICTIVE CARDIOMYOPATHY AND HYPEREOSINOPHILIC HEART DISEASE

In restrictive cardiomyopathy, the stiff ventricle has difficulty in filling, and manifestations of diastolic heart failure are evident. The most important conditions causing restrictive cardiomyopathy are sarcoidosis (*see* Figs. 5-18 and 5-19), hemochromatosis, amyloidosis (*see* Figs. 5-20 and 5-21), radiation heart disease, glycogen storage disease, and familial neuromuscular disorders (*see* Figs. 5-29 to 5-36). Restrictive cardiomyopathy may also be idiopathic.

FIGURE 5-23. The etiology of heart failure can virtually always be identified in patients with restrictive cardiomyopathy. The causes include sarcoidosis and amyloidosis, which have already been described [29]. (*Adapted from* Kushwaha *et al.* [29].)

CLASSIFICATION OF TYPES OF RESTRICTIVE CARDIOMYOPATHY ACCORDING TO CAUSE

MYOCARDIAL

Noninfiltrative
Idiopathic cardiomyopathy*   Scleroderma
Familial cardiomyopathy   Pseudoxanthoma elasticum
Hypertrophic cardiomyopathy   Diabetic cardiomyopathy
Infiltrative
Amyloidosis*   Hurler's disease
Sarcoidosis*   Fatty infiltration
Gaucher's disease
Storage diseases
Hemochromatosis   Glycogen storage disease
Fabry's disease

ENDOMYOCARDIAL

Endomyocardial fibrosis*   Radiation*
Hypereosinophilic syndrome   Toxic effects of anthracycline*
Carcinoid heart disease   Drugs causing fibrous
Metastatic cancers   endocarditis (serotonin,
                                       methysergide,
                                       ergotamine, mercurial
                                       agents, bisulfan)

*This condition is more likely than the others to be encountered in clinical practice.

IDIOPATHIC RESTRICTIVE CARDIOMYOPATHY

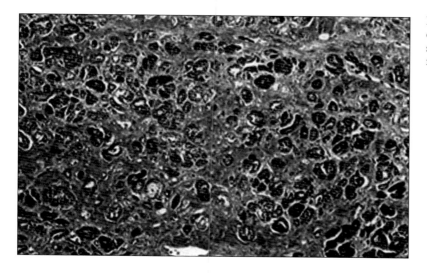

FIGURE 5-24. Idiopathic restricted cardiomyopathy. Cross-sectional view of myocytes surrounded by fibrous tissue (Mallory-azan stain). Whereas severe interstitial fibrosis is seen here, fibrous tissue surrounds each myocyte (predominantly endomysial fibrosis).

SEQUENTIAL PATHOPHYSIOLOGY
Impaired LV relaxation and reduced LV early diastolic filling
Reduced LV compliance: elevated LV end-diastolic pressure; accentuated a-wave with E/A <1 by Doppler echocardiography; absence of square root sign
Elevation of LV diastolic and left atrial pressures: pseudonormalization of LV filling pattern by Doppler echocardiography; square root sign may be present
Development of atrial fibrillation and pulmonary congestion
Pulmonary hypertension
Elevation of right ventricular diastolic and right atrial pressures
Tricuspid regurgitation: right and left atrial pressures become equal

FIGURE 5-25. The sequential pathophysiologic changes in restrictive cardiomyopathy. The differences between the early and late stages are well documented in amyloid heart disease [28,30]. Pseudo-normalization of transmitral flow by Doppler echocardiography is seen when left atrial pressure is elevated [30–32]. Elevation of right atrial pressure with severe tricuspid regurgitation is seen in patients in advanced stages [33]. E/A—ratio of the peak early diastolic (E) to atrial (A) contraction transmitral flow velocities; LV—left ventricular.

HYPEREOSINOPHILIC HEART DISEASE (LÖFFLER'S SYNDROME)

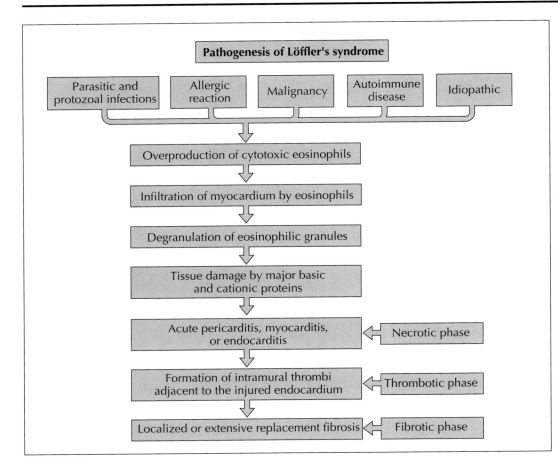

FIGURE 5-26. The pathogenesis of Löffler's syndrome. Tissue damage is caused by major basic and cationic proteins derived from cytotoxic eosinophils [34–38]. These cytotoxic proteins may stay in the myocardium for a prolonged period and produce continuous tissue damage. At the fibrotic phase, various types of heart diseases, such as endomyocardial fibrosis, dilated cardiomyopathy, atrioventricular block, or valvular regurgitation can be seen according to the difference of the most dominantly involved site.

CLINICAL MANIFESTATIONS

Necrotic phase

Manifestations of acute endo-, myo-, or pericarditis with hypereosinophilia

Thrombotic phase

Cavity obliteration with intramural thrombi with or without hypereosinophilia (common in the tropics and rare in the temperate zone)

Fibrotic phase

Atrioventricular block

Valvular regurgitation

Heart failure with restrictive physiology (ranging from diastolic dysfunction to endomyocardial fibrosis) or systolic dysfunction

Absence of hypereosinophilia

FIGURE 5-27. The clinical manifestations of Löffler's syndrome and endomyocardial fibrosis [34,37]. The necrotic phase is acute, lasting for months. The thrombotic phase is subacute, lasting for months to 2 years. The fibrotic phase is chronic, and lasts for years.

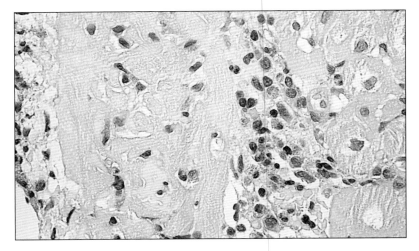

FIGURE 5-28. Histologic view of a biopsy specimen (same patient as in Fig. 5-35) showed massive infiltration of eosinophils in the myocardium as well as in the endocardium (hematoxylin and eosin).

CLINICAL MANIFESTATIONS WITH CARDIAC INVOLVEMENT

MUSCULAR DYSTROPHY

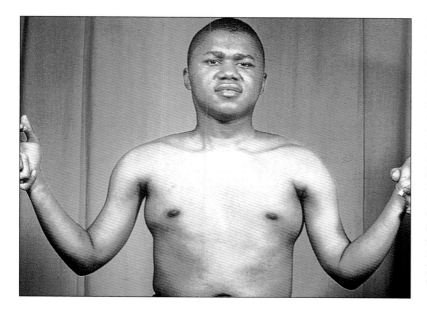

FIGURE 5-29. A 17-year-old boy with Duchenne muscular dystrophy demonstrating striking enlargement (hypertrophy-pseudohypertrophy) of the deltoid and pectoralis major muscles. There is also enlargement of the calves, which is the earliest clinical expression (phenotype) of human Duchenne dystrophy in skeletal muscle. Such calf enlargement has been called "pseudohypertrophy" because of extensive infiltration if not replacement by connective tissue and fat. However, before age 2 years, connective tissue and fat can be minimal, so calf enlargement is due to true hypertrophy rather than pseudohypertrophy. Exceptionally, regional muscle enlargement (hypertrophy-pseudohypertrophy) in Duchenne dystrophy can be striking in muscle groups other than the calves, as is illustrated here. Animal models shed further light on hypertrophy, at least in striated muscle. Dystrophin-deficient mice and cats do not experience overt clinical dystrophy but instead manifest hypertrophy of striated muscle in both the early and late stages of the disease. Especially striking is the systemic striated muscle hypertrophy in dystrophin-deficient cats that have a paucity of overt muscle necrosis but remarkable hypertrophy of individual muscle fibers. The hypertrophy-pseudohypertrophy distribution shown in this patient is rare in humans with Duchenne dystrophy, but is typical of the dystrophin-deficient cat.

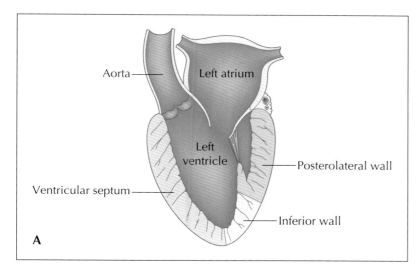

A

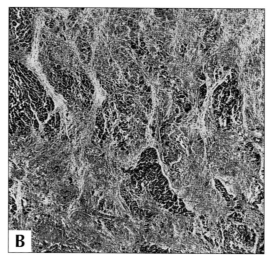

B

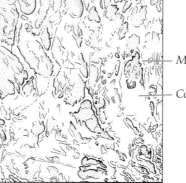

Myocardial fibers

Connective tissue

FIGURE 5-30. **A,** The posterolateral (infra-atrial) involvement of the left ventricle in Duchenne dystrophy. **B,** Posterobasal portion of the left ventricular wall. In contrast to the posterobasal wall, which shows extensive connective tissue proliferation with scattered islands of myocardial fibers, no fibrous scars are present in the ventricular septum (hematoxylin and eosin, × 25). A reduction in or loss of electromotive force caused by the location of myocardial dystrophy in the posterobasal and contiguous lateral left ventricular walls is believed to be responsible for the characteristic scalar electrocardiogram, and is represented by tall right precordial R waves and deep but narrow Q waves in leads 1, aVL, and the left precordium. Duchenne dystrophy emerges as a unique form of heart disease characterized by a genetically determined predilection for specific regions of myocardium.

CARDIOMYOPATHY, MYOCARDITIS, AND PERICARDIAL DISEASE

167

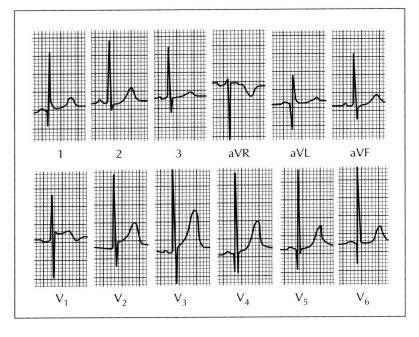

FIGURE 5-31. Typical electrocardiogram of Duchenne muscular dystrophy in a 10-year-old boy. The P-R interval is short (0.10 seconds in lead 2). The QRS complex shows an anterior shift in the right precordial leads (tall R waves) and deep but narrow Q waves in leads 1, aVL, and V_{4-6}. A reduction in or loss of electromotive force caused by myocardial dystrophy in the postero-basal and contiguous lateral left ventricular walls is believed to be responsible for the QRS pattern. The standard scalar electrocardiogram is the simplest and most reliable tool for detecting cardiac involvement in Duchenne dystrophy. Abnormal electrocardiograms are present even in early childhood. Tall right precordial R waves and increased R:S amplitude ratios, together with deep Q waves in leads 1, aVL, and V_{5-6}, are characteristic of classic, rapidly progressive X-linked Duchenne dystrophy.

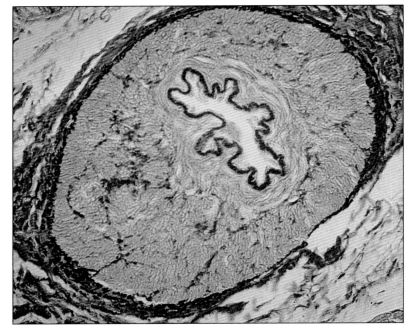

FIGURE 5-32. Histologic section of small intramural coronary arteries in the left atria of patient with Duchenne dystrophy. Striking hypertrophy of medial smooth muscle with luminal narrowing (Verhoeff-von Gieson elastic tissue stains, × 260). The coronary arteriopathy is characterized principally by striking hypertrophy of the media with luminal narrowing, and less commonly by coexisting cystic degeneration. The dystrophin content of vascular smooth muscle cells (shown here) is similar to that of striated myofibers. The smooth muscle form of dystrophin is believed to be slightly smaller than the predominant striated muscle dystrophin, implying that a smaller form might represent a vascular smooth muscle isoform. A fundamental question is why dystrophin deficiency in the vascular smooth muscle of Duchenne dystrophy (in contrast to striated muscle) expresses itself chiefly as hypertrophy rather than necrosis.

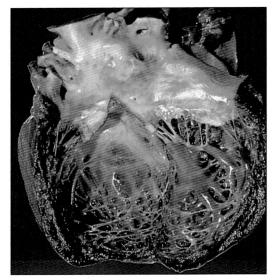

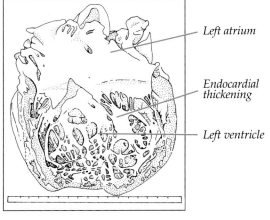

Left atrium

Endocardial thickening

Left ventricle

FIGURE 5-33. Gross and microscopic cardiac pathologic specimen from a 45-year-old man with late-onset, slowly progressive Becker muscular dystrophy. The left atrium was also dilated. No significant coronary artery disease was identified. In Becker dystrophy, the protein product of the gene is present but is abnormal in molecular weight, while in Duchenne dystrophy the protein product is absent or scanty but of normal molecular weight. In contrast to Duchenne dystrophy, cardiac involvement in Becker dystrophy involves all four chambers, with dilatation and failure of the ventricles in addition to abnormalities of the His bundle and infranodal conduction that express themselves as fascicular block and complete heart block.

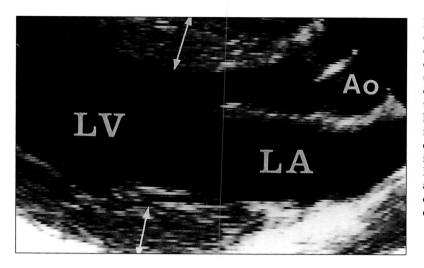

FIGURE 5-34. Two-dimensional echocardiogram (parasternal long axis diastolic frames) from a 14-year-old girl with Friedreich's ataxia and concentric hypertrophy (*arrows*) of the left ventricle (LV). The most common echocardiographic finding in Friedreich's ataxia is concentric (symmetric) left ventricular hypertrophy. Asymmetric septal hypertrophy occurs less frequently, and is occasionally accompanied by a left ventricular to aortic systolic gradient. Septal cellular disarray, which is the histologic hallmark of genetic hypertrophic cardiomyopathy, has not been identified in necropsy studies of Friedreich's ataxia—an observation that may in part explain why the potentially malignant ventricular arrhythmias that prevail in genetic hypertrophic cardiomyopathy are essentially unknown in Friedreich's ataxia. In hypertrophic cardiomyopathy of Friedreich's ataxia, systolic ventricular function is normal, not supernormal, and diastolic function is not deranged as in genetic hypertrophic cardiomyopathy. Ao—aorta; LA—left atrium.

OTHER NEUROLOGIC DISORDERS

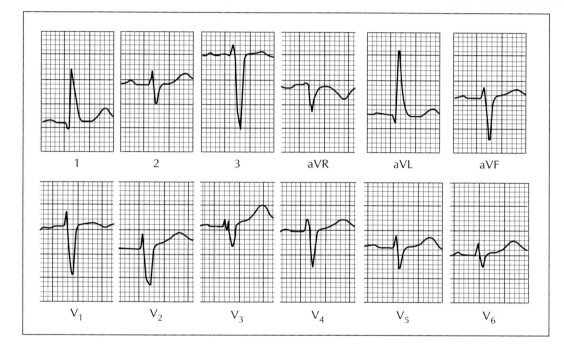

FIGURE 5-35. Typical electrocardiogram from an adult man with myotonic muscular dystrophy. There is P-R interval prolongation (0.20 seconds) and left anterior fascicular block. Cardiac involvement is relatively selective in myotonic dystrophy, primarily targeting specialized tissues, and more specifically the His-Purkinje system. The most common electrocardiographic abnormalities—prolongation of the P-R interval, left anterior fascicular block, and increased QRS duration—reflect the His-Purkinje disease that can progress rapidly, culminating in fatal Stokes-Adams episodes unless anticipated by pacemaker insertion.

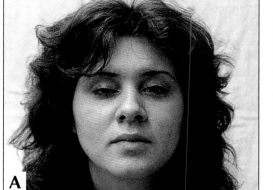
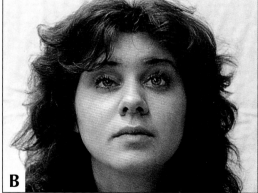

FIGURE 5-36. Kearns-Sayre syndrome is a mitochondrial myopathy expressed as external ophthalmoplegia, pigmentary retinopathy, and cardiac involvement that typically afflicts specialized conduction tissues culminating in complete heart block [39]. This 18-year-old girl with Kearns-Sayre syndrome and bilateral asymmetric ptosis had pigmentary retinopathy and an electrocardiogram that progressed from normal to bifascicular block. **A,** The asymmetric ptosis is present when the patient looks straight ahead. **B,** Ptosis of the right lid persists during upward gaze.

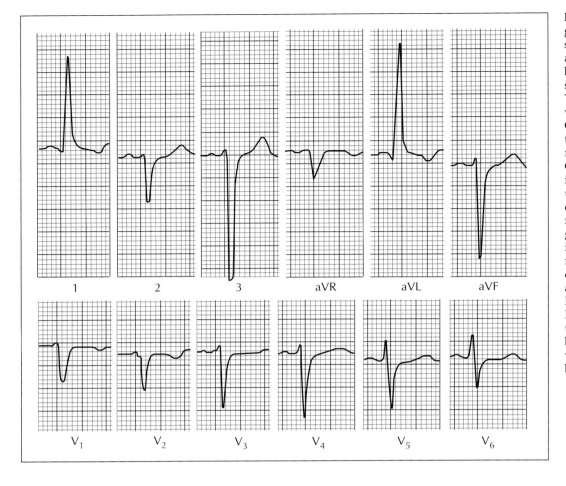

FIGURE 5-37. Twelve-lead scalar electrocardiogram from a 14-year-old girl with Kearns-Sayre syndrome. There is left anterior fascicular block and right bundle branch block (bifascicular block); 4 years earlier, the electrocardiogram showed isolated left anterior fascicular block. The patient had bilateral asymmetric ptosis that was especially apparent on upward gaze. Ophthalmologic examination disclosed pigmentary retinopathy. Skeletal muscle biopsy identified ragged red fibers in the trichrome stain. Clinically overt myocardial disease is exceptional in Kearns-Sayre syndrome, despite the fact that ultrastructural abnormalities, especially in mitochondria, are well established. Two derangements of the specialized conduction pathways generally coexist: 1) gradually progressive impairment of infranodal conduction (left anterior hemiblock, right bundle branch block, and complete heart block), and 2) enhancement of atrioventricular nodal conduction. The morphologic basis for impaired infranodal conduction lies in the extensive changes in distal portions of the His bundle extending to the origins of the bundle branches. Evidence of enhanced atrioventricular nodal conduction has been identified by His bundle electrograms.

GENETIC AND INHERITED DISORDERS

GENE MUTATIONS CAUSING DILATED CARDIOMYOPATHY

CHROMOSOME	PROTEIN	DISEASE	INHERITANCE
1p1–q21	Lamins A and C	Dilated cardiomyopathy	Autosomal dominant
1q11–21	Unknown	Dilated cardiomyopathy*†	Autosomal dominant
1q11–23	Lamins A and C	Autosomal dominant Emery-Dreifuss muscular dystrophy	Autosomal dominant
1q32	Unknown	Dilated cardiomyopathy	Autosomal dominant
2q11–22	Unknown	Dilated cardiomyopathy	Autosomal dominant
2q31	Unknown	Dilated cardiomyopathy	Autosomal dominant
3p22–25	Unknown	Dilated cardiomyopathy	Autosomal dominant
6q23	Unknown	Dilated cardiomyopathy*	Autosomal dominant
9q13–22	Unknown	Dilated cardiomyopathy	Autosomal dominant
10q21–23	Unknown	Dilated cardiomyopathy	Autosomal dominant
10q22	Metavinculin	Dilated cardiomyopathy	Unknown
15q14	Actin	Dilated cardiomyopathy	Autosomal dominant
17q12–21.33	alpha-Sarcoglycan (adhalin)	Dilated cardiomyopathy*	Autosomal recessive
Xq28	Emerin	Emery-Dreifuss muscular dystrophy	X-linked
Xp21	Dystrophin	X-linked dilated cardiomyopathy	X-linked
Xp21	Dystrophin	Becker type muscular dystrophy	X-linked
Xp21	Dystrophin	Duchenne type muscular dystrophy	X-linked

*This form is associated with limb-girdle muscular dystrophy.
†Although the loci on chromosome 1q are similar to those for Emery-Dreifuss muscular dystrophy, the disease form is distinct.

FIGURE 5-38. Specific genetic mutations are increasingly being associated with both hypertrophic and dilated cardiomyopathy. Familial (genetic) dilated cardiomyopathy may account for 20% of all patients presenting with cardiomyopathy [40].

ETIOLOGY AND EPIDEMIOLOGY

ETIOLOGIES OF HUMAN MYOCARDITIS: INFECTIOUS

Viral
  Coxsackievirus (A and B)
  Echovirus
  Influenza
  Cytomegalovirus
  Hepatitis
  Mumps
  Herpes simplex
  Rabies
  EBV
  HIV
Rickettsial
  Q fever
  Rocky Mountain spotted fever
  Scrub typhus
Fungal
  Cryptococcus
  Candidiasis
  Histoplasmosis
  Aspergillus

Protozoal and metazoal
  Trypanosomiasis
  Toxoplasmosis
  Malaria
  Schistosomiasis
  Trichinosis
Bacterial
  Diphtheria
  Tuberculosis
  Legionella
  Brucella
  Clostridium
  Salmonella/shigella
  Meningococcus
  Yersinia
Spirochetal
  Borellia (Lyme)

FIGURE 5-39. Infectious causes of myocarditis. Strictly speaking, the Dallas criteria are confined to cases of idiopathic myocarditis rather than cases secondary to specific infectious or noninfectious causes. The presence of cardiotropic viruses is rarely confirmed, however, and the clinical significance of such viruses is still debated. Thus, most cases of myocarditis are clinically idiopathic and likely represent the largest subgroup of cases of human myocarditis. EBV—Epstein-Barr virus.

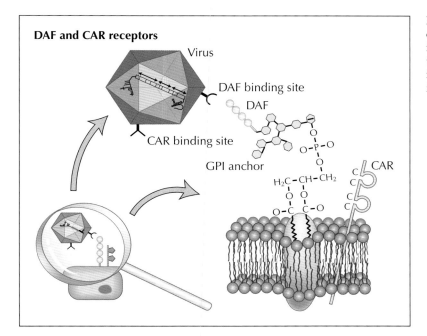

DAF and CAR receptors

FIGURE 5-40. Viral receptors on myocardial cells. Viruses enter the heart cells through receptors on the myocyte membrane. This is best characterized with the coxsackie adenoviral receptor (CAR), immunoglobulins that colocalize in target cell membranes. The CAR binds to the virus, and in the presence of coreceptors such as delay activating factor (DAF), facilitates virus entry into the cell [41]. GPI—glycosylphosphatidylinositol.

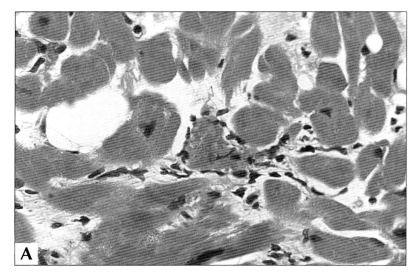

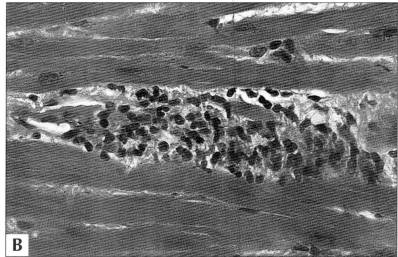

FIGURE 5-41. Histopathologic features of endomyocardial biopsy samples from patients with myocarditis. **A,** High-power photomicrograph of an endomyocardial biopsy sample stained with hematoxylin and eosin, highlighting one isolated necrotic myocyte surrounded by a mixed inflammatory infiltrate. **B,** A small cluster of longitudinally oriented myocytes engulfed in a dense inflammatory infiltrate composed primarily of mononuclear cells. Typically, outside the focus of active myocarditis, the adjacent myocardium appears relatively preserved. Interstitial inflammatory cells surround the myocytes, which no longer have crisp cellular outlines. The interstitial space between affected myocytes contains granular basophilic material that contains fibrin and fibrinogen, a likely consequence of microvascular injury. The inflammatory

cells extend from the central core of necrotic myocytes into the adjacent myocardium. In 1986 and 1987 Aretz *et al.* [42,43], in an attempt to establish a uniform histologic classification for the diagnosis of myocarditis on endomyocardial biopsy, published a classification proposed by eight cardiac pathologists (the Dallas panel). Two separate classifications were described, one for the first biopsy and one for subsequent biopsies. On the first biopsy, *active myocarditis* was defined as a process characterized by an inflammatory infiltrate of the myocardium with necrosis or degeneration of adjacent myocytes not typical of the ischemic damage associated with coronary artery disease. The diagnosis of active myocarditis therefore requires the presence of myocardial inflammation as well as adjacent myocyte damage.

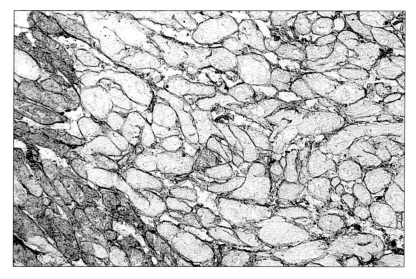

FIGURE 5-42. Myocardial immunoglobulin G deposition 14 days post-coxsackie-virus B3 infection. The diffuse reactivity on myocyte sarcolemmal membranes suggests that in the setting of induced expression of

major histocompatibility complex (MHC) antigens (either by primary viral infection or by secondary release of cytokines by cardiac-infiltrating cells), antibodies bind to self-peptides on the myocyte cell surface. Investigative studies have shown that in addition to myosin, other intracellular proteins (such as the two mitochondrial proteins known to be autoantigens in human myocarditis: the adenine nucleotide translocator [ANT] and the branched-chain ketoacid dehydrogenase [BCKD] complex) are transported to the myocyte cell surface during the course of chronic myocarditis. These proteins are thus presented to the immune system in the context of MHC [44]. Studies by Huber and Moraska [45] have raised the possibility that nonviral insults that produce myocarditis may similarly induce cardiac-specific autoimmunity. Adriamycin-treated mice developed myocarditis and cytolytic T lymphocytes as well as antibodies specifically reactive to only drug-treated myocytes. Thus, the antigenicity of a myocyte may change sufficiently to induce immune reactivity to new antigenic epitopes regardless of the type of toxic insult. Whether these autoantibodies are directly involved in the pathogenesis of cardiac injury or whether they represent an epiphenomenon of ongoing myocardial injury is still the subject of debate. In addition, whether autoantibodies recognize intracellular proteins (such as myosin, ANT, and BCKD) transported to the surface of myocytes and expressed as peptides that have been part of the MHC or normal membrane constituents, which cross-react with antigenic epitopes of these intracellular proteins, is not known.

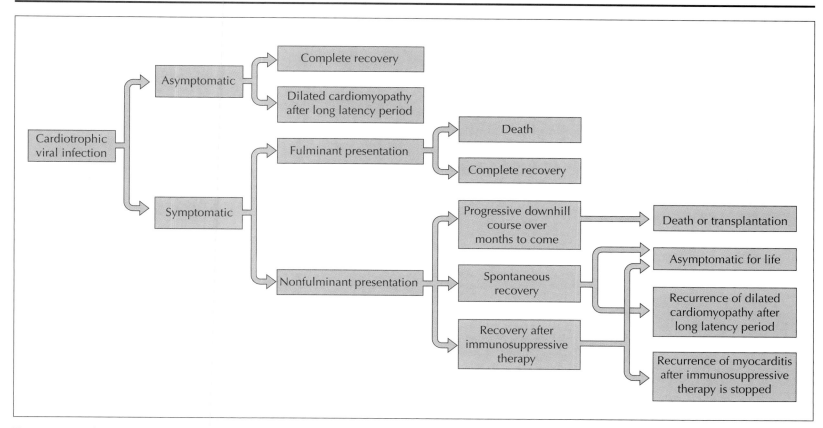

FIGURE 5-43. The natural history of human myocarditis. Most patients with mild symptoms of acute myocarditis are not seen by cardiologists and most of these patients appear to recover fully. Of the patients with symptomatic heart disease typically seen by cardiologists, a small number have fulminant presentations and either die in the acute stage or appear to recover fully. Of the remaining patients with myocarditis, a few are characterized by a progressive downhill course over a period of months to years that ends in death from heart failure or intractable arrhythmias [46,47]. Some spontaneously recover and remain asymptomatic for life, and others have an asymptomatic period followed by development of dilated cardiomyopathy. The heterogeneity of clinical presentations and natural history in human myocarditis probably reflect the genetic predisposition of the individual, the virulence of the cardiotropic virus, and environmental factors. With the advent of molecular viral probes, it will be critical to relate the presence of persistent enterovirus RNA with the patterns of the natural history of myocarditis.

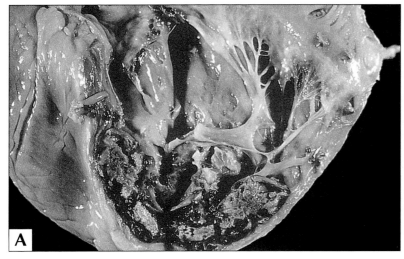

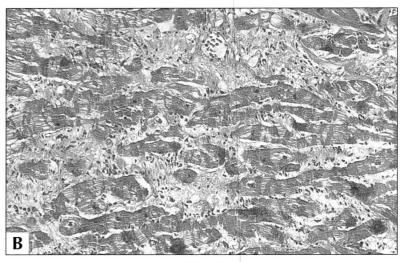

FIGURE 5-44. A, Gross autopsy specimen of a heart with fulminant myocarditis. The right ventricle is cut along the long axis to demonstrate an apical mural thrombus. Fulminant myocarditis is characterized by a nonspecific, severe influenza-like illness and the distinct onset of cardiac involvement. The patient's condition deteriorates rapidly, and the disorder frequently results in profound hemodynamic compromise and multisystem failure. Endomyocardial biopsies from fulminant myocarditis patients demonstrate unequivocal active myocarditis and are particularly notable for very extensive inflammatory infiltrates and numerous foci of myocyte necrosis. Within 1 month, the patients usually recover left ventricular function completely or die [48]. In contrast, acute myocarditis describes the clinical spectrum of the largest group of patients with active or borderline myocarditis. These patients have minimally dilated, hypokinetic left ventricles on presentation. The onset of cardiac symptoms is frequently indistinct, and some patients provide a vague history consistent with (but not diagnostic of) an antecedent viral illness. Active or borderline myocarditis is present on initial (but not subsequent) endomyocardial biopsies. Some patients in this group appear to respond to immunosuppressive therapy [49], while others experience either partial recovery of ventricular function or continue to deteriorate to end-stage dilated cardiomyopathy. **B,** Masson's trichrome (which stains collagen blue) of an endomyocardial biopsy of a patient with chronic active myocarditis. Note the extensive collagen deposition characteristically seen in end-stage dilated cardiomyopathy. Patients with chronic active myocarditis usually have a vague clinical presentation. Such patients have a slowly progressive course that inevitably deteriorates but may be punctuated by brief, often-dramatic but unsustained responses to immunosuppressive therapy. Serial endomyocardial biopsies demonstrate ongoing myocarditis with the development of extensive interstitial fibrosis. Inflammatory infiltrates in this subgroup of myocarditis patients may contain multinucleated giant cells.

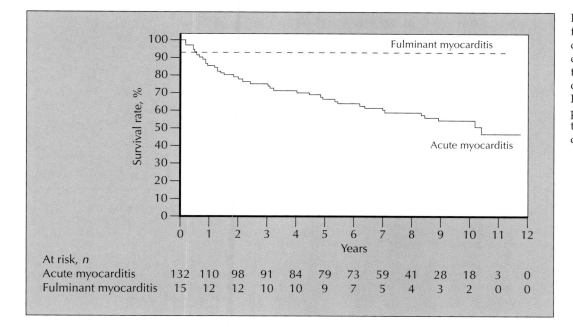

FIGURE 5-45. The outcome of patients with fulminant versus acute myocarditis is dramatically different. Those with fulminant myocarditis die acutely or survive without additional evidence of left ventricular compromise or symptoms of congestive heart failure. Patients with acute myocarditis display a progressive mortality rate that is similar to that of patients with idiopathic dilated cardiomyopathy [50].

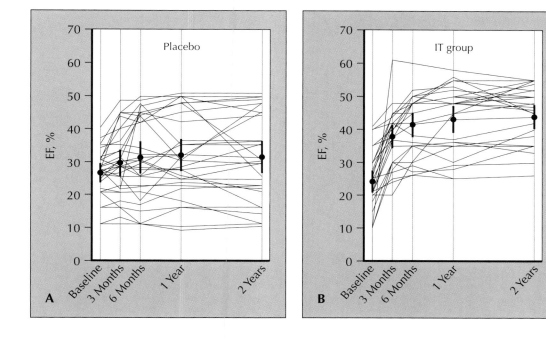

FIGURE 5-46. Response of patients with myocarditis to immunosuppressive therapy. *Myocarditis* was defined as an expression of human leukocyte antigen (HLA) on endomyocardial biopsy specimens as opposed to using the Dallas criteria of lymphocytic infiltrate and asociated myocyte destruction. **A** and **B**, Using HLA expression criteria, patients were treated with immunosuppressive agents versus placebo for 3 months. Although there was no significant difference in the primary endpoint of death, heart transplantation, and hospital readmission between the two groups, immunosuppression improved ejection fraction during the course of treatment (3 months), which was maintained for 2 years. At the end of the follow-up period, 71.4% of patients in the immunosuppressive group versus 30.8% in the placebo group were improved [51]. Others have demontrated that viral persistence may identify patients with myocarditis who do not respond to immunosuppressive therapy [52]. These studies challenge the current thinking that immunosuppressive theapy provides no benefit to patients with myocarditis. EF—ejection fraction.

I Family history

Familial disease confirmed at necropsy or surgery

Minor

Family history or premature sudden death (< 35 years) caused by suspected ARVC

Family history (clinical diagnosis based on present criteria)

II ECG depolarization/conduction abnormalities

Major

Epsilon waves or localized prolongation (≥ 110 ms) of the QRS complex in the right precordial leads (V_1–V_3)

Minor

Late potentials seen on signal-averaged ECG

III EEG repolarization abnormalities

Minor

Inverted T waves in right precordial leads (V_2 and V_3) in people > 12 years and in the absence of right bundle branch block

IV Arrhythmias

Minor

Sustained or nonsustained left bundle branch block type ventricular tachycardia documented on the ECG, Holter monitoring, or during exercise testing

Frequent ventricular extrasystoles (more than 1000/24 hr on Holter monitoring)

V Global and/or regional dysfunction and structural alterations*

Major

Severe dilatation and reduction of right ventricular ejection fraction with no (or only mild) left ventricular involvement

Localized right ventricular aneurysms (akinetic or dyskinetic areas with diastolic bulgings)

Severe segmental dilatation of the right ventricle

Minor

Mild global right ventricular dilatation and/or ejection fraction reduction with normal left ventricle

Mild segmental dilatation of the right ventricle

Regional right ventricular hypokinesia

VI Tissue characteristics of walls

Major

Fibrofatty replacement of myocardium on endomyocardial biopsy

*Detected by ECG, angiography, magnetic resonance imaging, or radionuclide scintigraphy.

FIGURE 5-47. Criteria for the diagnosis of arrhythmogenic right ventricular cardiomyopathy (dysplasia). Arrhythmogenic right ventricular dysplasia is increasingly being recognized as a cause of sudden death. Based on this classification, the presence of two major criteria or one major criteria plus two minor criteria, or four minor criteria from different groups may be used to establish the diagnosis [53,54]. ARVC—arrhythmogenic right ventricular cardiomyopathy; ECG—electrocardiogram.

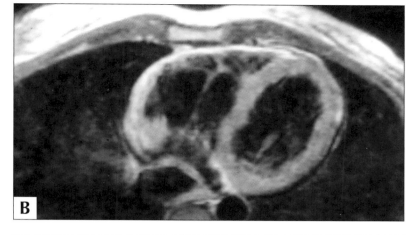

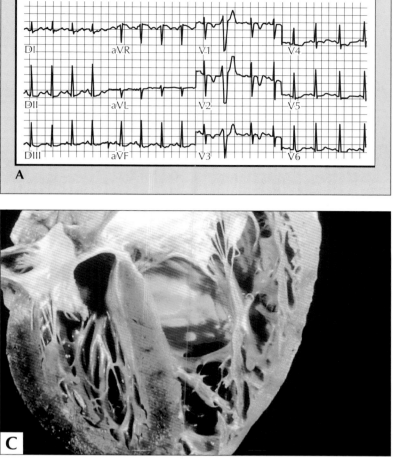

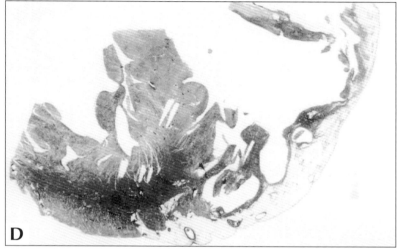

FIGURE 5-48. Means of diagnosing arrhythmogenic dysplasia. **A**, Electrocardiogram. Note the typical abnormalities consisting of inverted T waves in V_1 to V_4 and isolated premature ventricular contractions with a left bundle branch block morphology. **B**, Magnetic resonance imaging. The right ventricle is dilated with bright signals from the thinned and fatty infiltrated right ventricular free wall. **C**, Histologic confirmation. Transmural fibrofatty replacement of the right ventricular free wall. Morphologic features in a 25-year-old man who died suddenly from arrhythmo-genic right ventricular cardiomyopathy. This is a four-chamber view cut of the heart speciment showing the transmural fatty replacement of the right ventricular free wall and the translucent infundibulum. **D**, Panoramic histologic section of the heart noted in **C** displaying myocardial atrophy in the right ventricle affecting the primarily the free wall. Increased fat or fibrous material, beyond normal limits, helps to establish the diagnosis in those submitted to right ventricular endomyocardial biopsy.

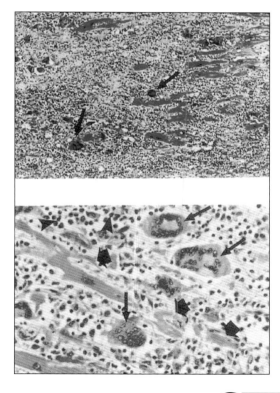

FIGURE 5-49. Giant cell myocarditis. Multinucleated giant cells (*long arrows*) are seen adjacent to degenerating myocytes (*short arrows*). The cellular infiltrate contains lymphocytes, histiocytes, and collections of eosinophils (*arrowheads*) (hematoxylin and eosin, X 400) [55,56].

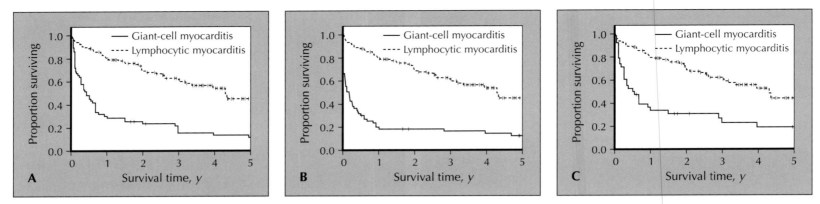

FIGURE 5-50. A–C, Survival curves in giant cell myocarditis versus lymphocytic myocarditis. These Kaplan-Meier suvival curves show the duration of survival from the onset of symptoms until death in patients with giant cell myocarditis compared with those afflicted with stand lymphocytic myocarditis. Note the substantially worse survival for those with giant cell myocarditis.

PERICARDIAL DISEASE

The most important clinical manifestations of pericardial disease are cardiac tamponade, acute pericarditis, and chronic constrictive pericarditis.

CARDIAC TAMPONADE

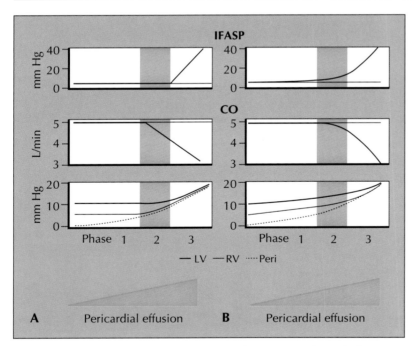

FIGURE 5-51. Hemodynamic changes in cardiac tamponade, including pericardial (Peri), right ventricular (RV), and left ventricular (LV) pressures and the inspiratory fall in arterial systolic pressure (IFASP) and cardiac output (CO), with increasing pericardial effusion in any given patient depicted by the increasing height of the triangle from left to right. *Shaded vertical area* indicates phase 2. **A,** The original concept. **B,** The revised concept, in which LV diastolic pressure does not equilibrate with RV diastolic pressure and pericardial pressure until phase 3. In phase 1, pericardial pressure rises but does not equilibrate with RV and LV diastolic pressures. There is no pulsus paradoxus. In phase 2, RV diastolic pressures equilibrate but not with LV diastolic pressure, which remains higher. Pulsus paradoxus is often present. In phase 3, left and right diastolic pressures equilibrate with pericardial pressure, and pulsus paradoxus is nearly always present. (*Adapted from* Reddy *et al.* [57].)

ECHOCARDIOGRAPHIC FINDINGS IN CARDIAC TAMPONADE

RA diastolic collapse

RV early diastolic collapse

LA collapse

Abnormal inspiratory increase in tricuspid valve flow and >15% inspiratory decrease of mitral valve flow

Abnormal inspiratory increase of RV dimension with abnormal inspiratory decrease of LV dimension

Inspiratory decrease of mitral valve DE excursion and EF slope

Inferior vena caval plethora (failure to decrease proximal diameter by ≥50% on sniff or deep inspiration)

LV pseudohypertrophy

Swinging heart

FIGURE 5-52. Right atrial (RA) collapse and right ventricular (RV) diastolic collapse are the most sensitive echocardiographic signs of cardiac tamponade. However, these signs may be absent when there is elevation of right heart pressures, RV or RA hypertrophy with reduced compliance, or with regional tamponade of the left heart. LA—left atrial; LV—left ventricular.

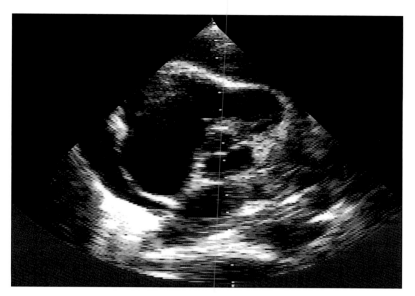

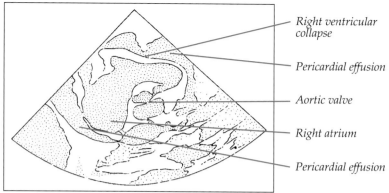

FIGURE 5-53. Two-dimensional echocardiogram, parasternal short-axis view, showing right ventricular diastolic collapse in a patient with a large pericardial effusion and cardiac tamponade. (*Courtesy of* Brian Hoit, MD.)

Right ventricular collapse

Pericardial effusion

Aortic valve

Right atrium

Pericardial effusion

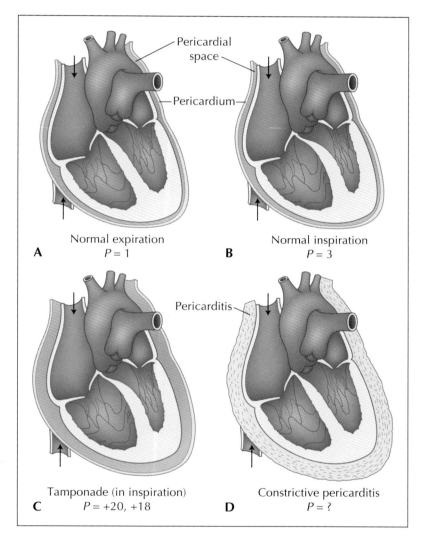

Pericardial space

Pericardium

A Normal expiration
$P = 1$

B Normal inspiration
$P = 3$

Pericarditis

C Tamponade (in inspiration)
$P = +20, +18$

D Constrictive pericarditis
$P = ?$

FIGURE 5-54. A comparison of the hemodynamic effects and the effects of respiration on cardiac tamponade compared with constrictive pericarditis. **A** and **B**, Normal physiology. In *A*, *arrows* in the venae cavae indicate systemic venous return. During inspiration, intrathoracic pressure declines, causing the pericardial pressure to fall from 1 to -3 mm Hg. Venous return increases (*arrows* in *B*), causing an increase in the size of the right heart at the expense of the left ventricle, which becomes smaller. The latter effect is caused in part by bowing of the interventricular septum from right to left. The upper lead lines indicate the parietal pericardium; the lower ones indicate the pericardial space, which normally may contain up to 25 mL of pericardial fluid. **C** and **D,** Compressive cardiac disorders. During inspiration in cardiac tamponade (*C*), venous return increases (*arrows*) and pericardial pressure falls from 20 to 18 mm Hg. Right heart volume increases slightly because of septal bulging. In constrictive pericarditis (*D*), inspiration does not increase venous return (*arrows*). The pericardial space is obliterated and therefore intrathoracic pressure changes are not transmitted to the heart. During inspiration the septum does not bow toward the left. (*Adapted from* Shabetai [58].)

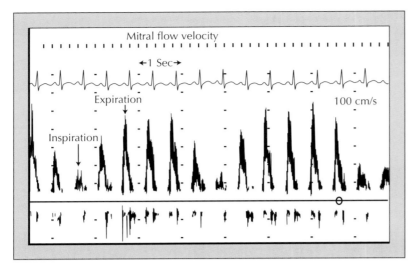

FIGURE 5-55. Doppler echocardiogram demonstrating abnormal inspiratory decrease in mitral flow velocity in cardiac tamponade. The normal decrease is less than 15%. Abnormal inspiratory decreases in mitral flow velocity also occur in constrictive pericarditis, right ventricular infarction, and chronic obstructive airway disease. (*Adapted from* Hoit [59].)

ACUTE PERICARDITIS

A. CAUSES OF ACUTE PERICARDITIS

Malignant tumor
Idiopathic pericarditis
Uremia
Bacterial infection
Anticoagulant therapy
Dissecting aortic aneurysm
Diagnostic procedures
Connective tissue disease
Postpericardiotomy syndrome
Trauma
Tuberculosis
Others
  Radiation
  Drugs inducing lupuslike syndrome
  Myxedema
  Chylopericardium
  Postmyocardial infarction syndrome (Dressler's)
  Fungal infections
  AIDS-related pericarditis

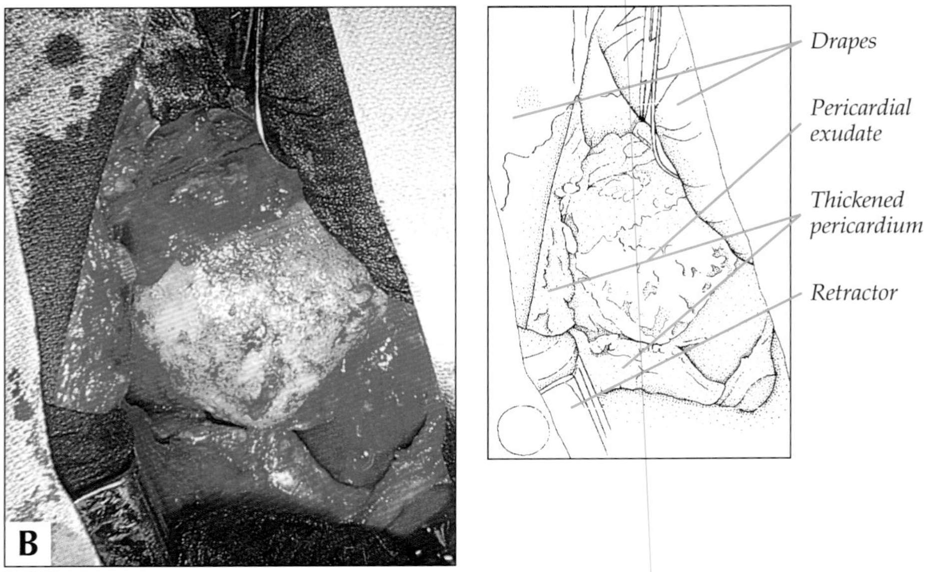

FIGURE 5-56. A, In most hospital series, malignant tumors are the most common cause of acute pericarditis, and idiopathic pericarditis is the second most common. These two causes, together with chronic renal failure, infection, and connective tissue disease, comprise about 50% of cases. In some inner-city hospitals, acquired immunodeficiency syndrome (AIDS)–related pericarditis has become one of the most common causes [60]. **B,** The exposed heart of a patient with pneumococcal pericarditis, showing purulent exudate and thickened pericardium.

PRESENTING FEATURES OF ACUTE PERICARDITIS

Chest pain of pleuropericardial quality
Dull, oppressive chest pain
Pericardial rub
Dyspnea or tachycardia
Unexplained fever or toxicity

Cardiac tamponade with elevated venous pressure
Incidental finding on electrocardiogram, echocardiogram, or chest radiogram

FIGURE 5-57. Acute pericarditis is usually recognized by the presenting findings of chest pain or pericardial rub, but may be first recognized by echocardiographic evidence of pericardial effusion or changes on the chest radiogram or electrocardiogram. Some cases present with cardiac tamponade, dyspnea, tachycardia, and elevated venous pressure, simulating congestive heart failure

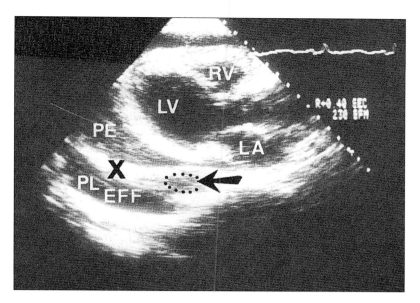

FIGURE 5-58. Two-dimensional echocardiogram (parasternal long-axis view) in a patient with pericardial and pleural effusions. A large pericardial effusion (PE) is present posterior to the left ventricle (LV) and left atrium (LA). A left pleural effusion (PL EFF) is seen as an echo-free space posterior to the pericardial effusion and partitioned from it by a linear echo (X) representing the pericardium. The most important landmark in distinguishing pleural from pericardial effusions is the descending thoracic aorta (*outlined, arrow*). Pericardial fluid accumulates anterior to the pericardial border, insinuating itself between the aorta and the heart; the left pleural effusion, conversely, resides exclusively posterior to the descending aorta. RV—right ventricle. (*From* Fowler [61]; with permission.)

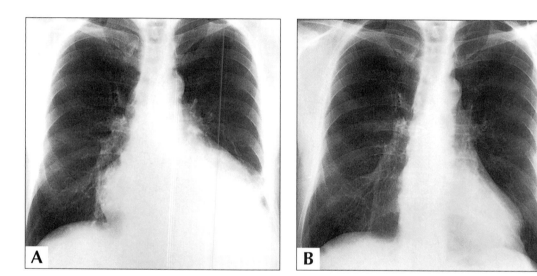

FIGURE 5-59. Chest radiographs of a patient with relapsing idiopathic pericarditis [62]. **A,** Enlarged cardiopericardial silhouette with a left pleural effusion. **B,** Essentially normal radiograph made during a remission following prednisone therapy. Pleural effusions occur commonly in idiopathic pericarditis and usually are either on the left or bilateral.

CONSTRICTIVE PERICARDITIS

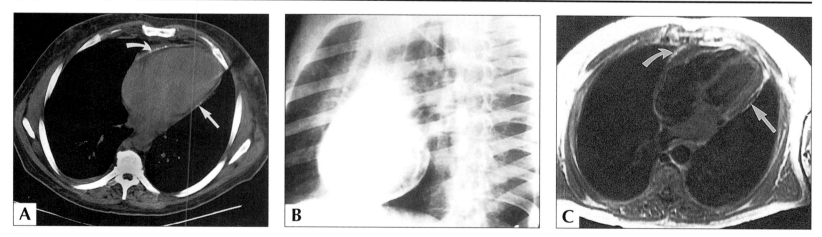

FIGURE 5-60. **A,** Computed tomography of the chest showing thickened pericardium and calcification (*arrows*) in a patient with constrictive pericarditis. **B,** Extensive pericardial calcification may occur with chronic pericarditis without constriction. The typical hemodynamic pattern must also be present to make the diagnosis of constrictive pericarditis. **C,** Magnetic resonance imaging from a patient with constrictive pericarditis. Note a dark area of thickened pericardium over the left ventricle (*straight arrow*) and a light area of pericardial fat over the right ventricle (*curved arrow*). (Part A *from* Fowler [60]; with permission.)

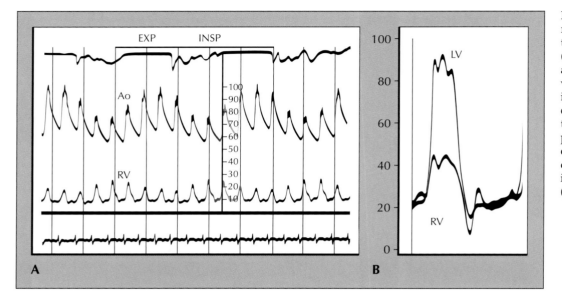

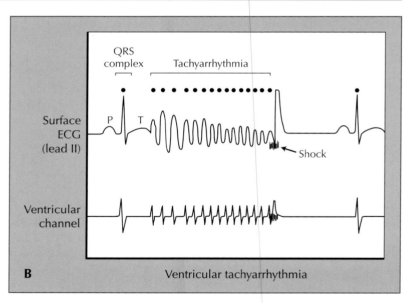

FIGURE 5-61. Contrasting pattern of a ventricular pressure pulse recording in cardiac tamponade (A) and in constrictive pericarditis (B) [54]. In constrictive pericarditis, there is a dip and plateau pattern (square-root sign) in both ventricular pressure pulse tracings with equalization of right (RV) and left ventricular (LV) end-diastolic pressures. In cardiac tamponade, there is no pronounced diastolic dip in the RV pressure pulse. The patient with cardiac tamponade demonstrates a pronounced inspiratory decline of aortic pressure (Ao). Pressure scale is in mm Hg. EXP—expiration; INSP—inspiration. (*Adapted from* Shabetai *et al.* [63].)

DEVICE THERAPY FOR ADVANCED HEART DISEASE

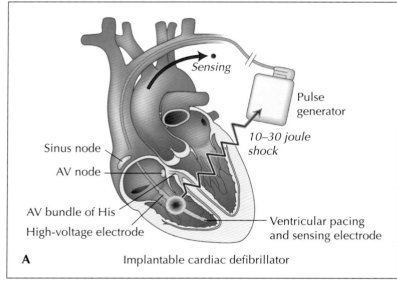

FIGURE 5-62. Schematic of an implantable cardiac defibrillator (ICD) and ventricular tachyarrhythmia. A, ICD. A lead is placed in the right ventricular apex. The ICD monitors the heart rate via a pacing and sensing electrode. B, If the patient develops a ventricular tach- yarrhythmia, the rapid ventricular activity is sensed by the ICD and a shock is delivered between a large proximal, high voltage electrode and the ICD pulse generator, returning the patient to normal sinus rhythm [64].

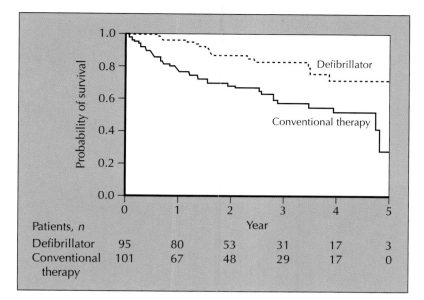

FIGURE 5-63. Kaplan-Meier analysis of the probability of survival according to assigned treatment. Probability of survival in patients randomly assigned to defibrillator versus conventional therapy (Multicenter Automatic Defibrillator Implantation Trial – 1 [MADIT]). Patients selected had New York Heart Association class 1–3 heart failure with prior myocardial infarction and a left ventricular ejection fraction below 35%. Each candidate had a documented episode of asymptomatic unsustained ventricular tachycardia and inducible nonsuppressible ventricular tachyarrhythmia on electrophysiologic study. This patient population demonstrated that prophylactic therapy with an implantable defibrillator leads to improved survival compared with conventional therapy [65].

Patients, n						
Defibrillator	95	80	53	31	17	3
Conventional therapy	101	67	48	29	17	0

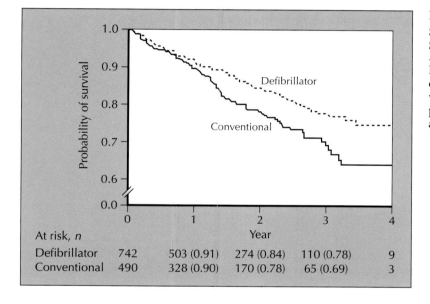

FIGURE 5-64. Kaplan-Meier estimates of the probability of survival in the group assigned to receive an implantable defibrillator compared with the group assigned to receive conventional medical therapy in the Multicenter Automatic Defibrillator Implantation Trial – 2 (MADIT 2). Patients in the MADIT 2 trial qualified by having a recent myocardial infarction and an ejection fraction of 30% or below. Even without evidence of nonsustained ventricular tachycardia or inducible ventricular tachycardia by electrophysiologic testing, the superiority of a prophylactic defibrillator was again demonstrated [16].

At risk, n				
Defibrillator	742	503 (0.91)	274 (0.84)	110 (0.78)	9
Conventional	490	328 (0.90)	170 (0.78)	65 (0.69)	3

FIGURE 5-65. Cardiac resynchronization therapy requires the placement of three pacing leads in the heart as depicted. Two leads allow pacing of the right atrium and the right ventricle, as has been standard for atrial-ventricular pacing. A third lead is advanced through the coronary sinus into a venous branch that runs along the free wall of the left ventricle, allowing early activation of the left ventricular lateral wall. In patients with cardiomyopathy and QRS interval greater than 130 milliseconds with left bundle branch block pattern, this resynchronization of ventricular contraction improves ventricular performance and ejection fraction [67].

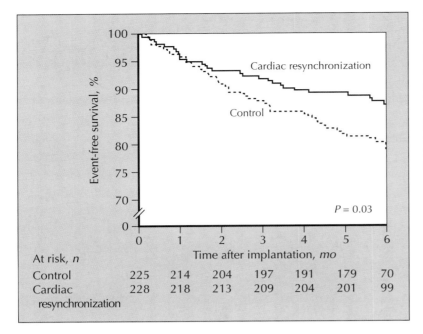

FIGURE 5-66. Kaplan-Meier estimates of the time to death or hospitalization for worsening heart failure in patients assigned to resynchronization therapy compared with control. Qualifying patients had moderate to severe heart failure symptoms with an ejection fraction of 35% or less and a QRS interval of 130 milliseconds or more. In addition to the improved survival noted, patients in the cardiac resynchronization group had an improved 6-minute walk test, functional class, quality of life or time on treadmill, and ejection fraction. Fewer resynchronization patients were hospitalized or received intravenous medications for heart failure. Of note, 8% of the patients could not have the device implanted for technical reasons. In these instances, a left thoracotomy may be necessary to implant the lead on the lateral wall (in appropriate candidates) [68–70].

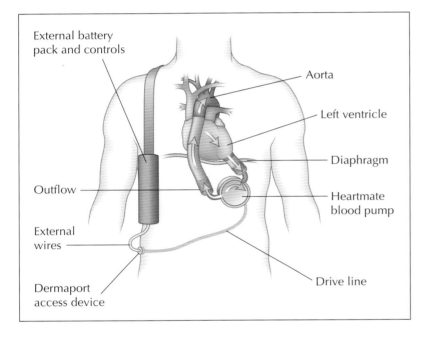

FIGURE 5-67. A wearable left ventricular assist device and its components. The inflow canula is placed in the apex of the left ventricle and blood is drawn into the blood pump. The inflow conduit has a valve allowing one-way flow. The outflow conduit also has a valve and the blood pump forces blood through the valve into the ascending aorta. The pumping chamber is placed in the abdominal wall. A single transcutaneous line carries the electrical cable and air vent to the battery pack that is worn externally [71].

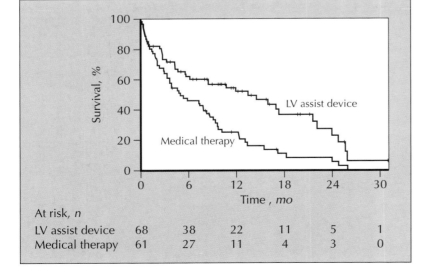

FIGURE 6-68. Kaplan-Meier analysis of survival in a group of patients that received a left ventricular assist device compared with a group that received optimal medical therapy. Patients were selected who were ineligible for cardiac transplantation and received the ventricular assist device as "destination" therapy. The rates of survival at 1 year were 52% in the device group and 25% in the optimal medical group; at 2 years the rates were 23% and 8%, respectively. The device group had 2.4 times the serious adverse event rate compared with the optimal medical group. These complications included infection, bleeding, and malfunction of the device. The quality of life was nonetheless improved at 1 year in the device group [72,73].

REFERENCES

1. Kamisago M, Sharma SD, DePalma SR, *et al.*: Mutations in sarcomere protein genes as a cause of dilated cardiomyopathy. *N Engl J Med* 2000, 343:1688–1696.

2. Wigle ED, Sasson Z, Henderson MA, *et al.*: Hypertrophic cardiomyopathy. The importance of the site and the extent of hypertrophy: a review. *Prog Cardiovasc Dis* 1985, 28:1–85.

3. Shah PM, Taylor RD, Wong M: Abnormal mitral valve coaptation in hypertrophic obstructive cardiomyopathy: proposed role in systolic anterior motion of mitral valve. *Am J Cardiol* 1981, 48:258–262.

4. Grigg LE, Wigle ED, Williams WG, *et al.*: Transesophageal Doppler echocardiography in obstructive hypertrophic cardiomyopathy: clarification of pathophysiology and importance in intraoperative decision making. *J Am Coll Cardiol* 1992, 20:42–52.

5. Braunwald E: Hypertrophic cardiomyopathy – the benefits of a multidisciplinary approach. *N Engl J Med* 2002, 347:1306–1307.

6. McDonald K, McWilliams E, O'Keeffe B, *et al.*: Functional assessment of patients treated with permanent dual chamber pacing as a primary treatment for hypertrophic cardiomyopathy. *Eur Heart J* 1988, 9:893–898.

7. Fananapazir L, Cannon RO, Tripodi D, *et al.*: Impact of dual-chamber permanent pacing in patients with obstructive hypertrophic and cardiomyopathy with symptoms refractory to verapamil and beta-adrenergic blocker therapy. *Circulation* 1992, 85:2149–2161.

8. Wigle ED, Chrysohou A, Bigelow W: Results of ventriculomyotomy in muscular subaortic stenosis. *Am J Cardiol* 1963, 11:572–586.

9. Maron BJ, Epstein SE, Morrow AG: Symptomatic status and prognosis of patients after operation for hypertrophic obstructive cardiomyopathy: efficacy of ventricular septal myotomy and myectomy. *Eur Heart J* 1983, 4(suppl F):175–185.

10. Beahrs MM, Tajik AJ, Seward JB, *et al.*: Hypertrophic obstructive cardiomyopathy: 10–21 year follow-up after partial septal myectomy. *Am J Cardiol* 1983, 51:1160–1166.

11. Williams WG, Wigle ED, Rakowski H, *et al.*: Results of surgery for idiopathic hypertrophic obstructive cardiomyopathy (IHSS). *Circulation* 1987, 76:V104–V108.

12. Spirito P, Bellone P, Harris KM, *et al.*: Magnitude of left ventricular hypertrophy and risk of sudden death in hypertrophic cardiomyopathy. *N Engl J Med* 2000, 342:1778–1785.

13. Maron BJ, Shen WK, Link MS, *et al.*: Efficacy of implantable cardioverter-defibrillators for the prevention of sudden death in patients with hypertrophic cardiomyopathy. *N Engl J Med* 2000, 342:365–373.

14. Manolio TA, Baughman KL, Rodeheffer R, *et al.*: Prevalence and etiology of idiopathic dilated cardiomyopathy. *Am J Cardiol* 1992, 69:1458–1466.

15. Abelmann WH: Classification and natural history of primary myocardial disease. *Prog Cardiovasc Dis* 1985, 127:73–94.

16. Felker GM, Thompson RE, Hare JM, *et al.*: Underlying causes and long-term survival in patients with initially unexplained cardiomyopathy. *N Engl J Med* 2000, 342:1077–1084.

17. Wallis DE, O'Connell JB, Henkin RE, *et al.*: Segmental wall motion abnormalities in dilated cardiomyopathy: a common finding and good prognostic sign. *J Am Coll Cardiol* 1984, 4:674–679.

18. Fitzpatrick TB, Eisen AZ, Wolff K, *et al.*: *Dermatology in General Medicine*, vol 2, ed 4. New York: McGraw-Hill; 1993:2412.

19. McAlister HF, Klementowicz PT, Andrews C, *et al.*: Lyme carditis: an important cause of reversible heart block. *Ann Intern Med* 1989, 110:339–345.

20. Van der Linde MR, Crijns HJCM, de Konig J, *et al.*: Range of atrioventricular disturbances in Lyme borreliosis: a report of four cases and review of other published reports. *Br Heart J* 1990, 63:162–168.

21. Steere AC: A 58-year-old man with a diagnosis of chronic Lyme disease. *JAMA* 2002, 288:1002–1010.

22. Roberts WC, McAlister HA, Ferrano VJ: Sarcoidosis of the heart. *Am J Med* 1977, 63:86–108.

23. Shammas RL, Movahed A: Sarcoidosis of the heart. *Clin Cardiol* 1993, 16:462–472.

24. Uretsky BF: Diagnostic considerations in the adult patient with cardiomyopathy or congestive heart failure. In *Cardiovascular Clinics*. Edited by Shaver JA. Philadelphia: FA Davis; 1988:35–56.

25. Sekiguchi M, Numao Y, Nunoda S, *et al.*: Clinical histopathological profile of sarcoidosis of the heart and acute idiopathic myocarditis: concepts through a study employing endomyocardial biopsy. *Jpn Circ J* 1980, 44:249–263.

26. Gertz MA, Kyle RA: Primary systemic amyloidosis: a diagnostic primer. *Mayo Clin Proc* 1989, 64:1505–1519.

27. Falk RH: Cardiac amyloidosis. In *Progress in Cardiology*. Edited by Zipes DP, Rowlands DJ. Philadelphia: Lea & Febiger; 1989:143–153.

28. Klein AL, Hatle LK, Burstow DJ, *et al.*: Doppler characterization of left ventricular diastolic function in cardiac amyloidosis. *J Am Coll Cardiol* 1989, 13:1017–1026.

29. Kushwaha SS, Fallon JT, Fuster V: Restrictive cardiomyopathy [review]. *N Engl J Med* 1997, 336:267–276.

30. Hongo M, Fuji T, Hirayama J, *et al.*: Radionuclide angiographic assessment of left ventricular diastolic filling in amyloid heart disease: a study of patients with familial amyloid polyneuropathy. *J Am Coll Cardiol* 1989, 13:48–53.

31. Bessen M, Gardin JM: Evaluation of left ventricular diastolic function. *Cardiol Clin* 1990, 8:315–332.

32. Appleton CP, Hatle LK, Popp RL: Demonstration of restrictive ventricular physiology by Doppler echocardiography. *J Am Coll Cardiol* 1988, 11:757–768.

33. Hirota Y, Shimizu G, Kita Y, *et al.*: Spectrum of restrictive cardiomyopathy: report of the national survey in Japan. *Am Heart J* 1990, 120:188–194.

34. Spry CJF, Tai PC: clinical studies on endomyocardial fibrosis in patients with hypereosinophilia: a historical review. In *Cardiomyopathy Update 3. Restrictive Cardiomyopathy and Arrhythmias*. Edited by Olsen EGJ, Sekiguchi M. Tokyo: University of Tokyo Press; 1990:81–98.

35. Vijayaraghavan G, Sadanandan S, Cherian G: Endomyocardial fibrosis in India: an overview. In *Cardiomyopathy Update 3. Restrictive Cardiomyopathy and Arrhythmias*. Edited by Olsen EGJ, Sekiguchi M. Tokyo: University of Tokyo Press; 1990:9–20.

36. Nakayama Y, Kohriyama T, Yamamoto S, *et al.*: Electron microscopic and immunohistochemical studies on endomyocardial biopsies from a patient with eosinophilic endomyocardial disease. *Heart Vessel* 1985, 1(suppl 1):250–255.

37. Olsen EGJ: Morphological overview and pathogenetic mechanism in endomyocardial fibrosis associated with eosinophilia. In *Cardiomyopathy Update 3. Restrictive Cardiomyopathy and Arrhythmias*. Edited by Olsen EGJ, Sekiguchi M. Tokyo: University of Tokyo Press; 1990:1–8.

38. Andy JJ: The relationship of microfilaria and other helminthic worms to tropical endomyocardial fibrosis: a review. In *Cardiomyopathy Update 3. Restrictive Cardiomyopathy and Arrhythmias*. Edited by Olsen EGJ, Sekiguchi M. Tokyo: University of Tokyo Press; 1990:21–34.

39. Roberts NK, Perloff JK, Kark RAP: Cardiac conduction in the Kearns-Sayre syndrome (a neuromuscular disorder associated with progressive external ophthalmoplegia and pigmentary retinopathy). *Am J Cardiol* 1979, 44:1396–1400.

40. Graham RM, Owens WA: Pathogenesis of inherited forms of dilated cardiomyopathy. *N Engl J Med* 1999, 341, 1759–1762.

41. Liu PP, Mason JW: Advances in the understanding of myocarditis. *Circulation* 2001, 104:1076–1082.

42. Aretz HT: Myocarditis: the Dallas criteria. *Hum Pathol* 1987, 18:619–624.

43. Aretz HT, Billingham ME, Edwards WD, *et al.*: A histopathologic definition and classification. *Am J Cardiovasc Pathol* 1986, 1:3–14.

44. Neumann DA, Rose NR, Ansari AA, *et al.*: Induction of heart auto-antibodies in mice with coxsackievrius B3- and cardiac myosin-induced autoimmune myocarditis. *J Immunol* 1994, 152:343–350.

45. Huber SA, Moraska A: Cytolytic T lymphocytes and antibodies to myocytes in adriamycin-treated BALB/c mice. *Am J Pathol* 1992, 140:233–242.

46. Strain JE, Grose RM, Factor SM, *et al.*: Results of endomyocardial biopsy in patients with spontaneous ventricular tachycardia but without apparent structural heart disease. *Circulation* 1983, 68:1171–1181.

47. Smith WG: Coxsackie B myopericarditis in adults. *Am Heart J* 1980, 80:34–36.

48. Rockman HA, Adamson RM, Dembitsky WP, *et al.*: Acute fulminant myocarditis: long-term follow-up after circulatory support with left ventricular assist device. *Am Heart J* 1991, 121:922–926.

49. Jones SR, Herskowitz A, Hutchins GM, *et al*.: Effects of immunosuppressive therapy in biopsy-proved myocarditis and borderline myocarditis on left ventricular function. *Am J Cardiol* 1991, 68:370–376.

50. McCarthy RE, Boehmer JP, Hruban RH, *et al*.: Long-term outcome of fulminant myocarditis as compared with acute (nonfulminant) myocarditis. *N Engl J Med* 2000, 342:690–695.

51. Wojnicz R, Nowalany-Kozielska E, Wojciechowska C, *et al*.: Randomized, placebo-controlled study for immunosuppressive treatment of inflammatory dilated cardiomyopathy: two-year follow-up results. *Circulation* 2001, 104:39–45.

52. Frustaci A, Chimenti C, Calabrese F, *et al*.: Immunosuppressive therapy for active lymphocytic myocarditis: virological and immunologic profile of responders versus nonresponders. *Circulation* 2003, 107:857–863.

53. Corrado D, Basso C, Thiene G: Arrhythmogenic right ventricular cardiomyopathy: diagnosis, prognosis, and treatment. *Heart* 2000, 83:588–595.

54. Goldschlager N, Epstein A, Grubb BP, *et al*.: Etiologic considerations in the patient with syncope and an apparently normal heart. *Arch Intern Med* 2003, 163:151–162.

55. Cooper LT Jr, Berry GJ, Shabetai R: Idiopathic giant-cell myocarditis – natural history and treatment. Multicenter Giant Cell Myocarditis Study Group Investigators. *N Engl J Med* 1997, 336:1860–1866.

56. Menghini VV, Savcenko V, Olson LJ, *et al*.: Combined immunosuppression for the treatment of idopathic giant cell myocarditis. *Mayo Clin Proc* 1999, 74:1221–1226.

57. Reddy PS, Curtiss EI, Uritsky BF: Spectrum of hemodynamic changes in cardiac tamponade. *Am J Cardiol* 1990, 66:1487–1491.

58. Shabetai R: *The Pericardium*. New York: Grune and Stratton; 1981.

59. Hoit BD: Imaging the pericardium. In *Diseases of the Pericardium: Cardiology Clinics*, vol 8. Philadelphia: WB Saunders; 1990:587–600.

60. Fowler NO: Pericardial disease. *Heart Dis Stroke* 1992, 1:85–94.

61. Fowler NO: *The Pericardium in Health and Disease*. Mount Kisco, NY: Futura Publishing Co; 1985.

62. Fowler NO: Recurrent pericarditis. In *Diseases of the Pericardium: Cardiology Clinics*, vol 8. Edited by Shabetai R. Philadelphia: WB Saunders; 1990:621–626.

63. Shabetai R, Fowler NO, Guntheroth WG: The hemodynamics of cardiac tamponade and constrictive pericarditis. *Am J Cardiol* 1970, 26:480–489.

64. Kusumoto FM, Goldschlager N: Device therapy for cardiac arrhythmias. *JAMA* 2002, 287:1848–1852.

65. Moss AJ, Hall WJ, Cannon DS, *et al*.: Improved survival with an implanted defibrillator in patients with coronary disease at high risk for ventricular arrhythmia. Multicenter Automatic Defibrillator Implantation Trial Investigators. *N Engl J Med* 1996, 335:1933–1940.

66. Moss AJ, Zareba W, Wall WJ, *et al*.: Prophylactic implantation of a defibrillator in patients with myocardial infarction and reduced ejection fraction. *N Engl J Med* 2002, 346:877–883.

67. Hare JM: Cardiac resynchronization therapy for heart failure. *N Engl J Med* 2002, 346:1902–1905.

68. Abraham WT, Fisher WG, Smith AL, *et al*.: Cardiac resynchronization in chronic heart failure. *N Engl J Med* 2002, 346:1845–1853.

69. Cazeau S, Leclercq C, Lavergne T, *et al*.: Effects of multisite biventricular pacing in patients with heart failure and intraventricular conduction delay. *N Engl J Med* 2001, 344:873–880.

70. Linde C, Leclercq C, Rex S, *et al*.: Long-term benefits of biventricular pacing in congestive heart failure: results from the Multisite Stimulation in Cardiomyopathy (MUSTIC) trial. *J Am Coll Cardiol* 2002, 40:111–118.

71. Goldstein DJ, Oz MC, Rose EA: Implantable left ventricular assist devices. *N Engl J Med* 1998, 339:1522–1533.

72. Rose EA, Gelijns AC, Moskowitz AJ, *et al*.: Long-term mechanical left ventricular assistance for end-stage heart failure. *N Engl J Med* 2001, 345:1435–1443.

73. Hunt SA, Frazier OH: Mechanical circulatory support and cardiac transplantation. *Circulation* 1998, 97:2079–2090.

ARRHYTHMIAS

Edited by Byron K. Lee and Melvin Scheinman

James L. Cockrell, Laurence M. Epstein, Adam Fitzpatrick, Kathryn A. Glatter, Harlan R. Grogin, Edmund C. Keung, Randall J. Lee, Michael D. Lesh, Andreana Siu

CHAPTER 6

CONDUCTION AND EXCITATION: NORMAL PATHWAY OF ELECTRICAL CONDUCTION

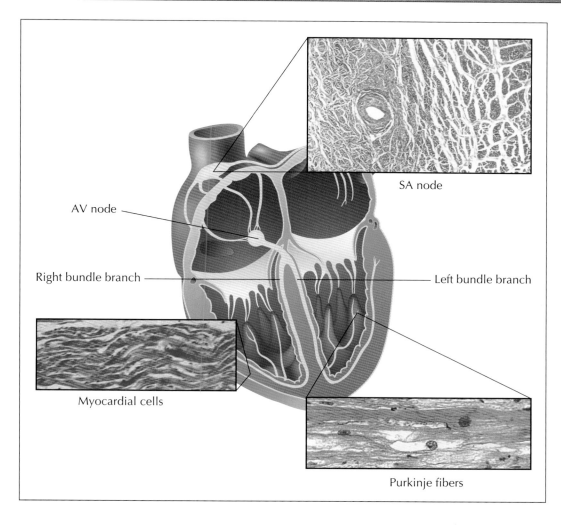

FIGURE 6-1. Normal pathway of electrical conduction in the heart. Note the differences between the conductive and the contractile tissue of the heart (*insets*). The sinus nodal cells are smaller and interwoven so as to form a network of cells grouped together by the surrounding fibrous matrix. They contain relatively few myofilaments compared with "working" myocardial cells. The Purkinje fibers are composed of short, cylindrical cells that are irregularly shaped. The ultrastructure of an irregularly shaped cell, which increases cell-to-cell contact, and the large gap junctions at both the ends and sides of the cells provide the membrane properties of rapid impulse conduction. AV—atrioventricular; SA—sinoatrial.

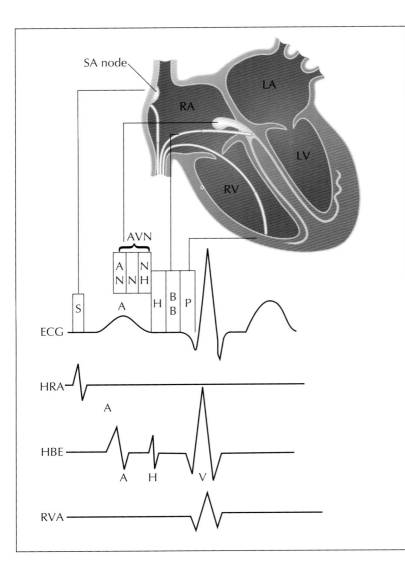

FIGURE 6-2. Sequence of activation through the conduction system relative to surface electrocardiogram (ECG) events and intracardiac electrograms. The intracardiac catheters are positioned in the high right atrium (to record atrial intracardiac ECGs), the low atrioseptal right atrium (RA; to record the His bundle ECG), and the right ventricular (RV) apex (to record the ventricular intracardiac ECG). Note the activation of the sinoatrial (SA) node prior to the onset of the P wave. Conduction through the AV node begins well before atrial depolarization is completed, while conduction through the His-Purkinje system precedes contraction of the ventricles (reflected as the QRS complex). Intracardiac ECGs confirm the activation sequence and timing of the conduction system. Note that the atrial activity in the atrial intracardiac ECG precedes the atrial activity in the His bundle recording, as atrial conduction begins high in the SA node. A—atrial conduction; AN—nodal conduction; AVN—AV nodal conduction; BB—bundle branch conduction; H—His bundle conduction; HBE—His-bundle ECG; HRA—high RA intracardiac ECG; LA—left atrium; LV—left ventricle; N—nodal conduction; NH—nodal–His conduction; P—Purkinje fiber conduction; RVA—RV apex ECG; S—SA node conduction; V—ventricular conduction. (*Adapted from* Marriot and Conover [1].)

CELLULAR ELECTROPHYSIOLOGY

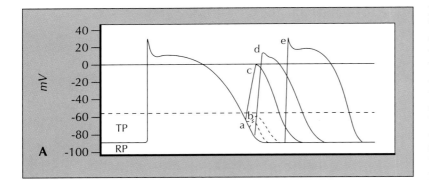

FIGURE 6-3. **A,** A normal action potential and its relative refractory period. This diagram represents a normal action potential and the responses elicited by stimuli applied at different stages of repolarization. The amplitude and upstroke velocity of the elicited responses are directly related to the membrane potential stimuli applied early during repolarization. As *a* and *b* arise from such a low level of membrane potential, they are too small to propagate graded or local responses. The earliest propagated action potential is response *c*, which defines the end of the effective refractory period (ERP). However, response *c* propagates slowly due to its low amplitude and low upstroke velocity. Response *d* is elicited during the supernormal period (SNP) of excitability and its rates of rise and amplitude are greater than those of *c* because it arises from a higher membrane potential. However, it still propagates more slowly than the normal response *e*, which occurs after complete repolarization and therefore has a normal rate of depolarization and amplitude. Response *e* propagates rapidly [2].

Continued on next page

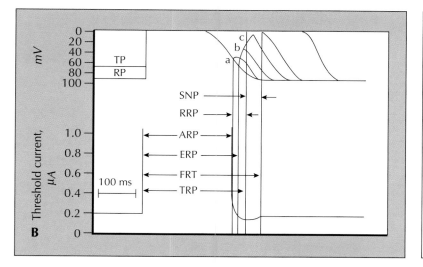

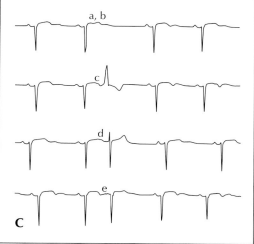

FIGURE 6-3. *(Continued)* **B,** The refractory periods in respect to the action potential. The fiber becomes inexcitable beginning with the inscription of phase 0 of the action potential. Recovery of excitability progresses slowly during phase 3 of repolarization. A period of supernormal excitability, in which a submaximal stimulus can elicit a propagated action potential, occurs at the terminal portion of phase 3. The diagram also illustrates the absolute refractory period (ARP), ERP, relative refractory period (RRP), total refractory period (TRP), full recovery time (FRT), and the SNP of excitability. The threshold currents are indicated in microamperes (μA). Vertical lines demonstrate the relationship of the refractory period to the elicited responses during repolarization. This diagram demonstrates the time course relationships among repolarization, refractoriness, and excitability.

C, The electrocardiographic strips of atrial premature beats are examples of stimuli during the different periods of repolarization. Beats *a* and *b* occur during the total refractory period and are either not conducted or result in a nonconducted atrial premature beat. Beats *c* and *d* occur with aberration, since recovery is incomplete. Beat *c*, being earlier, is conducted more aberrantly. Beat *e* occurs after full recovery and is conducted normally. (Part A *adapted from* Singer and Ten Eick [2]; part B *adapted from* Mandel [3].)

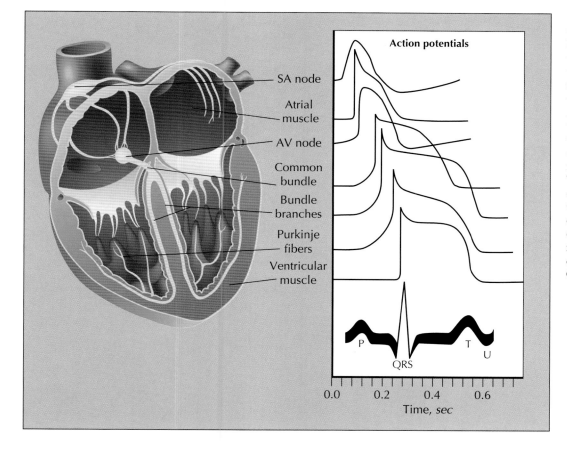

FIGURE 6-4. Localized variations in the action potential of the heart's electrical system. Cardiac action potentials from different locations in the heart have different shapes, leading to different electrophysiologic properties. The SA node and AV node depolarize in response to the slow inward current of calcium and sodium. All other cardiac cells depolarize in response to the rapid inward current of sodium ions. Note the progressive increase in the action potential duration beginning at the AV node and reaching its maximum in the Purkinje fiber. This results in the functional refractory period of the ventricular tissue being dependent on the effective refractory period of the Purkinje cell. Furthermore, specialized cells depolarize during phase 4, whereas atrial and ventricular muscle does not. (*Adapted from* CIBA Pharmaceutical Company Division of CIBA-GEIGY Corporation [4].)

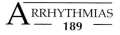

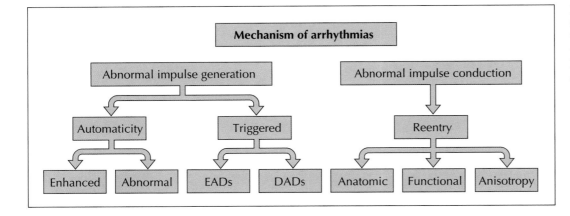

FIGURE 6-5. Mechanism of arrhythmias. Mechanistically, arrhythmias can be separated into those due to abnormal impulse generation and those due to abnormal impulse conduction. EAD—early after-depolarization; DAD—delayed after-depolarization.

AUTOMATICITY

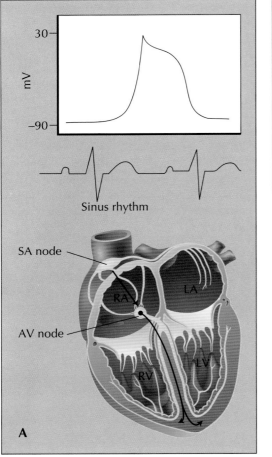

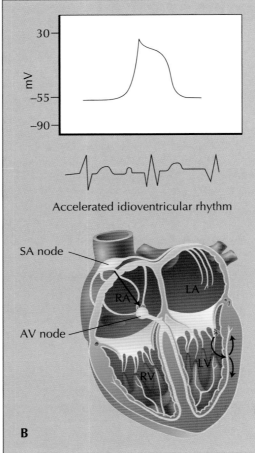

FIGURE 6-6. Abnormal automaticity occurs when spontaneous depolarizations are generated in partially depolarized tissue (reduced maximum diastolic potential or resting membrane potential) as a result of some pathologic process such as ischemia. Arrhythmias that may arise because of abnormal automaticity are certain types of ectopic atrial tachycardias, accelerated idioventricular rhythms, and ventricular tachycardias (especially within the first 72 hours after a myocardial infarction). Compared are normal ventricular tissue (**A**) and ischemic ventricular tissue (*asterisk* in **B**). Shown are the action potentials along with a schematic drawing of the possible conduction throughout the heart and the resultant rhythms. LA—left atrium; LV—left ventricle; RA—right atrium; RV—right ventricle.

TRIGGERED ARRHYTHMIAS

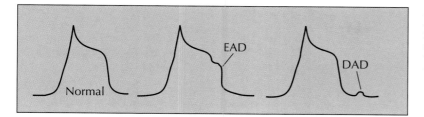

FIGURE 6-7. Triggered activity arises as a consequence of increased positive ions within the cardiac cell, leading to distortion of the action potential (after-depolarization). After-depolarizations can occur in the late phase 3 (early after-depolarization [EAD]) or early phase 4 (delayed after-depolarization [DAD]).

REENTRY

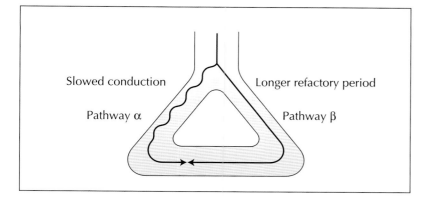

FIGURE 6-8. Prerequisites for reentry arrhythmias include: (1) an anatomic circuit with two pathways eventually joined by a common tissue, (2) the two pathways have different electrophysiologic properties, and (3) a section within the circuit (pathway β) has a longer refractory period than the pathway α, thus permitting unidirectional block.

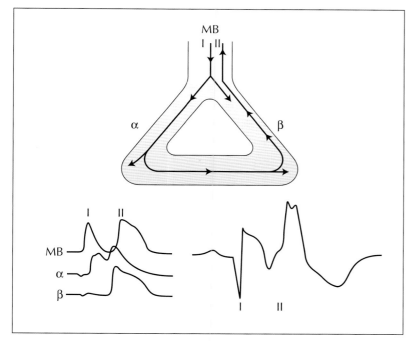

FIGURE 6-9. The sequence of activation within the reentry circuit, indicated by arrows I and II. Arrow I indicates an impulse of sinus origin entering the circuit. Arrow II is the reentry impulse leaving the loop. Under the reentry circuit are action potentials recorded from myocardial branches (MB) α and β together with an example of how an electrocardiogram might appear. Impulse I would cause ventricular depolarization and impulse II would cause a ventricular extrasystole. (*Adapted from* Wit and Bigger [5].)

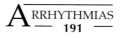

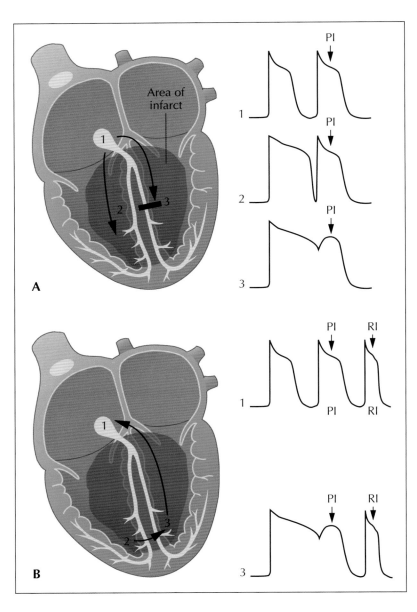

FIGURE 6-10. Mechanism for reentry resulting from dispersion of refractoriness in the subendocardial Purkinje fiber network over an area of extensive myocardial infarction. This figure shows the endocardial surface of the left ventricular anterior papillary muscle. The color area in each diagram is the scar resulting from the myocardial infarct that is covered by a blanket of the surviving Purkinje fibers. As depicted, Purkinje fibers in different regions have markedly different action potentials with respect to duration and refractory periods. Action potentials are recorded from normal tissue (site 1) and from subendocardial Purkinje fibers with prolonged repolarization phases (sites 2 and 3), surviving in the infarct. In **A**, premature impulse (PI) occurs at the infarct border (site 1) and conducts into the infarcted regions as indicated by the large arrows. Note that the action potentials are prolonged. The action potential at site 3 is longer than at site 2 in the infarcted area. Consequently, premature impulses can excite cells at site 2, but conduction blocks at site 3. **B,** The continuation of these events after the premature impulse conducts through site 2 and activates the cells at site 3. As a reentering impulse (RI), it then proceeds to its site of origin (site 1), which also re-excites as a reentry impulse (RI). (*Adapted from* Wit *et al.* [6].)

ANTIARRHYTHMIC DRUGS

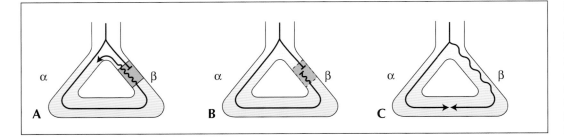

FIGURE 6-11. Effect of antiarrhythmic drugs on reentry. The question of how antiarrhythmic drugs suppress arrhythmias must be addressed by considering arrhythmia mechanisms. Most arrhythmias based on abnormal conduction involve reentry circuits, as illustrated in **A** (described in Figs. 6-8 and 6-9). The *shaded area* represents the depolarized tissue in which conduction block occurs, and retrograde conduction is slow enough to allow the cells in limb α to recover and propagate the reentrant impulse. Antiarrhythmic drugs can eliminate reentry tachyarrhythmias by impairing conduction sufficiently to cause interruption of conduction through the circuit (**B**) or by improving conduction in limb β, which prevents the development of conduction block (**C**). Class I drugs prevent reentry by causing a greater amount of slow conduction in depolarized tissue, thus producing conduction block in both the forward and reverse directions in limb β.

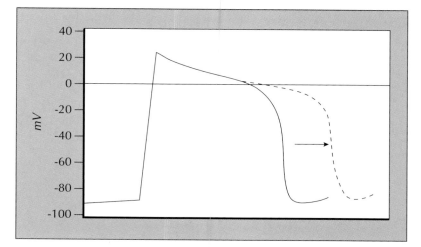

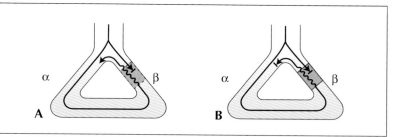

FIGURE 6-13. The probable effect of a drug with Class III antiarrhythmic action on a reentry circuit. Class III drugs can affect a prototypic reentry circuit (**A**; described in Figs. 6-8 and 6-9) by sufficiently prolonging the refractory period of path α, thus preventing reentry from occurring (**B**).

FIGURE 6-12. Class III antiarrhythmics. Class III action consists of prolongation of the action potential duration, which leads to a prolongation of refractoriness. The diagram represents a normal action potential of a Purkinje cell (*solid line*) and the effects of d-sotalol (*dotted line*) on the action potential duration.

SINUS NODE DISORDERS

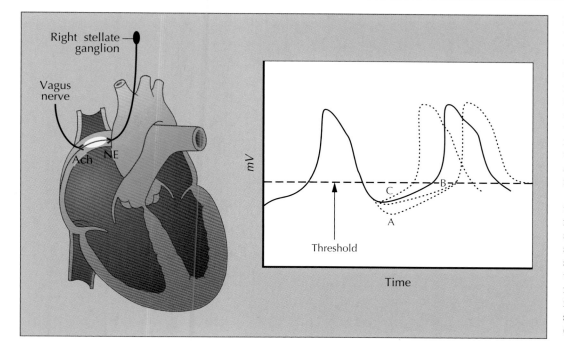

FIGURE 6-14. Autonomic nervous system inputs to the sinus node. Parasympathetic stimulation via the vagus nerve results in the release of acetylcholine (Ach). This produces a *negative* chronotropic response due to a decrease in the maximum diastolic potential (hyperpolarization) (A) and a decrease in the slope of phase and depolarization (B). Sympathetic stimulation via the right stellate ganglion results in norepinephrine (NE) release from the postsynaptic nerve terminals within the sinus node. This produces a *positive* chronotropic response mainly by an increase in the rate of phase 4 depolarization (C).

Modulation of the sinus rate is therefore due to the interactions of the two limbs of the autonomic nervous system (parasympathetic and sympathetic). During sleep and in response to some stimuli (nausea, and in some people, the sight of blood or pain, for example), parasympathetic stimulation predominates, and the heart rate slows. During exercise and in response to fright or to some kinds of pain, sympathetic stimulation predominates, and the heart races. (*Adapted from* Talano *et al.* [7].)

TYPES OF SINUS NODE DYSFUNCTION

CONDITIONS ASSOCIATED WITH SINUS NODE DYSFUNCTION

INTRINSIC

Aging
Hypertension
Coronary artery disease
Rheumatic heart disease
Cardiomyopathies
Pericarditis
Congenital heart abnormalities
Collagen vascular disease
Amyloidosis
Trauma
  Surgical
    Closure of ASD (sinus venosus type)
    Mustard procedure
    Placement of caval cannula
Tumor
Irradiation

EXTRINSIC

Hypothermia
Electrolyte abnormalities
Hypothyroidism
Abnormalities of autonomic nervous
  system (carotid hypersensitivity)
Hyperbilirubinemia
Drugs
  Cardiac glycosides
  β-Adrenergic receptor blockers
  Calcium-channel blockers
  Methyldopa
  Reserpine
  Lithium carbonate
  Cimetidine
  Amitriptyline
  Phenothiazines

FIGURE 6-15. Conditions associated with sinus node dysfunction. Sinus node dysfunction may be due to a pathologic process that directly involves the sinus node (intrinsic) or other processes and drugs that have secondary effects on the sinus node (extrinsic). ASD—atrial septal defect.

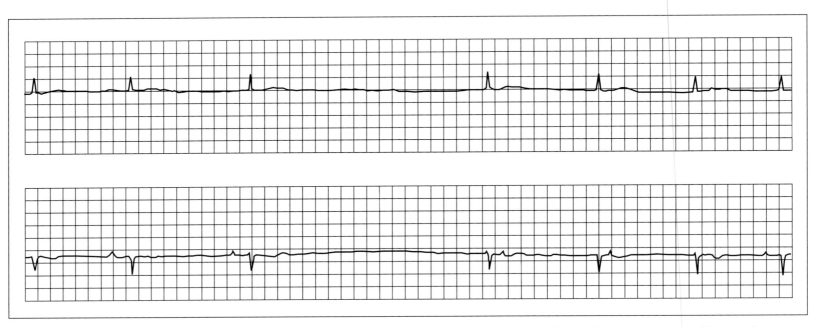

FIGURE 6-16. Failure of impulse generation. Sinus node dysfunction can be manifested as a failure of impulse generation. This can result in sinus bradycardia (defined as sinus rhythm < 60 bpm) or sinus arrest. However, this rate is considered normal during sleep or in a trained person at rest. Sinus bradycardia is clinically significant only if it results in failure to meet the patient's metabolic demands. This may result in physical signs such as hypotension or congestive heart failure or symptoms of fatigue, shortness of breath, exercise intolerance, angina, lightheadedness, or even syncope.

Simultaneous leads V_5 (*top*) and V_1 (*bottom*) of a Holter recording from an 85-year-old woman with a history of syncope. Both sinus bradycardia (38 bpm) and sinus arrest (4.2-second pause) with a junctional escape rhythm are represented. (*Adapted from* Evans [8].)

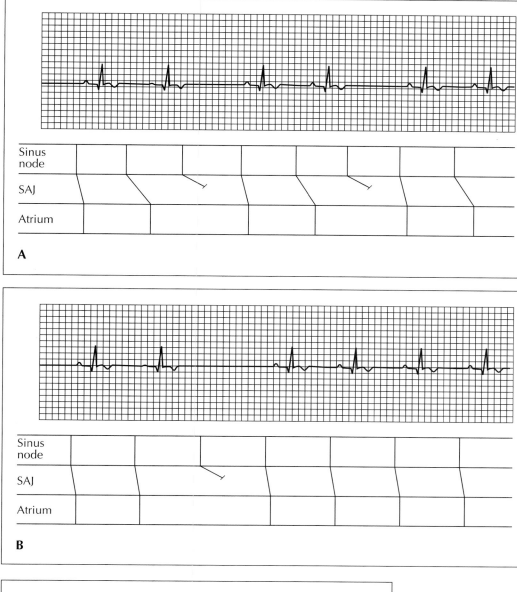

A

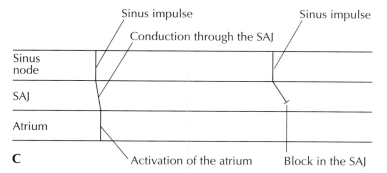

B

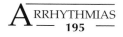

C

FIGURE 6-17. Abnormalities of impulse conduction. Sinus pauses can be due to sinoatrial exit block of the impulse generated from the primary pacemaker cells in the node itself or at the sinoatrial junction.

Block may be manifested in one of two forms. **A,** A typical Wenckebach pattern, with progressive slowing of conduction (in the sinoatrial junction [SAJ]), resulting in progressive shortening of the P-wave–P-wave interval, ending in a sinus pause (blocked impulse). The pause is less than twice the shortest atrial cycle length. **B,** Sudden block, with no prior evidence of conduction slowing, may be observed. In this setting the pause is equal to twice the atrial cycle length (Mobitz II SA block). In *A,* Wenckebach block in the SAJ can be seen. There is progressive slowing (represented by a deceased slope) of conduction in the SAJ prior to block (beats 3 and 6). In *B,* there is no change in conduction through the SAJ. Block (beat 3) occurs suddenly. **C,** A ladder diagram with explanation. Through-out this chapter, ladder diagrams are used to demonstrate electrophysiologic phenomena. Each horizontal area represents a region within the heart. Impulse origin and conduction are represented by the vertical (or slanting) lines. Conduction block is represented by a vertical line with a perpendicular ine at the end of it.

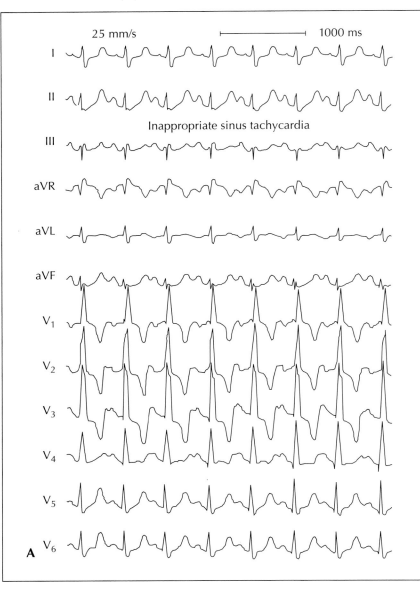

Inappropriate sinus tachycardia

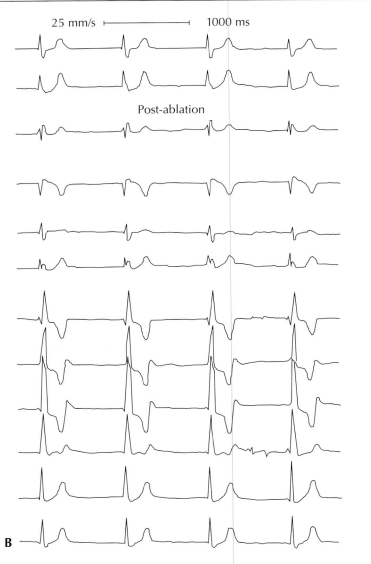

Post-ablation

FIGURE 6-18. Inappropriate sinus tachycardia often can be difficult to treat, and in many cases even combination drug therapy fails to control this arrhythmia adequately [9]. Transcatheter sinus node ablation and/or modification using radiofrequency energy appears to be a treatment option in patients with this refractory arrhythmia. **A,** A 12-lead electro-cardiogram from a patient with drug-resistant inappropriate sinus tachycardia. **B,** Following sinus node ablation the patient initially had a junctional rhythm, but within a week a stable atrial rhythm that appropriately responded to exercise was evident.

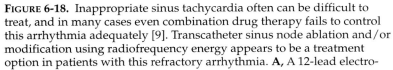

PHARMACOLOGIC INTERVENTIONS FOR ASSESSMENT OF SINUS NODE DISORDERS

DRUG	DOSAGE	RESPONSE		COMMENTS
		NORMAL	ABNORMAL	
Atropine	1.0 mg	> 17% decrease in cycle length	< 25% increase in sinus rate	Relatively easy, safe; helpful only if positive
	0.04 mg/kg	> 15% increase in HR		
	0.03 mg/kg	HR >90 bpm		
	0.04 mg/kg	HR >85 bpm		
Isoproterenol	3 mg/min	> 25% increase in HR	< 25% increase in sinus rate	Helpful if positive; may be dangerous in patients with ventricular arrhythmias or CAD
	Variable	Based on dose required for 20% increase in HR		
Propranolol	0.2 mg/kg	≥ 12% decrease in HR	> 20% decrease in sinus rate	May be dangerous in patients with marked bradycardia or decreased LV function
	0.1 mg/kg	≥ 12% decrease in HR		
Atropine + propranolol	0.04 mg/kg + 0.2 mg/kg	IHR=118.1-(0.57 × age); SD depends on age	> 10% decrease in age-predicted rate	Wide variability
	0.03 mg/kg + 0.15 mg/kg	IHR=118.1-(0.57 × age); SD depends on age		

FIGURE 6-19. Pharmacologic interventions for the assessment of sinus node disorders. A variety of pharmacologic interventions can be used to assess sinus node competence. Included in this table are agents that either enhance or block autonomic activity in the heart. Although abnormal responses may suggest sinus node dysfunction, these interventions are neither sensitive nor specific. CAD—coronary artery disease; HR—heart rate; IHR—intrinsic heart rate; LV—left ventricular; SD—standard deviation [7,10,11].

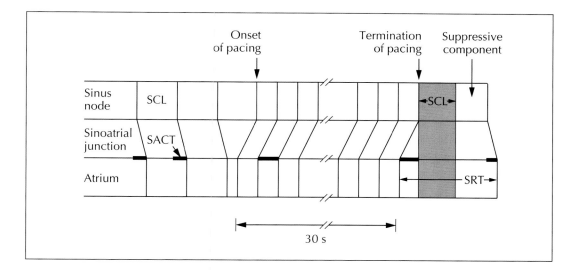

FIGURE 6-20. Sinus node recovery time (SRT). By pacing the atrium at rates progressively faster than the sinus rate (atrial decremental pacing), the SRT can be determined. Rapid stimulation of the sinus node may suppress intrinsic automaticity, resulting in a delay in the post-pacing response. This ladder diagram depicts events during decremental atrial pacing to assess sinus recovery time. At the termination of pacing, the SRT, as determined from recordings in the atria, actually consists of three elements: retrograde atriosinus conduction, the intranodal cycle length (which is an interval equal to the basic sinus cycle length [SCL] plus an interval resulting from overdrive suppression), and antegrade sinoatrial conduction. The length of sinoatrial conduction time (SACT) is emphasized periodically with a thickening of the rung between the sinoatrial junction and the atrium. (*Adapted from* Reiffel [12].)

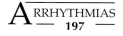

THERAPEUTIC OPTIONS FOR SINUS NODE DISORDERS

DIAGNOSIS	THERAPY
Symptomatic sinus node dysfunction (bradycardia, chronotropic incompetence, sinus arrest, sinoatrial exit block)	AAIR pacing when no evidence of AV conduction disease DDDR pacing with evidence of AV conduction disease
Tachy-brady syndrome	Type I or III antiarrhythmics to treat atrial arrhythmias β-Blockers, calcium-channel blockers, and/or digoxin to control ventricular response VVI or DDD pacing for bradycardic episodes (drug used to treat atrial arrhythmia may worsen bradyarrhythmias and precipitate the need for cardiac pacing) AV junction ablation with DDDR or VVIR pacing in patients whose ventricular response is difficult to control
Sinus node reentry	β-Blockers, calcium-channel blockers Type I and III antiarrhythmics Catheter ablation (sinus node modification)
Inappropriate sinus tachycardia	β-Blockers, calcium-channel blockers Catheter ablation (sinus node ablation/modification)
Carotid sinus hypersensitivity	Pindolol, Norpace Cardiac pacing Avoidance of tight collars

FIGURE 6-21. Therapeutic options for sinus node disorders. Pacing nodes are standard. AAIR—rate-responsive atrial pacing; AV—atrioventricular; DDD—dual chamber pacing; DDDR—rate-responsive dual chamber pacing; VVI—ventricular pacing; VVIR—rate-responsive ventricular pacing.

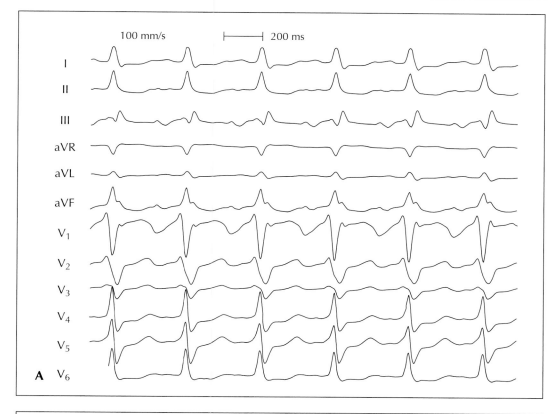

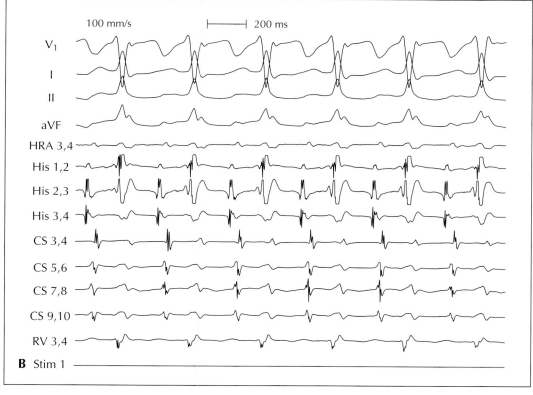

FIGURE 6-22. Atrial tachycardia. **A**, 12-lead electrocardiogram (ECG) of an atrial tachycardia. This ECG shows a narrow complex tachycardia with a rate of 130 beats per minute. Note the upright P waves in leads II, III, aVL, and aVF, and negative P wave in lead V_1. The relationship between the P wave and the QRS complex is consistent with a long RP tachycardia. The differential diagnosis of a long RP tachycardia includes atypical atrioventricular (AV) node reentry, a slowly conducting bypass tract, or an atrial tachycardia. From the intracardiac recordings in **B** we clearly see the atrial and ventricular ECG relationship. Atrial intracardiac electrograms from the coronary sinus (CS) catheter, along the left atrioventricular groove, come after the right septal (His bundle) electrograms. Tachycardia initiation required isoproterenol and was induced with programmed stimulation. Surface leads are V_1, I, II, and aVF. Intracardiac leads include high right atrium (HRA 3,4), His bundle recording (His 1,2–His 3,4), CS recordings (CS 3,4–CS 9,10), and right ventricular apex.

Continued on next page

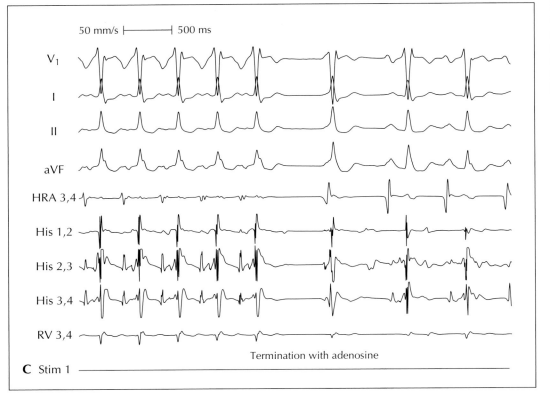

50 mm/s ├────┤ 500 ms

V₁

I

II

aVF

HRA 3,4

His 1,2

His 2,3

His 3,4

RV 3,4

Termination with adenosine

C Stim 1

FIGURE 6-22. *(Continued)* In **C** the tachycardia was terminated with adenosine. There was no evidence for an accessory pathway or dual AV nodes. These findings are consistent with an adenosine-sensitive atrial tachycardia. Note, the first beat after the tachycardia is terminated in a junctional beat [13].

MECHANISMS

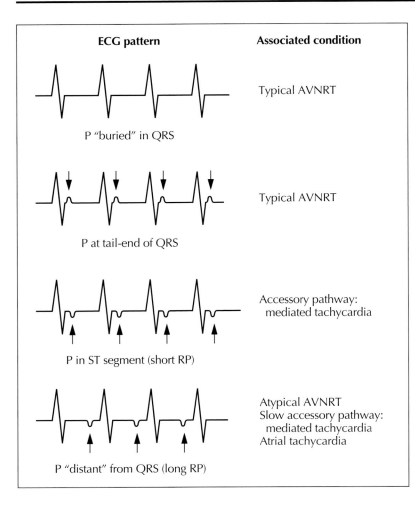

ECG pattern	Associated condition
P "buried" in QRS	Typical AVNRT
P at tail-end of QRS	Typical AVNRT
P in ST segment (short RP)	Accessory pathway: mediated tachycardia
P "distant" from QRS (long RP)	Atypical AVNRT Slow accessory pathway: mediated tachycardia Atrial tachycardia

FIGURE 6-23. Electrocardiographic patterns of narrow complex tachycardias. The most important clue to the mechanism of a narrow complex tachycardia is the relationship of the P wave to the QRS complex. No visible P wave often means that the P wave is buried in the QRS complex. This is usually due to typical atrioventricular (AV) nodal reentry. With typical AV nodal reentry, the P wave may also be located just at the start or end of the QRS complex, giving a qRs or Rsr' pattern. When the P wave is located close to the previous QRS complex, it is identified as a short-RP tachycardia. This is often seen with accessory pathway–mediated tachycardia and is due to retrograde atrial activation over the accessory pathway. The P wave may also be far from the previous QRS complex and classified as a long-RP tachycardia. If the P wave is inverted, it may be the result of atypical AV node reentry, or it may be using a slowly conducting accessory pathway in the retrograde direction. AVNRT—atrioventricular snodal reentry tachycardia; ECG—electrocardiogram [14].

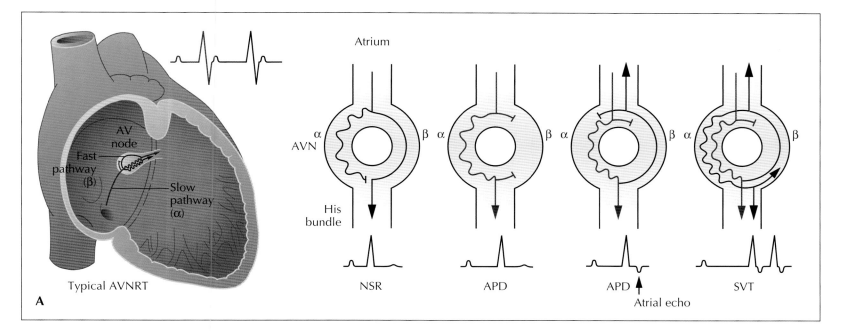

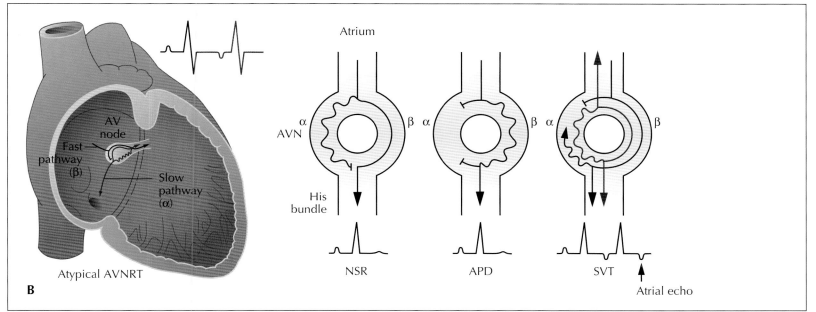

FIGURE 6-24. Schema for typical and atypical atrioventricular node reentrant tachycardia (AVNRT). Typical atrioventricular (AV) node reentry is shown in **A**. An impulse from the atrium enters the AV node and travels down both the slow and fast pathways. It quickly travels down the fast pathway resulting in activation of the ventricles with a short PR interval and results in the blocking of the impulse from the slow pathway when it reaches the terminal portion of the AV node since the tissue is still refractory. An atrial premature depolarization (APD) results in the conduction of the impulse down the slow pathway and thus longer PR interval. It blocks in the fast pathway since that tissue has a longer refractory period. If the tissue of the fast pathway regains conduction, the impulse after traveling down the slow pathway can return retrogradely back to the atrium via the fast pathway resulting in an atrial echo beat. A key component of the circuit is that the retrograde impulse finds the fast pathway no longer refractory. For this to occur, there must be a suitable delay in antegrade conduction over the slow pathway. The QRS complex

is narrow because the ventricle is being activated via the normal HPS. Retrograde activation over the fast pathway happens quickly, and on the surface electrocardiogram, the retrograde P wave is usually "buried" or at the tail end of the QRS complex. This can give the appearance of a "pseudo" right bundle branch pattern in lead V_1. This is a short-RP tachycardia. **B** demonstrates that when the circuit is reversed, as during atypical AV node reentry, antegrade conduction occurs over the fast pathway and retrograde conduction over the slow pathway. In atypical AV node reentry, an APD is conducted over the fast pathway. The PR interval remains short. If there is retrograde activation over the slow pathway to the atrium, then SVT may be initiated. The QRS complex remains narrow because activation of the ventricle is still via the normal HPS. Retrograde atrial activation over the slow pathway takes longer compared with conduction over the fast pathway, resulting in a long-RP interval. This is a long-RP tachycardia. α—slow pathway; β—fast pathway. NSR–sinus rhythm; SVT–supraventricular tachycardia.

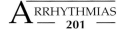

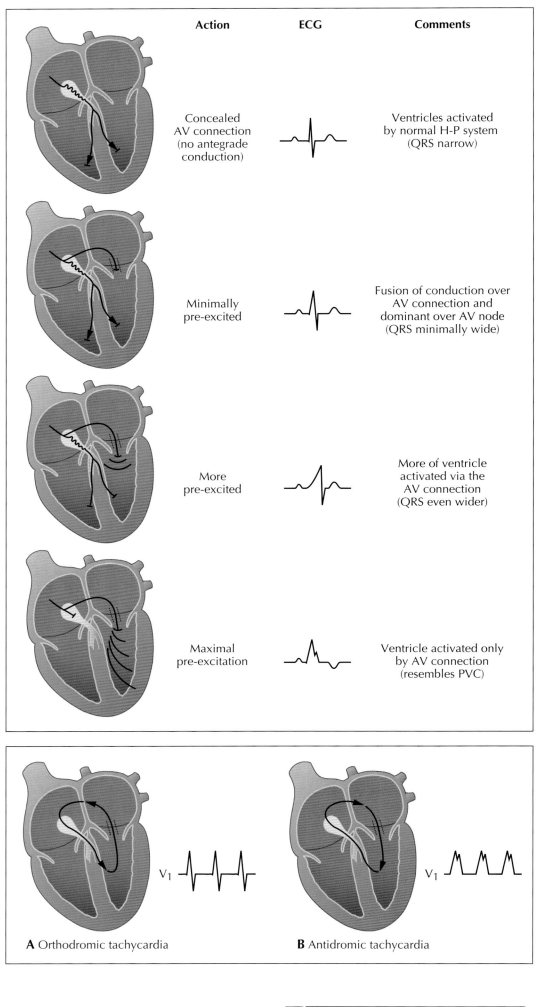

Action	ECG	Comments
Concealed AV connection (no antegrade conduction)		Ventricles activated by normal H-P system (QRS narrow)
Minimally pre-excited		Fusion of conduction over AV connection and dominant over AV node (QRS minimally wide)
More pre-excited		More of ventricle activated via the AV connection (QRS even wider)
Maximal pre-excitation		Ventricle activated only by AV connection (resembles PVC)

A Orthodromic tachycardia   V₁

B Antidromic tachycardia   V₁

FIGURE 6-25. Conduction over an accessory pathway. The morphology of a QRS complex in patients with an accessory pathway (AP) is an excellent example of fusion. Conduction over an AP is influenced by drugs, sympathetic states, and its location along the atrioventricular annulus. If there is no antegrade conduction, the AP may still conduct in the retrograde direction but is considered concealed, because it is not apparent on the ECG. When conduction over the AP is minimal and atrioventricular (AV) node conduction predominates, the QRS becomes a fusion of conduction over the AV node–His-Purkinje system and the AP. When conduction to the ventricle over the AP predominates compared with AV nodal conduction, the QRS represents a fusion of conduction over the AV node–HPS and the AP, but the larger the portion of the ventricle activated by the AP, the wider the QRS complex appears. If ventricular activation is only over the AP, as with maximally preexcited tachycardias, it is difficult to distinguish the complex from ventricular tachycardia. H-P—His Purkinje; LA—left atrium; LV—left ventricle; PVC—premature ventricular complex; RA—right atrium; RV—right ventricle.

FIGURE 6-26. Tachycardia circuits using an accessory pathway. When antegrade conduction is over the atrioventricular (AV node–His-Purkinje system (HPS) and retrograde conduction is over the AP, the QRS complex is narrow and is called an orthodromic AV reentry tachycardia (**A**). The retrograde P wave is further away from the QRS complex compared with typical AV node reentry, because the time (and distance) it takes to travel over the HPS and the AP is longer than the retrograde fast pathway conduction in AV node reentry. Most orthodromic tachycardias are short-RP tachycardias. When conduction is antegrade over the AP with retrograde conduction over the AV node, *ie*, an antidromic tachycardia, the QRS morphology is wide because of ventricular activation spread through muscle to muscle connections. The appearance of the QRS complex demonstrates maximal preexcitation (**B**).

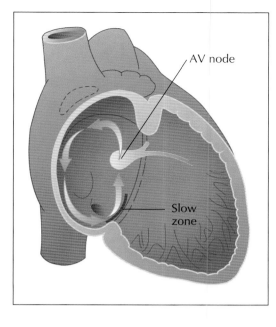

FIGURE 6-27. Atrial flutter circuit. With atrioventricular (AV) nodal reentry, AV reentry utilizing an accessory pathway, and a reentrant atrial tachycardia, there is usually a defined circuit which, if interrupted, can terminate the tachycardia. We now have learned that atrial flutter is a macro reentrant circuit in the right atrium. The circuit involves conduction in a counterclockwise (or clockwise) direction from the low posterior right atrium near the tricuspid valve annulus (TA), the posteroseptal region near the coronary sinus os, the interatrial septum, the high lateral right atrium, and down the crista terminalis to the isthmus between the inferior vena cava and the TA. The region of the posterior right atrium is thought to be the slow zone of conduction in the circuit. Evidence that supports this theory consists of data showing that atrial flutter can be entrained with atrial pacing. This has led to the development of techniques allowing electrophysiologists to ablate the critical regions of the circuit causing atrial flutter, thus, rendering the circuit inoperable [15].

ATRIAL FIBRILLATION

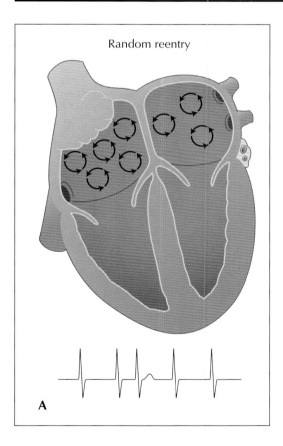

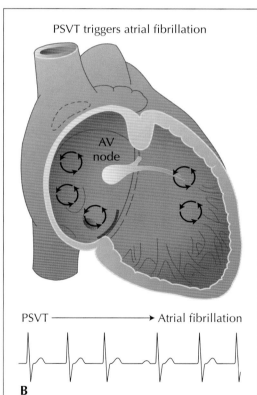

FIGURE 6-28. Mechanisms of atrial fibrillation (AF). AF is the most common sustained arrhythmia and is particularly prevalent in the elderly. While atrial flutter has one reentrant circuit, AF demonstrates multiple random reentrant circuits. This leads to clot formation and systemic embolic events. Thus, most patients with persistent or permanent AF require anticoagulation. Patients with "lone AF" (no structural heart disease or hypertension and under age 60) are considered to have a lower risk of stroke. **A**, Random reentry. AF is thought to be due to multiple wavelets produced by functional or anatomic reentry [16]. **B**, Paroxysmal supraventricular tachycardia (PSVT) can trigger AF. Ablation of the PSVT may, in some cases, prevent AF recurrence [17].

Continued on next page

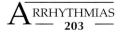

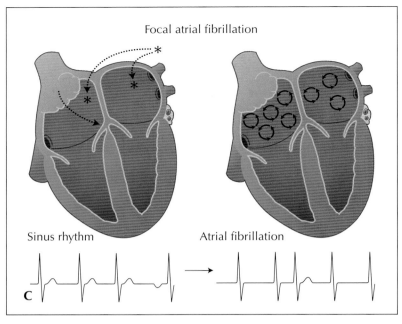

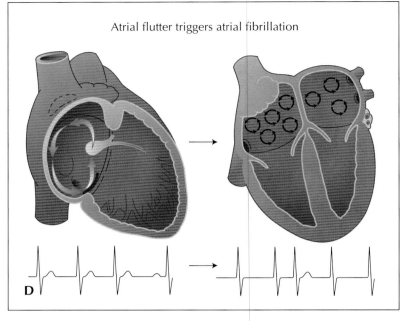

FIGURE 6-28. *(Continued)* **C,** Focal atrial premature complexes usually originating from pulmonary veins can initiate AF [18,19]. Ablation of these arrhythmogenic focal triggers can restore rhythm. This finding opens an exciting era in electrophysiology with the possibility of curing

AF by ablation. **D,** Atrial flutter (AFL) triggers AF. There is a relationship between the more organized reentrant AFL arrhythmia and AF [20,21]. Certain class IC drugs (such as propafenone) can convert AF to AFL. Additionally, the two rhythms often coexist in the same patient.

TREATMENT MODALITIES FOR ATRIAL FIBRILLATION

Pharmacologic therapy: goal is to restore sinus rhythm or rate control
    AV nodal blocking agents: β-blockers, calcium channel blockers,
      digoxin
    Class IA: procainamide, disopyramide
    Class IC: flecainide, propafenone
    Class III: amiodarone, sotalol, dofetilide
Acute cardioversion
    Electrical
    Chemical: ibutilide or ibutilide + chronic amiodarone
Catheter ablation
    Complete AV node ablation + pacemaker
    Focal pulmonary vein ablation
    Pulmonary vein isolation
    Catheter maze procedure (right and/or left atria)
Surgery
    Maze procedure

FIGURE 6-29. Treatment of atrial fibrillation (AF). Many drugs are available for rate control of AF. Acute cardioversion can be attempted by electrical means (monophasic or biphasic shocking waveforms) [22] or by chemical means with ibutilide (class III drug) [23,24] or ibutilide and amiodarone [25]. Dofetilide is a new class III drug that can be used for cardioversion in patients with congestive heart failure [26]. Using ibutilide or dofetilide in patients with renal failure increases the incidence of torsade de pointes. Anticoagulation should be maintained for one month after cardioversion. Complete atrial ventricular (AV) node ablation and placement of a permanent pacemaker can be performed for rate control. Other catheter ablation techniques include ablation of atrial premature beats from pulmonary veins that trigger focal AF [18,19]. The catheter Maze procedure places drag lesions in the right and/or left atria to restore sinus rhythm.

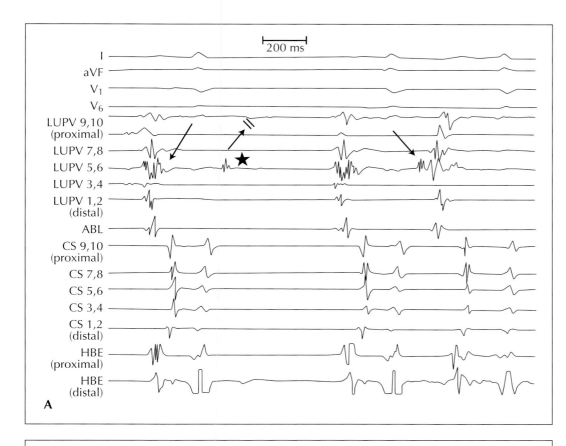

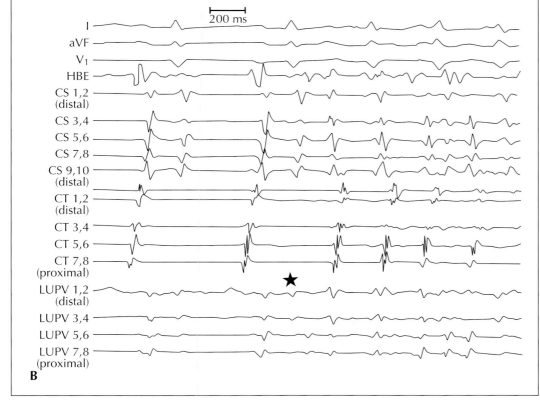

Figure 6-30. Focal origin of atrial fibrillation (AF). **A**, Intracardiac electrocardiograms demonstrating pulmonary vein potentials. A 38-year-old man with paroxysmal AF underwent an ablation procedure for focal AF. *Arrows*, a pulmonary vein potential that follows the left atrial activation in the first (sinus) beat but precedes left atrial activation in the premature beat; *star*, a blocked premature beat originating in the left upper pulmonary vein (LUPV). The pulmonary veins are wrapped in atrial myocardium that extends for several centimeters into the pulmonary veins. Such atrial tissue can become arrhythmogenic foci that fire rapidly and initiate AF. The upper pulmonary veins are common origins for these foci. **B**, Intracardiac electrocardiograms during an ablation procedure for focal AF in a 35-year-old man with paroxysmal AF. Note that an atrial premature complex (*star*) originating from the LUPV initiates sustained AF. Elimination of this focal trigger by radiofrequency ablation appears to restore sinus rhythm in the patient over long-term follow-up. The finding of focal triggers to AF has heralded an exciting new era in arrhythmia management. Potential complications of focal AF ablations include tamponade (due to transseptal puncture), pulmonary vein stenosis, and stroke. ABL—ablating catheter; CS—coronary sinus; CT—crista terminalis (in lateral right atrium); HBE—His bundle electrogram; LUPV—left upper pulmonary vein.

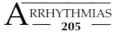

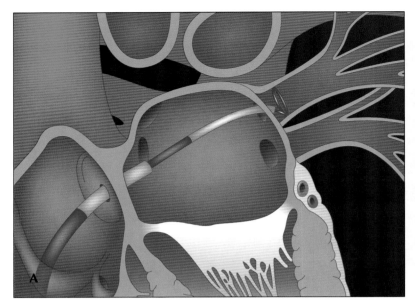

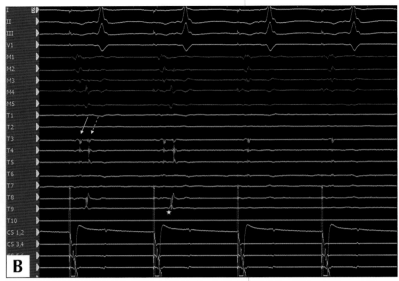

FIGURE 6-31. Atrial fibrillation (AF) ablation using the pulmonary vein isolation technique. AF has been shown to often be triggered by ectopy coming from the pulmonary veins [27]. Currently, a common approach to atrial fibrillation ablation is electrically isolating the pulmonary veins so that the ectopy cannot conduct into atrium and initiate AF. **A,** Mapping of a pulmonary vein is often done by placing a loop shaped catheter at its ostium. This shows the electrical signals from the connections extending from the atrium to the pulmonary vein. **B,** T1–T10 are intracardiac electrograms from the loop shaped catheter. Pacing delineates the far field atrial potential (*arrow*) from the local pulmonary vein potential (*dashed arrow*). The earliest local pulmonary vein potential seen at T9 (star) indicates the location of an electrical connection from the atrium to the pulmonary vein. Ablation near T9 eliminates all the local pulmonary vein potentials in the final two beats.

CLASS III ANTIARRHYTHMIC DRUGS

IBUTILIDE

Inhibits I_{Kr} channels (outward repolarizing current)

Enhances slow inward sodium current

Prolongs QT interval

Intravenous formulation only

Useful for terminating acute onset atrial fibrillation or flutter

Post-cardiac surgery atrial arrhythmias

Facilitates transthoracic electrical cardioversion

Can be used to treat rapid atrial fibrillation with Wolff-Parkinson-White syndrome

Causes torsades de pointes

DOFETILIDE

Inhibits I_{Kr} channels

Intravenous and oral formulation

Prolongs QT interval

Useful for conversion of atrial arrhythmias and maintenance of sinus rhythm

Can be used in high-risk patients with heart failure or post-myocardial infarction

Causes torsades de pointes—narrow therapeutic window

AZIMILIDE

Inhibits both I_{Kr} and I_{Ks} channels

Intravenous and oral formulation

Prolongs QT interval

Useful for atrial arrhythmias

Causes torsades de pointes

FIGURE 6-32. New class III antiarrhythmic drugs. Ibutilide, dofetilide, and azimilide represent potassium-channel blocking agents useful for cardioversion of atrial fibrillation and flutter [23,24,26,28]. All three drugs increase the atrial refractory period and exhibit reverse-use dependence, or greater drug effect at slow heart rates. As a general class effect, they prolong the QT interval and can exhibit proarrhythmic effects including torsades de pointes. Risk factors for torsades de pointes with these drugs include hypokalemia, female gender, the presence of heart failure, and renal failure.

DIAGNOSIS

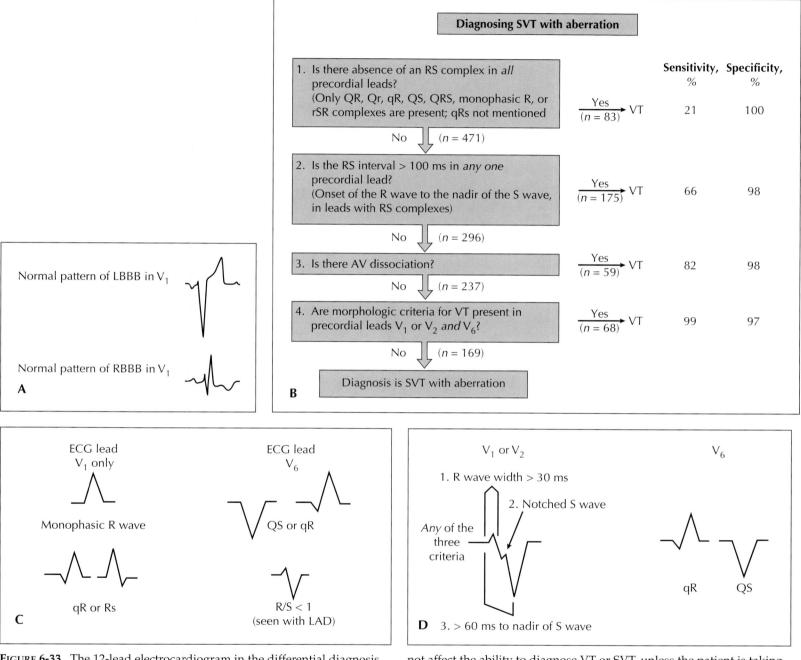

Diagnosing SVT with aberration

	Sensitivity, %	Specificity, %
1. Is there absence of an RS complex in *all* precordial leads? (Only QR, Qr, qR, QS, QRS, monophasic R, or rSR complexes are present; qRs not mentioned — Yes $(n = 83)$ → VT	21	100
No $(n = 471)$		
2. Is the RS interval > 100 ms in *any one* precordial lead? (Onset of the R wave to the nadir of the S wave, in leads with RS complexes) — Yes $(n = 175)$ → VT	66	98
No $(n = 296)$		
3. Is there AV dissociation? — Yes $(n = 59)$ → VT	82	98
No $(n = 237)$		
4. Are morphologic criteria for VT present in precordial leads V_1 or V_2 *and* V_6? — Yes $(n = 68)$ → VT	99	97
No $(n = 169)$		

Diagnosis is SVT with aberration

Normal pattern of LBBB in V_1

Normal pattern of RBBB in V_1

A

B

ECG lead V_1 only

Monophasic R wave

qR or Rs

ECG lead V_6

QS or qR

R/S < 1 (seen with LAD)

C

V_1 or V_2

1. R wave width > 30 ms

2. Notched S wave

Any of the three criteria

D 3. > 60 ms to nadir of S wave

V_6

qR   QS

FIGURE 6-33. The 12-lead electrocardiogram in the differential diagnosis of wide complex tachycardia. Brugada *el al.* [29] analyzed 384 cases of ventricular tachycardia (VT) and 170 cases of supraventricular tachycardia (SVT) with aberrancy, representing 554 patients with tachycardia (those taking antiarrhythmic medications were excluded). They then devised a systematic approach for diagnosing wide QRS complex tachycardia with regular rhythmicity. **A,** The first step is to exclude sinus tachycardia or atrial tachycardia with right bundle branch block (RBBB) or left bundle branch block (LBBB). This can usually be done by finding P waves in lead V_1: the ST segment and T wave are always smooth, unless distorted by a P wave. However, missing this diagnosis should not affect the ability to diagnose VT or SVT, unless the patient is taking QRS-lengthening drugs. **B,** Steps in diagnosis of SVT with aberration. A *yes* answer at any point indicates that no further steps need to be taken. When the answer is *no*, proceed to the next step. The cumulative sensitivity using this method is 97% and specificity is 99%. **C,** Morphologic criteria favoring diagnosis of VT in the presence of RBBB-type QRS complexes (dominant *positive* in V_1). Both leads must meet these criteria in order to diagnose VT. **D,** Morpho-logic criteria used to diagnose VT in the presence of LBBB-type QRS complexes (dominant *negative* in V_1). Both leads must meet these criteria to diagnose VT. (*Adapted from* Brugada *et al.* [29].)

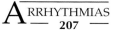

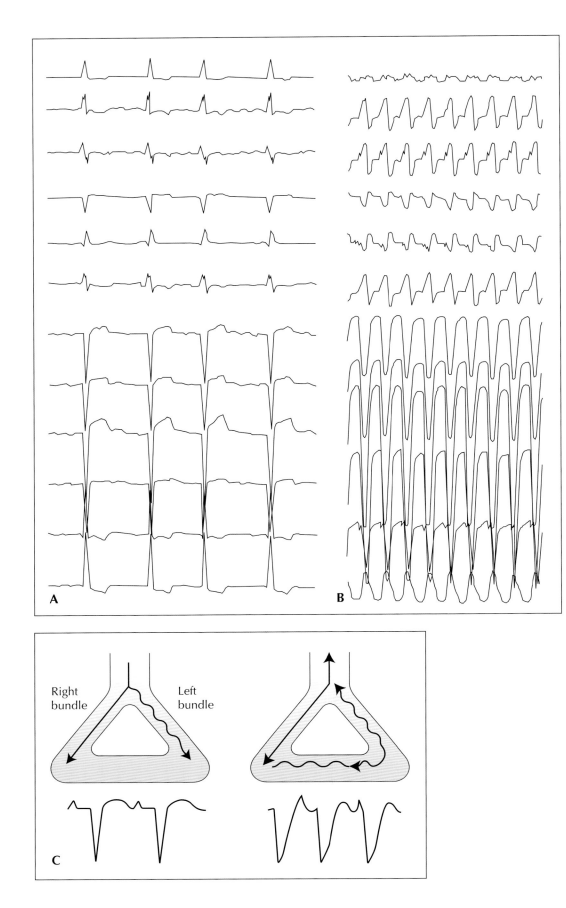

FIGURE 6-34. Aborted sudden death in a 65-year-old man. The patient had an ischemic cardiomyopathy with a left ventricular ejection fraction of 20%, although myocardial infarction was ruled out and he had no current signs of ischemia. **A,** The 12-lead electrocardiogram (ECG) shows sinus rhythm with an incomplete left bundle branch block. **B,** At electrophysiologic (EP) testing, a wide complex tachycardia was induced at the rate of 250 beats per minute, which was accompanied by almost immediate loss of consciousness requiring cardioversion. The QRS morphology of the tachycardia is similar to, although slightly wider than, sinus rhythm, so a diagnosis of supraventricular tachycardia with aberration might be considered. However, ECG analysis confirmed a diagnosis of bundle branch (so-called macro reentrant) ventricular tachycardia (BBR-VT). **C,** Pathophysiology includes a diseased left bundle (LB) and ventricular muscle. During tachycardia, an impulse proceeds down the right bundle (RB; hence the left bundle morphology), across the diseased intraventricular system, and up the LB. Because the His-Purkinje system is involved, these tachycardias are almost always quite rapid (> 200 bpm) and patients with BBR-VT present with syncope or aborted sudden death. Hallmarks include LB intraventricular conduction defect in sinus, LB morphology in VT, idiopathic or ischemic dilated cardiomyopathy, long His to ventricle (HV) interval at EP study, and importantly, BBR-VT that can be cured with radiofrequency catheter ablation of the RB. A pacemaker usually is not required.

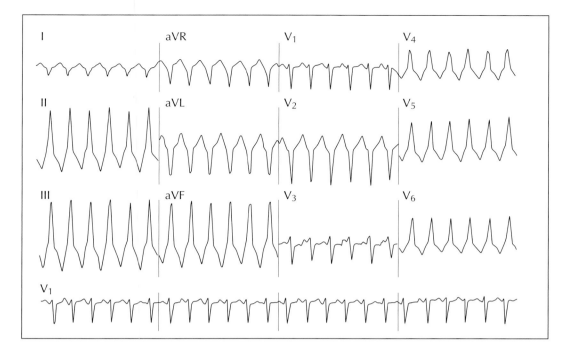

FIGURE 6-35. Right ventricular outflow tract (RVOT) ventricular tachycardia (VT). This 12-lead EKG from a healthy 22-year-old woman who experienced frequent palpitations with exercise shows the typical pattern for RVOT VT, *ie*, a left-bundle branch block type pattern, right axis deviation, and an inferior axis [30]. The QS pattern in leads I and aVL suggests a septal origin to the VT. Such VTs occur in patients with structurally normal hearts and are due to cAMP-mediated triggered activity. They are frequently adenosine-sensitive. These VTs are important to recognize because they can be cured by radiofrequency ablation, as opposed to VT associated with idiopathic or ischemic cardiomyopathies. Other forms of idiopathic VT (*ie*, VT with a structurally normal heart) may arise from left septal foci.

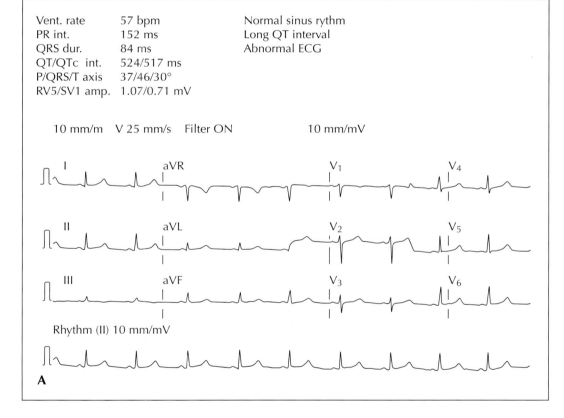

Vent. rate	57 bpm	Normal sinus rythm
PR int.	152 ms	Long QT interval
QRS dur.	84 ms	Abnormal ECG
QT/QTc int.	524/517 ms	
P/QRS/T axis	37/46/30°	
RV5/SV1 amp.	1.07/0.71 mV	

10 mm/m   V 25 mm/s   Filter ON   10 mm/mV

Rhythm (II) 10 mm/mV

A

FIGURE 6-36. Long QT. **A**, Baseline 12-lead electrocardiogram (ECG) for an asymptomatic 38-year-old woman with Long QT syndrome (LQTS) taking no medications. Her corrected QT interval (QTc) measured 517 ms. Two of her sisters died suddenly in their forties associated with periods of exertion and strong emotion. All three were subsequently genotyped for a defect in the KVLQT1 gene (I_{Ks} defect). Three female cousins also died suddenly in their thirties. A dual-chamber pacemaker-defibrillator was implanted, and beta-blocker therapy was initiated.

Continued on next page

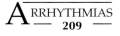

B. LONG QT SYNDROME GENOTYPE–PHENOTYPE CORRELATIONS

TYPE	ION CHANNEL MUTATION/ CHROMOSOME LOCATION	ARRHYTHMIA TRIGGER	INCIDENCE OF KNOWN GENOTYPES
LQT1	I_{Ks}/chromosome 11	Exercise, swimming, strong emotion, rarely auditory stimuli	≈50%
LQT2	I_{Kr} ("HERG")/chromosome 7	Auditory stimuli, abrupt arousal from sleep	≈45%
LQT3	SCN5A (sodium)/chromosome 3	Usually not related to exercise; may occur during sleep	≈5%
LQT4	Ankyrin/chromosome 4 Alters calcium signaling and several ion channels and pumps	?	?
LQT5	minK/chromosome 21 Interacts to form I_{Ks}	Exercise, swimming, strong emotion, rarely auditory stimuli	?
LQT6	MiRP1/chromosome 21 Interacts to form I_{Kr}	Auditory stimuli, abrupt arousal from sleep	?

FIGURE 6-36. *(Continued)* **B,** Only half of all patients with LQTS can be currently genotyped because their mutations have not yet been identified. LQTS is an autosomal dominant genetic disorder (Romano-Ward syndrome) with incomplete penetrance [31–33]. Up to 30% of patients with LQTS have normal or only borderline prolonged QT intervals, which can make diagnosis difficult. If both parents carry the defective gene for the I_{Ks} channel and pass it on, the child will have a severe form of LQTS associated with congenital hearing loss (Jervell-Lange-Nielsen syndrome). Treatment options include beta-blocker therapy, dual-chamber pacemaker, and/or dual-chamber pacemaker-defibrillator therapy [34].

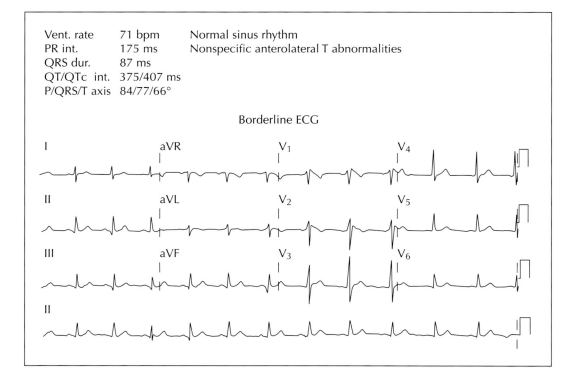

Vent. rate	71 bpm	Normal sinus rhythm
PR int.	175 ms	Nonspecific anterolateral T abnormalities
QRS dur.	87 ms	
QT/QTc int.	375/407 ms	
P/QRS/T axis	84/77/66°	

Borderline ECG

FIGURE 6-37. A 12-lead electrocardiogram (ECG) obtained from a 57-year-old man without structural heart disease who survived a cardiac arrest. The ECG has features that suggest Brugada's syndrome, including persistent ST elevation in leads V_1–V_3, right bundle branch block-type pattern, prominent J wave (positive deflection at the end of the QRS complex), and inverted T waves. The prevalence of primary ventricular fibrillation in symptomatic individuals is 40%–60%, and defibrillator implantation is often recommended for these patients. Brugada's syndrome appears to be a genetic disorder caused by mutations in SCN5A, the cardiac sodium channel [35,36]. Flecainide or other sodium channel blocker drugs can unmask the typical ECG phenotype in these patients.

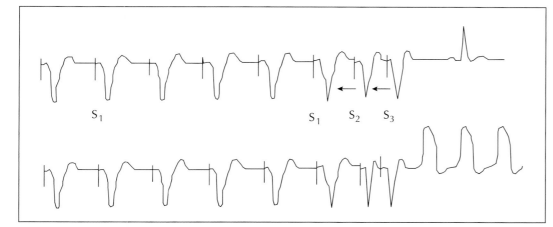

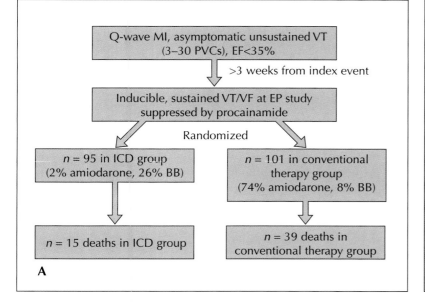

at a basic drive rate (S_1) are introduced, followed by one, two, or three premature extra beats (S_2,S_3,S_4). These extra beats are placed at programmed intervals, and the intervals are shortened by scanning diastole until refractoriness. This technique has a sensitivity and specificity of over 90% for the induction of reentrant sustained monomorphic VT in patients with healed myocardial infarction (MI). However, it is not sensitive in patients whose VT is due to acute MI, reversible ischemia, electrolyte disturbances, or other etiologies. The induction of nonsustained VT, polymorphic VT, or ventricular fibrillation has reduced specificity, especially if induced with aggressive stimulation with very early premature beats. Repeat PES following drug administration in patients with inducible sustained VT may be used to help predict drug efficacy.

FIGURE 6-38. Programmed electrical stimulation (PES). PES can be used in the diagnosis and management of ventricular tachycardia (VT) by inserting a catheter into the right ventricle. Although this is the typical application, the left ventricle can also be used. Eight or more beats

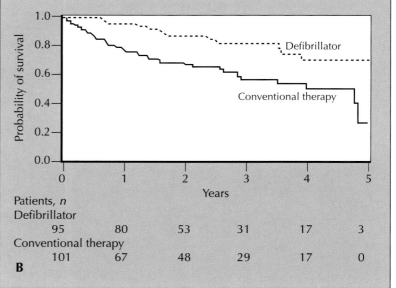

FIGURE 6-39. Multicenter Automatic Defibrillator Implantation Trial (MADIT). **A,** MADIT was a primary prevention study where high-risk patients with known coronary artery disease and asymptomatic unsustained ventricular tachycardia (VT) not suppressible by procainamide were randomly assigned to receive an implantable cardioverter/defibrillator (ICD) or conventional medical therapy, which consisted mainly of amiodarone therapy. **B,** There was a significant difference in survival between the two treatment groups ($P = 0.009$), with fewer deaths reported in the ICD group at follow-up after 27 months. BB—beta-blocker; EP—electrophysiology; EF—ejection fraction; MI—myocardial infarction; PVC—premature ventricular complexes; VF—ventricular fibrillation. (*Adapted from* Moss *et al.* [37].)

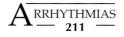

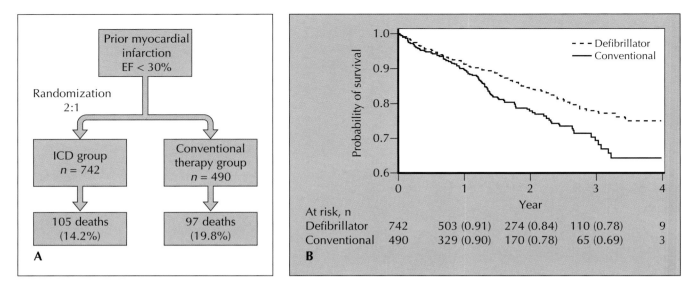

A

Prior myocardial
infarction
EF < 30%

Randomization
2:1

ICD group
n = 742

Conventional
therapy group
n = 490

105 deaths
(14.2%)

97 deaths
(19.8%)

B

At risk, n					
Defibrillator	742	503 (0.91)	274 (0.84)	110 (0.78)	9
Conventional	490	329 (0.90)	170 (0.78)	65 (0.69)	3

FIGURE 6-40. Multicenter Automatic Defibrillator Implantation Trial II (MADIT II). **A**, MADIT II was a primary prevention study where patients post–myocardial infarction with ejection fraction less than 30% were randomized to receive an implantable cardioverter defibrillator (ICD) or conventional medical therapy. **B**, There was a significant difference in survival between the two treatment groups, with a hazard ratio for the risk of death from any cause in the ICD group compared with the conventional medical therapy group of 0.69 (95% CI, 0.51–0.93; $P = 0.016$). (*Adapted from* Moss *et al.* [38].)

TREATMENT OPTIONS FOR SYMPTOMATIC SUSTAINED VT OR VF NOT DUE TO A REVERSIBLE CAUSE

NO STRUCTURAL HEART DISEASE

Calcium-channel blockers

β-blockers

Class I or III agents (propafenone, sotalol, amidarone)

RF catheter ablation

IDIOPATHIC CARDIOMYOPATHY

Drugs (especially amiodarone)

Implanted defibrillator with ATP

Catheter ablation for bundle branch reentrant VT, if present

PRIOR MYOCARDIAL INFARCTION

Class III agents (sotalol if preserved EF; amiodarone)

Catheter ablation

Implanted defibrillator with ATP

LONG QT SYNDROME

β-blockers and dual-chamber pacing to shorten QT interval

Implanted defibrillator with atrial pacing

FIGURE 6-41. Treatment options for patients with ventricular tachycardia (VT) or ventricular fibrillation (VF). The therapy recommended depends on presentation and substrate. ATP—antitachycardia pacing; EF—ejection fraction; RF—radiofrequency.

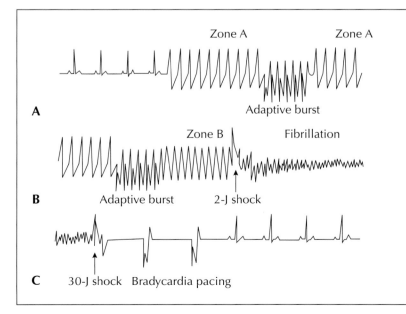

A

Zone A   Zone A

Adaptive burst

B

Zone B   Fibrillation

Adaptive burst   2-J shock

C

30-J shock   Bradycardia pacing

FIGURE 6-42. Incorporation of tiered or *zone* therapy in newer implantable devices for selective antitachycardia pacing, lower energy cardioversion, or high-energy defibrillation. Recordings show idealized tiered anti-tachycardia therapy. **A,** Onset of ventricular tachycardia (VT) with slower rate (zone A). Overdrive pacing is initiated with an adaptive burst, but tachycardia resumes with the same rate. **B,** Repeat burst pacing leads to acceleration of VT rate (zone B), and a low-energy (2 J) cardio-version shock leads to ventricular fibrillation (VF). **C,** VF is effectively terminated with 30-J shock delivery. (*Adapted from* Akhtar *et al.* [39].)

INDICATIONS FOR AICD

CLASS I

Cardiac arrest due to VF or VT not due to a transient or reversible cause

Spontaneous sustained VT

Syncope of undetermined origin with clinically relevant, hemodynamically significant sustained VT or VF induced at electrophysiologic study when drug therapy is ineffective, not tolerated, or not preferred

Nonsustained VT with coronary disease, prior MI, LV dysfunction, and inducible VF or sustained VT at electrophysiologic study that is not suppressible by a class I anti-arrhythmic drug

CLASS IIA

None

CLASS IIB

Cardiac arrest presumed to be due to VF when electrophysiologic testing is precluded by other medical conditions

Severe symptoms attributable to sustained ventricular tachyarrhythmias while awaiting cardiac transplantation

Familial or inherited conditions with a high risk for life-threatening ventricular tachy-arrhymias such as long QT syndrome or hypertrophic cardiomyopathy

Nonsustained VT with coronary artery disease, prior MI, and LV dysfunction, and inducible sustained VT or VF at electrophysiologic study

Recurrent syncope of undetermined etiology in the presence of ventricular dysfunction and inducible ventricular arrhythmias at electrophysiologic study when other causes of syncope have been excluded

FIGURE 6-43. Indications for using an automatic implantable cardioverter defibrillator (AICD). LV—left ventricular; MI—myocardial infarction; VF—ventricular fibrillation; VT—ventricular tachycardia.(*Adapted from* Gregoratos *et al.* [40].)

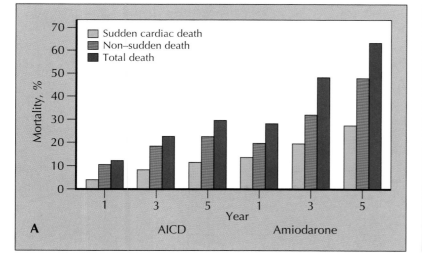

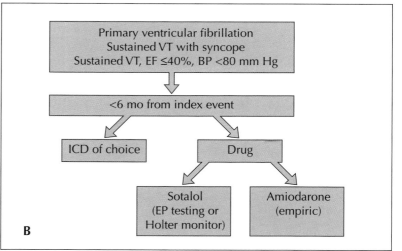

FIGURE 6-44. Automatic implantable cardioverter/defibrillator (AICD) versus drug therapy. The results of studies shown in **A** indicate that AICD therapy is associated with a lower incidence of sudden and nonsudden death compared with treatment with amiodarone, which is probably the most effective antiarrhythmic drug available. Caution must be exercised, however, in comparing studies that probably did not enroll comparable patient groups. It is still unknown whether amiodarone (or sotalol, another effective class III drug) or AICD is best in a matched cohort of patients with sustained ventricular tachycardia (VT) or ventricular fibril-lation (VF). **B,** The Antiarrhythmic Drug Versus Implanted Defibrillator (AVID) Trial, sponsored by the National Institutes of Health, was an important secondary prevention trial studying implantable cardio-verter/defibrillator (ICD) versus drug therapy for patients with hemo-dynamically unstable VT or VF. A total of 1016 high-risk patients were randomized to an ICD versus drug therapy (amiodarone or sotalol). At two years' follow-up, 82% of the patients in the drug therapy group were taking amiodarone; only 9% were using sotalol. ICD therapy conferred a survival benefit comparable to the drug therapy group. BP—blood pressure; EF—ejection fraction; EP—electrophysiology. (Panel A *adapted from* Winkle *et al.* [41].)

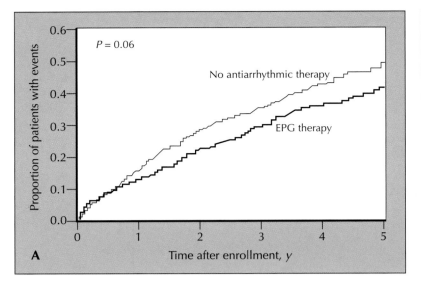

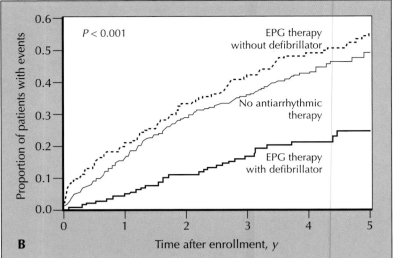

FIGURE 6-45. Use of electrophysiology (EP)-guided therapy. **A** and **B**, The Multicenter Unsustained Tachycardia Trial (MUSTT) study examined the hypothesis that EP-guided therapy would decrease the risk of sudden cardiac death in high-risk patients [39]. Study participants had a history of coronary artery disease, EF < 40%, and asymptomatic unsustained ventricular tachycardia (VT). Those patients with inducible monomorphic VT, polymorphic VT, or ventricular fibrillation at EP study were random- ized to EP-guided therapy (which included anti-arrhythmic drug or implantable cardioverter/defibrillator therapy) or to no anti-arrhythmic drug therapy. *Panel A* demonstrates that EP-guided therapy was not supe- rior to the no-therapy group in long-term follow-up. *Panel B* shows that therapy with defibrillator conferred the greatest survival benefit in this study. EF—ejection fraction. (*Adapted from* Buxton *et al.* [42].)

RANDOMIZED TRIALS OF ICD VS. DRUG THERAPY

TRIAL	TREATMENT GROUPS	PATIENTS	RESULTS
AVID	Amiodarone or EP-guided sotalol therapy vs ICD	SCD survivors VT + syncope + EF ≤40%	Lower mortality with ICD
CASH	Amiodarone vs β-blocker vs propafenone vs ICD	SCD survivors with inducible VT/VF	Lower mortality with ICD
CIDS	Amiodarone vs ICD	SCD survivors VT + syncope Symptomatic VT + EF ≤35%	No mortality benefit for ICD
CABG-Patch	CABG alone vs CABG + ICD	Elective CABG, positive SAECG, EF ≤35%	No mortality benefit for ICD
MADIT	Medical therapy vs ICD	NSVT, QWMI, EF ≤35%, inducible VT/VF at EP study	Lower mortality with ICD
MUSTT	No therapy vs. ICD vs drugs	CAD, asymptomatic NSVT, EF ≤40%	Lower mortality with ICD

FIGURE 6-46. Randomized trials of implantable cardioverter/defibrillator (ICD) versus drug therapy. Several large-scale prospective trials have compared ICD therapy to medical therapy as either primary or secondary prevention of sudden death. AVID—Antiarrhythmic Versus Implantable Defibrillator; CAD—coronary artery disease; CASH—Cardiac Arrest Hamburg Study; CABG—coronary artery bypass graft; CIDS—Canadian Implantable Defibrillator Study; EF—ejection fraction; EP—electrophysi- ology; MADIT—Multicenter Automatic Defibrillator Implantation Trial; MUSTT—Multicenter Unsustained Tachycardia Trial; NSVT—non- sustained VT; QWMI—Q-wave myocardial infarction; SAECG—signal- averaged electrocardiogram; SCD—sudden cardiac death; VT—ventric- ular tachycardia [42–46].

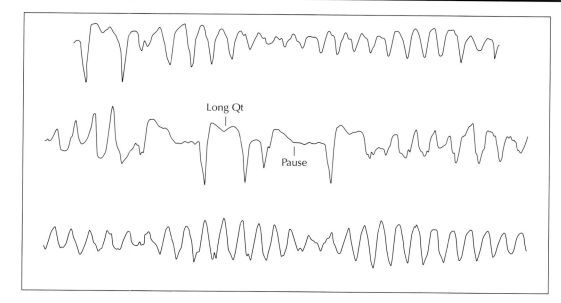

FIGURE 6-47. Torsades de pointes. When viewed in a single lead, torsades de pointes may appear monomorphic, thus multiple simultaneous leads should be obtained. The prolonged QT or QTU interval is the common denominator and may be congenital or acquired. In the top strip there is a polymorphic ventricular tachycardia that seems to undulate around a fixed baseline. The continuation of this strip is seen in the middle strip. Note that the arrhythmia self-terminates, a frequent characteristic of torsades de pointes. However, it is reinitiated after a characteristic pause followed by a shortly coupled premature ventricular complex. The arrhythmia continues in the bottom strip with its undulating nature.

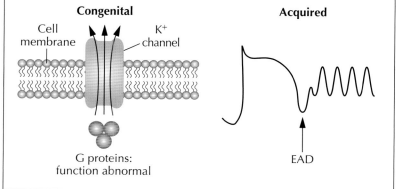

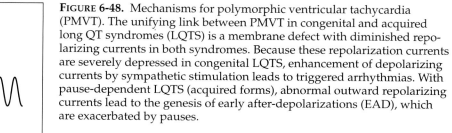

FIGURE 6-48. Mechanisms for polymorphic ventricular tachycardia (PMVT). The unifying link between PMVT in congenital and acquired long QT syndromes (LQTS) is a membrane defect with diminished repolarizing currents in both syndromes. Because these repolarization currents are severely depressed in congenital LQTS, enhancement of depolarizing currents by sympathetic stimulation leads to triggered arrhythmias. With pause-dependent LQTS (acquired forms), abnormal outward repolarizing currents lead to the genesis of early after-depolarizations (EAD), which are exacerbated by pauses.

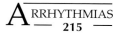

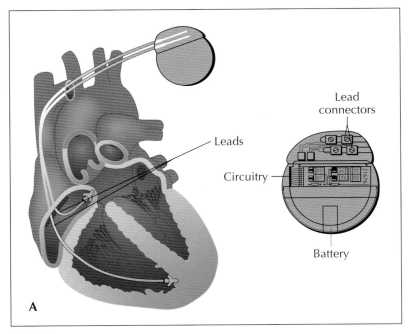

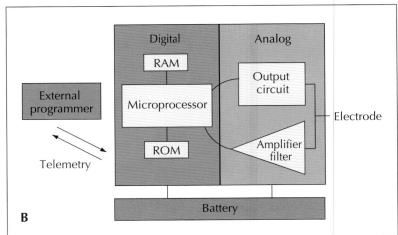

FIGURE 6-49. The pulse generator design. While early designs included a few hand-soldered transistors, resistors, and capacitors, the present devices include highly advanced, highly integrated microcircuits and microprocessors (**A**) resembling that found in personal computers. The microprocessor performs the logic chores of the pacemaker, including storage of programmable settings and interpretation and response to various sensed and paced cardiac electrical events, as well as the control of radiofrequency telemetry communications with external programmers. The microprocessor is dependent on a highly precise timer circuit based on a crystal oscillator.

Many devices (**B**) employ both "read only memory" (ROM), which contains the pacing algorithm, and "read and write memory" (RAM) for data, including programmed settings, device identification, and storage of a wide array of measured data values.

While the pacing algorithm and memory functions of the pacemaker represent the digital side of the device, certain analog elements, including filters and amplifiers for detecting intrinsic cardiac activity and controlling pacing output levels at appropriate intervals as instructed by the microprocessor, are necessary components as well.

All of these components are mounted on a circuit board and placed along with the battery within a hermetically sealed container, usually a titanium canister, for protection from the hostile environment of body fluids.

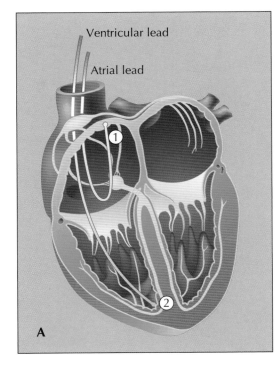

FIGURE 6-50. Pacemaker sensing. In addition to generating impulses to capture myocardium, pacemakers have the capacity to sense intrinsic cardiac activity. Electrical activity from intrinsic myocardial events is detected on the electrode lead system at sites ① and ② in **A** and is recorded as local electrogram ① and ② in **B**.

Continued on next page

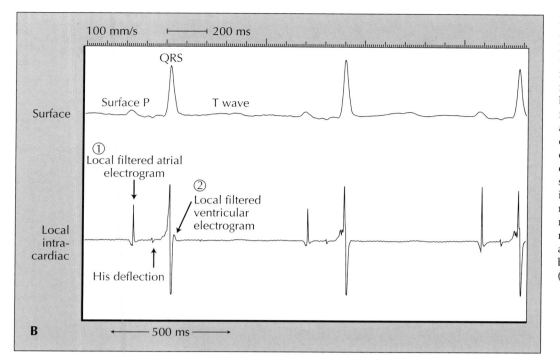

100 mm/s   ⊢———⊣ 200 ms

Surface

Surface P   QRS   T wave

① Local filtered atrial electrogram

② Local filtered ventricular electrogram

Local intra-cardiac

His deflection

B   ←——— 500 ms ———→

FIGURE 6-50. *(Continued)* These signals are amplified from biologic levels (millivolts) to levels commonly employed in electronic circuits (volts). Extraneous far-field electrical activity, including environmental "noise," skeletal muscle activity, and T waves, is filtered out by band-pass filters designed to "pass" those frequencies from signals that represent local activity and to progressively attenuate all others. The frequency band-width from signals of local myocardial electrical activity typically demonstrates associated slew rates (changes in signal amplitude with respect to time and an index of signal frequency content) that can be measured clinically. Typical slew rates are in the range of 0.5V to 3V/sec and are optimal for most pulse generator sensing systems. The amplified, filtered complex is then "sensed" by the pacing system if it is of a predetermined (programmable) amplitude.

NASPE/BPEG GENERIC (NBG) PACEMAKER CODE*

POSITION	I	II	III	IV	V
CATEGORY	CHAMBER(S) PACED	CHAMBER(S) SENSED	RESPONSE TO SENSING	PROGRAMMABILITY, RATE MODULATION	ANTITACHYARRHYTHMIA FUNCTIONS
	O=None	O=None	O=None	O=None	O=None
	A=Atrium	A=Atrium	T=Triggered	P=Simple programmable	P=Pacing (antitachyarrhythmia)
	V=Ventricle	V=Ventricle	I=Inhibited	M=Multiprogrammable	S=Shock
	D=Dual (A+V)	D=Dual (A+V)	D=Dual (T+I)	C=Communicating	D=Dual (P+S)
	S=Single (A or V)†	S=Single (A or V)†		R=Rate modulation	

*Positions I through III are used exclusively for antibradyarrhythmia functions.
†Manufacturer's designation only.

FIGURE 6-51. Modes of cardiac pacing. The mode of cardiac pacing refers to the way in which the pacemaker interacts with the underlying cardiac rhythm. The various modes may be described by the shorthand code suggested by the North American Society of Pacing and Electrophysiology (NASPE) and the British Pacing and Electrophysiology Group (BPEG) Pacemaker Code, 1987. (*Adapted from* Bernstein *et al.* [47]).

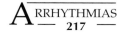

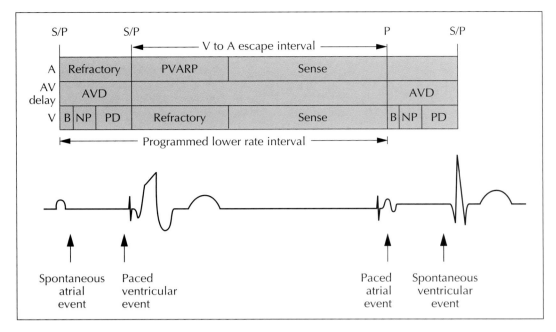

FIGURE 6-52. Dual-chamber timing cycle. Either a pace or a sense event occurring in the atrium initiates an atrioventricular (AV) delay period. This AV period is concluded by a ventricular stimulus or may be interrupted by sensing an intrinsic ventricular event. Refractory periods are initiated in both channels following either event. The refractory periods are in turn followed by sense periods in both chambers. The sense period is concluded by a pace event in the atrium or may be interrupted by sense events in either chamber. Unlike the single-chamber timing cycle, the escape interval in a dual-chamber pacemaker is shortened by the programmed AV delay period.

The ventricular channel timing system illustrated also incorporates "nonphysiologic AV delay" or "ventricular safety" pacing. The ventricular channel AV delay events (AVD) consist of three phases. First is the blanking period (B), which is a time of absolute refractoriness. The next is the nonphysiologic AV delay period (NP), ending 100 to 110 ms after an atrial event. Events sensed during this time initiate a ventricular stimulus at the conclusion of the nonphysiologic AVD phase and recycle the atrial and ventricular timing cycles. The final portion of the AVD is the physiologic period (PD). Sensed events during this period result in inhibition of ventricular channel output and initiation of a new timing cycle.

The rationale for shortened nonphysiologic AV delay ventricular safety pacing is that sensed events within the nonphysiologic AV delay are not the result of normal conduction stemming from the preceding atrial event (sensed or paced) to the ventricles. Therefore, such activity may represent either premature ventricular activity or extraneous sensed atrial activity (crosstalk). Since the system is unable to differentiate between these two possibilities, early ventricular activation "safety" pacing avoids pacing during the ventricular vulnerable period, and inappropriate ventricular channel output inhibition with crosstalk. A—atrial channel events; PVARP—post-ventricular atrial refractory period; P—pace event; S/P—sensing or pace event; V—ventricular channel events.

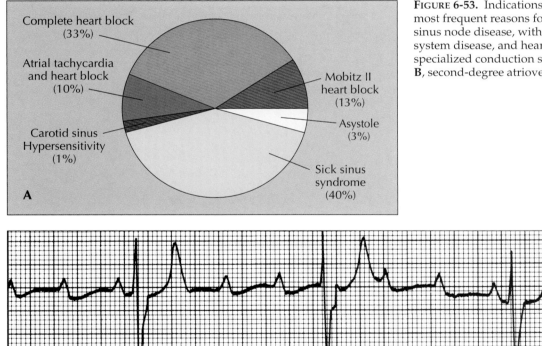

A

FIGURE 6-53. Indications for permanent pacemaker implantation. In **A**, the most frequent reasons for cardiac pacing at present are shown, including sinus node disease, with or without additional specialized conduction system disease, and heart block due to disease at some level along the specialized conduction system. The diagnostic ECG findings are shown in **B**, second-degree atrioventricular block with 2:1 conduction;

Continued on next page

B

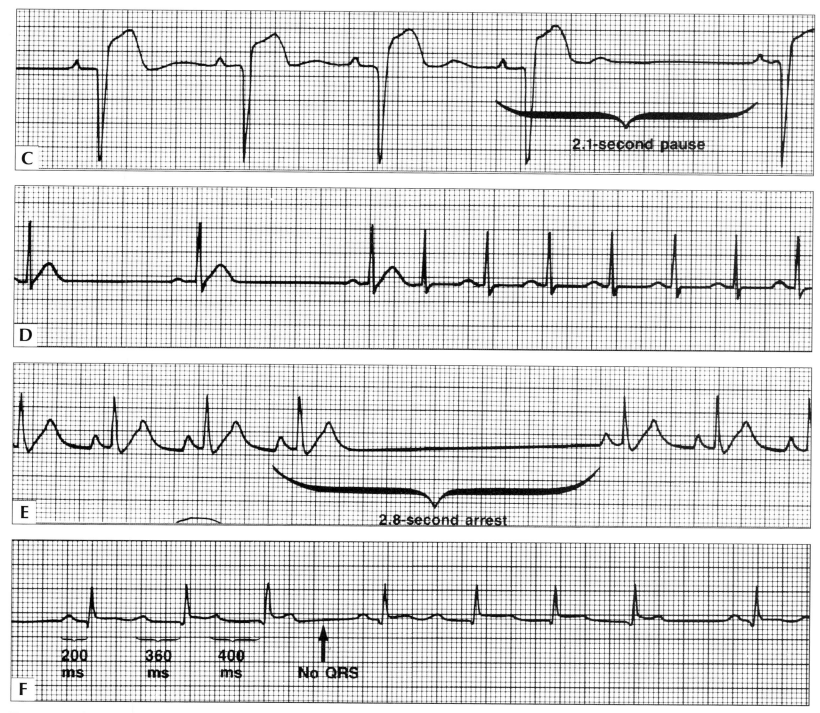

FIGURE 6-53. *(Continued)* **C**, asystole; **D**, sick sinus syndrome; **E**, carotid sinus hypersensitivity; and **F**, atrial tachycardia and atrioventricular Wenkebach conduction. (Panel A *adapted from* VA National Registry, June 1989–June 1990 [48]; B–F *Courtesy of* Ross Fletcher, MD, Washington, DC.)

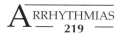

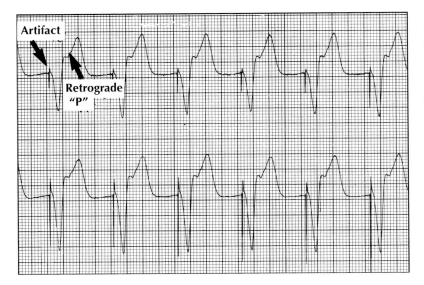

FIGURE 6-54. Pacemaker syndrome. Symptoms of syncope or dizziness associated with hypotension following single-chamber ventricular-based (VVI) pacing are less frequent today as a result of the more widespread use of atrial-based pacing systems. When present, the syndrome occurs predominantly in the setting of intact retrograde (ventricle-to-atrium) conduction as shown here. VVI pacing may result in atrial mechanical systole at the time of closed atrioventricular valves, producing elevated atrial pressures, reduced transmitral blood flow and cardiac output, together with atrial stretch-mediated systemic and pulmonary reflexes, resulting in inappropriate peripheral vascular vasodilation.

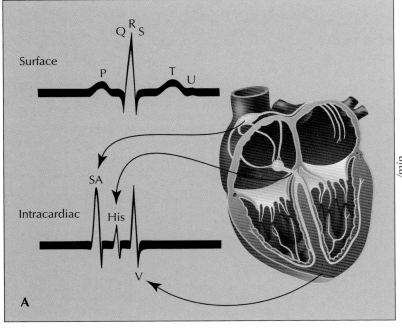

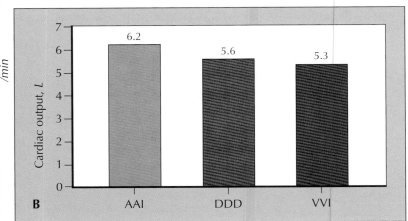

FIGURE 6-55. The importance of the sequence of ventricular activation. In **A**, the intact specialized interventricular conduction system results in the rapid, ordered, and precisely timed activation of both left and right cardiac chambers and regional (septal) segments as well as the natural repolarization sequence, resulting in optimal stroke volume.

Documentation of various pacing methods has highlighted the importance of the ventricular activation sequence [49] and the potential limita-

tions inherent with long-term pacing from the right ventricular apex. Pacing modes that allow for ventricular activation using the native specialized conduction system (AAI and DDD) result in greater cardiac output at rest and exercise as shown in **B**, perhaps largely due to intact septal activation and right-left heart synchrony. AAI—atrial pacing, sensing, inhibition; His—His bundle; SA—sinoatrial node; V—ventricular; VVI—ventricular pacing, sensing, inhibition.

CARDIAC PACING AND SURVIVAL

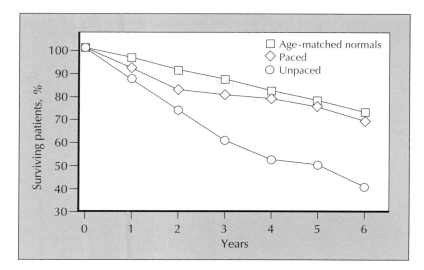

FIGURE 6-56. Heart block. Prior to the availability of pacemakers, survival among patients with third-degree heart block was dismal, approaching only 50% at 1 year and only 10% to 25% survival by 5 years [50]. Survival among patients with second-degree heart block is about 50% at 5 years compared with over 75% survival among patients receiving pacemakers [51].

RATE-ADAPTIVE PACING

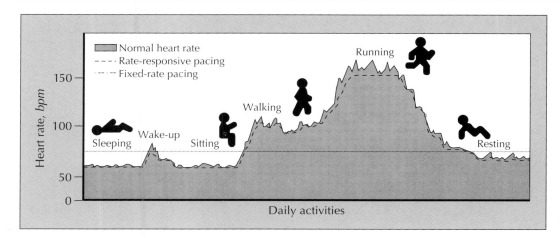

FIGURE 6-57. Adjusting heart rate to activity. Since the landmark achievement 35 years ago of restoring a stable cardiac rhythm with fixed-rate ventricular pacing (*straight dotted line*), efforts have focused on attempts to faithfully duplicate the rate responsiveness and physiologic characteristics of the native cardiac electrical pacemaking system. In the normal heart, rate

(chronotropic) response accounts for a significant amount of the total cardiac reserve output in response to metabolic requirements with exercise (*shaded area*). A significant number, perhaps 50%, of patients receiving pacemakers today show variable amounts of chronotropic incompetence and may potentially benefit from pacing systems that offer chronotropic, rate-adaptive support. In addition, a significant number (estimated at 5% per year) of patients receiving pacing systems initially for heart block, develop rate-incompetence during follow-up and would benefit from such capability as well. The ideal pacemaker would duplicate the impressive responsiveness of the autonomic and cardiac nervous system, sinus node, and specialized interventricular conduction system to meet the full array of physiologic requirements (dotted line). (*Adapted from* Medtronic, Inc., Minneapolis, MN.)

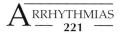

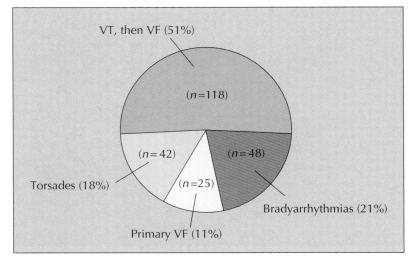

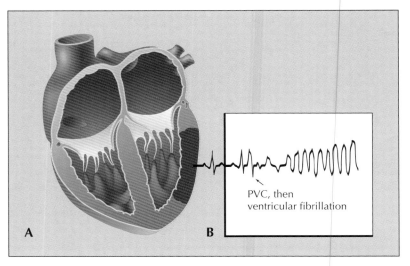

FIGURE 6-58. Cardiac arrhythmia at the time of sudden death. The cardiac rhythm present at the time of sudden death is usually ventricular tachycardia (VT) or fibrillation (VF) [31] as detected by ambulatory monitoring. The cardiac arrhythmogenic substrate is generally chronic, with various degrees of myocardial fibrosis such as that following myocardial infarction. This predisposes to lethal events following otherwise benign triggering events. (*Adapted from* Bayes de Luna *et al.* [52].)

FIGURE 6-59. Substrate for malignant arrhythmias. **A**, Evidence of healed or recent myocardial infarction (shaded area) and significant coronary artery atherosclerosis [53], even in the absence of a suggestive clinical history [54], have been frequent findings at autopsy following sudden death. **B** shows premature ventricular contraction (PVC), resulting in ventricular fibrillation.

PREVENTION

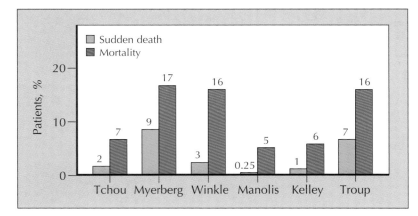

FIGURE 6-60. Improved survival after implantable cardioverter defibrillator therapy. The implantable defibrillator has had a remarkable impact on improving the freedom from recurrent sudden death relative to historical experiences, ranging from 91% at 1 year to 96% at 5 years, in a number of clinical studies. Overall survival has been reported to range from 95% at 1 year to 60% at 3 years. Most deaths are due to congestive heart failure and a much smaller proportion are due to bradyarrhythmias, electromechanical dissociation, or device failure [55–57]. (*Adapted from* Moss [57].)

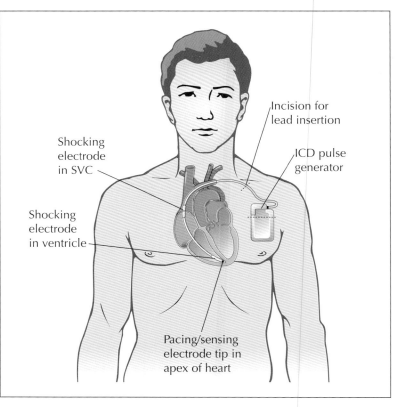

FIGURE 6-61. Pectoral implantable cardioverter/defibrillator (ICD). The ICD uses the defibrillation coils placed in the right ventricle apex and superior vena cava (SVC) with the titanium case of the pulse generator. Vascular access for the ICD leads is usually obtained via the left subclavian or cephalic vein. Typical volume for an ICD is 40 mL; typical weight is 80 g.

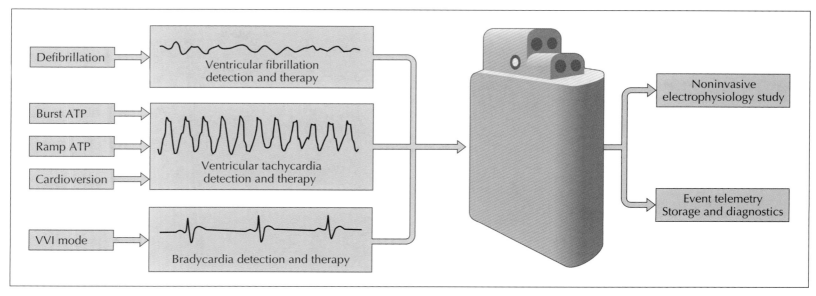

FIGURE 6-62. Tiered-therapy defibrillators. In addition to defibrillation, the implantable defibrillator has the capacity for several "tiered" functions including bradycardia pacing, antitachycardia pacing, and cardioversion. Therapy may be specifically programmed for individual patient needs and may include one or more "heart rate zones" based on both electrophysiologic testing and device-based testing after implantation. ATP—antitachycardia pacing; VVI—ventricular pacing, sensing, inhibiting. (*Adapted from* Medtronic, Inc., Minneapolis, MN.)

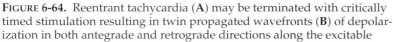

FIGURE 6-63. Antitachycardia pacing. Effective antitachycardia pacing burst patterns include those with between-burst decrement (SCAN) with or without an additional within-burst decrement (RAMP) pattern. In a randomized, controlled trial reported by Newman and colleagues [58], laboratory administration of adaptive SCAN or RAMP antitachycardia pacing patterns had a similar efficacy of 85% and 90% successful conversion among 29 patients with 65 inducible ventricular tachycardias. Acceleration due to antitachycardia pacing was observed in 7 (5 SCAN, 2 RAMP) of 65 (11%) tachycardias. Failure to convert tachycardia was associated with a shorter tachycardia cycle length. Basic cycle length = 240–340 ms; delay = 36 ms. ATP—antitachycardia pacing.

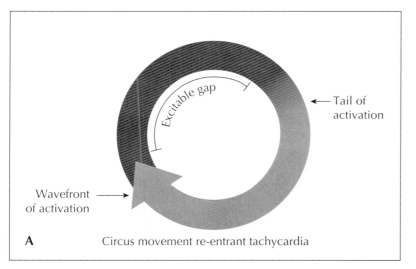

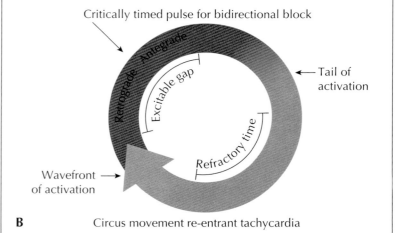

FIGURE 6-64. Reentrant tachycardia (**A**) may be terminated with critically timed stimulation resulting in twin propagated wavefronts (**B**) of depolarization in both antegrade and retrograde directions along the excitable reentrant pathway, resulting in bidirectional block to terminate the reentrant arrhythmia.

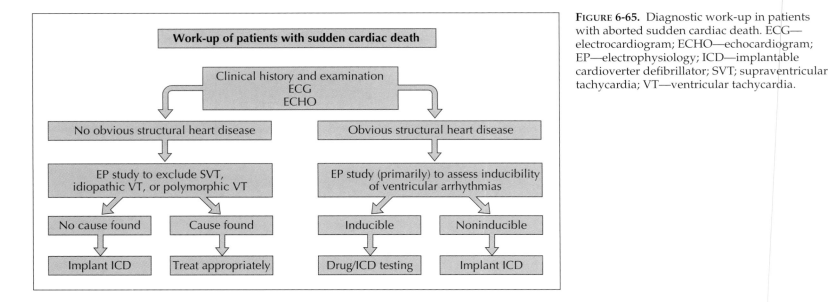

Work-up of patients with sudden cardiac death

Clinical history and examination
ECG
ECHO

No obvious structural heart disease

Obvious structural heart disease

EP study to exclude SVT, idiopathic VT, or polymorphic VT

EP study (primarily) to assess inducibility of ventricular arrhythmias

No cause found

Cause found

Inducible

Noninducible

Implant ICD

Treat appropriately

Drug/ICD testing

Implant ICD

FIGURE 6-65. Diagnostic work-up in patients with aborted sudden cardiac death. ECG—electrocardiogram; ECHO—echocardiogram; EP—electrophysiology; ICD—implantable cardioverter defibrillator; SVT; supraventricular tachycardia; VT—ventricular tachycardia.

CARDIAC RESYNCHRONIZATION THERAPY FOR HEART FAILURE

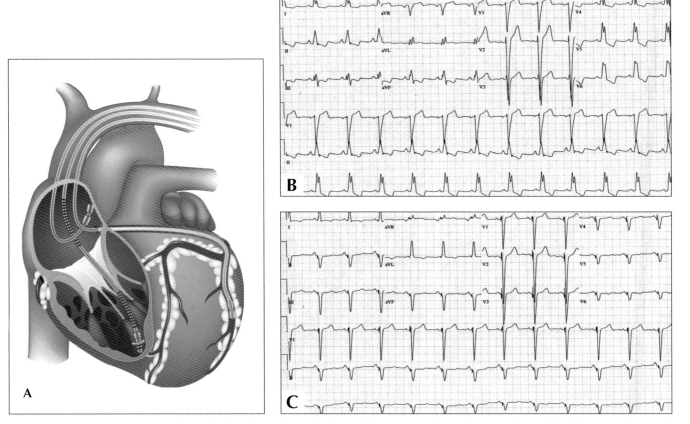

FIGURE 6-66. Cardiac pacing for heart failure. Several studies have shown that cardiac resynchronization therapy (CRT) can improve symptoms in a subset of patients with heart failure [59,60]. CRT is typically achieved by implanting pacing devices with a lead in the right atrium, right ventricle, and lateral branch of the coronary sinus (**A**). The lead in the lateral branch of the coronary sinus is placed to allow pacing of the left ventricle. Pacing of the right ventricle and the left ventricle simultaneously appears to improve ventricular hemodynamics. An electrocardiogram (ECG) from a patient with ischemic cardiomyopathy before CRT (**B**) shows a left bundle branch pattern. Approximately 30% of patients with chronic heart failure have conduction delays [61,62]. The ECG after the CRT device has been implanted (**C**) shows narrowing of the QRS.

CATHETER ABLATION

OVERVIEW OF CATHETER ABLATION

TYPE OF ARRHYTHMIA	SUCCESS RATE FOR CATHETER ABLATION (%)	ACCESS
WPW	85–95 (Right-sided) 95+ (Left-sided)	Transseptal or retrograde aortic approach for left-sided accessory pathways. Femoral right internal jugular or right subclavian for right-sided pathways.
AV node reentry	95+	Femoral
Atrial fibrillation: AV junction	95+	Femoral
Atrial flutter	80–90 for "typical atrial flutter"; 50–60 for "atypical atrial flutter"	Femoral
Atrial tachycardia	70–80	Femoral for right-sided atrial tachycardia; transseptal for left-sided atrial tachycardia
Paroxysmal atrial fibrillation	70–80	Transseptal

FIGURE 6-67. Summary of catheter ablation outcomes. In a number of large series [63,64], catheter ablation was used for treatment of the Wolff-Parkinson-White (WPW) syndrome. Approaches for left-sided accessory pathways have been highly successful. Transseptal approaches are highly useful in patients with aortic valve replacements, disease of the aortic arch, or congenital heart disease (associated with atrial septal defect). Patients with right-sided accessory pathways and Ebstein's anomaly may benefit from coronary artery mapping [65]. With atrioventricular (AV) node modification, the preferred approach is ablation of the slow AV nodal pathway rather than the fast pathway. With slow pathway modification, there is a less than 1% risk of requiring a permanent pacemaker [51]. Complete AV junction ablation requires the placement of a permanent pacemaker and anticoagulation for chronic atrial fibrillation. The His bundle may need to be ablated from the left ventricular septum if necessary. AV modification is a means of altering AV node conduction without causing complete AV node block, thus making a permanent pacemaker unnecessary [66]. There is now investigation into reproducing the surgical Maze procedure with catheter techniques for cure of atrial fibrillation. The complications of an invasive procedure include bleeding, infection, emboli, and blood clots. The risk of tamponade (from catheter perforation), stroke, or death is less than 1%.

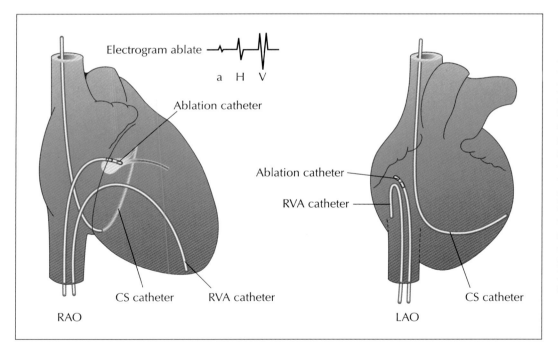

FIGURE 6-68. Right anterior oblique (RAO)/left anterior oblique (LAO) schematics for an atrioventricular (AV) junctional ablation. Using the femoral approach, the ablation catheter is placed to obtain the largest His and septal atrial signal possible. If the catheter is placed too distally, application of radiofrequency energy will cause right bundle branch block but not complete atrioventricular (AV) block. Therefore, a large atrial signal demonstrates that the proximal His bundle is being recorded. Compared with a slow junctional tachycardia with an AV node modification, there is usually a rapid junctional tachycardia prior to complete heart block. A ventricular electrode catheter is mandatory for pacing after the successful ablation. Although biplane images are shown here, an AV junctional ablation can usually be performed with an anteroposterior image. CS—coronary sinus; His—His bundle; RA—right atrium; RV—right ventricle; TV—tricuspid valve. Catheters: Abl, CS, RVA.

REFERENCES

1. Marriot HJC, Conover MH (eds): *Advanced Concepts in Arrhythmias*. St. Louis: CV Mosby; 1983:13–15.

2. Singer DH, Ten Eick RE: Pharmacology of cardiac arrhythmias. *Prog Cardiovasc Dis* 1969, 11(6):488–514.

3. Mandel WJ: *Cardiac Arrhythmias*. Philadelphia: JB Lippincott, 1995; 55–87.

4. CIBA Pharmaceutical Company Division of CIBA-GEIGY Corporation: The CIBA Collection of Medical Illustrations by Frank H. Netter, MD, 1969.

5. Wit AL, Bigger JT: Possible electrophysiologic mechanism for lethal arrhythmias accompanying myocardial ischemia and infarction. *Circulation* 1975, 3(Suppl 51, 52):96.

6. Wit AL, Rosen MR, Hoffman BF: Electrophysiology and pharmacology of cardiac arrhythmias. II: Relationship of normal and abnormal electrical activity of cardiac fibers to the genesis of arrhythmias. B. Reentry. *Am Heart J* 1974, 88:799.

7. Talano JV, Euler D, Randall WC, *et al.*: Sinus node dysfunction: an overview with emphasis on autonomic and pharmacologic considerations. *Am J Med* 1978, 64:773–781.

8. Evans T: *Electrocardiographic Test Set: Basic Electrocardiography and Cardiac Arrhythmias*, ed 2. Copyright © 1993 by Thomas Evans.

9. Man KC, Knight B, Tse HF, *et al.*: Radiofrequency catheter ablation of inappropriate sinus tachycardia guided by activation mapping. *J Am Coll Cardiol* 2000, 35:451–457.

10. Tchou PJ, Chung MK: Sick sinus syndrome and hypersensitive carotid sinus syndrome. In *Cardiac Electrophysiology: From Cell to Bedside*. Edited by Zipes DP, Jalife J. Philadelphia: W.B. Saunders; 2000:862–873.

11. Mandel WJ, Jordan JL, Karagueuzian HS: Disorders of sinus function. *Curr Treat Options Cardiovasc Med* 1999; 1:179–186.

12. Reiffel JA: Electrophysiologic evaluation of sinus node function. *Clin Cardiol* 1986, 4:401–416.

13. Glatter KA, Cheng J, Dorostkar P, *et al.*: Electrophysiologic effects of adenosine in patients with supraventricular tachycardia. *Circulation* 1999, 99:1034–1040.

14. Xie B, Thakur RK, Shah CP, *et al.*: Clinical differentiation of narrow QRS complex tachycardias. *Emerg Med Clin North Am* 1998, 16:295–330.

15. Daoud EG, Morady F: Pathophysiology of atrial flutter. *Annu Rev Med* 1998, 49:77–83.

16. Janse MJ: Mechanisms of atrial fibrillation. In *Cardiac Electrophysiology: From Cell to Bedside*. Edited by Zipes DP, Jalife J. Philadelphia: W.B. Saunders; 2000:476–481.

17. Brugada J, Mont L, Matas M, *et al.*: Atrial fibrillation induced by atrioventricular nodal reentrant tachycardia. *Am J Cardiol* 1997, 79:681–682.

18. Haissaguerre M, Jais P, Shah DC, *et al.*: Spontaneous initiation of atrial fibrillation by ectopic beats originating in the pulmonary veins. *N Engl J Med* 1998, 339:659–66.

19. Tsai CF, Tai CT, Hsieh MH, *et al.*: Initiation of atrial fibrillation by ectopic beats originating from the superior vena cava. *Circulation* 2000, 102:67–74.

20. Schumacher B, Jung W, Schmidt H, *et al.*: Transverse conduction capabilities of the crista terminalis in patients with atrial flutter and atrial fibrillation. *J Am Coll Cardiol* 1999, 34:363–73.

21. Chen PS, Athill CA, Ikeda T, *et al.*: Mechanisms of atrial fibrillation and flutter and implications for management. *Am J Cardiol* 1999, 84(9A):125R–130R.

22. Mittal S, Ayati S, Stein KM, *et al.*: Transthoracic cardioversion of atrial fibrillation: comparison of rectilinear biphasic versus damped sine wave monophasic shocks. *Circulation* 2000, 101:1282–1287.

23. VanderLugt JT, Mattioni T, Denker S, *et al.*: Efficacy and safety of ibutilide fumerate for the conversion of atrial arrhythmias after cardiac surgery. *Circulation* 1999, 100:369–375.

24. Oral H, Souza JJ, Michaud GF, *et al.*: Facilitating transthoracic cardioversion of atrial fibrillation with ibutilide pretreatment. *N Engl J Med* 1999, 340:1849–1854.

25. Glatter K, Yang Y, Chatterjee K, *et al.*: Chemical cardioversion of atrial fibrillation or flutter with ibutilide in patients receiving amiodarone therapy. *Circulation* 2001, 103:253–257.

26. Mounsey JP, DiMarco JP: Dofetilide. *Circulation* 2000, 102:2665–2672.

27. Haissaguerre M, Jais P, Shah DC, *et al.*: Spontaneous initiation of atrial fibrillation by ectopic beats originating in the pulmonary veins. *N Engl J Med* 1998, 339:659–666.

28. Pritchett ELC, Page RL, Connolly SJ, *et al.*: Antiarrhythmic effects of azimilide in atrial fibrillation: efficacy and dose-response. *J Am Coll Cardiol* 2000, 36:794–802.

29. Brugada P, Brugada J, Mont L, *et al.*: A new approach to the differential diagnosis of a regular tachycardia with a wide QRS complex. *Circulation* 1991, 83:1649–1659.

30. Lerman BB, Stein KM, Markowitz SM, *et al.*: Ventricular arrhythmias in normal hearts. *Cardiol Clin* 2000, 18:265–291.

31. Vincent GM: Long QT syndrome. *Cardiol Clin* 2000, 18:309–325.

32. Roden DM, Spooner PM: Inherited Long QT syndromes. *J Cardiovasc Electrophysiol* 1999, 10:1664–1683.

33. Mohler PJ, Schott JJ, Gramolini AO, *et al.*: Ankyrin-B mutation causes type 4 long-QT cardiac arrhythmia sudden cardiac death. *Nature* 2003, 421:634–639.

34. Dorostkar PC, Eldar M, Belhassen B, Scheinman MM: Long-term follow-up of patients with Long-QT syndrome treated with beta-blockers and continuous pacing. *Circulation* 1999, 100:2431–2436.

35. Priori SG, Napolitano C, Gasparini M, *et al.*: Clinical and genetic heterogeneity of right bundle branch block and ST-segment elevation syndrome. *Circulation* 2000, 102:2509–2515.

36. Gussak I, Antzelevitch C, Bjerregaard P, *et al.*: The Brugada syndrome: Clinical, electrophysiologic and genetic aspects. *J Am Coll Cardiol* 1999, 33:5–15.

37. Moss AJ, Hall WJ, Cannom DS, *et al.*: Improved survival with an implanted defibrillator in patients with coronary disease at high risk for ventricular arrhythmia. *N Engl J Med* 1996, 335:1933–1940.

38. Moss AJ, Zareba W, Hall WJ, *et al.*: Prophylactic implantation of a defibrillator in patients with myocardial infarction and reduced ejection fraction. *N Engl J Med* 2002, 346:877–883.

39. Akhtar M, Garan H, Lehmann H, Troup PJ: Sudden cardiac death: management of high-risk patients. *Ann Intern Med* 1991, 114:499–512.

40. Gregoratos G, Abrams J, Epstein AE, *et al.*: ACC/AHA/NASPE 2002 guideline update for implantation of cardiac pacemakers and antiarrhythmic devices: summary article. A report of the American College of Cardiology/American Heart Association Task Force on Practice Guidelines (ACC/AHA/NASPE Committee to Update the 1998 Pacemaker Guidelines). *J Cardiovasc Electrophysiol* 2002, 13:1183–1199.

41. Winkle RA, Mead RH, Ruder MA, *et al.*: Long-term outcome with the automatic implantable cardioverter-defibrillator. *J Am Coll Cardiol* 1989, 13:1353–1361.

42. Buxton AE, Lee KL, Fisher JD, *et al.*: A randomized study of the prevention of sudden death in patients with coronary artery disease. *N Engl J Med* 1999, 341:1882–1890.

43. The AVID Investigators: A comparison of antiarrhythmic-drug therapy with implantable defibrillators in patients resuscitated from near-fatal ventricular arrhythmias. *N Engl J Med* 1997, 337:1576–1583.

44. Kuck KH, Cappato R, Siebels J, *et al.*: Randomized comparison of antiarrhythmic drug therapy with implantable defibrillators in patients resuscitated from cardiac arrest. *Circulation* 2000, 102:748–754.

45. Naccarelli GV, Wolbrette DL, Dell'Orfano JT, *et al.*: A decade of clinical trial developments in postmyocardial infarction, congestive heart failure, and sustained ventricular tachyarrhythmia patients. *J Cardiovasc Electrophysiol* 1998, 9:864–891.

46. Bigger JT Jr: Prophylactic use of implanted cardiac defibrillators in patients at high risk for ventricular arrhythmias after coronary-artery bypass graft surgery. *N Engl J Med* 1997, 337:1569–1575.

47. Bernstein AD, Camm AJ, Fletcher RD, *et al.*: The NASPE/BPEG generic pacemaker code for antibradyarrhythmia and adaptive-rate pacing and antitachyarrhythmia devices. *PACE* 1987, 10:794.

48. VA National Registry. June 1989–June 1990.

49. Rosenqvist M, Isaz K, Botvinick EH, *et al.*: Relative importance of activation sequence compared to atrioventricular sequence in left ventricular function. *Am J Cardiol* 1991, 67:148–156.

50. Johansson BW: Longevity in complete heart block. *Ann NY Acad Sci* 1969, 167:1031–1037.

51. Shaw DB, Kekwick CA, Veal D, *et al.*: Survival in second degree AV block. *Br Heart J* 1990, 53:587–593.

52. Bayes de Luna AJ, Soldevila JG, Prat XV: Do silent myocardial ischemia and ventricular arrhythmias interact to result in sudden death? *Clin Cardiol* 1992, 10:449–459.

53. Myerberg RJ, Castellanos A: Cardiac arrest and sudden cardiac death. In *Heart Disease: A Textbook of Cardiovascular Medicine*, ed 5. Edited by Braunwald E. Philadelphia: WB Saunders; 1997:742–779.

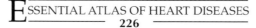

54. Newman WP 3d, Strong JP, Johnson WD, *et al.*: Community pathology of atherosclerosis and coronary heart disease in New Orleans. Morphologic findings in young black and white men. *Lab Invest* 1981, 44:496–501.

55. Fonarow GC, Feliciano Z, Boyle NG, *et al.*: Improved survival in patients with nonischemic advanced heart failure and syncope treated with an implantable cardioverter-defibrillator. *Am J Cardiol* 2000, 85:981–985.

56. Menon V, Steinberg JS, Akiyama T, *et al.*: Implantable cardioverter defibrillator discharge rates in patients with unexplained syncope, structural heart disease, and inducible ventricular tachycardia at electrophysiologic study. *Clin Cardiol* 2000, 23:195–200.

57. Moss AJ: Implantable cardioverter defibrillator therapy: the sickest patients benefit the most. *Circulation* 2000, 101:1638–1640.

58. Newman D, Dorian P, Hardy J: Randomized controlled comparison of antitachycardia pacing algorithms for the termination of ventricular tachycardia. *J Am Coll Cardiol* 1993, 21:1413–1418.

59. Cazeau S, LeClercq C, Lavergne T, *et al.*: Effects of multisite biventricular pacing in patients with heart failure and intraventricular conduction delay. *N Engl J Med* 2001, 344:873–880.

60. Abraham WT, Fisher WG, Smith AL, *et al.*: Cardiac resynchronization in chronic heart failure. *N Engl J Med* 2002, 346:1845–1953.

61. Aaronson KD, Schwartz JS, Chen TM, *et al.*: Development and prospective validation of a clinical index to predict survival in ambulatory patients referred for cardiac transplant evaluation. *Circulation* 1997, 95:2660–2667.

62. Farwell D, Patel NR, Hall A, *et al.*: How many people with heart failure are appropriate for biventricular resynchronization. *Eur Heart J* 2000, 21:1246–1250.

63. Jackman WM, Wang XZ, Friday KJ, *et al.*: Catheter ablation of accessory atrioventricular pathways (WPW syndrome) by radiofrequency current. *N Engl J Med* 1991, 324:1605.

64. Saad EB, Marrouche NF, Natale A: Ablation of focal atrial fibrillation. *Card Electrophysiol Rev* 2002, 6:389–396.

65. Van Hare GF: Radiofrequency ablation of accessory pathways associated with congenital heart disease. *Pacing Clin Electrophysiol* 1997, 20:2077–2081.

66. Scheinman MM, Huang S: The 1998 NASPE prospective catheter ablation registry. *Pacing Clin Electrophysiol* 2000, 23:1020–1028.

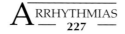

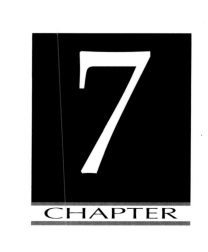

7 CHAPTER

HYPERTENSION

Edited by Norman K. Hollenberg

R. Wayne Alexander, John Amerena, Henry R. Black,
Emmanuel L. Bravo, Hans R. Brunner, Robert M. Carey,
William J. Elliott, Kathy K. Griendling, Randolph A. Hennigar,
Stevo Julius, Barry J. Materson, Kenneth Jamerson,
Helmy M. Siragy, Bernard Waeber, Alan B. Weder, Matthew R. Weir

PATHOGENESIS OF HYPERTENSION

GENETIC AND ENVIRONMENTAL FACTORS

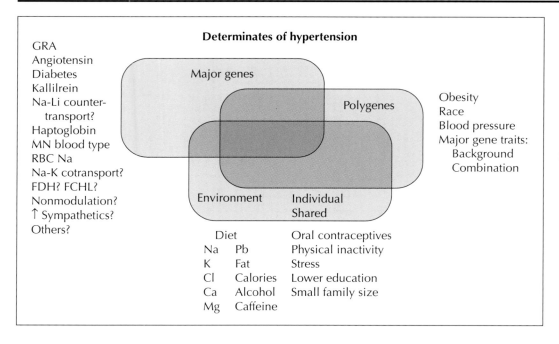

Determinates of hypertension

GRA
Angiotensin
Diabetes
Kallilrein
Na-Li counter-
   transport?
Haptoglobin
MN blood type
RBC Na
Na-K cotransport?
FDH? FCHL?
Nonmodulation?
↑ Sympathetics?
Others?

Major genes

Polygenes

Obesity
Race
Blood pressure
Major gene traits:
   Background
   Combination

Environment

Individual
Shared

Diet		Oral contraceptives
Na	Pb	Physical inactivity
K	Fat	Stress
Cl	Calories	Lower education
Ca	Alcohol	Small family size
Mg	Caffeine	

FIGURE 7-1. A model indicating the mechanisms by which essential hypertension could result from the combined effects of individual major genes that have a large impact on blood pressure, blended polygenes with small individual contributions, and environmental effects operating on individuals or within families. FCHL—familial combined hyperlipidemia; FDH—familial dyslipidemic hypertension; GRA— glucocorticoid-remediable aldosteronism. (*Courtesy of* Roger R. Williams, MD.)

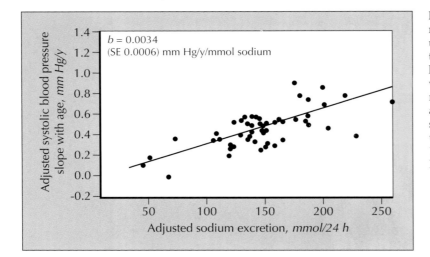

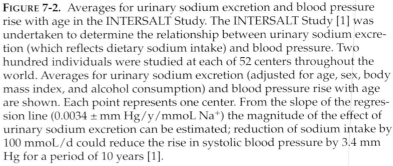

FIGURE 7-2. Averages for urinary sodium excretion and blood pressure rise with age in the INTERSALT Study. The INTERSALT Study [1] was undertaken to determine the relationship between urinary sodium excretion (which reflects dietary sodium intake) and blood pressure. Two hundred individuals were studied at each of 52 centers throughout the world. Averages for urinary sodium excretion (adjusted for age, sex, body mass index, and alcohol consumption) and blood pressure rise with age are shown. Each point represents one center. From the slope of the regression line (0.0034 ± mm Hg/y/mmoL Na+) the magnitude of the effect of urinary sodium excretion can be estimated; reduction of sodium intake by 100 mmoL/d could reduce the rise in systolic blood pressure by 3.4 mm Hg for a period of 10 years [1].

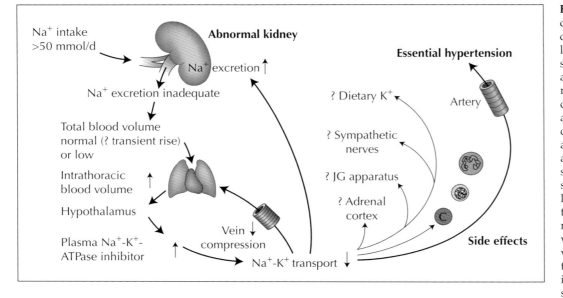

FIGURE 7-3. Hypothetical sequence of events demonstrating the role of sodium retention in cases of hypertension. An underlying genetic lesion may be expressed as a deficiency of sodium excretion, which becomes more apparent as sodium intake increases. The reduction in sodium excretion may initially cause a transient increase in total blood volume and a rise in intrathoracic blood volume. This change stimulates the hypothalamus to secrete a circulating sodium transport inhibitor, which adjusts renal sodium excretion, returning the sodium balance to normal. This balance is sustained only by a continuously high circulating sodium transport inhibitor, which raises the tone and reactivity of vascular smooth muscle. As a result, arterial pressure rises and venous compliance diminishes. Increased venous tone shifts blood from the periphery to the central vascular bed and thus raises intrathoracic pressure and perpetuates the stimulus for greater secretion of the sodium transport inhibitor. Total blood volume may be normal or low. JG—juxtaglomerular. (*Adapted from* de Wardener and MacGregor [2].)

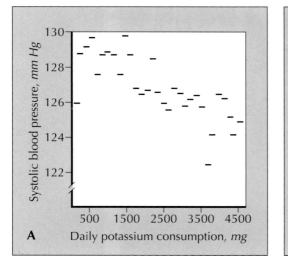

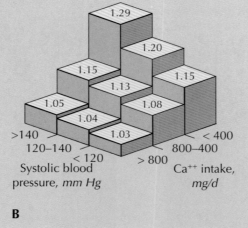

FIGURE 7-4. **A,** Dietary potassium intake is inversely related to systolic blood pressure. Displayed are values for systolic blood pressure and daily intake of potassium, as determined from dietary recall by participants in the NHANES-I cohort (a national population-based sample) [3]. **B,** Several dietary factors may interact to promote hypertension. The effect of dietary sodium and potassium on blood pressure may be conditioned by the contemporaneous intake of calcium. In this survey, continuous and graded relationships between blood pressure, dietary calcium, and the ratio of dietary sodium to potassium intake (numbers inside each bar) were found. Low calcium intake and an increased ratio of sodium to potassium intake were both associated with higher systolic blood pressure; the combination of both dietary habits was associated with the highest systolic blood pressure. (Part B *adapted from* Gruchow *et al.* [4].)

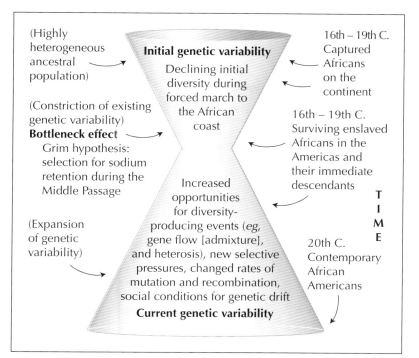

(Highly heterogeneous ancestral population)

Initial genetic variability

Declining initial diversity during forced march to the African coast

(Constriction of existing genetic variability)
Bottleneck effect
Grim hypothesis: selection for sodium retention during the Middle Passage

(Expansion of genetic variability)

Increased opportunities for diversity-producing events (*eg*, gene flow [admixture], and heterosis), new selective pressures, changed rates of mutation and recombination, social conditions for genetic drift
Current genetic variability

16th – 19th C. Captured Africans on the continent

16th – 19th C. Surviving enslaved Africans in the Americas and their immediate descendants

20th C. Contemporary African Americans

T I M E

FIGURE 7-5. The slavery hypothesis. Blacks of the Western Hemisphere have a high prevalence of hypertension and a tendency toward salt sensitivity. One possible explanation of these observations is the slavery hypothesis [5]. Intense selection pressure mediated by the stresses of restricted availability of dietary salt and excessive salt wasting from heat and diarrhea is hypothesized to have resulted in a complement of genes optimized to conserve salt. As selection pressure waned and the salt-conserving genotype was exposed to a high-salt environment, excessive salt conservation is thought to have resulted in a tendency toward salt-sensitive hypertension. It is not clear that such genotypic homogeneity could have persisted during subsequent outbreeding [6].

ADRENERGIC NERVOUS SYSTEM

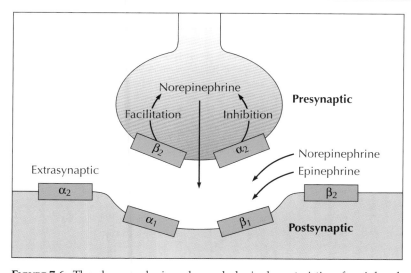

FIGURE 7-6. The pharmacologic and morphologic characteristics of peripheral adrenoreceptors. Nerve terminals within the autonomic nervous system are composed of several distinct receptor subtypes within and outside the synaptic cleft. These receptor subtypes have distinct and often opposing functional effects as well as different sensitivity to circulating catecholamines depending on their site and affinity. Stimulation of vascular postsynaptic α_1-receptors is predominantly by norepinephrine released locally (from the nerve terminal) and causes vasoconstriction. Extrasynaptic α_2-receptors, which are abundant in blood vessels, also cause vasoconstriction but are more responsive to circulating catecholamines (epinephrine > norepinephrine) because of their extrasynaptic location. Presynaptic α_2-receptors are more sensitive to locally released norepinephrine but decrease vasoconstriction by inhibiting further release of norepinephrine from the nerve terminal. Postsynaptic β_1-receptors are abundant in the heart and control heart rate and contractility while extrasynaptic β_2-receptors are predominantly located in resistance vessels in skeletal muscle and induce vasodilatation [7]. The overall physiologic effect of adrenergic receptor stimulation is determined by the degree of activation of the receptor subtypes and the balance between their opposing functional effects. (*Adapted from* Struyker Boudier [7].)

DISTRIBUTION AND PHYSIOLOGIC EFFECTS OF DIFFERENT ADRENERGIC RECEPTORS

TISSUE	RECEPTOR TYPE	EFFECT
Blood vessels	α_1 and α_2	Constriction
	β_2	Dilatation
Heart	β_1	Tachycardia; increased contractility
	α_1	Increased contractility
Bronchi	β_2	Relaxation
Thrombocytes	α_2	Aggregation
Kidneys	α_1 and α_2	Vasoconstriction
	β_1 and β_2	Renin release; inhibition tubular sodium reabsorption
Adipocytes	α_2	Inhibition lipolysis
	β_1, β_2, and β_3 (?)	Lipolysis

FIGURE 7-7. Adrenergic receptor subtype characterization by distribution and physiologic function. Subtypes of adrenergic receptors can be characterized by their distribution and physiologic function [7]. Along with variation in the distribution between organs there is variation in patterns of distribution within organs. For example, postsynaptic α_2-receptors are numerous in the peripheral vasculature but are present in greater numbers on the venous side of the circulation than on the arterial side. α-Receptors and β-receptors generally have opposite physiologic effects but in some organs, *eg*, the heart, the effects are complementary. β_3-Receptors have been described recently in adipose tissue but their physiologic role is uncertain, although a role in lipolysis has been postulated [8].

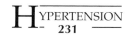

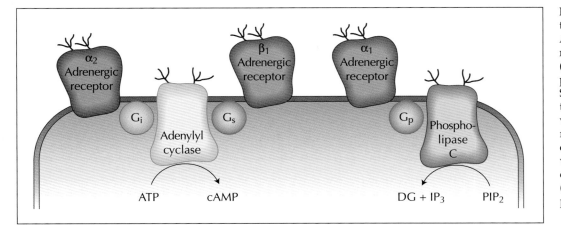

FIGURE 7-8. Types of adrenergic receptors and their functional relationship to G proteins. Adrenergic receptors are situated on the cellular membrane in close proximity to adenylyl cyclase (α_2 and β), phospholipase C (α_1), and the G protein subtypes G_i, G_s, and G_p, respectively [9]. Stimulation of β- or α_2-receptors leads to activation of G_s or G_i, which act as transducers to activate (G_s) or inhibit (G_i) adenylyl cyclase. This results in increased or decreased production of cAMP from ATP. α_1-Receptors work through G_p, which activates phospholipase C to promote conversion of phosphatidyl inositol bisphosphate (PIP_2) to diacyl glycerol (DG) and inositol triphosphate (IP_3). (*Adapted from* Linden and Gilman [9].)

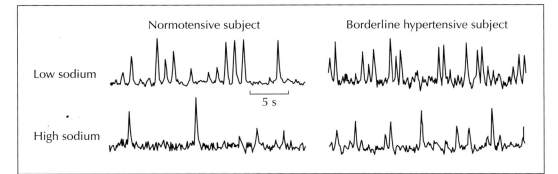

FIGURE 7-9. Microneurographic recordings in a normotensive and a borderline hypertensive subject. Microneurography permits recording of the rate of sympathetic bursts in the peroneal nerve. This method is excellent for evaluation of reflex responses within the same individual and it has been recognized recently to be a sufficiently sensitive and reproducible technique to allow comparison between groups. These recordings show increased rates of sympathetic bursts in the patient with borderline hypertension [10]. They also show a higher rate of discharge on a low-sodium diet in both normotensive and hypertensive subjects. (*Adapted from* Anderson *et al.* [10].)

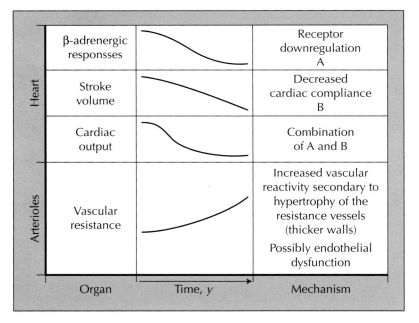

FIGURE 7-10. The proposed mechanism of hemodynamic transition in hypertension, showing the effects of decreased β-adrenergic responsiveness and decreased cardiac compliance/low stroke volume on the cardiac output. The cardiac output first decreases and then levels off. Later, if the patient develops congestive heart failure, the resting cardiac output decreases further. The process of structural amplification as a result of the hypertrophy of the arteriolar wall supports the increase of vascular resistance. With time the hemodynamics of hypertension change from an increase of the cardiac output to an increase of vascular resistance.

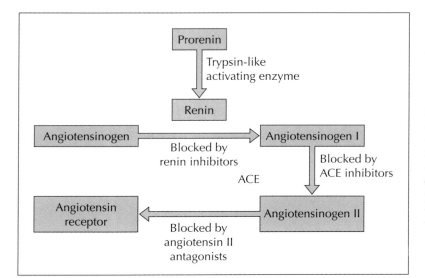

FIGURE 7-11. The renin-angiotensin system. Prorenin is converted to active renin by a trypsin-like activating enzyme. Renin enzymatically cleaves angiotensinogen to form the decapeptide angiotensin I; this step can be blocked by renin inhibitors. Angiotensin I is hydrolyzed to the octapeptide angiotensin II by angiotensin-converting enzyme (ACE); this step is blocked by ACE inhibitors. Angiotensin II acts at a specific receptor, and this interaction can be blocked by a variety of peptide or nonpeptide angiotensin II antagonists. Blockade of the renin-angiotensin system at each step results in an increase in the components proximal to the indicated step. For example, renin inhibitors, which block enzymatic cleavage of angiotensinogen to angiotensin I, increase the formation and release of renin; however, renin *activity* (ie, generation of angiotensin I) is decreased. ACE inhibition decreases angiotensin II and increases plasma renin activity and angiotensin I. Blockade of angiotensin receptors increases plasma renin activity as well as concentrations of angiotensins I and II.

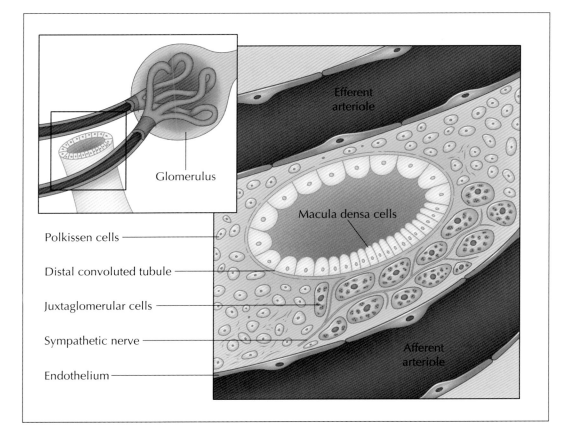

FIGURE 7-12. The juxtaglomerular apparatus, illustrating tubular and vascular components. The tubular component consists of 1) a specialized region of the distal convoluted tubule, which bends between the afferent and efferent arterioles, and 2) the macula densa, which contains cells that are sensitive to sodium chloride flux and control renin secretion. The macula densa cells can be identified by the proximity of their nuclei to each other. The vascular component consists of the afferent and efferent arterioles as well as the extraglomerular mesangium. The extraglomerular mesangium is a collection of small cells with pale nuclei, called Polkissen cells, the function of which is unknown. The juxtaglomerular cells, in which renin is synthesized, stored, and secreted, are vascular smooth muscle cells modified by the presence of secretory and lysosomal granules; juxtaglomerular cells are absent from the efferent arteriole. The macula densa cells have no basement membrane, allowing intimate contact of the juxtaglomerular cells with tubular cells. Renin is stored in and secreted from the granules of the juxtaglomerular cells. The vascular and tubular components are innervated by sympathetic nerves. Renal nerve stimulation increases renin secretion by norepinephrine-induced stimulation of β-adrenergic receptors. Juxtaglomerular cells also have angiotensin II receptors, the stimulation of which leads to inhibition of renin secretion.

MAJOR MECHANISMS OF RENIN RELEASE

Individual nephron signals
    Low macula densa sodium chloride (stimulates)
    Decreased afferent arteriolar pressure (stimulates)
Whole kidney modulating signals
    Angiotensin II negative feedback (inhibits)
    β-1 receptor stimulation (stimulates)
    Other humoral factors
        Vasopressin (inhibits)
        Atrial natriuretic peptide (inhibits)
        Dopamine DA-1 receptor (stimulates)
Local effectors
    Prostaglandins (stimulate)
    Nitric oxide (inhibits)
    Adenosine (inhibits)
    Kinins (stimulate)

FIGURE 7-13. Major mechanisms of renin release. Three major mechanisms are thought to govern renin release: 1) signals at the individual nephron, 2) signals involving the entire kidney, and 3) local effectors. Individual nephron signals include decreased sodium chloride load at the macula densa, which is the specialized group of distal tubular cells in approximation to the juxtaglomerular apparatus, and decreased afferent arteriolar pressure, which is probably mediated by a cellular stretch mechanism. Whole kidney signals include negative-feedback inhibition by angiotensin II at the juxtaglomerular cell, β_1-adrenergic receptor stimulation at the juxtaglomerular cell, and other hormonal factors. Local effectors include the prostaglandins E_2 and I_2, nitric oxide, adenosine, dopamine, and arginine vasopressin. The angiotensin II inhibitory feedback loop is thought to be the predominant and overriding mechanism that controls renin release in humans.

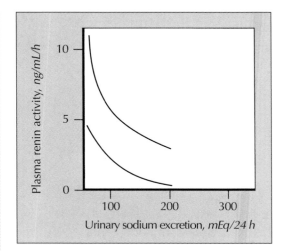

FIGURE 7-14. Relationship of plasma renin activity in ambulatory human subjects to the concurrent daily rate of urinary sodium excretion. The hyperbolic curves define the normal range. Approximately 25% of patients with untreated essential hypertension have low renin profiles, whereas approximately 15% have high renin profiles. Only 50% to 80% of patients with renovascular hypertension have elevated plasma renin activity. (*Adapted from* Brunner *et al.* [11].)

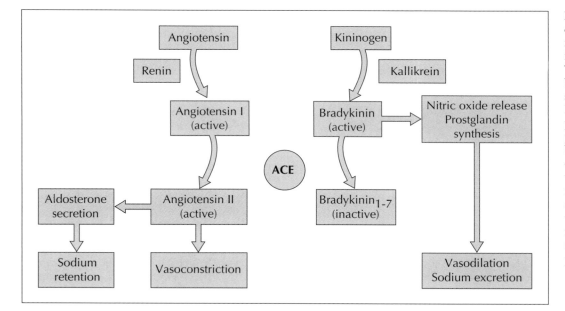

FIGURE 7-15. The actions of angiotensin-converting enzyme (ACE). The left side of the figure demonstrates how the enzyme converts inactive angiotensin I to active angiotensin II. The right side depicts how ACE metabolizes bradykinin, an active vasodilator and natriuretic substance, to bradykinin$_{1-7}$, an inactive metabolite. ACE therefore increases production of a potent vasoconstrictor, angiotensin II, while promoting the degradation of a vasodilator, bradykinin. Both actions of ACE increase vasoconstriction, and inhibition of ACE leads to vasodilation and natriuresis. Bradykinin is formed by the action of the enzyme kallikrein on substrate kininogen. Bradykinin acts as a vasodilator and natriuretic substance by releasing nitric oxide (an endothelium-derived relaxing factor) and stimulating formation of prostaglandins E_2 and I_2.

CLASSIFICATION CRITERIA OF ANGIOTENSIN RECEPTOR SUBTYPES

	AT_1	AT_2
Potency order	Angiotensin II > angiotensin III	Angiotensin II = angiotensin III
Selective antagonists	Losartan (DuPont-Merck, Wilmington, DE)	PD 123177 (Parke-Davis, Morris Plains, NJ)
	EXP 3174 (DuPont-Merck)	PD 123319 (Parke-Davis, Morris Plains, NJ)
	DuP 532 (DuPont-Merck)	CGP 42112A (Ciba-Geigy, Basel, Switzerland)
	L-158,809 (Merck, West Point, PA)	
	SKF 108566 (SmithKline Beecham, Philadelphia, PA)	
	GR 117289 (Glaxo, Research Triangle Park, NC)	
	SR 47436 (Sanofi, Montpelier, France)	
Effector pathways	↑ Phospholipase C	↓ Guanylate cyclase
	↑ Phospholipase D	
	↓ Adenylate cyclase	
Sensitivity to dithiothreitol (sulfhydryl reducing agents)	↓ Binding	↑ Binding
Effect of GppNHp	↓ Affinity	No change
	↑ Hill coefficient to no change ~1	

FIGURE 7-16 Classification criteria of angiotensin (AT) receptor subtypes. Pharmacologic and biologic evidence suggests the existence of heterogeneity in the angiotensin AT II receptor population. AT_1 receptors are those selectively blocked by biphenylimidazoles, such as the compound losartan (DUP 753), whereas AT_2 binding sites are blocked by tetrahydroimidazopyridines, typified by PD 123177. AT_1 receptors are more responsive to angiotensin II than to angiotensin III, are positively coupled to phospholipase C, and may be negatively coupled to adenylyl cyclase. AT_2 binding sites may be involved in modulation of the intracellular content of cGMP. Angiotensin II and angiotensin III are equally potent in binding to AT_2 receptors. AT_1 receptors mediate vascular smooth muscle contraction, aldosterone secretion, pressor and tachycardic responses, angiotensin II–induced water consumption, and hypertension in cases of renal artery stenosis. The physiologic effects of AT_2 receptor activation are unknown. GppNH—guanylyl-imidodiphosphate. (*Adapted from* Griendling *et al.* [12].)

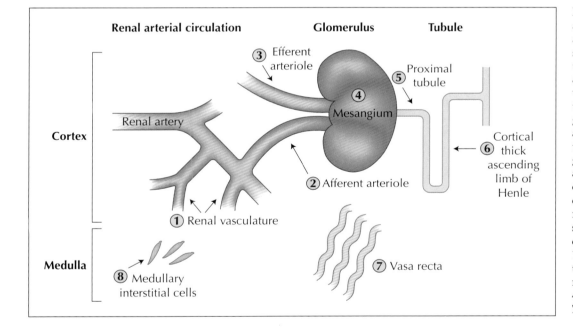

FIGURE 7-17. The renal tissue localization of angiotensin II receptors and the physiologic action stimulated by these receptors. Vasoconstriction occurs when angiotensin II acts at receptors in the arcuate and interlobular arteries, the afferent and efferent arterioles, and the medullary vasa recta. Angiotensin II preferentially constricts the efferent arteriole, thereby increasing glomerular filtration pressure; however, angiotensin II also acts on mesangial cell receptors to produce cellular contraction and reduce glomerular filtration. Angiotensin II receptors also are localized to the proximal tubule and the cortical thick ascending loop of Henle cells, which cause sodium resorption. Angiotensin II receptors recently have been found on renomedullary interstitial cell membranes, but the physiologic significance of these receptors is still unknown. 1—vasoconstriction; 2—limited vasoconstriction, and inhibition of renin synthesis and release; 3—preferential vasoconstriction; 4—contraction; 5 and 6—sodium reabsorption; 7—vasoconstriction; 8—unknown action.

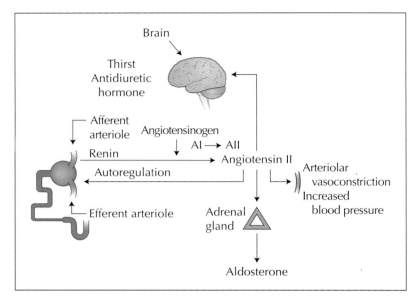

FIGURE 7-18. Effects of angiotensin II. Angiotensin II has three major effects: 1) arteriolar vasoconstriction; 2) renal sodium retention; and 3) increased aldosterone biosynthesis, all of which result in sodium retention. These effects work together to maintain arterial blood pressure as well as blood volume. Angiotensin II also stimulates the sympathetic nervous system, particularly the thirst center in the hypothalamus.

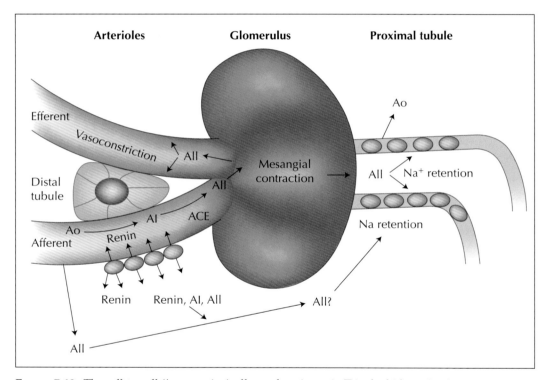

FIGURE 7-19. The cell-to-cell (*ie*, paracrine) effects of angiotensin II in the kidney. Angiotensinogen (Ao) either circulates to the kidney from the site of production in the liver or is synthesized in proximal tubular cells in the kidney. It is likely that renal interstitial angiotensinogen is derived predominantly from proximal tubular synthesis. Renin is synthesized and released from the juxtaglomerular cells into the afferent arteriolar lumen or into the renal interstitium. Angiotensin I (AI) is generated in the afferent arteriole and is converted to angiotensin II (AII) by angiotensin-converting enzyme (ACE). AII can cause mesangial cell contraction or efferent arteriolar constriction. AII can also be filtered at the glomerulus and may subsequently act at the proximal tubular cells to increase sodium reabsorption. In the renal interstitium, renin can cleave angiotensinogen to produce angiotensin peptides; these peptides may act at vascular and tubular structures. Angiotensin peptides may also be synthesized in and released from renal juxtaglomerular cells. Alternatively, the peptides may be taken up by renal cells from either interstitial fluid or the renal circulation.

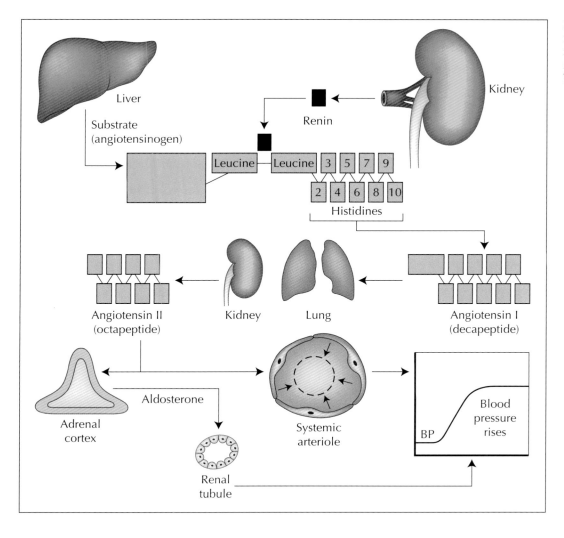

FIGURE 7-20. The circulating components of the renin-angiotensin system [13]. The circulating renin-angiotensin system plays a role in body fluid regulation, electrolyte homeostasis, and blood pressure control.

Liver

Substrate
(angiotensinogen)

Renin

Kidney

Leucine — Leucine — 3 5 7 9

2 4 6 8 10

Histidines

Angiotensin II
(octapeptide)

Kidney

Lung

Angiotensin I
(decapeptide)

Adrenal
cortex

Aldosterone

Renal
tubule

Systemic
arteriole

BP

Blood
pressure
rises

VASCULAR MECHANISMS

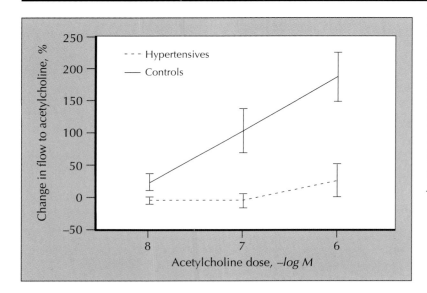

FIGURE 7-21. Evidence for defective endothelium-dependent relaxation in the coronary arteries of hypertensive subjects. Infusion of acetylcholine into the left anterior descending coronary artery of normal subjects leads to a dose-related increase in flow. The mechanism is presumably through the increased release of nitric oxide in the resistance circulation. In contrast, the increase in flow in response to acetylcholine infusion is markedly impaired in hypertensive subjects with ventricular hypertrophy. Maximal dilator capacity in response to nonendothelium-dependent dilators is not different between the two groups. The loss of this endothelial vasodilator mechanism probably contributes to disordered coronary flow regulation. Loss of endothelial-dependent vasodilator mechanisms could be associated more generally with the increase in vascular resistance in hypertension. (*Adapted from* Treasure *et al.* [14].)

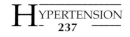

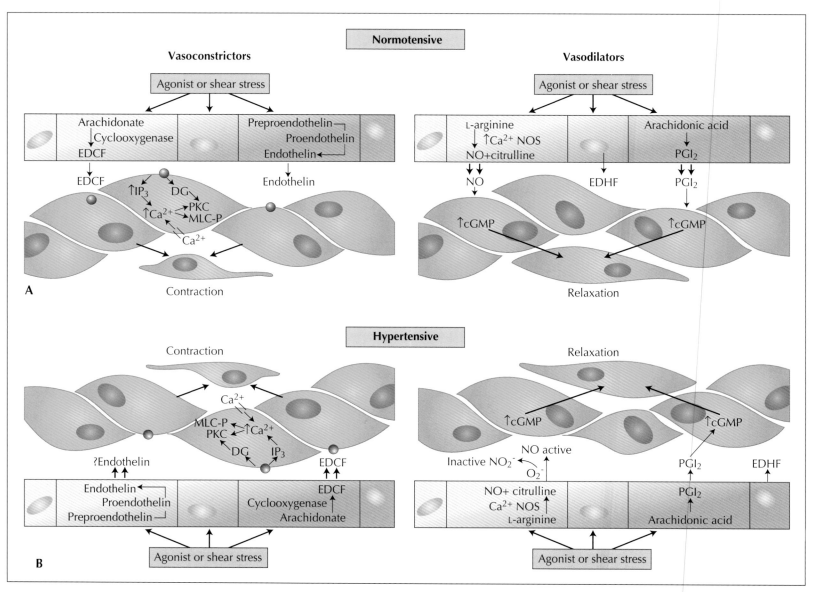

FIGURE 7-22. Endothelium-dependent vasodilator and vasoconstrictor mechanisms: modification in hypertension. Normal endothelial cells secrete both vasodilators, the most prominent of which are nitric oxide (NO), prostacyclin (PGI$_2$), and endothelium-derived hyperpolarizing factor (EDHF), and vasoconstrictors, including endothelin and endothelium-derived contracting factor (EDCF) [15]. Vessel tone is dependent on the balance between these factors and on the ability of the smooth muscle cell to respond to them.

A, In normotensive vessels there is a predominance of vasodilator secretion. These substances may also contribute to the inhibition of smooth muscle cell growth or hypertrophy. The relative concentrations of the vasoconstricting/vasodilating agents are indicated by the relative sizes of the arrows and bold type in the illustration.

B, In hypertension, release of vasoconstrictor substances may predominate [16]. In addition, vasodilator release may be decreased or, alternatively, the vasodilator itself may be inactivated by superoxide anion. Under certain circumstances, endothelin can also be growth-promoting, thereby

contributing to smooth muscle cell hypertrophy or hyperplasia and intimal thickening. The biochemical pathways activated by endothelial agonists and by contracting and relaxing factors acting on smooth muscle can also be affected in hypertension. NO, produced by the conversion of L-arginine to citrulline, traverses the endothelial cell membrane, and activates the smooth muscle cell guanylate cyclase to generate intracellular cyclic guanosine monophosphate. PGI$_2$ and EDCF are produced via cyclo-oxygenase action on arachidonic acid. PGI$_2$ relaxes vessels by increasing smooth muscle cell cyclic adenosine monophosphate; the mechanism of action of EDCF is unknown. Endothelin is made and modified by endothelium. It then stimulates the phospholipase C pathway in smooth muscle to produce the second messengers inositol trisphosphate (IP$_3$) and diacylglycerol (DG), which in turn activate the Ca^{2+} and protein kinase C (PKC) signaling pathways. This leads to phosphorylation of the myosin light chain (MLC-P), causing contraction. Alterations of any of these signals could easily augment contraction or decrease the ability of the vessel to dilate.

POTENTIAL MECHANISMS OF DEFECTIVE ENDOTHELIAL-DEPENDENT VASODILATION IN HYPERTENSION

Decreased production of nitric oxide

Increased degradation of nitric oxide by free radicals

Defective responsiveness of vascular smooth muscle to endothelial-dependent vasodilators

Increased production of endothelial-derived vasoconstrictors

FIGURE 7-23. Possible mechanisms responsible for defective endothelium-dependent vasodilatation in hypertension. As described earlier, nitric oxide is perhaps the most important of the endothelium-derived relaxing factors. Therefore, decreased production of nitric oxide or increased degradation by free radicals markedly impairs vasodilatation [17]. The smooth muscle itself may exhibit decreased responsiveness to ambient endothelium-derived vasodilators. Finally, an imbalance in the production of endothelium-derived relaxing and contracting factors to favor excess production of the latter may also contribute to defective vasodilatation.

MEMBRANE ION TRANSPORT AND/OR CONTENT ABNORMALITIES THAT HAVE BEEN REPORTED IN HUMAN ESSENTIAL HYPERTENSION

Increased Ca^{2+} concentration in platelets

Decreased Na^+-Ca^+ exchange

Decreased Ca^{2+}-ATPase activity

Decreased activity of the Na^+/K^+-ATPase leading to increased intracellular Na^+ concentration

Increased Na^+ content in red and white blood cells

Low Na^+/K^+/(^+2Cl-) cotransport activity

Increased Na^+-Li^+ countertransport

Increased Na^+-H^+ exchange

FIGURE 7-24. Membrane ion transport or content abnormalities that have been reported in human essential hypertension. Studies of ion transport and content in cells from hypertensive patients are numerous. Many ion transporters have been examined, and many have been found to be altered in platelets or erythrocytes of subsets of hypertensive patients. This table summarizes the abnormalities identified in various cell types in human essential hypertension. In the following figures, each will be considered separately.

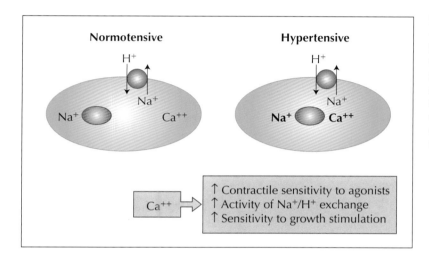

FIGURE 7-25. Unifying concept linking increased growth and contractility with ion abnormalities in vascular smooth muscle in hypertension. It has become apparent that human hypertension is associated with abnormalities of ion transport in vascular smooth muscle that result in an increase in intracellular Na^+ and Ca^{2+}. The increase in intracellular Ca^{2+} could enhance contractile sensitivity to agonists and increase activity of Na^+/H^+ exchanger. The resulting alkalinization, as well as the increased calcium, could lead to increased sensitivity to growth stimulation. Therefore, most of the important pathophysiologic features of the disease are potentially explainable in the context of abnormalities of ion transport.

SECONDARY HYPERTENSION

Approximately 5% of patients with hypertension have secondary hypertension, including renovascular hypertension, hypertension secondary to parenchymal renal disease, Cushing's syndrome, aldosterone-producing tumors, and pheochromocytoma.

RENOVASCULAR HYPERTENSION

CLINICAL CLUES SUGGESTING RENOVASCULAR HYPERTENSION

Systolic/diastolic epigastric, subcostal, or flank bruit

Accelerated or malignant hypertension

Unilateral small kidney discovered by any clinical study

Severe hypertension in child or young adult, or after age 50 y

Sudden development or worsening of hypertension at any age

Hypertension and unexplained impairment of renal function

Sudden worsening of renal function in hypertensive patient

Hypertension refractory to appropriate three-drug regimen

Impairment in renal function in response to angiotensin-converting enzyme inhibitor

Extensive occlusive disease in coronary, cerebral, and peripheral circulation

FIGURE 7-26. Causes of renal artery stenosis. Lesions of the renal arteries associated with hypertension can be divided into several categories. Atherosclerosis, which tends to occur in older individuals, and fibromuscular hyperplasia, which tends to occur in young women, are the most common causes of significant renal artery stenosis. Other causes are uncommon. Renal artery stenosis occurs in the absence of hypertension and may be present in a hypertensive patient without being the cause of the hypertension. Therefore, the functional significance of the renal artery lesion as a cause of hypertension must be validated by appropriate tests. The clinical characteristics listed here should raise the index of clinical suspicion for renovascular hypertension.

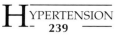

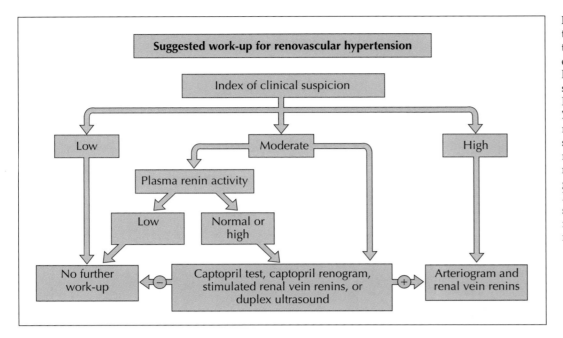

FIGURE 7-27. Work-up for renovascular hypertension. The work-up for renovascular hypertension depends on the index of clinical suspicion. In the absence of suggestive signs it is likely that test results would be inconclusive; in such cases, no work-up is recommended. Patients with suggestive clinical clues (*see* Fig. 7-26) have a 5% to 15% likelihood of having renovascular hypertension. Such patients can be screened with noninvasive studies and, if results are positive, confirmation of the diagnosis can be accomplished with renal arteriography and sampling of renin in the renal vein. If renovascular hypertension is strongly suggested, renal arteriography and sampling of renin in the renal vein are recommended, regardless of the results of noninvasive tests.

DIAGNOSTIC STUDIES FOR RENOVASCULAR HYPERTENSION

	SENSITIVITY, %	SPECIFICITY, %
Rapid sequence IVP	74	86
Isotope renography with ACE inhibition test	93	95
Peripheral vein PRA with ACE inhibition test (captopril test)	74	89
Renal vein ratio of PRA test (stenotic/contralateral):		
>1.3	85	40
>1.9	78	60
Peripheral vein PRA	92	96
Intravenous digital subtraction angiography	88	89
Doppler ultrasonography	86	93
Magnetic resonance imaging	97	95
Renal artery angiography	100	100

FIGURE 7-28. Indentification of renovascular hypertension. Three indicators have been defined and evaluated for the capacity to identify curable renovascular hypertension: 1) elevation of peripheral plasma renin activity (PRA) when considered in relation to 24-hour urinary sodium excretion; 2) suppression of renin secretion from the contralateral uninvolved kidney; and 3) abnormally increased renin in the renal vein as compared with the renin in the artery of the suspect kidney—this relationship has been shown to provide an index for the degree of ischemia in the suspect kidney. The sensitivity and selectivity of various tests are shown in this figure. ACE—angiotensin-converting enzyme; IVP—intravenous pyelography.

CAPTOPRIL TEST: CRITERIA FOR RENOVASCULAR HYPERTENSION

Stimulated PRA of ≥12 ng/mL/h
Absolute increase in PRA of ≥10 ng/mL/h
Increase in plasma renin activity PRA of ≥150% or ≥400% if baseline PRA is less than 3 ng/mL/h

FIGURE 7-29. The captopril test. The captopril test is used to identify patients with renovascular hypertension. The patient should consume a normal amount of salt and receive no diuretics. If possible, all antihypertensive medications should be withdrawn 3 weeks before the test. The patient should be seated for at least 3 minutes. Blood pressure should be measured at 20, 25, and 30 minutes, and the three readings averaged for a baseline. A blood sample is then drawn from a vein for measurement of baseline plasma renin activity (PRA). Captopril (50 mg diluted in 10 mL of water immediately before the test) is administered orally. Blood

pressure is measured 15, 30, 40, 45, 50, 55, and 60 minutes after administration of captopril; at 60 minutes, a blood sample is drawn from a vein for measurement of stimulated PRA. Three variables define the renin secretory response: 1) stimulated renin level, 60 minutes after captopril administration; 2) the absolute increase in PRA; and 3) the percent increase in PRA after captopril administration. The criteria for distinguishing renovascular hypertension from essential hypertension by the captopril test are shown.

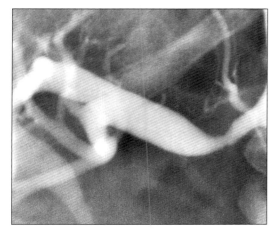

FIGURE 7-30. Selective renal arteriogram of a 43-year-old nonsmoking white man with a 2-year history of hypertension. The arteriogram shows 80% stenosis of the left renal artery with poststenotic dilatation caused by atherosclerotic vascular disease. Transluminal angioplasty or surgery can be successful in opening the artery and abrogating or curing the hypertension.

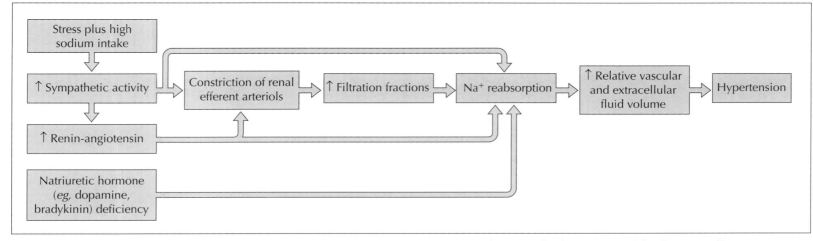

FIGURE 7-31. Mechanisms that can influence the kidney and lead to development of hypertension. The combination of physical or emotional stress and high sodium intake, especially in the absence of a natriuretic hormone, increases sympathetic nervous system activity. As a result, either directly or through stimulation of the renin-angiotensin system, renal efferent arterioles are constricted, causing fluid retention and development of hypertension. Natriuretic hormone deficiency or increased activity of the sympathetic nervous system or the renin-angiotensin system can increase sodium resorption and expand extracellular fluid volume, leading to hypertension. (*Adapted from* Kaplan [18].)

HYPERTENSIVE SYNDROMES SECONDARY TO CORTISOL EXCESS

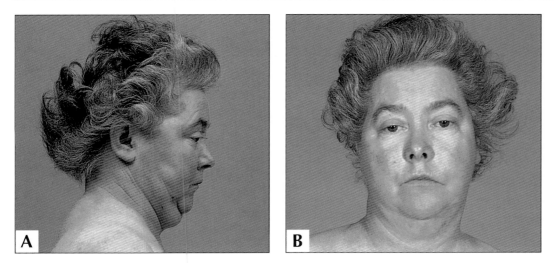

FIGURE 7-32. Physical features of Cushing's syndrome. The recognizable causes of Cushing's syndrome include Cushing's disease (72%), ectopic adrenocorticotropic hormone (ACTH) excess (12%), adrenal adenoma (8%), carcinoma (6%), and hyperplasia (4%). The typical clinical presentation of Cushing's syndrome includes truncal obesity, moon facies, hypertension, plethora, muscle weakness and fatigue, hirsutism, emotional disturbances, and typical purple skin striae. Carbohydrate intolerance or diabetes, amenorrhea, loss of libido, easy bruising, and spontaneous fracture of ribs and vertebrae may also be en-countered. Patients with ectopic ACTH excess may not have the typical manifestations of cortisol excess but may present with hyperpigmentation of the skin, severe hypertension, and marked hypokalemic alkalosis.

These images show the physical features of Cushing's syndrome: **A,** Side view of the patient revealing a buffalo hump. **B,** Facial features show the characteristic moon facies with a malar flush. Also obvious are the full supraclavicular fat pads. (*continued*)

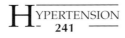

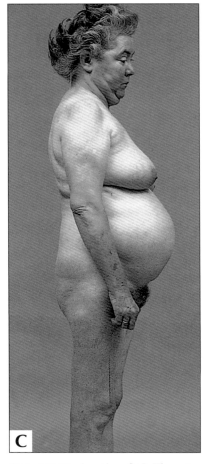

FIGURE 7-32. (*continued*) **C,** There is centripetal distribution of fat associated with significant atrophy of the thigh muscles.

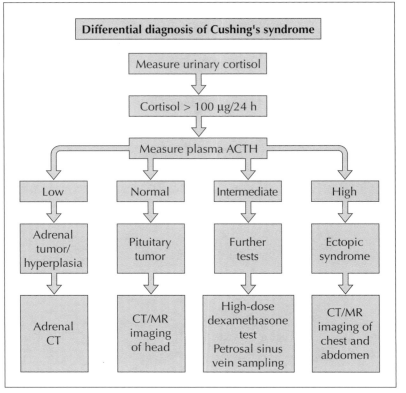

Differential diagnosis of Cushing's syndrome

Measure urinary cortisol
↓
Cortisol > 100 µg/24 h
↓
Measure plasma ACTH

Low	Normal	Intermediate	High
Adrenal tumor/ hyperplasia	Pituitary tumor	Further tests	Ectopic syndrome
Adrenal CT	CT/MR imaging of head	High-dose dexamethasone test Petrosal sinus vein sampling	CT/MR imaging of chest and abdomen

FIGURE 7-33. Differential diagnosis of Cushing's syndrome. Although it is cumbersome to perform, the determination of 24-hour urinary free cortisol is the best available test for documenting endogenous hypercortisolism. A level above 100 µg/24 h suggests excessive cortisol production. There are virtually no false-negative results. False-positive results may, however, be obtained in non-Cushing's hypercortisolemic states (*eg*, stress, chronic strenuous exercise, psychiatric states, glucocorticoid resistance, and malnutrition). If differentiation between pituitary and ectopic sources cannot be made based on plasma levels alone, pharmacologic manipulation of adrenocorticotropic hormone (ACTH) secretion should be performed (*ie*, high-dose dexamethasone suppression test or inferior petrosal sinus sampling for ACTH after corticotropin-releasing hormone administration).

The overnight dexamethasone suppression test requires only a blood collection for serum cortisol the morning after the patient has taken a 1.0-mg dose of dexamethasone at 11 PM of the previous evening. In normal subjects, cortisol levels at 8 AM will be suppressed to 5.0 µg/dL or less. When the presence of the syndrome has been verified by appropriate biochemical testing, the cause must be identified. Radioimmunoassay of plasma ACTH is the procedure of choice for pinpointing the basis of hypercortisolism. In patients with ACTH-independent Cushing's syndrome, ACTH levels have usually been suppressed to less than 5 pg/mL. In contrast, patients with the ACTH-dependent form tend to have either normal or elevated levels, usually greater than 10 pg/mL. In patients with Cushing's disease, ACTH release can be inhibited only at much higher doses of dexamethasone (2 mg every 6 hours for 2 days). The established criterion for the test is that suppression of the 24-hour urine and plasma steroids to less than 50% of baseline indicates pituitary Cushing's syndrome. Failure to suppress to less than 50% of baseline is considered consistent with an ectopic source of ACTH or ACTH-independent Cushing's syndrome.

Surgical resection of a pituitary or ectopic source of ACTH or of a cortisol-producing adrenocortical tumor is the treatment of choice for Cushing's syndrome. For pituitary Cushing's syndrome, transsphenoidal pituitary adenomectomy is the treatment of choice but total hypophysectomy may be required in patients with diffuse hyperplasia or large pituitary tumors. Bilateral adrenalectomy for Cushing's disease is universally successful in alleviating the hypercortisolemic state; however, 10% to 38% of individuals may later develop pituitary tumors and hyperpigmentation (Nelson's syndrome). Radiotherapy (*ie*, external pituitary irradiation, seeding the pituitary bed with yttrium or gold) has also been used with occasionally good results. The long-acting analogue SMS 201-995 (octreotide or sandostatin) has been used with varied success to treat ectopic ACTH syndromes; some benefit has been reported in Cushing's disease and Nelson's syndrome. Cyproheptadine has had limited success in the treatment of Cushing's disease. Ketoconazole, an inhibitor of several steroid biosynthetic pathways, has been used for rapid correction of hypercortisolism awaiting definitive intervention. Mitotane (o,p'-DDD), an insecticide derivative, induces destruction of the zonae reticularis and fasciculata with relative sparing of the zona glomerulosa. Mitotane has been used to treat Cushing's syndrome associated with adrenal carcinoma or to suppress cortisol secretion in Cushing's disease. CT—computed tomography; MR—magnetic resonance.

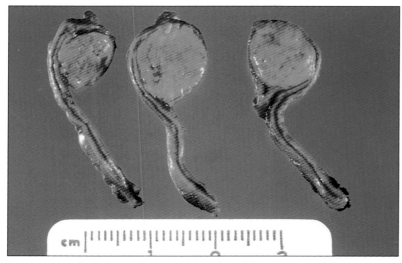

FIGURE 7-34. Pathologic characteristics of an aldosterone-producing tumor. Primary aldosteronism is an uncommon cause of hypertension, but is nevertheless an important disorder to recognize in hypertensive patients. First, the associated hypertension can be severe and cardiovascular and renal complications tend to occur. Second, removal of the tumor often results in

cure of hypertension or at the very least renders it more responsive to medical therapy. Third, knowledge of the presence of the disorder allows the physician to formulate a rational and specific therapeutic regimen, resulting in better compliance and better blood pressure control.

In the classic form of primary aldosteronism (Conn's syndrome), excessive aldosterone production results from a unilateral adrenocortical adenoma. In approximately one third of all patients, the adrenal glands may show hyperplasia of the zona glomerulosa, with or without micronodular changes (idiopathic hyperaldosteronism). Rarely, the syndrome can result from either an adrenal or ovarian carcinoma. In certain patients, the hypertension and biochemical abnormalities can be corrected by administration of dexamethasone. This form of aldosteronism in which aldosterone secretion is regulated by adrenocorticotropic hormone is hereditary and can be remedied by glucocorticoids. Recent studies demonstrate that this disorder is caused by a mutation in the zona fasciculata 11β-hydroxylase, which confers methyl oxidase activity. Such mutations result in ectopic expression of aldosterone synthase in adrenal fasciculata.

This image shows the pathologic characteristics of an aldosterone-producing tumor. Aldosterone-producing tumors arise from the zona glomerulosa cells of the adrenal cortex. Such tumors characteristically measure from 1 to 3 cm in diameter and are golden yellow on cross-section. The tumors are homogenous, and may or may not be encapsulated; atrophy of the adjacent adrenal cortical tissue may be seen.

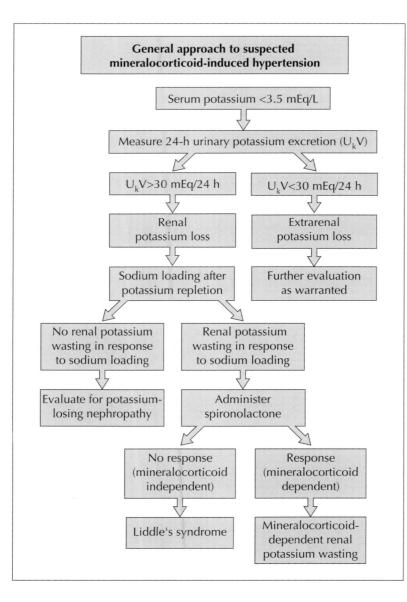

FIGURE 7-35. Algorithmic approach to suspected mineralocorticoid-induced hypertension, which is usually associated with spontaneous hypokalemia. Although hypokalemia is often simply a side effect of diuretics, evaluation is recommended under the following circumstances: diuretic therapy results in serum potassium less than 3.0 mEq/L even if levels normalize when diuretics are withdrawn; oral potassium supplementation and potassium-sparing agents fail to maintain serum potassium values greater than 3.5 mEq/L in a patient on diuretics; or serum potassium levels fail to normalize after 4 weeks of diuretic abstinence.

The initial assessment and subsequent studies should be designed to answer three questions: Is potassium loss renal or extrarenal? If renal, is it steroid or nonsteroid-dependent? If steroid-dependent, what is its cause? A 24-hour urinary potassium excretion greater than 30 mEq/24 h when the serum potassium is equal to or less than 3.0 mEq/L usually reflects renal potassium wasting. Correction of hypokalemia, especially in the face of continued high dietary sodium, by short-term administration (3 to 5 days) of the specific aldosterone-receptor antagonist, spironolactone, indicates that the renal potassium wasting is steroid-dependent.

Specific diagnostic tests should then be performed to confirm the diagnosis. Serum potassium levels of 3.4 mEq/L or less associated with urinary potassium excretion greater than 30 mEq/24 h indicates renal wasting, while lower excretion rates suggest extrarenal loss caused by diarrhea, vomiting, or laxative abuse. Renal wasting should be investigated further after adequate repletion of total body potassium with oral chloride potassium supplementation. Salt-loading (oral sodium of 250 mEq/24 h for 5 to 7 days) that results in hypokalemia with renal potassium wasting suggests an exaggerated exchange mechanism of sodium for potassium at distal tubular sites mediated by inappropriate secretion of electrolyte-active steroids. An exception to this rule is Liddle's syndrome, a familial, non-steroid-dependent renal potassium wasting disorder associated with hypokalemia and hypertension. Response to spironolactone (50 mg four times daily for 3 to 5 days) can demonstrate conclusively whether renal potassium wasting is truly mineralocorticoid-dependent. If spironolactone produces an elevation in the serum potassium level with concomitant reduction in urinary excretion, potassium wasting is probably mediated by electrolyte-active steroids.

The determination of dexamethasone responsiveness is the final step in the evaluation, to be undertaken if the physician suspects familial primary aldosteronism. This glucocorticoid-responsive aldosteronism should be suspected in patients with a family history of aldosteronism when imaging techniques fail to reveal anatomic abnormalities in the adrenal glands. Administration of dexamethasone, in doses of 0.5 mg four times daily, usually results in remission of hypertension and hypokalemia in 10 to 14 days. (*Adapted from* Bravo [19].)

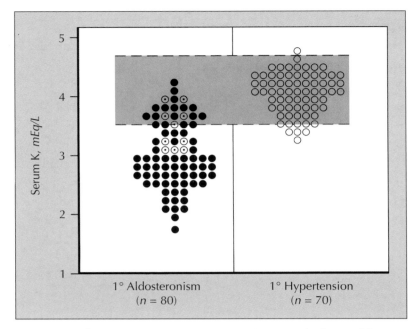

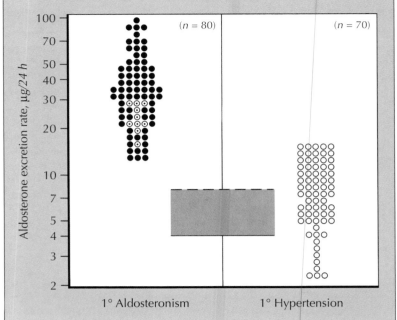

FIGURE 7-36. Serum potassium concentrations in cases of primary aldosteronism and essential hypertension. Patients were age- and sex-matched. No medication had been given for at least 2 weeks, and the patients were on an isocaloric diet containing 110 mEq of sodium and 80 mEq of potassium per day for 5 days. Blood was drawn between 8 AM and 9 AM after an overnight fast and at least 30 minutes of supine rest. Each point represents the mean of at least three determinations. For patients with primary aldosteronism, *solid circles* represent adenomas ($n = 70$) and *open circles with dotted centers* represent hyperplasia ($n = 10$). The *shaded area* represents 95% confidence intervals (3.5 to 4.6 mEq/L) of values obtained from 60 healthy subjects.

Twenty-two patients (27.5%) with primary aldosteronism (17 with tumors and five with hyperplasia) had fasting serum potassium values of 3.5 mEq/L or greater, while four (5.7%) subjects with essential hypertension had values below 3.5 mEq/L. Serum potassium values below 3.0 mEq/L were usually associated with the presence of a tumor. Ten patients (six of 17 with tumors and four of five with hyperplasia) remained persistently normokalemic, despite intake of high dietary sodium for 3 days. (*Adapted from* Bravo *et al.* [20].)

FIGURE 7-37. Aldosterone excretion rate after 3 days of high dietary sodium intake. Clinical conditions and patient identification are the same as in Fig. 6-16. Urine was collected on the third day of high sodium intake. The level of aldosterone in the urine was measured by a radioimunoassay technique as the pH 1.0 conjugate 18-glucuronide metabolite. The *shaded area* represents the mean (4.0 μg/24 h) and +2 SD (8.0 μg/24 h) of values obtained from 47 healthy subjects. No patient with primary aldosteronism had a value within the 95% normal range. Ten patients (14%) with primary hypertension had values that fell within the range obtained in patients with primary aldosteronism. Using a reference value of greater than 14 μg/24 h after a high sodium intake for 3 days, the sensitivity and specificity of the test were 96% and 93%, respectively. (*Adapted from* Bravo *et al.* [20].)

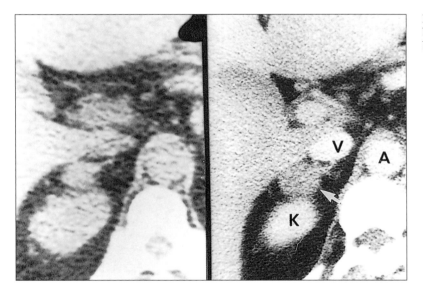

FIGURE 7-38. Computed tomography scan of a right adrenal tumor (*arrow*) before (*left*) and after (*right*) contrast injection. The tumor is located between the vena cava (v) and the upper pole of the kidney (k). A—aorta.

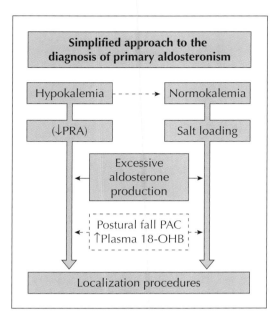

FIGURE 7-39. A simplified approach to the diagnosis of primary aldosteronism. Priority of evaluation should be given to patients with a history of spontaneous hypokalemia, marked sensitivity to potassium-wasting diuretics, or refractory hypertension in whom other causes of secondary hypertension (*ie*, renal parenchymal disease, renovascular disease, pheochromocytoma) have been eliminated. Patients with significant hypokalemia, suppressed plasma renin activity (PRA) (< 2 ng/mL), or an increased aldosterone excretion rate (> 14 µg/24 h) have unequivocal evidence of primary aldosteronism. Patients with equivocal findings will require salt loading. This evaluation can be accomplished on an outpatient basis by adding 10 to 12 g sodium chloride to the patient's daily diet in addition to determining the values of serum potassium concentration and 24-hour urinary excretion of sodium, potassium, and aldosterone after 7 days of high salt intake. A 24-hour urinary sodium value of at least 250 mEq gives some assurance that the patient has ingested the amount of salt prescribed.

Under these conditions, an aldosterone excretion rate greater than 14 µg/24 h suggests inappropriate aldosterone production. The development of hypokalemia or suppressed PRA are corroborative data, but their absence does not rule out a diagnosis of inappropriate aldosterone production. Demonstration of a postural decrease in plasma aldosterone concentration (PAC) and overnight recumbent plasma 18-hydroxycorticosterone (OHB) greater than 100 ng/dL indicate the presence of an adenoma. For localization, adrenal computed tomography should be performed first and considered diagnostic if an adrenal mass is clearly identified. When the results of computed tomography are inclusive adrenal venous sampling for aldosterone levels may be performed. (*Adapted from* Bravo [21].)

PHEOCHROMOCYTOMA

IMPORTANT FACTS ABOUT PHEOCHROMOCYTOMAS

About 30% of pheochromocytomas reported in the literature are found either at autopsy or at surgery for an unrelated problem

Thirty-five percent to 76% of pheochromocytomas discovered at autopsy are clinically unsuspected during life

The average age of diagnosis in those whose disease was discovered before death was 48.5 y, while the average in those diagnosed at autopsy was 65.8 y

Death was usually attributed to cardiovascular complications

FIGURE 7-40. Facts about pheochromocytoma. *Pheochromocytoma* is a tumor of neuroectodermal origin that produces excessive quantities of catecholamines, thereby causing hypertension with a constellation of signs and symptoms that can mimic several other acute medical and surgical disorders. Early recognition, accurate localization, and appropriate management of benign pheochromocytomas nearly always result in complete cure. If unrecognized, these tumors cause lethal disease that can lead to significant cardiovascular morbidity and mortality and particularly to sudden death during surgical and obstetric procedures.

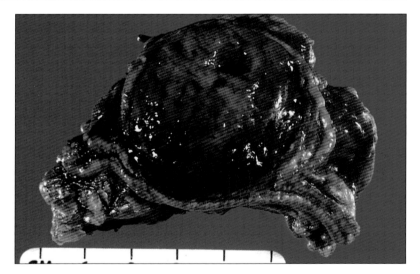

FIGURE 7-41. Typical gross pathologic features of an adrenal pheochromocytoma. The specimen is ovoid and encapsulated, surrounded by a rim of yellow tissue grossly resembling adrenal cortex. The lesion is rubbery to moderately firm and is pale gray to dusky brown. Pheochromocytomas have a strong affinity for chromium salts. Immersion in chromium salt fixative (Zenker's or potassium dichromate solution) changes the tumor from the usual pale-gray appearance to a dark-black color as cytoplasmic catecholamines are oxidized.

FIGURE 7-42. Priorities for detection of pheochromocytoma. The detection of pheochromocytoma requires a high degree of clinical alertness. Pheochromocytoma usually occurs as a sporadic event. These tumors, have, however, been associated with other clinical syndromes, such as von Recklinghausen's disease, von Hippel-Lindau's disease, Werner's syndrome (MEN type I), Sipple's syndrome (MEN type IIA), mucocutaneous neuroma (MEN type IIB), acromegaly, and Cushing's syndrome. Most patients present with labile hypertension, diaphoresis, headaches, and tachycardia with or without palpitations; however, as many as 30% of all reported cases were unsuspected during life and the tumors were found either at autopsy or during surgery for an unrelated condition.

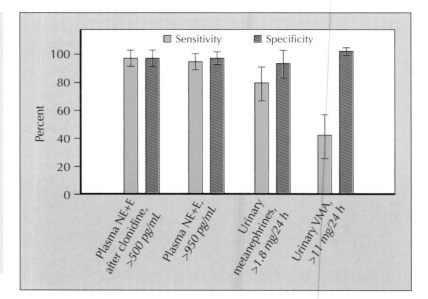

FIGURE 7-43. Sensitivity and specificity of various tests for pheochromocytoma. Measurement of plasma catecholamines appears to be the most sensitive test, and measurement of urinary vanillylmandelic acid (VMA) seems to be the least sensitive. When levels of catecholamines are elevated, all three tests provide excellent specificity. A combination test of plasma catecholamines and 24-hour urinary metanephrines provides nearly 100% accuracy (sensitivity and selectivity) in the diagnosis of pheochromocytoma. All values are mean ± 2 standard error. NE+E—norepinephrine plus epinephrine.

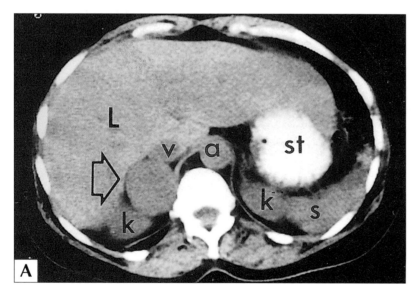

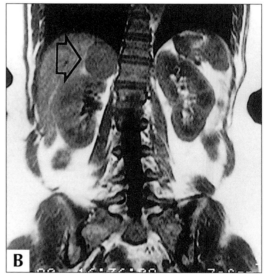

FIGURE 7-44. Three modalities used to localize pheochromocytomas. Computed tomography (CT) can accurately detect tumors larger than 1.0 cm and has a localization precision of approximately 98%, although it is only 70% specific. CT is the most widely applied and accepted modality for the anatomic localization of pheochromocytomas. Magnetic resonance (MR) imaging is equally sensitive to CT and lends itself to *in vivo* tissue characterization, which is not possible with CT. MR imaging is nearly 100% sensitive but is only 67% specific. Scintigraphic localization with radioiodinated ^{131}I-meta-iodobenzylguanidine (MIBG) provides both anatomic and functional characterization. Although this modality is less sensitive than CT and MR imaging, it has a specificity of 100%. Ninety-seven percent of pheochromocytomas are found in the abdominal region, with most found in the adrenal glands. Less likely sites are the thorax (2% to 3%) and the neck (1%). Multiple tumors may arise in 10% of adults. Familial pheochromocytomas are frequently bilateral or arise from multiple sites. Pheochromocytomas occurring in children are more commonly bilateral and more frequently lie outside the adrenal glands than in adults. Tumor localization not only serves to confirm the diagnosis of pheochromocytoma but also assists the surgeon in planning the surgical strategy. Advances in noninvasive imaging techniques now provide safe and reliable means of localizing pheochromocytomas regardless of their location.

A, CT of the adrenal glands (*arrow*). B and C, Coronal and sagittal MR imaging sections of the abdomen, respectively. Pheochromocytomas demonstrate high signal intensity on a T_2-weighted image, (*continued*)

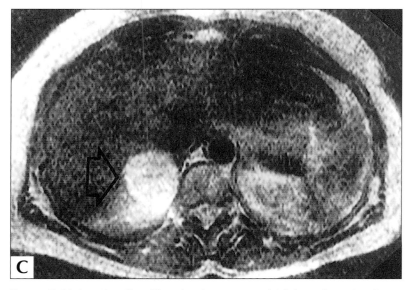

C

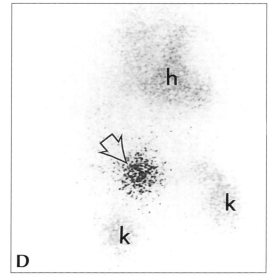

D

FIGURE 7-44. (*continued*) unlike a benign tumor, which has a low signal intensity. **D**, Scintigraphic localization of a pheochromocytoma (*arrow*) with radioiodinated 131I-MIBG. This modality provides both anatomic and functional characterization of a tumor. Because 131I-MIBG is actively concentrated in sympathomedullary tissue through the catecholamine pump, the administration of drugs that block the reuptake mechanism (*eg*, tricyclic antidepressants, guanethidine, labetalol) may result in false-negative results [22]. a—aorta; h—heart; k—kidney; L—liver; s—spleen; st—stomach; v—vena cava. (Part B *from* Bravo [23]; with permission.)

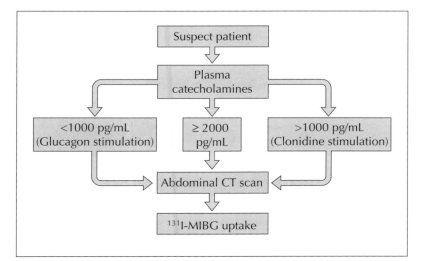

FIGURE 7-45. Diagnostic strategies in pheochromocytoma. Priority of evaluation is given to patients with the signs and symptoms detailed in Fig. 7-42. Concentrations of plasma norepinephrine and epinephrine are measured after the patient has rested in a supine position for at least 30 minutes. Caffeine and nicotine are prohibited for at least 3 hours before testing. Values of 2000 pg/mL or greater are considered pathognomonic for pheochromocytoma. Values between 1000 and 2000 pg/mL require a clonidine suppression test. Abdominal computed tomography (CT) or magnetic resonance imaging is then performed in patients with clinical and biochemical features suggestive of pheochromocytoma. Approximately 5% of patients may have plasma catecholamines of 1000 pg/mL or less. If the clinical presentation strongly suggests pheochromocytoma in these patients, further evaluation should be performed. Such evaluation may include measurement of urinary catecholamine metabolites or a glucagon stimulation test. For patients with arterial pressure greater than 160/100 mg Hg or if coexistent medical problems make sudden increases in blood pressure risky, pretreatment with 10 mg of oral nifedipine, 30 minutes before testing, will attenuate any increases in blood pressure without interfering with catecholamine release. MIBG—meta-iodobenzylguanidine.

NONPHARMACOLOGIC THERAPY

In most patients with hypertension, therapy should begin with or certainly include nonpharmacologic therapy.

TRIAL RESULTS ON EFFICACY OF INTERVENTIONS FOR PRIMARY PREVENTION OF HYPERTENSION

DOCUMENTED EFFICACY	LIMITED OR UNPROVED EFFICACY
Weight loss	Stress management
Reduced sodium intake	Potassium (pill supplementation)
Reduced alcohol consumption	Fish oil (pill supplementation)
	Calcium (pill supplementation)
Exercise	Magnesium (pill supplementation)
	Macronutrient alteration
	Fiber supplementation

FIGURE 7-46. Trial results on the efficacy of interventions for the primary prevention of hypertension. It is ideal to prevent hypertension from becoming clinically evident in genetically susceptible people. We have not yet learned how to select our own genes, but it is possible to manipulate our environment. Not surprisingly, the methods for primary prevention of hypertension are quite similar to those for nonpharmacologic treatment of established hypertension [24].

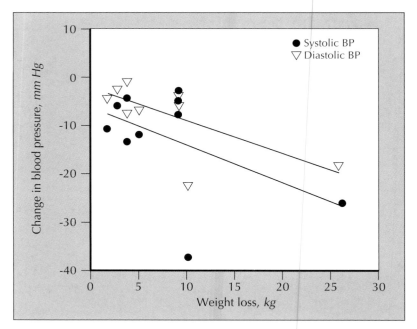

FIGURE 7-47. Regression of blood pressure (BP) following weight loss. Excellent studies have demonstrated that weight reduction, even without sodium restriction, is generally associated with substantial reductions in BP. Either the BP normalizes or the amount of drug required for normalization is reduced. The regression of change in systolic and diastolic BP on weight loss from 10 studies was reviewed by Johnston [25]. Although there is a great deal of scatter, greater weight loss does seem to correlate with greater reduction in BP ($r=0.50$ and $r=0.66$ for systolic and diastolic BP, respectively). The regression lines for systolic (lower) and diastolic (upper) pressures are nearly parallel.

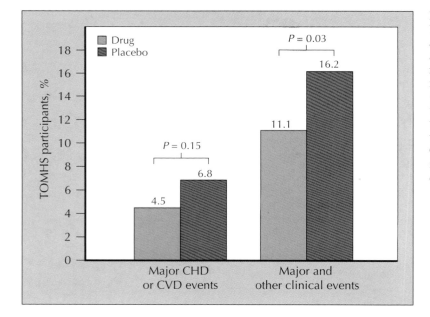

FIGURE 7-48. The Treatment of Mild Hypertension Study (TOMHS). Despite the substantial reduction in blood pressure (-9.1/-8.6 mm Hg) achieved in the TOMHS patients with nutritional-hygienic intervention alone, the greater reduction achieved by the addition of drug therapy to nutritional-hygienic intervention (-15.9/-12.3 mm Hg) was sufficient to reduce major coronary heart disease (CHD) and cerebrovascular disease (CVD) events more than that achieved by nutritional-hygienic intervention alone [26]. This difference did not achieve statistical significance, but when major and all other clinical events were combined, drug treatment was significantly more effective than nonpharmacologic therapy alone. Other clinical events included hospitalization for cerebral transient ischemic attacks, definite angina or intermittent claudication, and peripheral arterial occlusive disease.

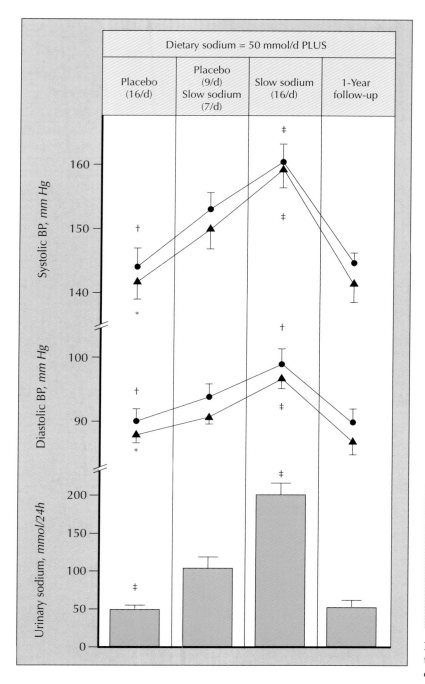

Dietary sodium = 50 mmol/d PLUS

| Placebo (16/d) | Placebo (9/d) Slow sodium (7/d) | Slow sodium (16/d) | 1-Year follow-up |

FIGURE 7-49. Data from one of many studies demonstrating the pressor effect of additional dietary sodium. These patients were placed on a sodium-restricted diet (about 50 mmol/d) to which either placebo or slow-release sodium tablets were added. Both systolic and diastolic blood pressures increased with the addition of sodium and returned to baseline when the supplement was discontinued. Patient samples included 19 patients (*closed circles*), three of whom required the addition of antihypertensive medications, and 16 patients (*closed triangles*) who were not taking medications. *Asterisks* indicate $P < 0.05$; *daggers* indicate $P < 0.01$; and *double daggers* indicate $P < 0.001$ compared with the phase of seven slow-release tablets per day. *T-bars* indicate standard error. (*Adapted from* MacGregor *et al.* [27].)

NONPHARMACOLOGIC (NUTRITIONAL-HYGIENIC) THERAPY

ADVANTAGES

May reduce blood pressure substantially without drugs

Enhances efficacy of drug therapy

May prevent or mitigate adverse drug effects (*eg*, hypokalemia, hyperlipidemia)

May regress left ventricular hypertrophy

DISADVANTAGES

Labor-intensive, expensive

Requires high patient and provider motivation

Requires continuous monitoring and reinforcement

May not protect against coronary artery disease and cardiovascular disease, including stroke, as well as does the addition of drugs

FIGURE 7-50. Nutritional-hygienic therapy. Nonpharmacologic (nutritional-hygienic) therapy is of great potential value. However, there are disadvantages to its use as well.

PRINCIPLES OF PHARMACOLOGIC THERAPY

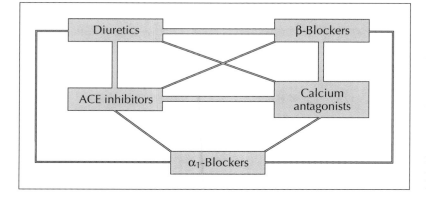

FIGURE 7-51. First-line antihypertensive drugs. Different classes of antihypertensive agents are proposed as first-line treatment for hypertension, *ie*, diuretics, β- (and α-) adrenergic blockers, angiotensin-converting enzyme (ACE) inhibitors, and calcium antagonists [28,29]. These agents reduce blood pressure by various mechanisms. They are therefore more or less effective, depending on the prevailing pathogenic factors in a given hypertensive patient. The angiotensin receptor blockers (ARBs) have been listed next to the ACE inhibitors. At the moment, they appear to be equivalent in efficacy with a lower frequency of adverse events and dropout associated with the ARBs. There is no reliable way to predict a positive response (*ie*, normalized blood pressure) to a specific therapeutic approach. A patient may respond favorably to one class of drugs exclusively or to several types of antihypertensive agents. Some patients may remain hypertensive regardless of the drug used as monotherapy. When necessary, different types of antihypertensive agents can be combined. Some drug associations are particularly effective (*thick lines*) [30].

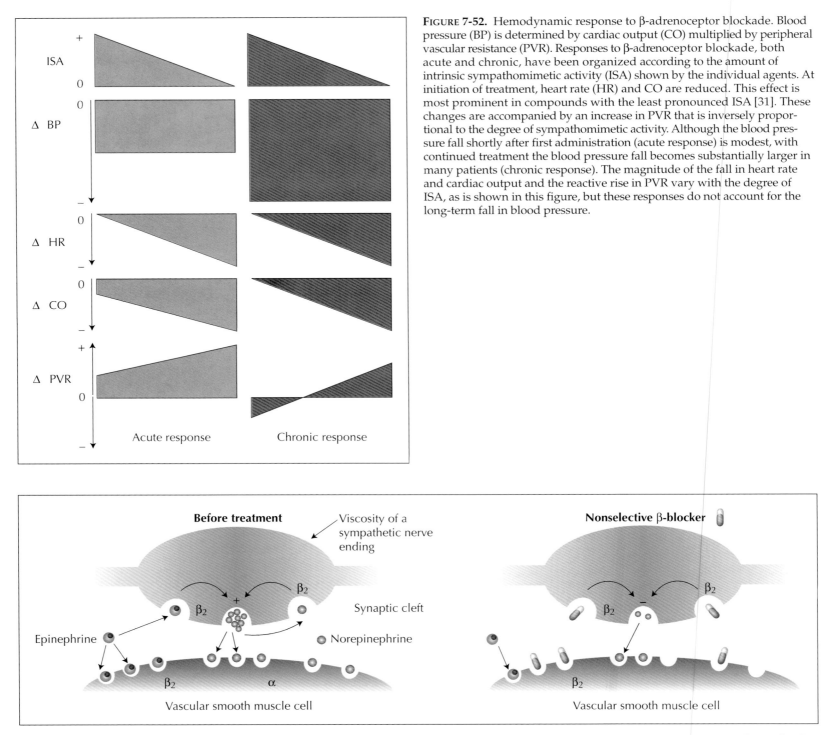

FIGURE 7-52. Hemodynamic response to β-adrenoceptor blockade. Blood pressure (BP) is determined by cardiac output (CO) multiplied by peripheral vascular resistance (PVR). Responses to β-adrenoceptor blockade, both acute and chronic, have been organized according to the amount of intrinsic sympathomimetic activity (ISA) shown by the individual agents. At initiation of treatment, heart rate (HR) and CO are reduced. This effect is most prominent in compounds with the least pronounced ISA [31]. These changes are accompanied by an increase in PVR that is inversely proportional to the degree of sympathomimetic activity. Although the blood pressure fall shortly after first administration (acute response) is modest, with continued treatment the blood pressure fall becomes substantially larger in many patients (chronic response). The magnitude of the fall in heart rate and cardiac output and the reactive rise in PVR vary with the degree of ISA, as is shown in this figure, but these responses do not account for the long-term fall in blood pressure.

FIGURE 7-53. Reduced release of norepinephrine during blockade of presynaptic β-adrenoceptors. β_2-adrenoceptors are located on varicosities of sympathetic nerve endings. Activation of these receptors enhances the neurally induced release of norepinephrine. Blockade of presynaptic β_2 receptors causes a decrease in norepinephrine discharge (*right panel*). This effect may be an important contributor to the antihypertensive action of β-blockers.

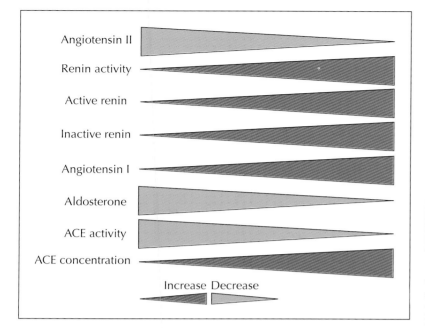

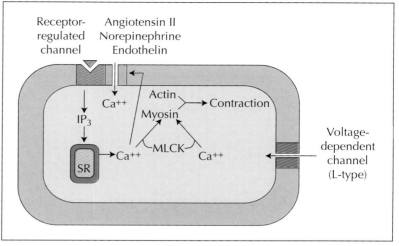

FIGURE 7-54. Effects of chronic angiotensin-converting enzyme (ACE) inhibition on the components of the renin-angiotensin system. Angiotensin II nearly disappears from the circulation during peak ACE inhibition [32]. Angiotensin II normally exerts a negative inhibitory feedback on renin secretion. During blockade of angiotensin II generation, plasma renin activity as well as active and inactive renin concentrations increase. The hyperreninemia is accompanied by a rise in plasma angiotensin I levels. Angiotensin II is a physiologic stimulus of aldosterone secretion. The plasma levels of this salt-retaining hormone are reduced during ACE inhibition. There is an induction of ACE synthesis during long-term treatment with ACE inhibitors.

FIGURE 7-55. Mechanism of action of calcium antagonists. Increased free calcium in the cytoplasm of vascular smooth muscle cells leads to vasoconstriction [33,34]. The calcium ion, after binding to calcium-binding proteins, activates a myosin light-chain kinase (MLCK), causing phosphorylation of myosin filaments followed by an interaction of these filaments with actin filaments and finally cell contraction. The calcium ion can enter the vascular smooth muscle cell by two main channels. The receptor-regulated channels cause, upon activation with an agonist (*eg*, angiotensin II, norepinephrine, endothelin), the formation of inositol trisphosphate (IP$_3$). This intracellular messenger triggers the release of calcium from the sarcoplasmic reticulum (SR). The rapid calcium mobilization by this pathway stimulates then sustains entry of calcium through the channel. Calcium antagonists block voltage-dependent channels. These channels allow the entry of calcium in response to cell depolarization.

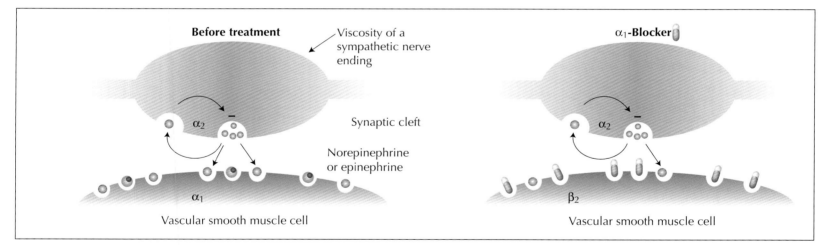

FIGURE 7-56. α$_1$-Adrenoceptor blocking agents. α$_1$-Blockers (doxazosin, prazosin, terazosin) lower blood pressure by preventing catecholamine-induced vasoconstriction [35]. In this illustration, norepinephrine released from the sympathetic nerve ending is depicted as *circles*, and the α$_1$-adrenergic blocking agent as an *oval*. The competitive action is confined to the vascular smooth muscle cell. These agents selectively block postsynaptic α$_1$-adrenoceptors. Catecholamines can still activate presynaptic α$_2$-receptors and thus exert an inhibitory action on norepinephrine release by the sympathetic nerve terminal. This probably accounts for the lack of reflex heart rate acceleration during α$_1$-adrenoceptor blockade. α$_1$-Blockers induce dilation of both arteries and veins. The effect on the capacitive system accounts for the prominent fall in postural blood pressure that occurs in some patients; this effect often limits the utility of these agents. α$_1$-Blockers are effective in reducing the symptoms of benign prostatic hypertrophy, which makes them an attractive choice in hypertensive elderly men with that disorder.

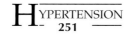

CLINICAL TRIALS OF DRUG THERAPY

VETERANS ADMINISTRATION STUDY

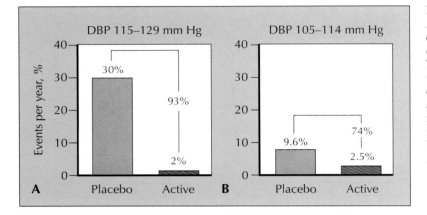

FIGURE 7-57. The Veterans Administration Study. The Veterans Administration Study in 1967 [36] was the first major therapeutic trial to establish the value of treating hypertension compared with placebo by demonstrating a 93% reduction in mortality and cardiovascular events. This study firmly established the value of treatment for patients with diastolic blood pressure (DBP) of 115 to 129 mm Hg (**A**). For patients with DBP of 105 to 114 mm Hg (**B**) a 74% reduction in events per year was observed after 5 years of follow-up. No statistically proven benefit for DBP in the range of 90 to 105 mm Hg was seen in these studies, nor did there appear to be any benefit in preventing coronary heart disease. (*Adapted from* the Veterans Administration Cooperative Study Group on Antihypertensive Agents [37].)

HYPERTENSION DETECTION AND FOLLOW-UP PROGRAM

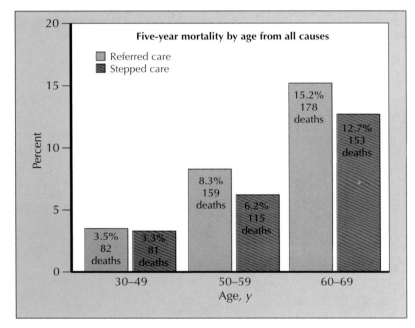

FIGURE 7-58. Five-year mortality rates by age. Five-year mortality rates by age in the Hypertension Detect-ion and Follow-up Program [38] revealed minimal benefit in those aged 30 to 49 years because of the low event rate. In the 50- to 59-year age group, the 25.3% benefit was significant. In the older age group (60 to 69 years) there was a smaller but still significant benefit of 16.4%, possibly due to the fact that more elderly patients were treated by referred care. (*Adapted from* the Hypertension Detection and Follow-Up Program Cooperative Group [38].)

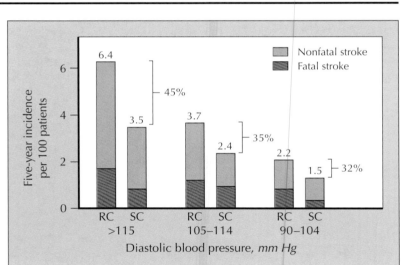

FIGURE 7-59. Effects of treatment in patients with mild to severe hypertension. Stroke reduction in the Hypertension Detection and Follow-up Program was greatest in the more severe hypertensives, especially for nonfatal stroke, but was demonstrable at all levels of hypertension. For those with a diastolic blood pressure of less than 100 mm Hg the benefit was statistically significant. Bracketed percentages represent the percent reduction in the endpoints of nonfatal or fatal stroke. RC—referred care; SC—stepped care. (*Adapted from* the Hypertension Detection and Follow-up Program Cooperative Group [39].)

BENEFIT OF TREATMENT OF HYPERTENSION

TRIAL	BLOOD PRESSURE RANGE, mm Hg	MORBIDITY/MORTALITY PER YEAR, %		REDUCTION IN EVENTS, %	BENEFIT OF THERAPY PER 100 PATIENT-YEARS
		TREATMENT	CONTROL		
VA 1967 [36]	115–129	2	30	93	28
VA 1970 [37]	105–114	2.5	9.6	74	7
Australian [40]	95–109	1.97	2.45	20	0.48
MRC [41]	90–109	0.14	0.26	54	0.12

FIGURE 7-60. Benefit of hypertension treatment. A summary overview of four major trials of antihypertensive treatment reveals a decline in benefit with treatment of milder degrees of hyper-tension. The benefit per 100 patients treated for 1 year falls from 28 persons to less than one. The implication of these results is clear: in mild hypertension, treatment must be maintained for many years in order to benefit the patient.

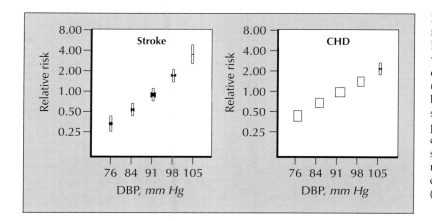

FIGURE 7-61. Diastolic blood pressure (DBP) versus relative risk of coronary heart disease (CHD) and stroke. The relationship between increasing levels of DBP and the risk of stroke and CHD is log-linear, based on observational studies of 420,000 individuals [42]. In these data there is no evidence of an increased risk associated with low levels of blood pressure (J curve). The risk of both stroke and CHD is substantially increased well below the conventional cut-point of 90 mm Hg. Stroke patients included seven prospective studies (843 events); CHD patients included nine prospective studies (4856 events). The slope of the curve for stroke is steep, confirming the fact that high blood pressure is the major risk factor for stroke. The slope of the curve for CHD is less steep because there are multiple risk factors for CHD. The data points in both curves show ±2 SE on the vertical axis and the blood pressure range on the horizontal axis. (*Adapted from* MacMahon *et al.* [42].)

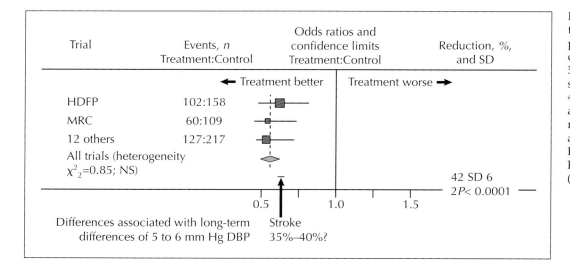

FIGURE 7-62. Meta-analysis of antihypertensive trials using diuretics. Meta-analysis of 14 antihypertensive trials using diuretics reveals an observed 42% reduction in stroke resulting from a 5 to 6 mm Hg reduction in diastolic blood pressure. This is consistent with a predicted benefit of 46% with a 7.5 mm Hg blood pressure reduction and confirms the usefulness of blood pressure reduction in stroke prevention. Horizontal lines are confidence limits around the means (*squares*). HDFP—Hypertension Detection and Follow-up Program; MRC—Medical Research Council. (*Adapted from* Collins *et al.* [43].)

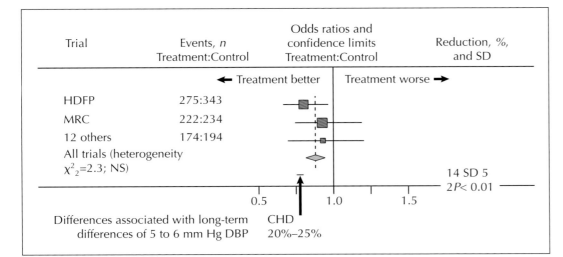

FIGURE 7-63. Meta-analysis of trials using diuretics and β-blockers. Despite a predicted benefit of 29% in coronary heart disease (CHD) events, the observed benefit was only 14% from the meta-analysis of 14 trials based on diuretic and β-blocker therapy. The reasons for this shortfall in benefit have been debated intensely. Whether other antihypertensive drugs might give different results is unknown. *Squares* indicate means. The size of the square indicates the amount of data. HDFP—Hypertension Detection and Follow-up Program; MRC—Medical Research Council. (*Adapted from* Collins *et al.* [43].)

EFFECTS OF ANTIHYPERTENSIVE AGENTS ON CORONARY RISK FACTORS

SIDE EFFECT	DIURETICS	β-BLOCKERS	α-BLOCKERS	CALCIUM CHANNEL BLOCKERS	ACE INHIBITORS
Blood pressure	+	+	+	+	+
Cholesterol	–	NS	+	NS	NS
HDL cholesterol	NS	–	NS	NS	NS
Glucose intolerance	–	–	+	NS	+
Hyperinsulinemia	–	–	+	NS	+
Physical activity	NS	–	+	NS	NS
Left ventricular hypertrophy	–	+	+	+	+

FIGURE 7-64. Effects of antihypertensive agents on coronary risk factors. The clinical importance of the adverse metabolic side effects of various antihypertensive agents is unknown. Those associated with diuretics and β-blockers might explain in part the lack of efficacy of these drugs in preventing the complication of coronary heart disease in hypertensive patients. Of special interest are the effects on serum lipids, insulin resistance, and glucose metabolism. It can be seen that the calcium blockers and angiotensin-converting enzyme (ACE) inhibitors are lipid-neutral and that the α-blockers have beneficial lipid effects. HDL—high-density lipoprotein; NS—not significant. (*Adapted from* Kaplan [44].)

A. EFFECTS OF THERAPY IN OLDER HYPERTENSIVE PATIENTS

	AUSTRALIAN [40]	EWPHE [45]	COOPE AND WARRENDER [46]
Patients, *n*	582	840	884
Age, *y*	60–69	>60	60–79
Mean entry blood pressure, *mm Hg*	165/101	182/101	197/100
Relative risk of event (treated vs control)			
Stroke	0.67	0.64	0.58*
CHD	0.82	0.80	1.03
CHF	—	0.78	0.68
All CVD	0.69	0.71*	0.76*

FIGURE 7-65. A and **B,** The results of seven clinical trials of antihypertensive therapy in the elderly. All showed a reduction in stroke, which was statistically significant in five of the trials. Although coronary heart disease (CHD) was reduced in six trials, statistical significance was achieved only in the Hypertension Detection and Follow-up Program (HDFP) and Systolic Hypertension in the Elderly Program (SHEP) trials. (*continued*)

B. EFFECTS OF THERAPY IN OLDER HYPERTENSIVE PATIENTS

	STOP [47]	MRC [48]	SHEP [49]	HDFP [45]
Patients, n	1627	4396	4736	2374
Age, y	70–84	65–74	60–≥80	60–69
Mean entry blood pressure, *mm Hg*	195/102	185/91	170/77	170/101
Relative risk of event (treated vs control)				
Stroke	0.53*	0.75*	0.67*	0.56*
CHD	0.87	0.81	0.73*	0.85*
CHF	0.49*	—	0.45*	—
All CVD	0.60*	0.83*	0.68*	0.84*

FIGURE 7-65. (*continued*) Whether hypertension in the elderly differs from hypertension in younger patients in terms of the relative weight of cardiovascular risk factors is unknown. This consideration might bear on the importance of the metabolic side effects of diuretics and β-blockers, making them more significant for younger hypertensives [28]. *Asterisks* indicate statistical significance. CHF—congestive heart failure; CVD—cardiovascular disease; EWPHE—European Working Party on High Blood Pressure in the Elderly; MRC—Medical Research Council; STOP—Swedish Trial in Old Patients.

FACTORS IN THE SELECTION OF ANTIHYPERTENSIVES

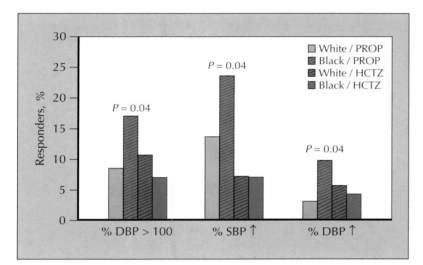

FIGURE 7-66. Treatment with propranolol (PROP) or hydrochlorothiazide (HCTZ). An effect of race on drug efficacy was noted in this study of 683 men who were randomly allocated to treatment with either PROP or HCTZ. There was no difference in systolic blood pressure (SBP) reduction between the two drugs in white patients, but HCTZ was highly superior in blacks (-20.3 vs -8.2 mm Hg). PROP reduced diastolic blood pressure (DBP) by 12.6 mm Hg compared with -10.9 mm Hg for HCTZ in whites. In contrast, HCTZ reduced DBP in blacks by 13 mm Hg compared with 9.5 mm Hg for PROP. More blacks achieved goal blood pressure with HCTZ than with PROP. PROP in blacks was associated with a significant number of patients whose blood pressure *increased* with treatment. (*Adapted from* the Veterans Administra-tion Cooperative Study Group on Antihypertensive Agents [50].)

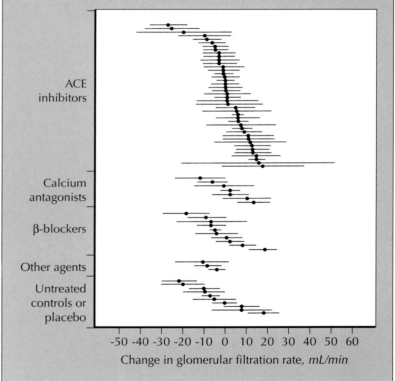

FIGURE 7-67. Effect on glomerularfiltratrion rate of antihypertensive agents. Kasiske *et al.* [51] reported a meta-analysis of 100 studies on the relative effect of different antihypertensive agents on proteinuria and renal function in hypertensive patients with diabetes. The meta-analysis confirmed that angiotensin-converting enzyme (ACE) inhibitors decrease proteinuria and preserve glomerular filtration rate in patients with diabetes, independent of changes in systemic blood pressure. In contrast, other antihypertensive agents had no effect on glomerular filtration rate, once the beneficial effects of mean arterial pressure reduction were taken into account. Thus, mean arterial pressure reduction from ACE inhibitor therapy caused a significantly greater improvement in glomerular filtra-tion rate than did a comparable pressure reduction from other agents. The relative increase in glomerular filtration rate after ACE inhibition was not significantly different in patients treated for short or prolonged periods of time. The authors further noted that the effects of ACE inhibitors on renal function were not limited to patients with type I or II diabetes, patients with hypertension, or patients with early or more advanced diabetic nephropathy. (*Adapted from* Kasiske *et al.* [51].)

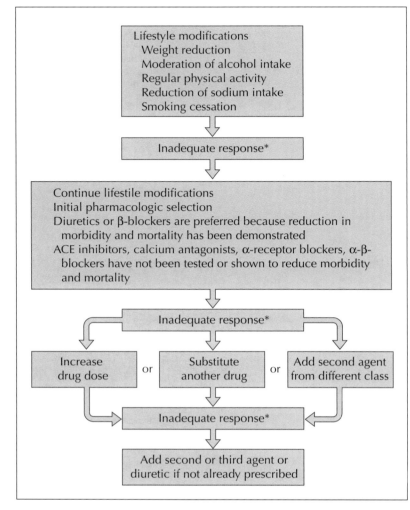

Lifestyle modifications
  Weight reduction
  Moderation of alcohol intake
  Regular physical activity
  Reduction of sodium intake
  Smoking cessation

↓

Inadequate response*

↓

Continue lifestile modifications
Initial pharmacologic selection
Diuretics or β-blockers are preferred because reduction in
  morbidity and mortality has been demonstrated
ACE inhibitors, calcium antagonists, α-receptor blockers, α-β-
  blockers have not been tested or shown to reduce morbidity
  and mortality

↓

Inadequate response*

Increase drug dose → or → Substitute another drug → or → Add second agent from different class

↓

Inadequate response*

↓

Add second or third agent or diuretic if not already prescribed

FIGURE 7-68. Treatment algorithm for hypertension. *Asterisks* indicate that response means the patient achieved goal blood pressure or is making considerable progress toward that goal. ACE—angiotensin-converting enzyme.

CLASSIFICATION OF BLOOD PRESSURE FOR ADULTS AGED 18 YEARS AND OLDER

Category	Systolic pressure, mm Hg	Diastolic pressure, mm Hg
Normal*	<130	<85
High normal	130–139	85–89
Hypertension[†]		
Stage 1 (mild)	140–159	90–99
Stage 2 (moderate)	160–179	100–109
Stage 3 (severe)	180–209	110–119
Stage 4 (very severe)	≥210	≥120

*Optimal blood pressure with respect to cardiovascular risk is <120/80 mm Hg. However, unusually low readings should be evaluated for clinical significance.

[†]Based on the average of ≥2 readings taken at each of two or more visits after an initial screening.

FIGURE 7-69. Classification of blood pressure for adults aged 18 years and older not taking antihypertensive drugs and not acutely ill. When systolic and diastolic pressures fall into different categories, the higher category should be selected to classify the individual's blood pressure status. For instance, 160/92 mm Hg should be classified as stage 2, and 180/120 mm Hg should be classified as stage 4. *Isolated systolic hypertension* is defined as a systolic blood pressure of 140 mm Hg or more and a diastolic blood pressure of less than 90 mm Hg and staged appropriately (*eg*, 170/85 mm Hg is categorized as stage 2 isolated systolic hypertension). In addition to classifying stages of hypertension on the basis of average blood pressure levels, the clinician should specify the presence or absence of target-organ disease and additional risk factors. For example, a patient with diabetes and a blood pressure of 142/94 mm Hg, plus left ventricular hypertrophy, should be classified as having "stage 1 hypertension with target-organ disease (left ventricular hypertrophy) and with another major risk factor (diabetes)." This specificity is important for risk classification and management.

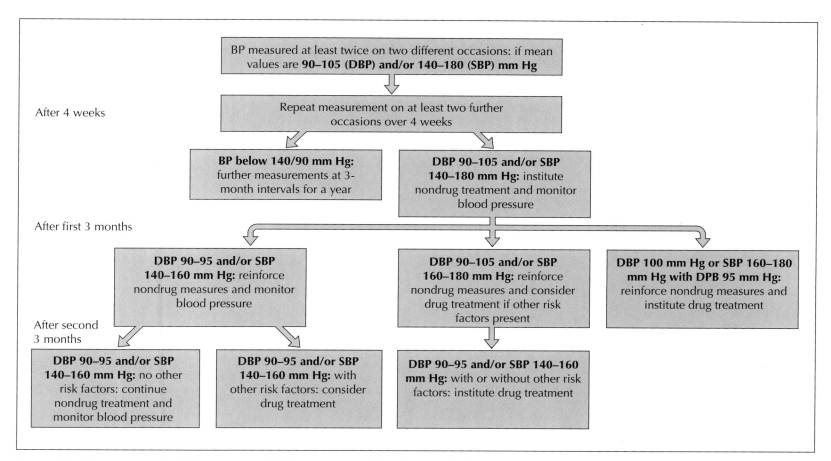

FIGURE 7-70. Management of mild hypertension. *Mild hypertension* is defined as diastolic blood pressure (DBP) of 90 to 105 mm Hg and/or systolic blood pressure (SBP) of 140 to 180 mm Hg. Drug treatment should be instituted more promptly in patients with evidence of substantial risk of cardiovascular disease or in patients with blood pressure above the mild hypertension range. Although the World Health Organization and Joint National Committee disagree on the definition of "mild" hypertension, both groups recommend non-drug treatment for 3 months before initiating drug treatment in this group. Many experts are sanguine about patient compliance with nondrug treatment, however, and would disagree with this recommendation. Although weight loss will correct hypertension in many who are overweight, and reduction in salt or alcohol intake will help if these are employed to excess, the ability of physicians to persuade patients to change their behavior—unless they have a strong support group and show evidence of being prepared to change their behavior—remains ambiguous.

RECOMMENDATIONS FOR FOLLOW-UP BASED ON INITIAL SET OF BLOOD PRESSURE MEASUREMENTS FOR ADULTS

INITIAL SCREENING BLOOD PRESSURE, mm Hg		FOLLOW-UP RECOMMENDED
SYSTOLIC	DIASTOLIC	
<130	<85	Recheck in 2 y
130–139	85–89	Recheck in 1 y
140–159	90–99	Confirm within 2 mo
160–179	100–109	Evaluate or refer to source of care within 1 mo
180–209	110–119	Evaluate or refer to source of care within 1 wk
≥210	≥120	Evaluate or refer to source of care immediately

FIGURE 7-71. Follow-up recommendations for adults based on initial blood pressure measurements. If the systolic and diastolic categories are different in the initial screening, recommendations for the shorter-term follow-up should be followed. That is, someone with a blood pressure of 160/85 mm Hg should be evaluated or referred to the source of care within 1 month. The scheduling of follow-up should be modified by reliable information about past blood pressure measurements, other cardiovascular risk factors, or target-organ disease. For patients with systolic pressures of 130 to 139 mm Hg and diastolic pressures of 85 to 89 mm Hg, the clinician should consider providing advice about lifestyle modifications.

SITUATIONS IN WHICH AUTOMATED NONINVASIVE AMBULATORY BLOOD PRESSURE MONITORING DEVICES MAY BE USEFUL

"Office" or "white-coat" hypertension: blood pressure repeatedly elevated in office setting but repeatedly normal out of office

Evaluation of drug resistance

Evaluation of nocturnal blood pressure changes

Episodic hypertension

Hypotensive symptoms associated with antihypertensive medications or autonomic dysfunction

Carotid sinus syncope and pacemaker syndromes

FIGURE 7-72. Situations in which automated noninvasive ambulatory blood pressure monitoring devices may be useful. For carotid sinus syncope and pacemaker syndromes, electrocardiographic monitoring should also be employed.

CAUSES OF LACK OF RESPONSIVENESS TO THERAPY

A

Nonadherence to therapy

Cost of medication

Instructions not clear and/or not given to patient in writing

Inadequate or no patient education

Lack of involvement of patient in treatment plan

Side effects of medication

Organic brain syndrome (*eg*, memory deficit)

Inconvenient dosing

B

Drug related causes
  Doses too low
  Inappropriate combinations (*eg*, two centrally acting adrenergic inhibitors)
  Rapid inactivation (*eg*, hydralazine)
  Drug interactions
    Nonsteroidal anti-inflammatory drugs
    Oral contraceptives
    Sympathomimetics
    Antidepressants
    Adrenal steroids
    Nasal decongestants
    Licorice-containing substances (*eg*, chewing tobacco)
    Cocaine
    Cyclosporine
    Erythropoietin

C

Associated conditions
  Increasing obesity
  Alcohol intake more than 1 oz/d of ethanol
Secondary hypertension
  Renal insufficiency
  Renovascular hypertension
  Pheochromocytoma
  Primary aldosteronism
Volume overload
  Inadequate diuretic therapy
  Excess sodium intake
  Fluid retention from reduction of blood pressure
  Progressive renal damage
Pseudohypertension

FIGURE 7-73. Causes of lack of responsiveness to antihypertensive therapy, including nonadherence (**A**), drug-related causes (**B**), and associated conditions (**C**).

HYPERTENSION IN PREGNANCY

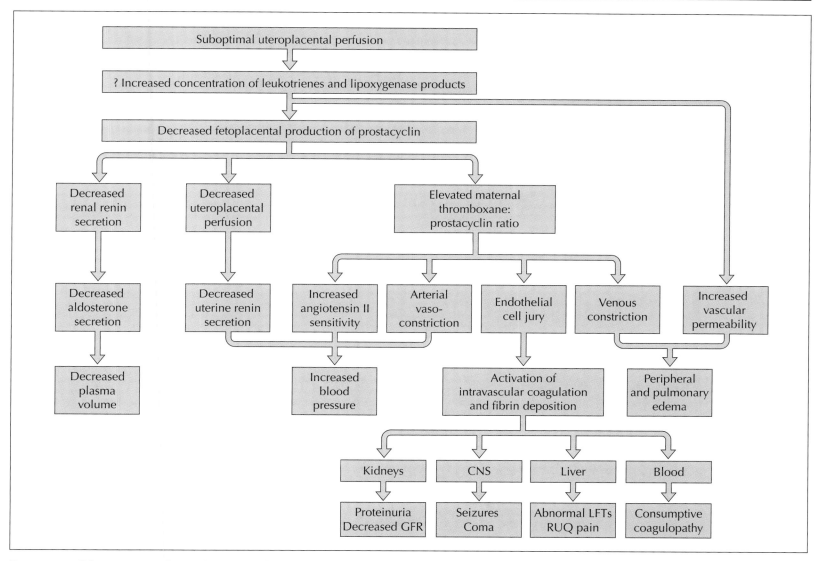

FIGURE 7-74. Scheme proposed to explain some of pathophysiologic factors thought to be operative in preeclampsia and their consequences [52]. Note that hypertension is but one feature of this complex illness. CNS—central nervous system; GFR—glomerular filtration rate; LFTs—liver function tests; RUQ—right upper quadrant.

CLASSIFICATION SCHEME FOR HYPERTENSION IN PREGNANCY

- Gestational hypertension or proteinuria

  Gestational hypertension: DBP > 110 once or 90 mm Hg twice, at least 4 h apart

  Gestational proteinuria: > 300 mg/24 h or two clean voided urines showing 2+ (1 g/L) dipstick proteinuria

  Gestational proteinuric hypertension (ie, preeclampsia)

- Chronic hypertension or chronic renal disease (*previously diagnosed*)

- Unclassified hypertension or proteinuria (usually from insufficient antenatal information)

- Eclampsia (convulsions during pregnancy or within 7 d of delivery not caused by convulsive disorders)

FIGURE 7-75. Classification of hypertensive disorders of pregnancy [53]. Knowledge of blood pressure before the 20th week of pregnancy is necessary to identify chronic hypertension. DBP—diastolic blood pressure.

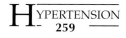

DRUG THERAPY OF HYPERTENSION IN PREGNANCY

Recommended	Methyldopa—initial drug of choice against which all other antihypertensive agents must be tested; used for the longest time in the treatment of hypertension of pregnancy, so it has the best long-term follow-up data supporting its lack of toxicity; also lowers the number of midtrimester abortions in hypertensive women compared with placebo
	Hydralazine—used extensively, usually with methyldopa, and considered safe for mother and fetus by most obstetricians
	β-blockers (typically atenolol and labetalol)—used with caution and concern about growth retardation, fetal bradycardia, and the ability of the fetus to withstand hypoxic stress
	Nifedipine—used in Europe but teratogenic in rats (at 30 × the recommended dose in humans); used mostly in preterm labor
Not recommended	Diuretics—cause volume depletion, which has been associated with poor fetal outcomes
Contraindicated	ACE inhibitors—associated with lethal acute renal failure in neonates of women treated in the third trimester

FIGURE 7-76. Drug therapy for hypertension in pregnancy, according to the Working Group on High Blood Pressure in Pregnancy [54]. Angiotensin-converting enzyme (ACE) inhibitors are contraindicated, and both dietary sodium restriction and the use of diuretics are controversial and not recommended unless such agents were necessary in the pregravid state.

HYPERTENSION IN CHILDREN AND THE ELDERLY

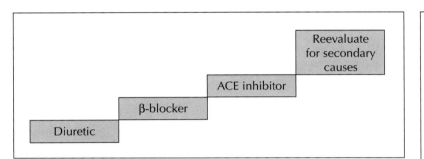

FIGURE 7-77. Treatment algorithm for hypertension in children, based on the 1987 Working Group Report [55]. This scheme closely follows earlier recommendations for using "stepped-care" therapy in adults. Since 1987, many pediatricians have also been considering the use of angiotensin-converting enzyme (ACE) inhibitors or calcium antagonists for the initial treatment of elevated blood pressures in children, particularly because many children develop impaired exercise tolerance with β-blockers and some physicians are concerned about the long-term metabolic effects of thiazide diuretics [56].

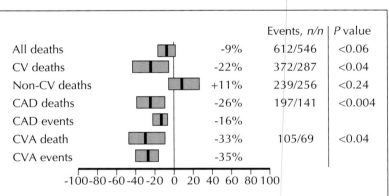

		Events, n/n	P value
All deaths	-9%	612/546	<0.06
CV deaths	-22%	372/287	<0.04
Non-CV deaths	+11%	239/256	<0.24
CAD deaths	-26%	197/141	<0.004
CAD events	-16%		
CVA death	-33%	105/69	<0.04
CVA events	-35%		

FIGURE 7-78. Results of a meta-analysis of six hypertension trials in the elderly, according to types of clinical event [57]. Unlike the situation in younger patients, the treatment groups (using diuretics and β-blocking agents) received nearly all of the expected beneficial reductions in fatal and nonfatal [58] cerebrovascular (CVA) and coronary artery diseases (CAD). Noncardiovascular (CV) deaths were not increased by effective antihypertensive therapy.

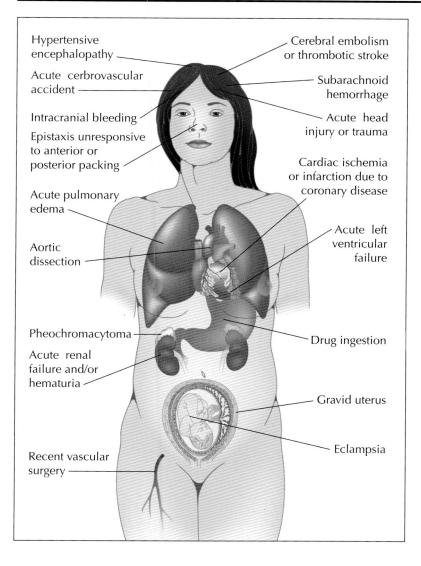

Hypertensive encephalopathy

Acute cerbrovascular accident

Intracranial bleeding

Epistaxis unresponsive to anterior or posterior packing

Acute pulmonary edema

Aortic dissection

Pheochromacytoma

Acute renal failure and/or hematuria

Recent vascular surgery

Cerebral embolism or thrombotic stroke

Subarachnoid hemorrhage

Acute head injury or trauma

Cardiac ischemia or infarction due to coronary disease

Acute left ventricular failure

Drug ingestion

Gravid uterus

Eclampsia

FIGURE 7-79. Common clinical conditions that are often considered hypertensive emergencies. Severe *acute* target organ damage is the major distinguishing factor between emergencies and urgencies.

A. PARENTERAL VASODILATORS

DRUG	DOSE	ONSET	CAUTIONS
Sodium nitroprusside	0.25–10 µg/kg/min as IV infusion; maximal dose for 10 min only	Instantaneous	Nausea, vomiting, muscle twitching; with prolonged use may cause thiocyanate intoxication, methemoglobinemia acidosis, cyanide poisoning; bags, bottles, and delivery sets must be light resistant
Nitroglycerin	5–100 µg as IV infusion	2–5 min	Headache, tachycardia, vomiting, flushing, methemoglobinemia; requires special delivery system due to drug binding to PVC tubing
Diazoxide	50–150 mg as IV bolus, repeated, or 15–30 mg/min by IV infusion	1–2 min	Hypotension, tachycardia, aggravation of angina pectoris, nausea and vomiting, hyperglycemia with repeated injections
Hydralazine	10–20 mg as IV bolus 10–40 mg IM	10 min 20–30 min	Tachycardia, headache, vomiting, aggravation of angina pectoris
Enalaprilat	0.625–1.25 mg every 6 h IV	15–60 min	Renal failure in patients with bilateral renal artery stenosis, hypotension

B. PARENTERAL ADRENERGIC INHIBITORS

DRUG	DOSE	ONSET	CAUTIONS
Phentolamine	5–15 mg as IV bolus	1–2 min	Tachycardia, orthostatic hypotension
Trimethaphan camsylate	1–4 mg/min as IV infusion	1–5 min	Paresis of bowel and bladder, orthostatic hypotension, blurred vision, dry mouth
Labetalol	20–80 mg as IV bolus every 10 min; 2 mg/min as IV infusion	5–10 min	Bronchoconstriction, heart block, orthostatic hypotension
Methyldopate	250–500 mg as IV infusion every 6 h	30–60 min	Drowsiness

C. ORAL AGENTS

DRUG	DOSE	ONSET	CAUTIONS
Nifedipine (not extended release)	10–20 mg PO, repeat after 30 min	15–30 min	Rapid, uncontrolled reduction in blood pressure may precipitate circulatory collapse in patients with aortic stenosis
Captopril	25 mg PO, repeat as required	15–30 min	Hypotension, renal failure in bilateral renal artery stenosis
Clonidine	0.1–0.2 mg PO, repeated every hour as required to a total dose of 0.6 mg	30–60 min	Hypotension, drowsiness, dry mouth
Labetalol	200–400 mg PO, repeat every 2–3 h	30 min–2 h	Bronchoconstriction, heart block, orthostatic hypotension

FIGURE 7-80. A–C, Emergencies and urgencies with various drugs in the management of hypertensive crises. It is sometimes appropriate to administer a diuretic agent with any of these drugs. PO—orally; PVC—polyvinyl chloride.

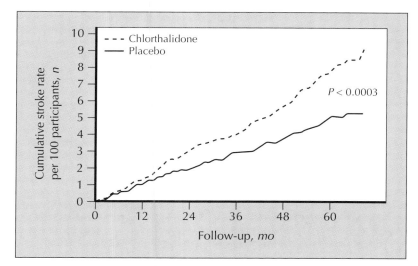

FIGURE 7-81. The occurrence of fatal and nonfatal strokes (the primary outcome measure) during the Systolic Hypertension in the Elderly Program [59]. In these elderly patients, compared with placebo, low-dose chlorthalidone therapy was statistically associated with decreased risk of stroke after an average of 4.5 years of therapy.

SECONDARY ENDPOINT REDUCTIONS IN THE SHEP TRIAL

Endpoint	Treated	Placebo	Reduction, % (95% CI)	P value
Nonfatal MI or CAD death	104	141	27(6–43)	< 0.05
CVA, nonfatal MI, or CAD death	199	289	33(20–44)	< 0.01
Any coronary event*	140	184	25(6–40)	< 0.05
Any cardiovascular event†	289	414	32(21–42)	< 0.01

*Coronary events included MI, sudden or rapid cardiac death, aortocoronary bypass surgery, or coronary angioplasty.
†Cardiovascular events included coronary event or stroke, transient ischemic attack, intracranial aneurysm, or carotid endarterectomy.

FIGURE 7-82. Reductions in other (secondary) endpoints during the Systolic Hypertension in the Elderly Program (SHEP) [59]. Reductions in all disorders were statistically significant and clearly show that the benefits of low-dose thiazide diuretic therapy in patients with coronary dysfunction extends far beyond reduction of fatal and nonfatal strokes. CAD—coronary artery disease; CI—confidence interval; CVA—cerebrovascular accident; MI—myocardial infarction.

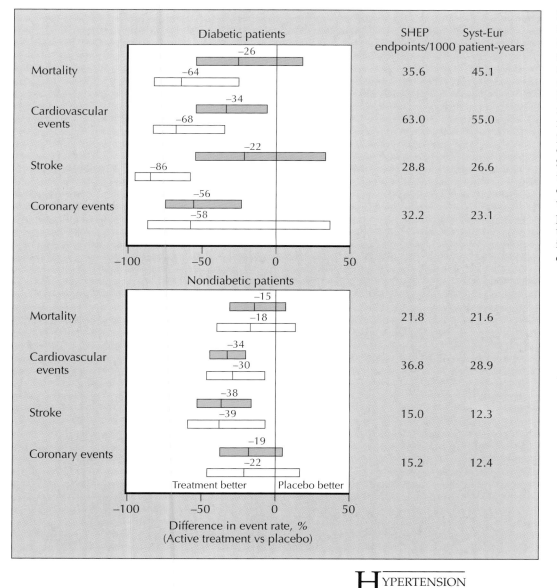

FIGURE 7-83. Comparison of the efficacy of two treatment regimens for isolated systolic hypertension in older diabetic and diuretic hypertensive patients. One regimen was diuretic-based and was used in the Systolic Hypertension in the Elderly (SHEP) trial. The other study, Syst-Eur, was calcium antagonist-based. Overall, the results were very similar, especially in the nondiabetic patients. Although some have pointed to a better response in the calcium channel blocker–based treatment arm in Syst-Eur to the use of the calcium antagonist, there are other differences that could have contributed: these differences include early versus scheduled termination, the percentage of patients on placebo at the end of the study, and the fact that the studies in the United States involve patients who are substantially more obese than those in the studies in Europe.

COMPARATIVE ANTIHYPERTENSIVE EFFICACY OF LOSARTAN

STUDY	YEAR	DRUG	ADDITIONAL REDUCTION IN DBP VERSUS LOSARTAN, mm Hg	P VALUE
Kassler-Taub [60]	1998	Irbesartan	-3.0	=0.01
Oparil et al. [61]	1998	Irbesartan	-3.0	<0.002
Andersson and Neldam [62]	1998	Candesartan	-3.7	=0.013
Hedner et al. [63]	1999	Valsartan	-0.8	NS
Maillon et al. [64]	1999	Telmisartan	-2.6–3.7	<0.05
Gradman et al. [65]	1999	Candesartan	-2.1	=0.016
Lacourciere and Asmar [66]	1999	Candesartan	-1.8	—

FIGURE 7-84. Comparative antihypertensive efficacy of losartan. Losartan was the first angiotensin II antagonist antihypertensive agent approved for clinical use in the United States and Europe. In seven studies [60–66] involving five different alternative angiotensin II receptor antagonists, without exception, these newer agents have shown greater efficacy than has losartan. The reputation that the class has of limited efficacy may reflect the experience with the first drug.

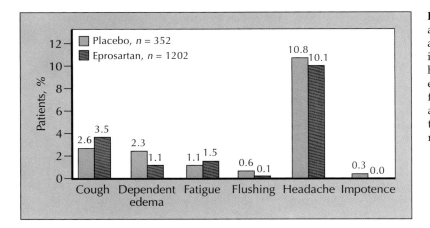

FIGURE 7-85. Selected adverse events reported among patients taking an angiotensin II antagonist, eprosartan, in placebo-controlled trials. Because adverse event reporting in this type of trial includes all events, the result is inflated numbers. Eprosartan and all of the angiotensin II antagonists have a side effect profile indistinguishable from placebo. This is a considerable therapeutic advantage for these agents. In many studies, the frequency of headache has been reduced sufficiently by treatment with an angiotensin receptor blocker to make it clear that headache, long denied to be an outcome of hypertension in most patients, almost certainly is responsible for headache in many. (*Adapted from* Hedner [67].)

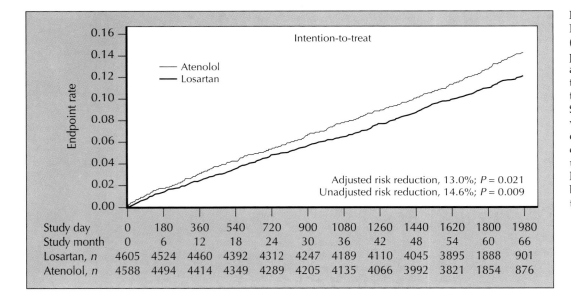

FIGURE 7-86. The Losartin Intervention for Endpoint reduction in hypertension study (LIFE). The LIFE study randomly assigned 9110 patients to receive either a β-blocker or angiotensin II receptor blocker as the baseline therapy (diuretics were allowed as add-on therapy). In this cohort of primarily older Scandinavian hypertensive subjects with left ventricular hypertrophy (LVH), there was an overall 16% reduction in combined cardiovascular disease events over the 4 years of follow-up. Interestingly, despite these subjects having higher risk of coronary events (all had LVH), the benefit was driven by reduction in stroke rather than heart disease [68].

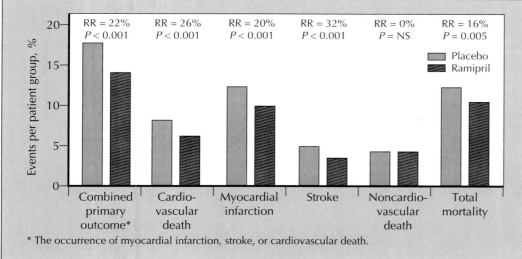

FIGURE 7-87. The Heart Outcomes Prevention Evaluation (HOPE) study. The HOPE study assessed the role of angiotensin-converting enzyme inhibition versus matching placebo in 9297 patients (≥ 55 years of age) who were at high risk for cardiovascular events, but who did not have left ventricular dysfunction or heart failure. Treatment with ramipril significantly reduced the rates of death from cardiovascular causes (6.1% vs 8.1%; $P < 0.001$), myocardial infarction (9.9% vs 12.3%; $P < 0.001$), heart failure (9% vs 11.5%; $P < 0.001$), and complications related to diabetes (6.4% vs 7.6%; $P = 0.03$). The HOPE study also found that improved outcome from ramipirl treatment was observed when patients were also treated with combination therapy. β-Blockers, diuretics, calcium channel blockers, lipid-lowering drugs, and aspirin were most commonly used safely and effectively [69].

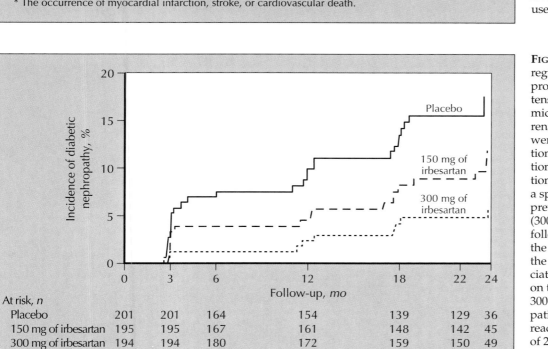

FIGURE 7-88. Advantages of antihypertensive regimens in preventing progression to clinical proteinuria. A total of 590 patients with hypertension (153/90 mm Hg), type 2 diabetes, microalbuminuria (56 µg/min), and normal renal function (serum creatinine 1.1 mg/dL) were randomly assigned to placebo plus conventional therapy, irbesartan 150 mg plus conventional therapy, or irbesartan 300 mg plus conventional therapy to see if there was an advantage of a specific antihypertensive regimen in preventing progression to clinical proteinuria (300 µg/min) over a 2-year period. The average follow-up blood pressure during the course of the study was approximately 143/83 mm Hg for the three groups. In this figure, one can appreciate the incidence of diabetic nephropathy based on the three therapies. Ten of 94 patients in the 300-mg irbesartan group (5.2%) and 19 of the 195 patients in the 150-mg irbesartan group (9.7%) reached clinical proteinuria, as compared with 30 of 201 patients in the placebo group: 14.9% (hazard ratios, 0.30; 95% CI, 0.14–0.61; $P < 0.001$) and 0.61% (95% CI, 0.34–1.09; $P = 0.08$), respectively. The angiotensin II receptor blocker irbesartan retards the progression to clinical proteinuria in hypertensive patients with type 2 diabetes and microalbuminuria independent of blood presure [70].

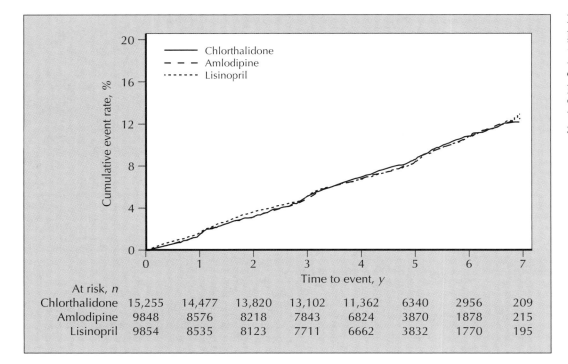

FIGURE 7-89. Cumulative event rate for the primary outcome in the Antihypertensive and Lipid-lowering Treatment to Prevent Heart Attack Trial (ALLHAT), which compared chlorthaladone, amlodipine, and lisinopril. The primary endpoint was fatal coronary heart disease or nonfatal myocardial infarction. There were no significant differences in the treatment groups [71].

At risk, n								
Chlorthalidone	15,255	14,477	13,820	13,102	11,362	6340	2956	209
Amlodipine	9848	8576	8218	7843	6824	3870	1878	215
Lisinopril	9854	8535	8123	7711	6662	3832	1770	195

CLASSIFICATION AND MANAGEMENT OF BP FOR ADULTS

				INITIAL DRUG THERAPY	
BP CLASSIFICATION	SBP*, MM HG	DBP*, MM HG	LIFESTYLE MODIFICATION	WITHOUT COMPELLING INDICATION	WITH COMPELLING INDICATIONS
Normal	< 120	and < 80	Encourage		
Prehypertension	120–139	or 80–89	Yes	No antihypertensive drug indicated	Drug(s) for compelling indications‡
Stage 1 hypertension	140–159	or 90–99	Yes	Thiazide-type diuretics for most; may consider ACE inhibitor, ARB, BB, CCB, or combination	Drug(s) for compelling indications‡
Stage 2 hypertension	≥ 160	or ≥ 100	Yes	Two-drug combination for most† (usually thiazide-type diurectic and ACE inhibitor or ARB or BB or CCB)	Other antihypertensive drugs (diuretics, ACE inhibitor, ARB, BB, CCB) as needed

*Treatment determined by highest BP category.
†Initial combined therapy should be used cautiously in those at risk for orthostatic hypotension.
‡Treat patients with chronic kidney disease or diabetes to BP goal of < 130/80 mm Hg.

FIGURE 7-90. Classification and management of blood pressure (BP) for adults. The recent publication of Joint National Committee (JNC)-7 reclassified hypertension with two important changes. The first involves the disappearance of stage 3 hypertension. Now stage 2 includes all blood pressure levels in which systolic blood pressure (SBP) exceeds 160 mm Hg or diastolic blood pressure (DBP) exceeds 100 mm Hg [72]. ACE—angiotensin-converting enzyme; ARB—angiotensin receptor blocker; BB—β-blocker; CCB—calcium channel blocker.

REFERENCES

1. INTERSALT Cooperative Research Group: INTERSALT: an international study of electrolyte excretion and blood pressure: results for 24 hour urinary sodium and potassium excretion. *BMJ* 1988, 297:319–328.

2. de Wardener HE, MacGregor GA: Natriuretic hormone and essential hypertension as an endocrine disease. In *Essential Hypertension as an Endocrine Disease*. Edited by Edwards CRW, Carey RM. London: Butterworths; 1985:132–157.

3. McCarron DA, Morris CD, Henry HJ, *et al.*: Blood pressure and nutrient intake in the United States. *Science* 1984, 224:1392–1398.

4. Gruchow HW, Sobocinski KA, Barboriak JJ: Calcium intake and the relationship of dietary sodium and potassium to blood pressure. *Am J Clin Nutr* 1988, 48:1463–1470.

5. Wilson TW, Grim CE: Biohistory of slavery and blood pressure differences in blacks today: a hypothesis. *Hypertension* 1991, 17(suppl I):I122–I128.

6. Jackson FLC: An evolutionary perspective on salt, hypertension, and human genetic variability. *Hypertension* 1991, 17(suppl I):I129–I132.

7. Struyker Boudier HAJ: Adrenergic mechanisms and pharmacotherapy of hypertension. In *Adrenergic Blood Pressure Regulation: Proceedings of a Symposium*. Edited by Birkenhäger WH, Folkow B, Struyker Boudier HAJ. Amsterdam, The Netherlands: Excerpta Medica; 1985:114–123.

8. Krief S, Lonnqvist F, Raimbaults, *et al.*: Tissue distribution of the beta-3 receptor m-RNA in man. *J Clin Invest* 1993, 91:344–349.

9. Linden ME, Gilman AG: G proteins. *Sci Am* 1992, 267:56–91.

10. Anderson EA, Sinkey CA, Lawton WJ, Mark AL: Elevated sympathetic nerve activity in borderline hypertensive humans: evidence from direct intra-neural recordings. *Hypertension* 1989, 14:177–183.

11. Brunner HR, Laragh JH, Baer L, *et al.*: Essential hypertension: renin and aldosterone, heart attack and stroke. *N Engl J Med* 1972, 286:441–449.

12. Griendling KK, Murphy TJ, Alexander RW: Molecular biology of the renin-angiotensin system. *Circulation* 1993, 87:1816–1828.

13. Chobanian AV: Hypertension. *CIBA Found Symp* 1982, 34:3–32.

14. Treasure CB, Klein JL, Vita JA, *et al.*: Hypertension and left ventricular hypertrophy are associated with impaired endothelium-mediated relaxation in human coronary resistance vessels. *Circulation* 1993, 87:86–93.

15. Griendling KK, Alexander RW: Cellular biology of blood vessels. In *Hurst's The Heart*. Edited by Schlant RC, Alexander RW, O'Rourke R, *et al.*: New York: McGraw-Hill; 1994:31–45.

16. Lüscher TF, Vanhoutte PM: Endothelium-dependent contraction to acetylcholine in the aorta of the spontaneously hypertensive rat. *Hypertension* 1986, 8:344–348.

17. Harrison D: The endothelial cell. *Heart Dis Stroke* 1992, 1:95–99.

18. Kaplan NM: Systemic hypertension: mechanisms and diagnosis. In *Heart Disease*. Edited by Braunwald E. Philadelphia: WB Saunders; 1988:819–883.

19. Bravo EL: What to do when potassium is low or high. *Diagnosis* 1988, 10:1–6.

20. Bravo EL, Tarazi RC, Dustan HP, *et al.*: The changing clinical spectrum of primary aldosteronism. *Am J Med* 1983, 74:641–651.

21. Bravo EL: Primary aldosteronism. *Urol Clin North Am* 1989, 16:433–473, 481–486.

22. Bravo EL, Gifford RW, Manger WM: Adrenal medullary tumors: pheochromocytoma. In *Endocrine Tumors*. Edited by Mazzaferri EL, Samaan NA. Boston: Blackwell Scientific Publications; 1993:426–447.

23. Bravo EL: Evolving concepts in the pathophysiology, diagnosis, and treatment of pheochromocytoma. *Endocr Rev* 1994, 15:356–368.

24. National High Blood Pressure Education Program Working Group: National High Blood Pressure Education Program working group report on primary prevention of hypertension. *Arch Intern Med* 1993, 153:186–208.

25. Johnston DW: The behavioral control of high blood pressure. *Curr Psychol Res Rev* 1987, 6:99–114.

26. Neaton JD, Grimm RH, Prineas RJ, *et al.*: The Treatment of Mild Hypertension Study Research Group. *JAMA* 1993, 270:713–724.

27. MacGregor GA, Markandu ND, Sagnella GA, *et al.*: Double-blind study of three sodium intakes and long-term effects of sodium restriction in essential hypertension. *Lancet* 1989, i:1244–1247.

28. The Fifth Report of the Joint National Committee on Detection, Evaluation, and Treatment of High Blood Pressure. *Arch Intern Med* 1993, 153:154–182.

29. 1993 Guidelines for the Management of Mild Hypertension. Memorandum from a World Health Organization/International Society of Hypertension meeting. *Hypertension* 1993, 22:392–403.

30. Chalmers J: The place of combination therapy in the treatment of hypertension in 1993. *Clin Exp Hypertens* 1993, 15:1299–1313.

31. Man in't Veld AJ, van den Meiracker A, Schalekamp MADH: The effect of beta-blockers on total peripheral resistance. *J Cardiovasc Pharmacol* 1986, 8(suppl 4):49–60.

32. Waeber B, Nussberger J, Juillerat L, Brunner HR: Angiotensin converting enzyme inhibition: discrepancy between antihypertensive effect and suppression of enzyme activity. *J Cardiovasc Pharmacol* 1989, 14(suppl 4):53–59.

33. Tonyz RM, Schiffrin EL: Signal transduction in hypertension: part I. *Curr Opin Nephrol Hypertens* 1993, 2:5–16.

34. Tonyz RM, Schiffrin EL: Signal transduction in hypertension: part II. *Curr Opin Nephrol Hypertens* 1993, 2:17–26.

35. Grimm RH: alpha$_1$-Antagonists in the treatment of hypertension. *Hypertension* 1989, 13(suppl I):131–136.

36. Veterans Administration Cooperative Study Group on Antihypertensive Agents: Effects of treatment on morbidity in hypertension: I. Results in patients with diastolic blood pressures averaging 115 through 129 mm Hg. *JAMA* 1967, 202:1028–1034.

37. Veterans Administration Cooperative Study Group on Antihypertensive Agents: Effects of treatment on morbidity in hypertension: II. Results in patients with diastolic blood pressure averaging 90 through 114 mm Hg. *JAMA* 1970, 213:1143–1252.

38. Hypertension Detection and Follow-up Program Cooperative Group: Five-year findings of the Hypertension Detection and Follow-up Program: I. Reductions in mortality in persons with high blood pressure including mild hypertension. *JAMA* 1979, 242:2562–2571.

39. Hypertension Detection and Follow-up Program Cooperative Group: Five-year findings of the Hypertension Detection and Follow-up Program: III. Reduction in stroke incidence among persons with high blood pressure. *JAMA* 1982, 247:633–638.

40. Australian National Blood Pressure Management Committee: The Australian National Therapeutic trial in mild hypertension. *Lancet* 1980, 1:1261–1267.

41. Medical Research Council Working Party: MRC trial of treatment of mild hypertension: principal results. *BMJ* 1985, 291:97–104.

42. MacMahon S, Peto S, Cutter J, *et al.*: Blood pressure, stroke and coronary heart disease: Part 1. Prolonged differences in blood pressure: prospective observational studies corrected for the regression dilution bias. *Lancet* 1990, 335:765–774.

43. Collins R, Peto R, MacMahon S, *et al.*: Blood pressure, stroke, and coronary heart disease. Part 2. Short-term reductions in blood-pressure: overview of randomized drug trials in their epidemiological context. *Lancet* 1990, 335:827–838.

44. Kaplan N: Changing hypertension treatment to reduce the overall cardiovascular risk. *J Hypertens* 1990, 8(suppl 7):S175.

45. Hypertension Detection and Follow-up Program Cooperative Group: Five-year findings of the Hypertension Detection and Follow-up Program: II. Mortality by race, sex and age. *JAMA* 1979, 242:2572–2576.

46. Coope J, Warrender TS: Randomized trial of treatment of hypertension in elderly patients in primary care. *BMJ* 1986, 293:1145–1151.

47. Dahlof B, Lindholm L, Hansson L, *et al.*: Morbidity and mortality in the Swedish Trial in Old Patients with Hypertension (STOP-Hypertension). *Lancet* 1991, 338:1281–1284.

48. MRC Working Party: Medical Research Council trial of treatment of hypertension in older adults: principal results. *BMJ* 1992, 1304:405–412.

49. SHEP Cooperative Research Group: Prevention of stroke by antihypertensive treatment in older persons with isolated systolic hypertension: final results of the Systolic Hypertension in the Elderly Program (SHEP). *JAMA* 1991, 265:3255–3264.

50. Veterans Administration Cooperative Study Group on Antihypertensive Agents: Comparison of propranolol and hydrochlorothiazide for the initial treatment of hypertension: I. Results of short-term titration with emphasis on racial differences in response. *JAMA* 1982, 248:1996–2003.

51. Kasiske BL, Kalel RSN, Ma JZ, *et al.*: Effect of antihypertensive therapy on the kidney in patients with diabetes: a meta-regression analysis. *Ann Intern Med* 1993, 118:129–138.

52. Friedman SA: Preeclampsia: a review of the role of prostaglandins. *Obstet Gynecol* 1988, 71:122–137.

53. Davey DA, MacGillivray I: The classification and definition of the hypertensive disorders of pregnancy. *Am J Obstet Gynecol* 1988, 158:892–898.

54. National High Blood Pressure Education Program: Working Group on High Blood Pressure in Pregnancy: Working group report on high blood pressure in pregnancy. *Am J Obstet Gynecol* 1990, 163:1689–1712.

55. Task Force on Blood Pressure Control in Children: Report of the Second Task Force on Blood Pressure Control in Children-1987. *Pediatrics* 1987, 79:1–25.

56. Sinaiko A: Pharmacologic management of childhood hypertension. *Pediatr Clin North Am* 1993, 40:195–212.

57. Thijs L, Fagard R, Lijnen P, *et al.*: A meta-analysis of outcome trials in elderly hypertensives [editorial]. *J Hypertens* 1992, 10:1103–1109.

58. Psaty BM, Furberg CD: Antihypertensive treatment trials: morbidity and mortality. In *Hypertension Primer*. Edited by Izzo JL Jr, Black HR. Dallas: American Heart Association; 1993:202–204.

59. SHEP Cooperative Research Group: Prevention of stroke by antihypertensive drug treatment in older persons with isolated systolic hypertension: final results of the Systolic Hypertension in the Elderly Program. *JAMA* 1991, 265:3255–3264.

60. Kassler-Taub K, Littlejohn T, Elliott W, *et al.*: Comparative efficacy of two angiotensin II receptor antagonists, irbesartan and losartan, in mild-to-moderate hypertension. *Am J Hypertens* 1998, 11:445–453.

61. Oparil S, Guthrie R, Lewin AJ, *et al.*: An elective-titration study of the comparative effectiveness of two angiotensin II-receptor blockers, irbesartan and losartan. *Clin Ther* 1998, 29:398–409.

62. Andersson OK, Neldam S: The antihypertensive effect and tolerability of candesartan cilexitil, a new generation angiotensin II antagonist in comparison with losartan. *Blood Pressure* 1998, 7:53–59.

63. Hedner T, Oparil S, Rasmussen K, *et al.*: A comparison of angiotensin II antagonists valsartan and losartan in the treatment of essential hypertension. *Am J Hypertens* 1999, 12:414–417.

64. Maillon J, Siche J, Lacourciere Y: ABPM comparison of the antihypertensive profiles of the selective angiotensin II receptor antagonists telmisartan and losartan in patients with mild-to-moderate hypertension. *J Hum Hypertens* 1999, 13:657–664.

65. Gradman AH, Lewin A, Bowling BT, *et al.*: Comparative effects of candesartan cilexitil and lsartan in patients with systemic hypertension. *Heart Disease* 1999, 1:52–57.

66. Lacourciere Y, Asmar R: A comparison of the efficacy and duration of action of candesartan cilexitil and losartan as assessed by clinic and ambulatory blood pressure after a missed dose, in truly hypertensive patients: a placebo-controlled, forced dose-titration study. *Am J Hypertens* 1999, 12:1181–1187.

67. Hedner T: Management of hypertension: the advent of a new angiotensin II receptor antagonist. *J Hypertens* 1999, 17(suppl):21–25.

68. Dahlöf B, Devereux BB, Kjeldsen SE, *et al.*, for the LIFE study group: Cardiovascular morbidity and mortality in the Losartan Intervention For Endpoint reduction study (LIFE): a randomised trial against atenolol. *Lancet* 2002, 359:995–1003.

69. Yusuf S, Sleight P, Pogue J, *et al.*, for the Heart Outcomes Prevention Evaluation Study Investigators: Effects of an angiotensin-converting enzyme inhibitor, ramipril, on cardiovascular events in high-risk patients. *N Engl J Med* 2000, 342:145–153.

70. Parving HH, Lenhert H, Brochner-Mortensen J, *et al.*: The effect of irbesartan on the development of diabetic nephropathy in patients with type 2 diabetes. *N Engl J Med* 2001, 345:870–878.

71. Major outcomes in high-risk hypertensive patients randomized to angiotensin-converting enzyme inhibitor or calcium channel blocker vs diuretic: the Antihypertensive and Lipid-lowering Treatment to Prevent Heart Attack Trial (ALLHAT). *JAMA* 2002, 288:2981–2997.

72. The Seventh Report of the Joint National Committee on Prevention, Detection, Evaluation, and Treatment of High Blood Pressure: the JNC 7 report. *JAMA* 2003, 289:2560–2572.

8 VALVULAR HEART DISEASE

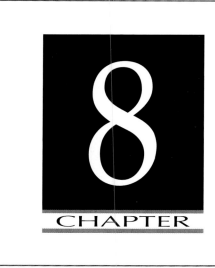

CHAPTER

Edited by Shahbudin H. Rahimtoola

*Manuel J. Antunes, Allen P. Burke, Blase A. Carabello,
Melvin D. Cheitlin, Andrew Farb, Gary L. Grunkemeier,
David T. Kawanishi, John S. MacGregor, Peter C. Nishan,
Rick A. Nishimura, Robert A. O'Rourke, Sumanth D. Prabhu,
Albert Starr, Renu Virmani*

MITRAL STENOSIS

PATHOPHYSIOLOGY

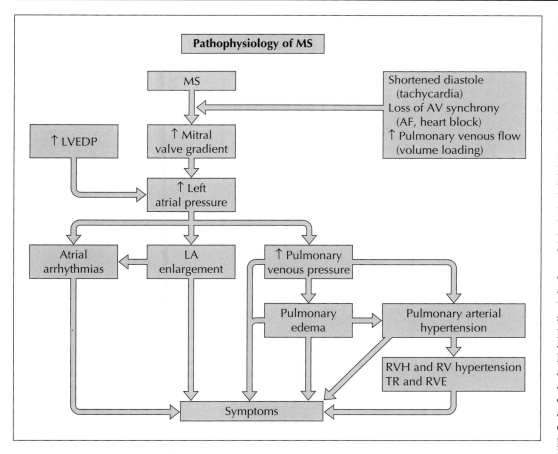

FIGURE 8-1. Pathophysiology of mitral stenosis (MS). MS results in a diastolic pressure gradient between the left atrium (LA) and the left ventricle (LV). The actual gradient depends on the mitral valve area (MVA) and the mitral valve *flow per diastolic second*. As a result, there is an elevation of LA pressure and, therefore, also of pulmonary venous pressure. Physiologic and pathologic changes—such as tachycardia and atrial fibrillation (AF) (which shorten diastole and may also result in loss of effective atrial contraction) or pregnancy, volume loading, and left-to-right shunts (at ventricular and aortopulmonary levels), which increase pulmonary venous flow—increase the mitral valve gradient and LA and pulmonary venous pressures. An increased LV end-diastolic pressure (LVEDP) also results in further increase of LA pressure.

An elevated LA pressure has several important effects, including enlargement of the LA, atrial arrhythmias, and an increase of pulmonary venous pressure. Pulmonary venous hypertension may result in pulmonary edema and pulmonary arterial hypertension. Pulmonary arterial hypertension and right ventricular (RV) hypertension result in RV hypertrophy (RVH) and may result in tricuspid regurgitation (TR) and RV enlargement (RVE). All of these changes contribute to producing symptoms. In addition, a fixed or even reduced cardiac output also contributes to the symptomatic state of the patient. AV—atrioventricular. (© Copyright SH Rahimtoola, MB, FRCP, MACP, MACC.)

PATHOLOGY

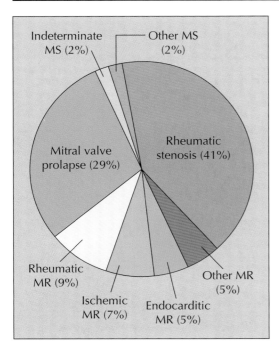

Figure 8-2. Causes of congenital and acquired mitral valve (MV) disease. Pathologic findings noted in MV excisions. MR—mitral regurgitation; MS—mitral stenosis. (*Adapted from* Dare *et al.* [1].)

PHYSICAL SIGNS

PHYSICAL SIGNS IN MS

EXAMINATION	SIGN
General	Low cardiac output: pink-purple facies, peripheral cyanosis, cool extremities
Arterial	Small-volume pulse
	Absent or reduced pulse in any vascular territory
Venous	Jugular venous distension
	Hepatojugular reflux
	Prominent *a* wave
	Prominent *v* wave
Cardiac palpation	Inconspicuous apical impulse
	Palpable mitral valve closure (S_1)
	Palpable diastolic thrill at apex
	Palpable pulmonic valve closure (P_2)
	RV lift
Cardiac	Accentuated S_1
Auscultation	Opening snap
	Diastolic rumbling murmur
	Presystolic murmur
	Accentuated P_2
	Pulmonic ejection click
	Pulmonic regurgitation (Graham-Steell) murmur
	RV S_4/S_3
Pulmonary	Egophony at tip of left scapula
	Rales

FIGURE 8-3. Physical signs of mitral stenosis (MS). In severe MS with a low cardiac output at rest, hypoperfusion may be suggested on general inspection of the patient; a characteristic pink-purple complexion was described by Wood [2]. The extremities may be cool and cyanotic. In such severe cases, the small stroke volume results in a perceptibly diminished pulse volume. An elevated right atrial (RA) pressure is apparent from distention of the jugular veins, or such distention may be elicited by compression of the abdomen. The elevated RA pressure is a result of fluid retention associated with heart failure, right ventricular (RV) hypertension, or tricuspid regurgitation. The *a* wave is prominent in the presence of RV hypertension and the *v* wave is prominent with tricuspid regurgitation.

Palpation of the precordium may reveal an inconspicuous apical impulse, and mitral valve closure may be felt (a palpable S_1). A loud diastolic rumbling murmur may be felt as a thrill at the apex; this can be better appreciated if the apex is brought more into proximity of the chest wall by placing the patient in the left lateral decubitus position. With pulmonary arterial hypertension or RV dilatation, a parasternal RV lift may be present. When the RV is markedly dilated, the left ventricular (LV) apical impulse may be displaced posteriorly and the RV impulse may be mistaken for the LV apex. Also in the presence of severe pulmonary arterial hypertension, pulmonic valve closure (P_2) may be palpable in the second left parasternal intercostal space.

On auscultation, a loud S_1, an opening snap, and a mid-diastolic rumbling murmur with presystolic accentuation are considered the cardinal signs of MS (*see* Fig. 8-4) [3,4]. With pulmonary arterial hypertension, the intensity of P_2 is increased; in severe pulmonary arterial hypertension, a pulmonary ejection click and a diastolic murmur of pulmonary valve regurgitation may be present (Graham Steell murmur). Auscultation of the posterior chest rarely reveals an area of egophony at the lower tip of the left scapula, a result of marked left atrial enlargement [5]. Rales may be present when there is pulmonary congestion or pulmonary edema.

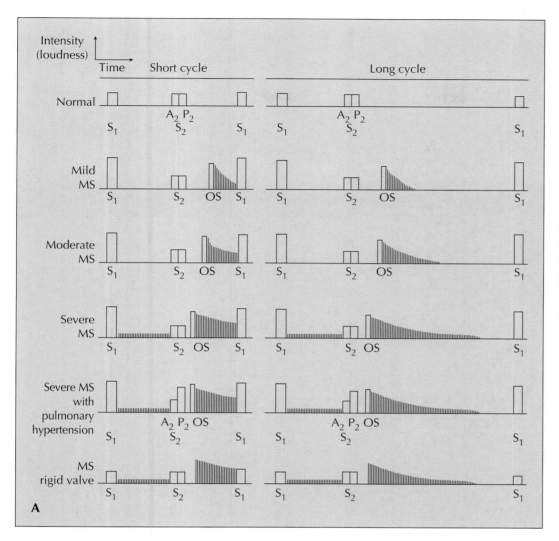

FIGURE 8-4. **A,** The classic auscultatory signs of mitral stenosis (MS) in atrial fibrillation (AF). The auscultatory findings are much more variable on a beat-to-beat basis in AF. The presystolic murmur is usually absent. The loud S_1 and the opening snap (OS) are still heard. In the short cycles, the duration of diastole is short and the mid-diastolic rumble occupies the whole of diastole (*left panel*). In the long cycles (*right panel*) the duration of the mid-diastolic murmur is related to the severity of MS (*panel A*). As the MS becomes more severe, the length of this murmur is increased. In AF, with a slow ventricular response and very long R-R intervals, the diastolic rumble may not occupy the whole diastolic period and the presystolic murmur is absent. Thus, one may get the impression that the MS is moderate rather than severe. Increasing the heart rate, *eg*, with brief physical exertion, may produce more characteristic auscultatory findings. Alternatively, when the ventricular rate in AF is rapid or in short cycles, the auscultatory findings may suggest a more severe degree of MS than is really the case (*left panel*).

Continued on next page

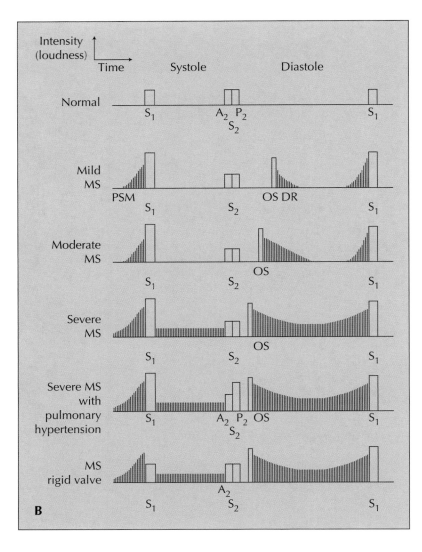

FIGURE 8-4. *(Continued)* **B,** The classic auscultatory signs of MS in patients in sinus rhythm. These include a presystolic murmur, a loud S_1, an OS, and a mid-diastolic murmur (DR, low-pitched, decrescendo diastolic rumble). These signs may be accentuated or at times may only be heard by placing the patient in the left lateral decubitus position.

Importantly, these signs are helpful in assessing the severity of the MS; as the MS becomes more severe, the S_2-OS interval is shortened and the length of the mid-diastolic rumble is increased. In mild MS, the S_2–OS interval is long and the diastolic murmur is short. In moderate MS, the S_2–OS interval is shorter and although the diastolic murmur is longer at rest, there is usually a gap between the end of the murmur and the onset of the presystolic murmur. When the MS is severe, the S_2–OS interval is short (usually 0.04 second) and the diastolic murmur is a full-length murmur. With pulmonary arterial hypertension, P_2 is increased in intensity. In the presence of a rigid mitral valve (with or without calcification), S_1 is soft and the OS is usually not heard. With severe MS and also with a rigid valve, a holosystolic murmur of mitral regurgitation is often present.

ECHOCARDIOGRAPHY

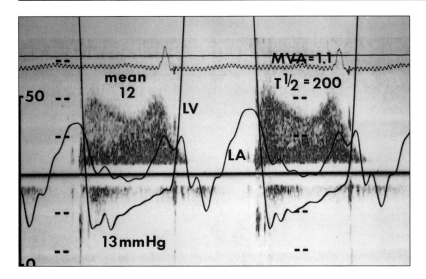

FIGURE 8-5. Continuous-wave Doppler tracing in mitral stenosis (MS). The continuous-wave velocity curve across the mitral valve provides an accurate measurement of the mean mitral gradient in patients with MS [6]. As opposed to the measurement of a mean aortic valve gradient, the measurement of the mean mitral valve gradient by Doppler ultrasound is simple to obtain from a technical standpoint. Thus a Doppler-derived mitral gradient is reliable and actually provides a more accurate measurement than conventional cardiac catheterization using pulmonary capillary wedge pressure [7]. Shown are the simultaneous pressure curves from direct left atrial (LA) and left ventricular (LV) measurements and the simultaneous mitral flow velocity curve in a patient with MS. There is an excellent correlation between the catheter-derived mean gradient of 13 mm Hg and the Doppler-derived mean gradient of 12 mm Hg. The mitral valve area (MVA) of 1.1 cm^2 is calculated from the diastolic half time ($t_{1/2}$). Doppler ultrasound can also be used to assess pulmonary pressures and the presence of coexistent mitral regurgitation in the patient with MS. (*From* Nishimura and Tajik [7]; with permission.)

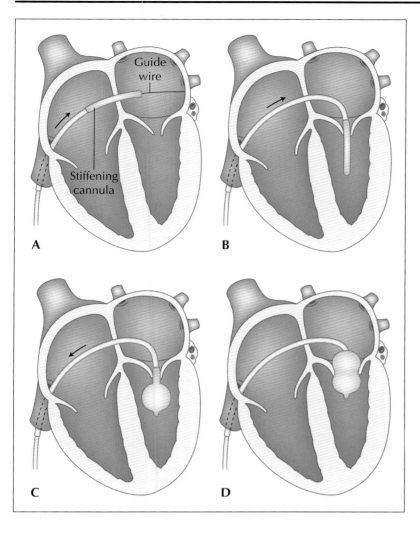

FIGURE 8-6. Inoue balloon technique for catheter balloon commissurotomy [8]. A transseptal puncture is performed (**A**) and the deflated Inoue balloon catheter is placed across the mitral valve into the left ventricle (**B**). Stepwise inflation of first the front then the rear of the Inoue balloon is performed (**C**). Inflation of the middle of the Inoue balloon and final expansion at the "waist" (**D**) suggests that enlargement of the valve orifice has occurred. The staged inflation of the various parts of this balloon are depicted. (*Adapted from* Inoue *et al.* [8].)

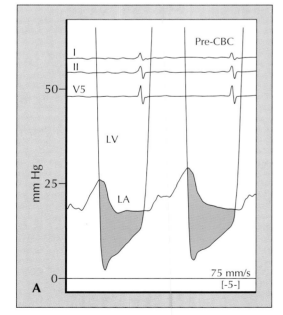

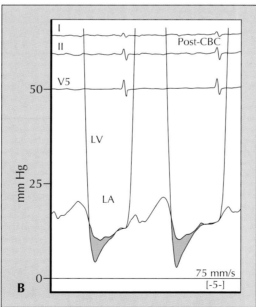

FIGURE 8-7. Left ventricular (LV) and left atrial (LA) pressures in a 58-year-old symptomatic woman with severe mitral stenosis and atrial fibrillation before (**A**) and after (**B**) catheter balloon commissurotomy (CBC). Pre-CBC, the mean valve gradient was 11 mm Hg, cardiac output was 4.4 L/min, and mitral valve area was 1.1 cm^2. Post-CBC mean valve gradient was 3 mm Hg, cardiac output was 5.4 L/min, and mitral valve area was 3.5 cm^2. In the pre-CBC tracings, there is a gradient (*shaded area*) throughout diastole, and in the post-CBC, there is no gradient in mid and late diastole in the R-R interval. Observe the changes in gradients (small in this instance) with changes in the R-R intervals.

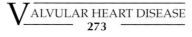

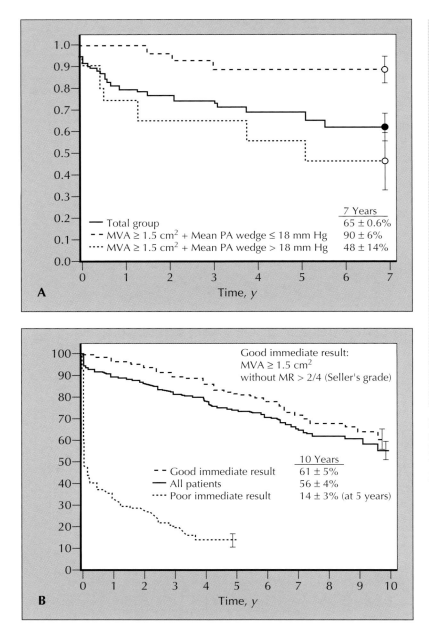

CBC

Hospital mortality rate in the past 10 years has been
close to zero

The success rate is 95% or greater

The MVA increases to an average 1.9 to 2.0 cm^2

There are reductions of MVG, LA (PA wedge), and PA
pressures, and an increase of CO; 60% of patients
improve to NYHA functional class (FC) I and 30% to
NYHA FC II, which has been objectively documented
by exercise tests

A good immediate result is obtained in approximately
89% of patients

A closed mitral commissurotomy in a nonrandomized
study in the 1950s and 1960s has shown an improved
survival in symptomatic patients (NYHA FC II and III-
IV) when compared with medical therapy

Surgical Valve Repair

If the valve is suitable for CBC, but there are contraindications for CBC, surgical valve repair is the procedure
of choice when appropriate skill and experience
are available

FIGURE 8-9. Summary of the results of catheter balloon commissuro-
tomy (CBC) for mitral stenosis. CO—cardiac output; LA—left atrium;
MVA—mitral valve area; MVG—mitral valve gradient; NYHA—New
York Heart Association; PA—pulmonary artery. (*Adapted from*
Rahimtoola *et al.* [11].)

FIGURE 8-8. Long-term outcomes after catheter balloon commissurotomy
(CBC) for mitral stenosis from two different centers. **A**, Event-free survival
(survival without mitral valve replacement, repeat CBC) [9]. **B**, Good functional results (freedom from cardiovascular deaths, mitral valve replacement, repeat dilatation, and New York Heart Association Functional Class I
or II) [10]. **A** and **B** demonstrate that patients who had a good result after
CBC had very good event-free survival up to 7 to 10 years [11]. (**A** *adapted
from* Orrange *et al.* [9]; **B** *adapted from* Iung *et al.* [10].) MR—mitral regurgitation; MVA—mitral valve area; PA—pulmonary artery.

SUMMARY OF THE RESULTS OF MITRAL VALVE REPLACEMENT

MVAs after MVR and CBC are similar

Operative mortality rate is 2%-7%

Prosthesis-related mortality averages 2.5% per year (range: 2%-3% per year), and prosthesis-related complications average 5% per year (range: 2%-6% per year)

Use of a mechanical valve necessitates use of anticoagulant therapy with its resultant problems and complications

The insertion of a bioprosthesis to avoid anticoagulation-related problems and complications is associated with structural valve deterioration. In young people (16-40 years of age), structural valve deterioration begins at ages 2-3 and is 60% or greater at 10 years. Even in people aged 41-60 years, bioprosthesis is associated with high structural valve deterioration up to 50%, and 50% of the late mortality is a consequence of structural valve deterioration

FIGURE 8-10. Summary of the results of mitral valve replacement (MVR). CBC—catheter balloon commissurotomy; MVA—mitral valve area. (*Adapted from* Rahimtoola *et al.* [11].)

INDICATIONS FOR CATHETER BALLOON COMMISSUROTOMY IN ASYMPTOMATIC PATIENTS WITH MITRAL STENOSIS

MVR vs CBC

The MVA should be 1 cm^2 or less, or > 1 to 1.5 cm^2 in selected patients; the valve should be suitable for CBC; there should be no contraindications for CBC; and a physician with appropriate skill and experience with CBC should be available

The indications are:

Pulmonary arterial hypertension

Episodic acute pulmonary edema

Atrial fibrillation/flutter (paroxysmal/permanent)

Embolism (systemic/pulmonary) and no thrombus in LA/inferior vena cava

Contemplating future pregnancy

Occupations that pose high risk to patient/public

FIGURE 8-11. Lists the suggested indications for catheter balloon commissurotomy (CBC) in asymptomatic patients with severe mitral stenosis (MS). LA—left atrium; MVA—mitral valve area; MVR—mitral valve replacement. (*Adapted from* Rahimtoola *et al.* [11].)

MITRAL REGURGITATION

PATHOLOGY

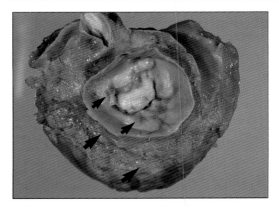

FIGURE 8-12. Mitral annular calcification (MAC). Seen primarily in patients older than 70 years and four times more common in women than men, MAC usually occurs at the angle between the base of the posterior mitral valve (MV) where it meets the left ventricular endocardium. MAC may be only barely detectable grossly or may involve the entire posterior leaflet, and extend onto the anterior leaflet, forming a "D." The aortic valve is also calcified in approximately 50% of cases [12]. Advanced degrees of MAC may result in mitral regurgitation.

This figure shows an atrial view of the MV with extensive calcification in the annular region with supravalvular extension (*arrows*) in a 72-year-old woman with mitral incompetence.

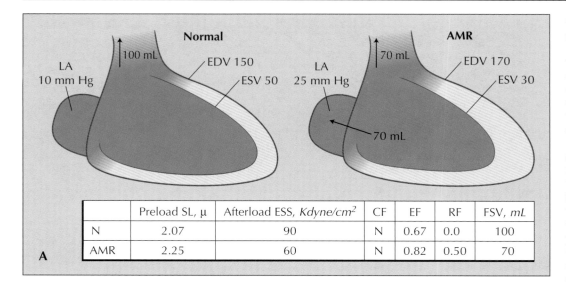

A

	Preload SL, μ	Afterload ESS, *Kdyne/cm²*	CF	EF	RF	FSV, *mL*
N	2.07	90	N	0.67	0.0	100
AMR	2.25	60	N	0.82	0.50	70

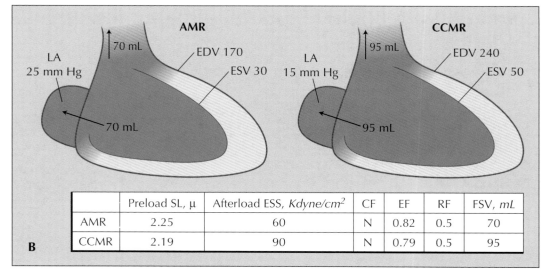

B

	Preload SL, μ	Afterload ESS, *Kdyne/cm²*	CF	EF	RF	FSV, *mL*
AMR	2.25	60	N	0.82	0.5	70
CCMR	2.19	90	N	0.79	0.5	95

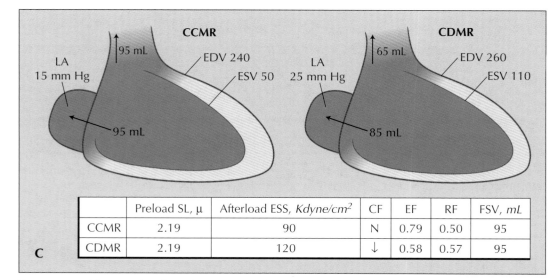

C

	Preload SL, μ	Afterload ESS, *Kdyne/cm²*	CF	EF	RF	FSV, *mL*
CCMR	2.19	90	N	0.79	0.50	95
CDMR	2.19	120	↓	0.58	0.57	95

FIGURE 8-13. Three pathophysiologic stages of mitral regurgitation (MR) [13]. **A,** The physiology of acute mitral regurgitation (AMR) is compared with that of normal (N) competent mitral valve. The acute volume overload of MR increases the sarcomere length (SL) of existing sarcomeres

toward maximum, producing a modest increase in end-diastolic volume (EDV) [14].

Simultaneously, the new pathway for left ventricular ejection into the left atrium (LA) effectively reduces the resistance to ejection (afterload), characterized as end-systolic stress (ESS) [15]. Reduced afterload allows the ventricle to eject more completely and thus end-systolic volume (ESV) is reduced.

Although contractile function (CF) has not changed, the changes in loading conditions increase total stroke volume in this example to 140 mL and increase ejection fraction (EF) to 82%. However, because 50% of the total stroke volume of the left ventricle is now entering the LA (regurgitant fraction [RF] = 0.5), LA pressure increases and forward stroke volume (FSV) decreases to 70 mL. At this point in the disease the patient will suffer from symptoms of congestive failure (fatigue and dyspnea) even though ventricular muscle function is normal.

B, If the patient in *panel A* tolerated the insult of AMR without the need for surgery and he were followed for several months, he might enter the chronic compensated mitral regurgitation (CCMR) phase, which is contrasted with the acute phase here. The major compensatory change is the development of eccentric cardiac hypertrophy in which the cardiocytes are elongated by the addition of sarcomeres in series [16]. The result is that EDV has increased from 170 mL during AMR to 240 mL in the CCMR. Total stroke volume is now 190 mL, allowing FSV to return nearly to normal. At the same time the LA has enlarged and can now better accommodate the volume overload and thus LA pressure has fallen significantly from the acute phase. CF is still relatively normal, which together with the compensatory hypertrophy and still favorable loading conditions, might allow the patient to be asymptomatic.

C, Although the patient may tolerate CCMR for years, eventually left ventricular CF deteriorates and the patient enters a chronic decompensated MR (CDMR) phase, which is compared with the compensated phase. Contractile dysfunction impairs left ventricular ejection, resulting in a larger ESV, in turn leading to a further increase in EDV. The increase in EDV may cause greater annular dilatation and misalignment of the papillary muscles, making the MR worse. The result of worsened muscle function and increased regurgitation is that both forward and total stroke volume fall. Increased left ventricular diastolic volume causes elevation of left ventricular end-diastolic pressure and LA pressure. The patient may again notice fatigue and dyspnea. Despite the presence of contractile dysfunction, EF remains in the normal range as a result of the still favorable loading conditions, although it is lower than in the compensated phase. (*Adapted from* Carabello [13].)

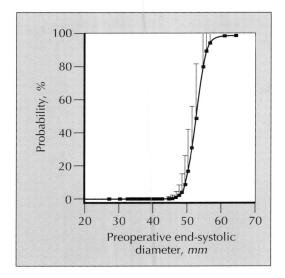

FIGURE 8-14. In patients with mitral regurgitation, the likelihood of postoperative death or persistence of severe heart failure is a function of the preoperative end-systolic diameter. The incidence of a poor postoperative outcome increased abruptly when the end-systolic diameter exceeded 45 mm [10]. (*Adapted from* Wisenbaugh *et al.* [17].)

ECHOCARDIOGRAPHY

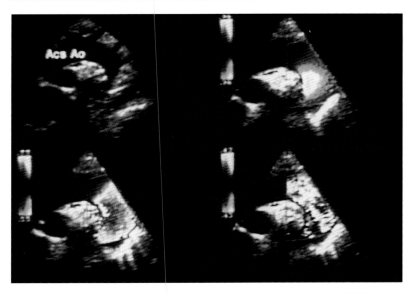

FIGURE 8-15. Determination of severity of mitral regurgitation (MR). It is difficult to determine the exact severity of MR on echocardiography. Two-dimensional echocardiographic findings suggest that severe MR

include a dilated hyperdynamic left ventricle or a flail mitral valve leaflet. Indirect clues to the severity of MR include the continuous-wave Doppler mitral regurgitation jet intensity, the initial mitral inflow velocity, the contour of the continuous-wave Doppler MR velocity curve, and interruption of pulmonary venous flow (*vide infra*). The area or extent of the jet into the left atrium on color-flow imaging was initially proposed as a method for determining the severity of MR [18]. However, subsequent reports showed that the color-flow jet area cannot be equated directly with the volume of regurgitation [19], because the jet area is also dependent on other physical factors such as the velocity of the jet. In addition, frequently eccentric jets impinge on adjacent structures, which decreases the appearance of the jet on color-flow imaging [20]. Finally, the jet area appearance may change with instrument adjustments in pulse repetition frequency, transducer frequency, filter setting (shown here), color maps, and gain level. Thus, the severity of MR cannot be based on the color-flow area alone but must be a culmination of all information provided by the clinical setting, two-dimensional echocardiographic findings, the color-flow jet, and the indirect Doppler findings. In experienced laboratories, a regurgitant fraction or volume can be calculated from volumetric flow rates [21]. Newer techniques such as amplitude-weighted continuous-wave signal intensity [22] and proximal isovelocity surface areas [23] show promise as future methods of further quantitating the severity of MR. Asc Ao—ascending aorta.

MANAGEMENT

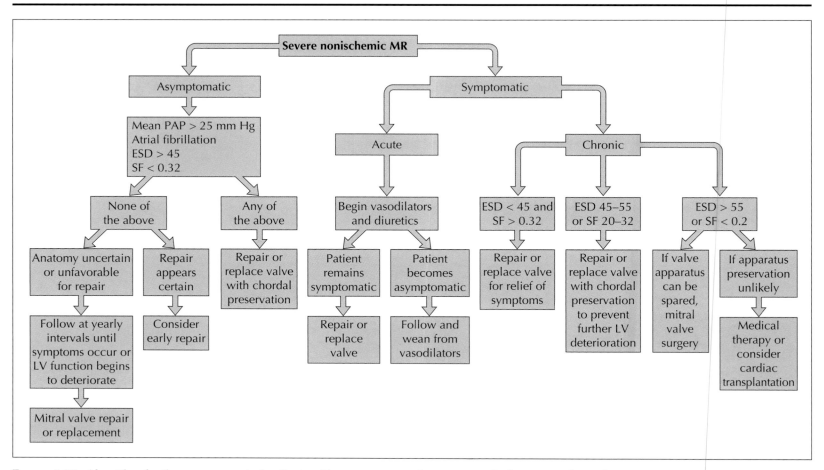

FIGURE 8-16. Algorithm for the management of patients with severe, nonischemic mitral regurgitation (MR). It is likely that preservation of the chordae tendineae and their effects on contractile function [24] allowed the entire ventricle to decrease in size postoperatively, reducing the radius (r) term in the stress equation (stress = P x r/2h, where *P* = pressure and *h* = wall thickness). Thus, wall stress actually fell when the chordae were preserved. Chordae tendineae are an integral part of the left ventricle (LV) and its systolic function. When the chordae tendineae are severed, LV function worsens; this tendency is exaggerated if preoperative muscle dysfunction is already present. When the chordae tendineae are preserved, LV ejection fraction is maintained both because afterload is reduced and because ventricular contractile performance is maintained at its preoperative level. These factors combined with a lower incidence of thromboembolism, the avoidance of anticoagulation, and a lower risk of late postoperative valve failure all lead to a reduced operative mortality rate and better long-term outcome for repair than for replacement with valve ablation.

It is important to note that not all valves can be repaired. Abnormalities involving the anterior leaflet of the mitral valve are more difficult to repair than those involving the posterior leaflet and severe rheumatic deformity may prevent an adequate repair. ESD—end-systolic dimension; PAP—pulmonary artery pressure; SF—shortening fraction.

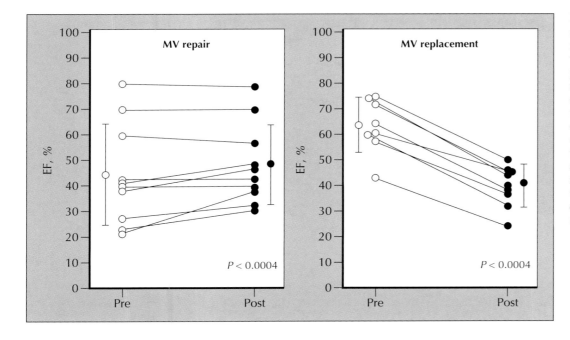

FIGURE 8-17. Reasons for mitral valve (MV) repair superiority over valve replacement. MV repair retains the patient's native mitral valve, which is more resistant to endocarditis than is a prosthetic valve. Additionally, the repaired native valve has a low risk for thromboembolism, obviating anticoagulation. Perhaps the most important reason for repair's superiority to replacement is shown in this figure that demonstrates preoperative (pre) and postoperative (post) ejection fraction for MV replacement and MV repair [25]. Ejection fraction fell after replacement but was preserved at its preoperative level after repair. These findings have been confirmed by additional studies [24,26,27]. (*Adapted from* Goldman *et al.* [25].)

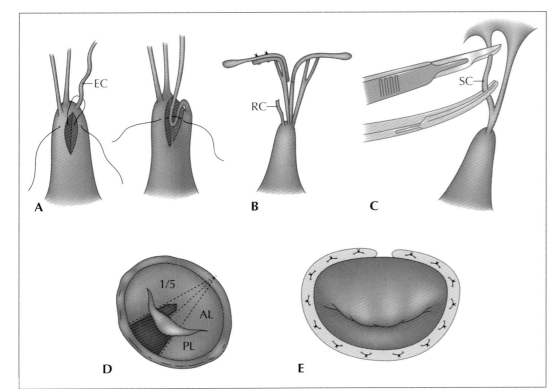

FIGURE 8-18. Reconstructive techniques. Because mitral valve disease, especially regurgitation, is usually multifactorial, that is, with simultaneous involvement of two or more components of the valve apparatus, several techniques of reconstruction must be applied, depending on the affected components, if a satisfactory result is to be achieved. **A,** Elongated chordae tendineae (EC) may be shortened by (among other techniques) burying the excessive length in the respective papillary muscle head. **B,** Ruptured chordae (RC) of the anterior leaflet (AL) may be replaced by transposing wormed chordae from the posterior leaflet (PL). **C,** Shortened chordae (SC), which retract the PL, may be excised. **D,** Flail segments of the PL, up to one third, may be resected; small triangular segments may very rarely be excised from the AL. **E,** In the last step, the dilated annulus is shortened and reshaped by implantation of a prosthetic ring. The mitral valve is seen as a functional unit and reconstructed accordingly.

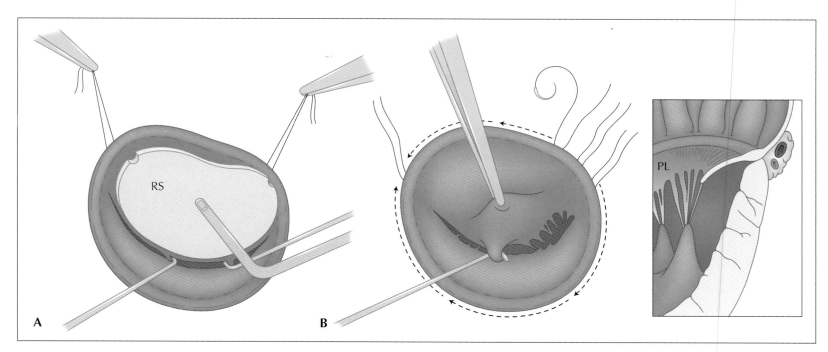

FIGURE 8-19. Annulus reshaping. Reduction of the size of the annulus and protection from disruption are obtained by all types of rings, but reshaping can only be achieved by preshaped rings. Because the shape of these rings approximates the systolic shape of the normal mitral valve, accurate sizing and positioning of the ring are essential. Otherwise, distortion with regurgitation may occur. **A,** The ring sizer (RS) is chosen appropriately to match the size of the anterior leaflet. **B,** The sutures (3–0 Ticron) must be precisely placed and distributed in the annulus, just outside the leaflet hinge to avoid interference with leaflet motion (**inset**). Similarly, precise distribution of the sutures through the ring is essential. Left ventricular outflow tract obstruction has been demonstrated after mitral valve repair, especially when a Carpentier ring has been implanted (although it has also occurred after repair with a flexible ring and without a ring). This is due to systolic anterior motion of the anterior leaflet, presumably due to excessive leaflet tissue. The prevalence of this complication is low and the obstruction decreases and may even disappear with time [28,29]. PL—posterior leaflet.

MITRAL VALVE PROLAPSE

PATHOLOGY

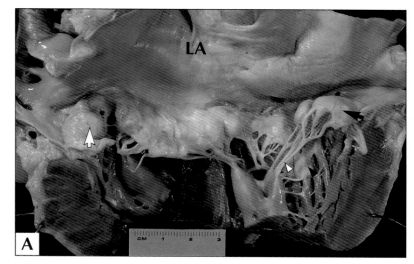

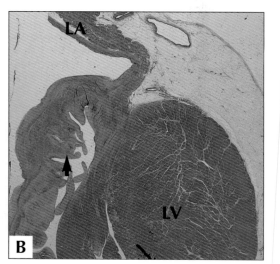

FIGURE 8-20. Mitral valve prolapse (MVP). The incidence of MVP in the general population is 3% to 5% and is higher in women. The majority of patients are asymptomatic. Symptomatic mitral regurgitation occurs in 10% to 15% of patients and is more common in men older than 50 years [12].

A, A 54-year-old white man died suddenly without previous cardiac history. Note the enlarged and billowing intermediate (*black arrow*) and medial (*white arrow*) scallop of the posterior mitral valve leaflet. *White arrowhead* denotes elongated chordal tendinae and *black arrowhead* denotes endocardial plaque.

B, Histologic section of the mitral valve shown in *panel A.* Note proteoglycan deposits (*green staining*) expanding the spongiosa and extending into the fibrosa. This Movat penta-chrome stain demonstrates elastic tissue (*black*), fibrous tissue (*yellow*), and proteoglycans (*blue-green*). *Arrow* denotes fibrosa. (Part A *from* Farb *et al.* [12]; with permission.)

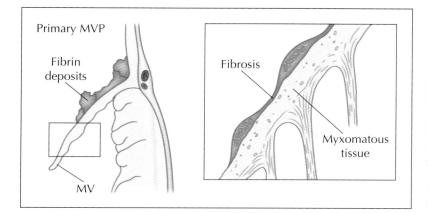

FIGURE 8-21. Histopathology of primary mitral valve prolapse (MVP). The normal mitral valve (MV) is composed of three layers: 1) the atrialis, a thin layer of collagen and elastic tissue along the atrial aspect of the leaflet; 2) the fibrosa (ventricularis), a denser layer of collagen along the ventricular aspect; and 3) the spongiosa, the fine myxomatous connective tissue layer between the two [30]. In primary MVP, as shown here, dissolution of collagen bundles occurs primarily with secondary myxomatous proliferation of the spongiosa and interruption of the fibrosa and fibrosis of the atrial and ventricular surfaces of the valve [30,31]. These secondary effects appear to occur as a response to repeated stress on the valve apparatus. Focal endothelial disruption occurs commonly and may provide a site for thrombus formation [32]. Fibrin deposits often form at the MV–left atrial angle. Similar histologic changes can occur in the chordae tendineae and result in chordal thinning and rupture. Myxomatous degeneration of the annulus can occur as well, especially in patients with connective tissue disorders, resulting in annular dilation and calcification and worsening of mitral regurgitation.

PHYSICAL EXAMINATION

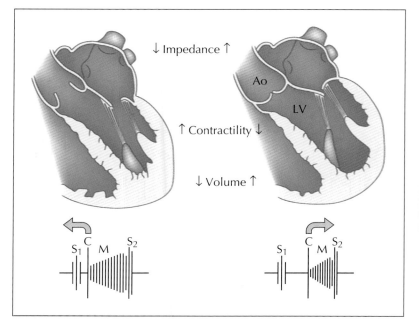

FIGURE 8-22. Dynamic auscultation. Mid-systolic clicks (C) may be secondary to factors aside from mitral valve prolapse (MVP). These include extracardiac causes, atrial septal aneurysms, and pericarditis. The mid-systolic click of MVP can be reliably distinguished from these by its temporal response to maneuvers that alter hemodynamic conditions. Any maneuver that decreases left ventricular (LV) volume (*eg*, decreased venous return, tachycardia, decreased outflow impedance, increased contractility) will worsen the mismatch in size between the enlarged mitral valve and LV chamber, resulting in prolapse earlier in systole and movement of the click and murmur (M) toward the first heart sound (S$_1$). Conversely, maneuvers that increase LV volume (*eg*, increased venous return, bradycardia, increased outflow impedance, decreased contractility) will delay the occurrence of prolapse, resulting in movement of the click and murmur toward the second heart sound (S$_2$). Ao—aorta. (*Adapted from* O'Rourke and Crawford [33].)

EFFECT OF VARIOUS MANEUVERS ON THE CLICK AND MURMUR OF MVP

MANEUVER	TIMING	MURMUR INTENSITY	MECHANISM
Standing	←	↑	↓VR
Squatting	→	↑↓	↑VR, ↓HR
Valsalva	←	↑↓	↓VR, ↑HR
Maximal handgrip	→	↑	↑AL, ↓HR
Amyl nitrite	←	↓	↓VR, ↓AL
β-blockers	→	↓	↓HR, ↓C

FIGURE 8-23. Effect of various maneuvers on the click and murmur of mitral valve prolapse (MVP). Although maneuvers that change left ventricular volume have consistent effects on the timing of the click and duration of the murmur, there may be divergent effects on the intensity of the murmur. For example, although amyl nitrite results in an earlier click and murmur, the decrease in systolic pressure results in less regurgitation and a softer murmur. Thus, in diagnosing MVP, changes in the timing of the click are usually more helpful than changes in the intensity of the murmur. ←—earlier; →—later; ↑—increase; ↓—decrease; ↑↓—variable; AL—afterload; C—contractility; HR—heart rate; VR—venous return.

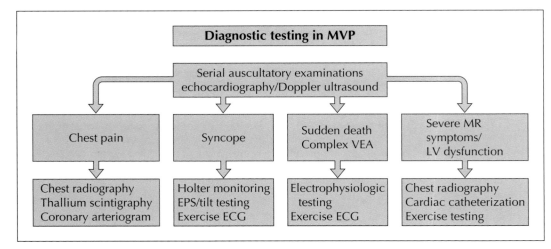

Diagnostic testing in MVP

Serial auscultatory examinations
echocardiography/Doppler ultrasound

Chest pain	Syncope	Sudden death Complex VEA	Severe MR symptoms/ LV dysfunction
Chest radiography Thallium scintigraphy Coronary arteriogram	Holter monitoring EPS/tilt testing Exercise ECG	Electrophysiologic testing Exercise ECG	Chest radiography Cardiac catheterization Exercise testing

FIGURE 8-24. Diagnostic testing in mitral valve prolapse (MVP). The diagnosis of MVP is based on the presence of typical auscultatory findings detected during carefully performed serial examinations. Echocardiography (M-mode, two-dimensional, and Doppler) is the single most useful test in the definition of MVP. It is used to assess natural history and prognosis, the presence of associated conditions (*eg*, atrial septal defect, hypertrophic cardiomyopathy), the need for antibiotic prophylaxis, and the degree of mitral regurgitation (MR). Echocardiography should *not* supplant the physical examination in the diagnosis of MVP; up to 10% of patients diagnosed with MVP by typical auscultatory findings will have a non-diagnostic two-dimensional echocardiogram [34].

Electrocardiography (ECG) is routinely performed to assess for ventricular preexcitation and resting ST- and T-wave abnormalities. The tests listed in the lowest level of the flow diagram are not required for the diagnosis of MVP, but they are useful in assessing certain symptoms and complications that can occur in this disorder. EPS—electrophysiology; LV—left ventricular; MR—mitral regurgitation; VEA—ventricular ectopic arrhythmia.

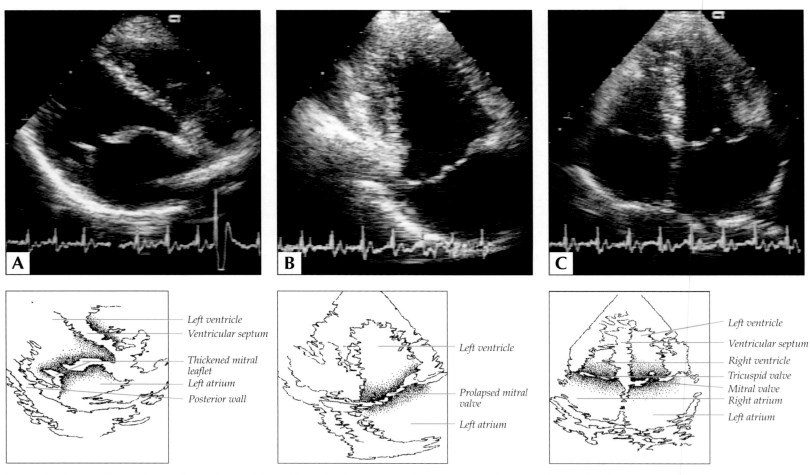

FIGURE 8-25. Two-dimensional echocardiographic and Doppler ultrasound images from a 55-year-old man with classic mitral valve prolapse and associated tricuspid valve prolapse. The parasternal long axis view shows significant leaflet thickening of both mitral leaflets (**A**). The apical long axis view shows prolapse of both leaflets and the coaptation point beyond the annular plane (**B**). The apical four-chamber view displays a systolic prolapse of both the mitral and tricuspid valves (**C**).

Continued on next page

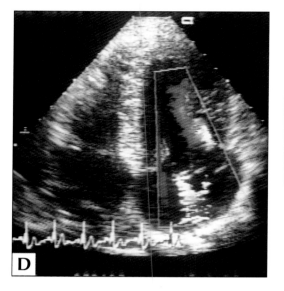 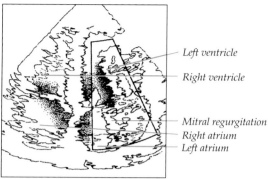

FIGURE 8-25. *(Continued)* Color flow Doppler mapping in the left atrium demonstrates central mitral regurgitation (**D**). Tricuspid regurgitation was noted as well (not shown).

Left ventricle

Right ventricle

Mitral regurgitation
Right atrium
Left atrium

MANAGEMENT

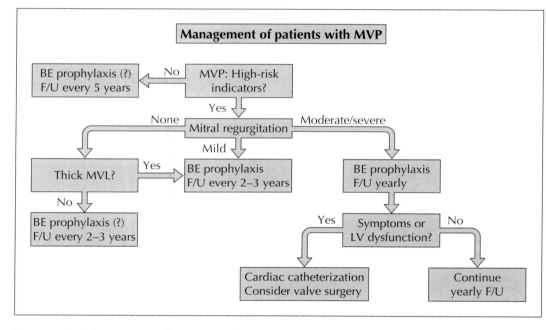

Management of patients with MVP

BE prophylaxis (?)
F/U every 5 years

← No — MVP: High-risk indicators?

↓ Yes

None — Mitral regurgitation — Moderate/severe

↓ Mild

Thick MVL? — Yes → BE prophylaxis F/U every 2–3 years

BE prophylaxis F/U yearly

No ↓

BE prophylaxis (?)
F/U every 2–3 years

Yes — Symptoms or LV dysfunction? — No

Cardiac catheterization
Consider valve surgery

Continue yearly F/U

FIGURE 8-26. Management of patients with mitral valve prolapse (MVP). High-risk characteristics in MVP patients are additive, that is, the more indicators present, the greater the total risk. The majority of patients with MVP are asymptomatic and have no or minimal high-risk indicators.

They are treated with reassurance and can lead a normal life [35,36]. Clinical and echocardiographic assessment every 5 years is reasonable to determine passage into a higher risk group. If any high-risk indicators are present, patients can be further stratified based on the presence of mitral regurgitation (MR). Some authorities advocate prophylaxis for bacterial endocarditis (BE) only if MVP is associated with MR or thickened mitral valve leaflets (MVL). However, given the variability of physical findings and the dynamic nature of MR in MVP, prophylaxis may be reasonable in all patients with MVP. Patients with MVP and severe MR should be managed in the same manner as patients with severe MR due to other causes. The decision to proceed with valve surgery is based on the presence of symptoms or impairment of left ventricular (LV) systolic function. Mitral valve reconstructive surgery can often be used in lieu of valve replacement to correct regurgitant floppy valves [37–39]. Compared with valve replacement, valve repair is associated with a lower operative and late mortality, lower long-term thromboembolic risk, and lower BE risk [37,39]. F/U—follow-up.

PATHOLOGY

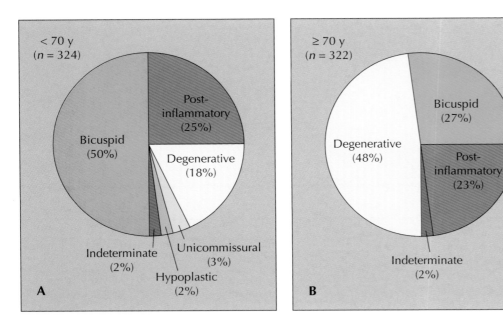

FIGURE 8-27. Causes of aortic stenosis (AS).
A, Among patients 70 years of age or younger,
calcification of congenitally bicuspid valves
accounted for half of the surgical cases of AS.
B, Conversely, degenerative calcification
accounted for almost half the cases of AS in
patients 70 years of age or older. (*Adapted from*
Passik *et al.* [40].)

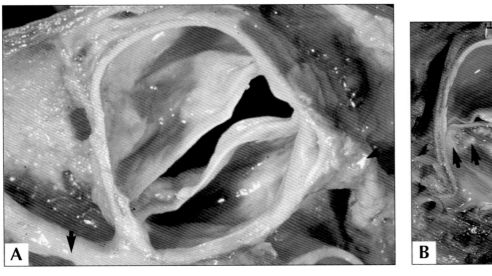

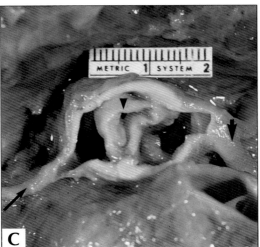

FIGURE 8-28. Congenital aortic valve (AV) disease. **A,** A normally functioning bicuspid AV with two commissures and the two leaflets, which are
almost equal in size in a 58-year-old man who died of metastatic lung
carcinoma. The commissures are located right and left and both coronary
ostia arise from the anterior aortic sinus. Note the absence of raphe in
either leaflet. The right coronary artery is denoted by an *arrow*; the left
coronary artery is denoted by an *arrowhead*.

B, A mildly calcified congenitally bicuspid AV in a 69-year-old man.
Note a nonstenotic functionally normal bicuspid valve with mild calcification (*arrows*) and a raphe (*arrowhead*) in the anterior leaflet.

C, A bicuspid dysplastic and fibrotic AV (*arrowhead*) from a 24-year-old
woman who had a commissurotomy 5 years before death. She was found
dead in the hospital while awaiting repeat surgery. The commissures are
located anterior and posterior and the leaflets are right and left with the right
coronary artery (*long arrow*) and the left coronary artery (*short arrow*) arising
from the right and left coronary sinuses. Patients with dysplastic bicuspid
valves usually become symptomatic early in life, whereas those with calcified
and fibrotic bicuspid valves usually present in the fifth to seventh decade.

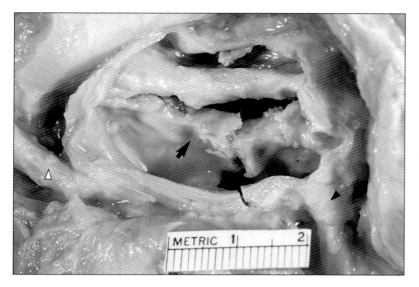

FIGURE 8-29. Bicuspid aortic valve (AV): congenital versus acquired. Congenital bicuspid stenotic AV with calcified and fibrotic raphe (*arrow*). The patient was in his fifth decade. Note that leaflets are anterior and posterior, and there is a rudimentary commissure in the anterior leaflet that does not reach the level of the true commissures. *Asterisk* shows calcified nodules; *black arrowhead* shows right commissure; *white arrowhead* shows left commissure.

Shown here is a calcified fibrotic congenital bicuspid aortic stenosis (AS) (*arrow*). No raphe is identified. Note the marked thickening of the valve leaflets, which are similar in size. The patient was a woman in her 40s with symptomatic AS. *White arrowhead* shows right coronary artery; *black arrowhead* shows left coronary artery.

PATHOPHYSIOLOGY

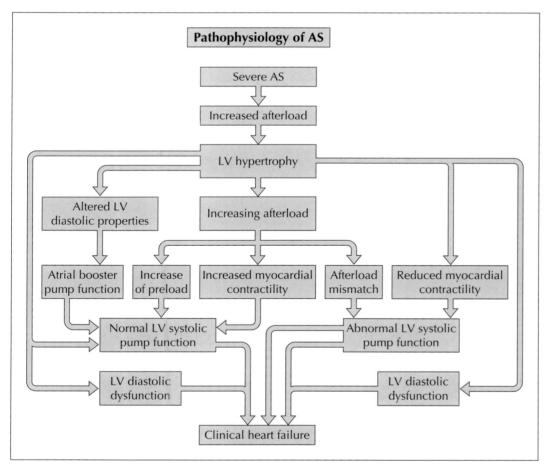

FIGURE 8-30. Pathophysiology of aortic stenosis (AS). With reduction in the aortic valve area (AVA), energy is dissipated during the transport of blood from the left ventricle (LV) to the aorta. The AVA has to be reduced by 50% of normal before a measurable gradient can be demonstrated. When a pressure gradient develops between the LV and the ascending aorta, LV pressure rises and LV wall stress (afterload) increases. This could result in an impairment of LV function. The heart responds by becoming hypertrophied and myocardial stress remains normal. LV mass in patients with severe AS undergoing valve replacement averages 229 g/m^2 (normal mass, 105 g/m^2) [41]; at autopsy, LVs weighing as much as 1000 g have been reported. LV volume remains within the normal range; therefore, there is considerable thickening of the LV wall. As a result of the LV hypertrophy, LV systolic pump function remains normal. LV hypertrophy may alter the LV diastolic properties and there is increased resistance to LV filling. As a result, LV end-diastolic pressure is elevated; but this cannot be used as a measure of LV failure. Powerful atrial contraction produces the required LV filling [42,43] and fiber length (atrial booster pump function). Because atrial systole occupies only a small part of the cardiac cycle, there is only a transient increase in left atrial pressure; therefore, mean left atrial pressure remains in the normal range [42] or is only minimally increased.

As LV afterload continues to increase, the LV uses two additional compensatory mechanisms, namely, increase of preload and increase of myocardial contractility. Both of these help maintain normal LV systolic pump function.

When the limit of the preload reserve has been reached (afterload mismatch) [44] or myocardial contractility is reduced, LV systolic pump function becomes abnormal.

Clinical heart failure is usually a result of abnormal LV systolic pump function; diastolic dysfunction may also be present in some patients. Clinical heart failure in those with normal systolic pump function is a result of LV diastolic dysfunction. (© Copyright SH Rahimtoola, MB, FRCP, MACP, MACC.)

PHYSICAL EXAMINATION

PHYSICAL EXAMINATION IN AS

	SEVERITY OF AS		
	MILD	MODERATE	SEVERE
Arterial pulse	Normal	Slowly rising	Parvus et tardus
Jugular venous pulse	Normal	Normal	Usually normal
Carotid thrill	±	±	±
Cardiac impulse	Normal	Heaving	Heaving, sustained
Precordial thrill	±	±	Palpable *a* wave
			Usually ++
Auscultation			
S_4	-	±	++
ESC	+	±	-
Peak of ESM	Early systole	Mid systole	Late systole
S_2	Normal	Normal or single	Single or paradoxic

FIGURE 8-31. Physical examination. The findings on physical examination in patients with mild aortic stenosis (AS) are an ejection systolic click (ESC) and ejection systolic murmur (ESM) that peak in early systole. The ESC may be absent if the valve is calcified or is rigid. These patients may have a carotid or precordial thrill.

Patients with severe AS display characteristic physical findings. The arterial pulse, which is best felt over the carotid or the suprasternal notch, shows a slowly rising pulse that takes longer to reach peak (parvus et tardus). The jugular venous pulse is normal and a carotid thrill may be present. The cardiac impulse is left ventricular (LV) in type; it is heaving and sustained. Often a powerful presystolic wave (*a* wave) is felt. A precordial systolic thrill is often present. On auscultation, there is an S_4 gallop, the ESC is absent, the ESM peaks in late systole, and the S_2 is single. S_2 is at times paradoxic, but this usually occurs in the presence of associated left bundle branch block or LV failure. In addition, there is usually a faint diastolic murmur of minimal aortic regurgitation. In the presence of congestive heart failure, the jugular venous pressure is often increased, the LV is dilated, there is an S_3, and the ESM may be very soft or absent. Frequently, a holosystolic murmur of mitral regurgitation is present. The findings on physical examination resemble those of heart failure from a variety of causes, *eg*, a cardiomyopathy, rather than AS. The physical findings in moderate AS are between those seen in mild and severe AS.

ECHOCARDIOGRAPHY

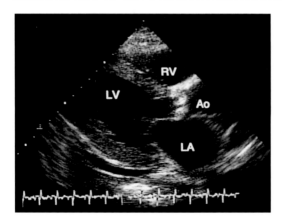

FIGURE 8-32. Calcific aortic stenosis (AS). In a patient with calcific AS, the aortic valve appears echo dense and immobile, as shown in the parasternal long-axis view. Two-dimensional echocardiographic imaging is a highly sensitive method for determining the presence of AS. However, the severity of AS cannot be determined reliably from the two-dimensional image alone. In the presence of calcification, it is frequently difficult to visualize the number of aortic valve cusps. Other information that should be obtained from the two-dimensional echocardiogram is the response of the left ventricle (LV) to the pressure overload (chamber size, ventricular hypertrophy, and ventricular systolic function), as well as other concomitant valve disease. Ao—aorta; LA—left atrium; RA—right atrium; RV—right ventricle.

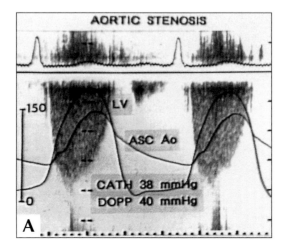

FIGURE 8-33. Aortic valve gradient in aortic stenosis (AS). Doppler ultrasound provides an accurate, noninvasive method for measurement of the aortic valve gradient in patients with AS [45]. The instantaneous pressure gradient between the left ventricle (LV) and aorta can be measured by applying the modified Bernoulli equation (pressure gradient = $4 \times$ [velocity]^2) to the continuous-wave Doppler signal across the aortic valve. The mean aortic valve gradient, the most useful measurement of the degree of obstruction, can be obtained by averaging the instantaneous pressure gradients and can be performed on-line quickly with the calculation packages in the newer echocardiographic instruments.

In the assessment of patients with AS, it is of critical importance to interrogate the valve from multiple windows to ensure that the Doppler beam is parallel to the velocity jet [7,45,46]. A deviation of greater than 20° will result in a clinically significant underestimation of the pressure gradient. The Doppler examination can underestimate an aortic valve gradient but should not overestimate the gradient (except in the rare instances of severe anemia or coexistent LV outflow obstruction). Thus, the results should be correlated with the two-dimensional echocardiographic findings, as well as with the clinical findings. **A,** Simultaneous measurement of the aortic valve mean gradient demonstrates the excellent correlation between the gradient derived from cardiac catheterization (CATH) and continuous-wave Doppler ultrasound (DOPP).

Continued on next page

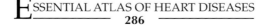

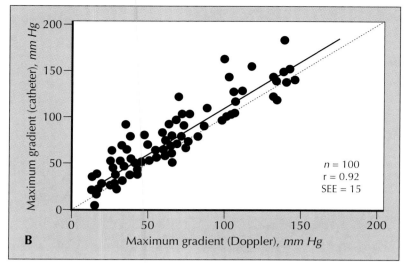

FIGURE 8-33. *(Continued)* **B,** Correlation between Doppler- and catheter-derived instantaneous aortic valve pressure gradient. The regression equation, catheter gradient = 10.3 + 0.97 × Doppler gradient, is represented by the *solid line* [46]. Asc Ao—ascending aorta; SEE—standard error of the estimate. (*Adapted from* Currie *et al.* [45].)

MANAGEMENT

INDICATIONS FOR SURGERY FOR PATIENTS WITH SEVERE ATRIAL STENOSIS

All symptomatic patients
    LV dysfunction normal: as soon as possible
    LV dysfunction: urgent
    Heart failure: emergent
Asymptomatic patients
    All patients
    Alternative strategy
        Patients undergoing surgery for CAD and aorta and other valves
        LV dysfunction
        Progressive decline of LVEF
        Marked or excessive LV hypertrophy:
            ≥ 11 to 12 mm in smaller people (*eg,* women)
            ≥ 13 to 14 mm in larger people (*eg,* men)
        Patients ages ≥ 60 to 65 years
        Arrhythmias
            Ventricular or atrial tachyarrhythmias
            AV block > 1° AV block
        "Very" severe AS ≤ 0.7 cm^2; 0.4 cm^2/m^2
        Abnormal response to exercise
            Hypotension or no or minimal increase in BP
            Ischemia
            LV dysfunction
            Arrhythmias

FIGURE 8-34. Indications for surgery for severe atrial stenosis (AS). Symptomatic patients with severe AS should have aortic valve surgery (usually valve replacement) unless there is a specific contraindication to its performance. The urgency of surgery depends on the state of left ventricular (LV) function and the severity of the symptoms. For example, if there is LV dysfunction, the procedure is urgent; in the presence of heart failure or cardiogenic shock, it is usually an emergency.

Probably all asymptomatic patients with severe AS should have valve surgery. An alternative strategy is to perform surgery on all patients with aortic valve areas of 0.75 cm^2 or less. In patients with small or large body size an equivalent value after correcting for body size may need to be determined. For patients with valve areas of 0.76 to 1.0 cm^2, surgery is performed in those at "higher risk." These include patients with LV dysfunction, associated significantly obstructive coronary artery disease (CAD), age 60 to 65 years or older, severe LV hypertrophy, painless ischemia, significant arrhythmias, and significant LV dysfunction on exercise. AV—atrioventricular; BP—blood pressure; LVEF—left ventricular ejection fraction. (© Copyright SH Rahimtoola, MB, FRCP, MAC, MACC.)

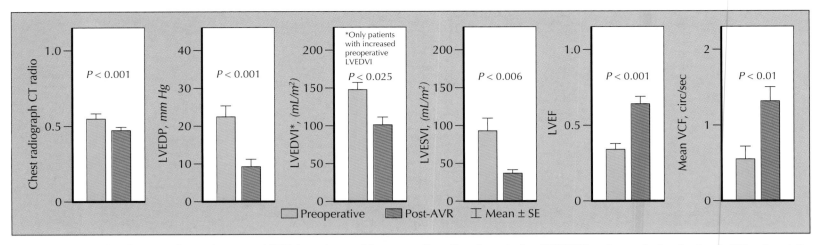

| □ Preoperative | ■ Post-AVR | ⊥ Mean ± SE |

FIGURE 8-35. Results of aortic valve replacement (AVR) in patients with severe aortic stenosis, left ventricular (LV) systolic dysfunction, and clinical heart failure. AVR has a marked beneficial effect [47]. There is a reduction in the cardiothoracic (CT) ratio on the chest radiograph and a large reduction in LV end-diastolic pressure (LVEDP). Patients in whom the LV end-diastolic volumes were increased preoperatively showed reductions in LV end-diastolic volume index (LVEDVI) and a marked reduction in LV end-systolic volume index (LVESVI). There is improvement in LV systolic pump function as demonstrated by increases in LV ejection fraction (LVEF) and mean velocity of circumferential fiber shortening (V_{cf}). circ—circumferences. (*Adapted from* Smith *et al.* [48].)

PREDICTORS OF POOR OUTCOME AFTER AORTIC VALVE REPLACEMENT FOR AORTIC STENOSIS

Age
Female gender
Emergency surgery
Coronary artery disease
Previous CABG surgery
Hypertension

Left ventricular dysfunction (EF >45% or 50%)
Heart failure
Atrial fibrillation
Concurrent mitral valve replacement or repair
Renal failure

FIGURE 8-36. Predictors of poor outcome after aortic valve replacement for aortic stenosis. CABG—coronary artery bypass grafting; EF—ejection fraction.

SUGGESTED INDICATIONS FOR CATHETER BALLOON VALVULOPLASTY IN PATIENTS WITH CALCIFIC SEVERE AS*

Bridge procedure to eventual AVR
  Cardiogenic shock
  Moderate to severe heart failure
  Emergent/urgent need for noncardiac therapeutic procedures
    (*eg*, operation)
Patient with limited life span
  Noncardiac reasons (*eg*, carcinoma)
  Cardiac reason(s) other than AS
Others
  Patient at extremely high risk for AVR
  AVR not desirable for noncardiac reasons or cardiac causes other
    than aortic stenosis
  Patient refuses surgery
Therapeutic test in rare instances: Patients with small stroke volume
    and small valve gradient with valve stenosis suspected
    to be severe but severity is in doubt even after provocative
    diagnostic tests

*Caution should be exercised in recommending this procedure in asymptomatic patients.

FIGURE 8-37. Indications for catheter balloon valvuloplasty (CBV). In older patients with severe calcific aortic stenosis (AS), CBV is largely a palliative procedure [49]. The major indication is as a "bridge" procedure to subsequent early aortic valve replacement (AVR). It is of benefit in patients in cardiogenic shock, those in moderate to severe heart failure, and those who are in emergent or urgent need for a noncardiac therapeutic procedure, *eg*, an abdominal operation. The modest improvement in aortic valve area usually improves the hemodynamics and the clinical state of the patients in cardiogenic shock and heart failure so that they become better candidates for subsequent early AVR. However, it must be emphasized that CBV is considered to be a palliative procedure and AVR should not be unduly delayed. CBV also makes the patients better candidates for emergent noncardiac surgery. The second main group of indications is for patients with a limited life span, either due to noncardiac disease (*eg*, carcinoma with a short life expectancy) or cardiac disease other than AS. The third major group includes those whom the surgeon and cardiologist consider to be at "extremely" high risk for AVR or in whom AVR is considered not desirable because of noncardiac or cardiac reasons other than AS. Finally, it can be considered in the occasional patient who refuses cardiac surgery.

On rare occasions, CBV can be considered as a "therapeutic" test. A small group of patients with left ventricular dysfunction have a small stroke volume and a small gradient with valve stenosis suspected to be severe on clinical grounds. If the severity of AS is in doubt after provocative diagnostic tests, then CBV can be considered as a procedure that will determine whether improving the aortic valve area modestly results in a significant improvement of stroke volume and a major increase of valve gradient. If it does, then the patient should undergo AVR; if it does not, then the patient most likely has left ventricular dysfunction due to causes other than AS. (*Adapted from* Rahimtoola [49].)

ACUTE AORTIC REGURGITATION

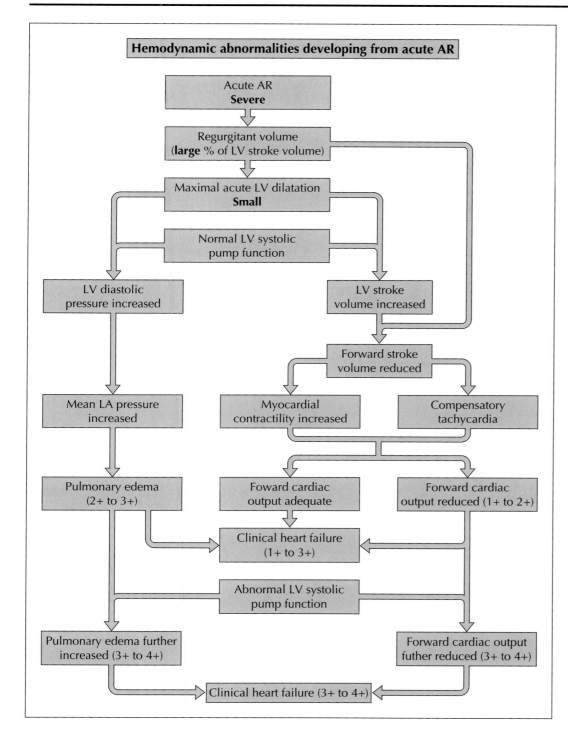

Hemodynamic abnormalities developing from acute AR

Acute AR
Severe

↓

Regurgitant volume
(**large** % of LV stroke volume)

↓

Maximal acute LV dilatation
Small

↓

Normal LV systolic
pump function

LV diastolic
pressure increased

LV stroke
volume increased

↓

Forward stroke
volume reduced

Mean LA pressure
increased

Myocardial
contractility increased

Compensatory
tachycardia

Pulmonary edema
(2+ to 3+)

Foward cardiac
output adequate

Forward cardiac
output reduced (1+ to 2+)

↓

Clinical heart failure
(1+ to 3+)

Abnormal LV systolic
pump function

Pulmonary edema further
increased (3+ to 4+)

Forward cardiac output
futher reduced (3+ to 4+)

↓

Clinical heart failure (3+ to 4+)

FIGURE 8-38. Hemodynamic abnormalities. Mild acute aortic regurgitation (AR) (*eg,* when associated with systemic hypertension) produces little or no hemodynamic abnormality. Increasing severity of regurgitation produces greater degrees of hemodynamic abnormalities, and severe AR often produces the clinical picture of heart failure.

Severe acute AR results in a large volume of regurgitant blood in the left ventricle (LV) in diastole. In an acute situation, the LV end-diastolic volume can only increase mildly (no more than 20% to 30%) and the LV diastolic pressure-volume relationships are particularly important. The LV systolic pump function is initially normal. The increased LV diastolic pressure results in increases in mean left atrial (LA) and pulmonary venous pressures and produces varying degrees of pulmonary edema [50]. The normal LV systolic pump function in the presence of LV dilatation results in an increase in LV stroke volume. However, a large percentage of the LV stroke volume is returned to the LV in diastole; as a result, the forward stroke volume is reduced. The LV uses two mechanisms, an increase of myocardial contractility and, importantly, a compensatory tachycardia to maintain an adequate forward cardiac output. As a result, initially the forward cardiac output may be appropriate. However, if the compensatory mechanisms are inadequate, forward cardiac output is reduced. The pulmonary edema with or without an adequate cardiac output produces the picture of clinical heart failure. Subsequently, LV systolic pump function may become abnormal; when that occurs, the pulmonary edema is further increased and the forward cardiac output is further reduced, leading to more severe manifestations of clinical heart failure. (© Copyright SH Rahimtoola, MB, FRCP, MACP, MACC.)

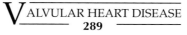

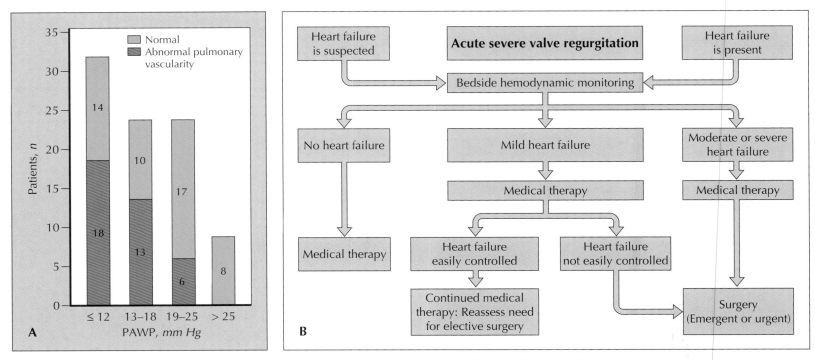

FIGURE 8-39. Hemodynamic parameters. In acute disorders affecting the left ventricle, including aortic regurgitation (AR), there may be a phase lag of up to 72 hours between the rise in left atrial and pulmonary venous pressures and the appearance of pulmonary edema on the chest radiograph, thus making the chest radiograph unreliable in this situation. **A,** Data from patients with acute myocardial infarction [51]. Of 32 patients who had pulmonary artery wedge pressures (PAWP) of 12 mm Hg or less, 14 had radiographic changes that were interpreted as pulmonary edema. Treatment with diuretics in such patients could result in a fall in cardiac output [52]. Of 31 patients with PAWP of 19 mm Hg or greater, six had normal chest radiographs. In such patients, volume loading for a reduced cardiac output or hypotension may result in a further increase in left atrial pressure and pulmonary edema.

Furthermore, the optimization of filling pressures and cardiac output may not be made accurately in acute heart failure without measuring their actual value. Thus, use of balloon flotation catheters for hemodynamic monitoring is recommended in almost all patients. **B,** This procedure can be used to determine the therapies that should be instituted.

If the AR is mild and there are no significant hemodynamic abnormalities, the balloon flotation catheter can be withdrawn. If the AR is moderate to severe and significant hemodynamic abnormalities are present, the balloon flotation catheter is left in place to guide therapy in the management of these acutely ill patients [53]. If the hemodynamic abnormalities are mild, the patient is treated medically. If these abnormalities are easily controlled, medical therapy is continued and periodic reassessments are made to determine the need for elective surgery. If the hemodynamic abnormalities are not easily corrected or the hemodynamic abnormalities initially are moderate or severe, surgery is undertaken either emergently or urgently. (Part A *adapted from* Kostuk *et al.* [51]; part B *adapted from* Rahimtoola [53].)

TIMING OF SURGERY IN HEART FAILURE DUE TO ACUTE AR

LESION	TIMING OF SURGERY
Dissection of aorta	Emergent
Infective endocarditis	Emergent, urgent, elective
Prosthetic valve dysfunction	Emergent, urgent, elective
Trauma	Emergent, urgent, elective

FIGURE 8-40. Timing of surgery. Surgical therapy (valve replacement or valve repair) is the cornerstone of the most definitive therapy currently available for heart failure in patients with acute aortic regurgitation (AR) [53–55]. If the AR is due to the dissection of the aorta, cardiac surgery is an emergency even if the AR is mild or moderate, because the AR indicates involvement of the dissection down to the region of the aortic valve root/ annulus. The indications for surgery in infective endocarditis usually depend on whether there is clinical heart failure, the type of infecting organism, and the response to therapy. Infective endocarditis due to special organisms (*eg*, fungi) can only rarely be controlled by pharmacologic therapy, and surgery is almost always needed. For these and some other conditions, valve surgery may be needed even if the AR is only mild or moderate. However, it must be recognized that in 90% to 95% of patients needing surgery for endocarditis, the indication for valve surgery is heart failure. When the heart failure is a result of prosthetic valve dysfunction or trauma, the need for surgery can be an emergency, an urgent situation, or elective.

Prosthetic valves are inherently stenotic. When AR is added, it produces a pressure plus volume overload on the left ventricle (LV) that the LV cannot handle very well acutely. Furthermore, valve regurgitation may be a sign of degeneration of biologic prosthetic valves or of prosthetic endocarditis; in both conditions, valve surgery is usually needed even if the valve regurgitation is mild to moderate. Trauma may result in AR from valve damage or dissection of the aorta. If trauma produces dissection of the aorta and AR, the need for surgery may be emergent.

In some patients, the heart failure can be easily controlled completely with pharmacologic therapy. The LV and left atrium are able to dilate and adapt to the volume overload; there are no hemodynamic abnormalities and LV function is normal. In such instances, surgical therapy may be delayed, perhaps for a considerable period of time.

CHRONIC AORTIC REGURGITATION

Echocardiography

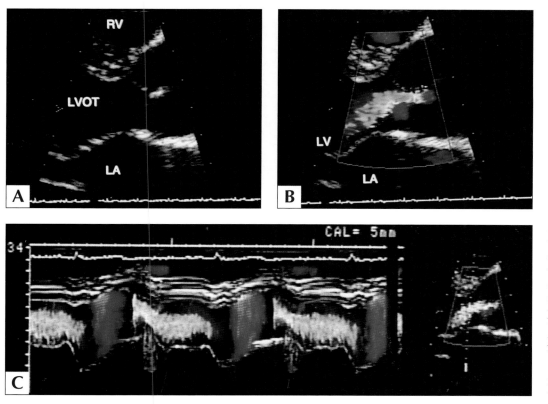

FIGURE 8-41. Doppler ultrasound imaging in the determination of the severity of aortic regurgitation (AR). The severity of AR can be assessed by several echocardiographic methods. The left ventricular (LV) size and function reflect the ventricular response to volume overload and should be considered when assessing the severity of the regurgitation. There are indirect Doppler findings, such as the diastolic half time, pulsed-wave Doppler interrogation of the descending aorta, LV outflow velocity, and mitral inflow velocity curve, which are useful in assessing the severity of regurgitation [56]. In the absence of mitral regurgitation, quantitative Doppler ultrasound measurements of regurgitant volume and regurgitant fraction can be obtained by experienced laboratories [21]. Color-flow imaging, which superimposes a color-coded display of the intracardiac velocities directly on the real-time two-dimensional image, has been used as a semiquantitative approach for determination of the severity of regurgitation in patients with central jets [57]. For AR, it is not the extent of the jet into the LV cavity but rather the width (or area) of the jet in the LV outflow tract (LVOT) that correlates with the severity of regurgitation.

A and **B**, Mild-to-moderate AR with the regurgitant jet width occupying 30% of the LVOT on the parasternal long-axis view. A color M-mode can be placed through the jet to further define the width of the jet in relation to the width of the LVOT (**C**). This method cannot be used when there is an eccentric jet of AR. LA—left atrium; RV—right ventricle.

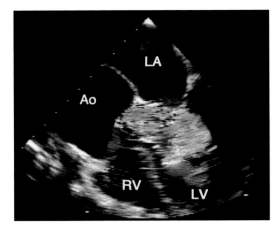

FIGURE 8-42. Transesophageal echocardiography (TEE) in the diagnosis of aortic regurgitation (AR). In this patient, severe AR is seen in the apex down the long-axis view of TEE as the regurgitant jet by color-flow imaging occupies nearly 100% of the left ventricular (LV) outflow tract. Ao—aorta; LA—left atrium; RV—right ventricle.

Pathophysiology

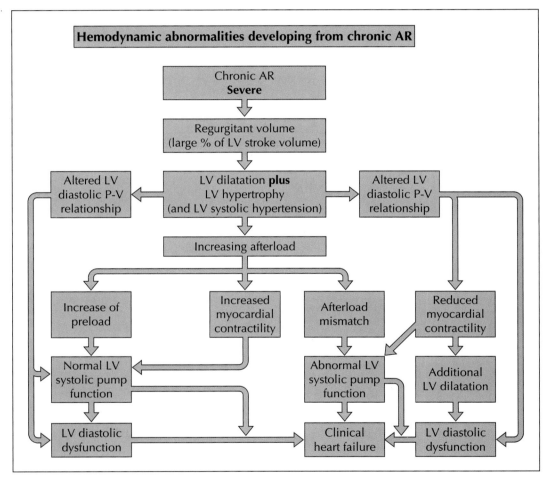

FIGURE 8-43. Hemodynamic abnormalities. Severe chronic aortic regurgitation (AR) results in a large regurgitant volume (a large percentage of left ventricular [LV] stroke volume). The LV responds by dilating (average LV end-diastolic volume in patients undergoing surgery, 205 mL/m²) [58]; the dilatation is proportional to the regurgitant volume. The subsequent large LV stroke volume results in the production of LV systolic hypertension. Both of these increase LV wall stress (afterload), which could result in an impairment of LV function. The heart responds by becoming hypertrophied (average LV mass in patients undergoing valve surgery 222 g/m²) [58]; myocardial stress remains normal and LV systolic pump function remains normal. There is an alteration of the LV diastolic pressure-volume (P-V) relationship. However, some patients with normal LV systolic pump function become symptomatic because of the abnormal LV diastolic function.

As LV afterload (a result of LV dilatation, hypertrophy, and systolic hypertension) continues to increase, the LV uses two additional compensatory mechanisms, namely, increase of preload and increase of myocardial contractility. Both of these help maintain normal LV systolic pump function.

When the limit of preload reserve has been reached (afterload mismatch) [44] or myocardial contractility is reduced, LV systolic pump function becomes abnormal. The additional LV dilatation also results in further alteration of the LV diastolic P-V relationship.

Clinical heart failure is usually a result of the abnormal LV systolic pump function; diastolic dysfunction may also be present in some patients. Clinical heart failure in those with normal LV systolic pump function is a result of LV diastolic dysfunction. (© Copyright SH Rahimtoola, MB, FRCP, MACP, MACC.)

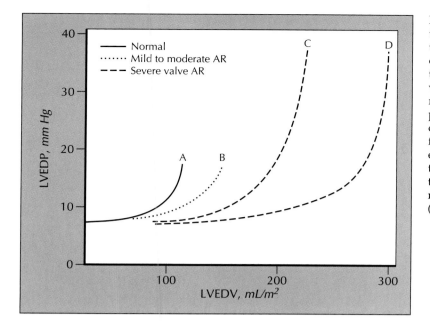

FIGURE 8-44. Left ventricular (LV) diastolic pressure-volume (P-V) relationships: effects of chronic valve regurgitation. In chronic aortic regurgitation (AR), as opposed to acute AR, the AR becomes severe over a period of time; and therefore, the LV diastolic P-V relationships are different from those seen in acute AR. If the AR is mild to moderate, the LV end-diastolic volume (LVEDV) is increased moderately, the LV diastolic P-V curve is moved to the right (curve B) of normal (curve A), and the LV end-diastolic pressure (LVEDP) is usually normal. In severe AR, the LV diastolic P-V curves are moved to the right (curves C and D). If the LV systolic pump function is normal, the LVEDV can be quite large without significant elevation of LVEDP (curve C). However, if the LVEDV increases further, the LVEDP will be increased. If LV systolic pump dysfunction supervenes, the LV diastolic P-V curve relationships are moved even further to the right (curve D) with quite marked LV dilatation and increases in LVEDP. (Adapted from Rahimtoola [53].)

Natural History

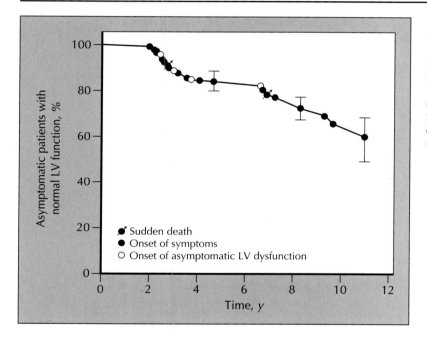

FIGURE 8-45. Natural history. The classic natural history study of Bonow et al. [59] from the National Institutes of Health prospectively evaluated 104 patients with severe aortic regurgitation who were initially asymptomatic and had normal left ventricular (LV) systolic pump function at rest. At the end of 11 years, 42% of them had become either symptomatic (19 patients), or had developed LV dysfunction (four patients) or had died suddenly (two patients); 11 of the 19 patients who had become symptomatic also developed LV dysfunction. In other words, the development of the adverse cardiac events occurs at a rate of just under 4% per year. (Adapted from Bonow et al. [59].)

Medical Management

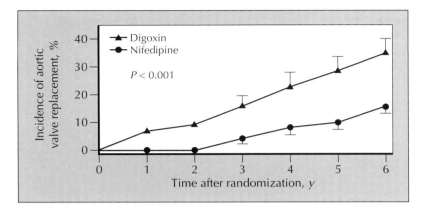

FIGURE 8-46. Long-term nifedipine therapy. The role of *long-term* slow-release nifedipine therapy in *asymptomatic* patients with severe aortic regurgitation (AR) and normal left ventricular (LV) systolic pump function was evaluated in 143 asymptomatic patients in a prospective randomized trial. The patients were followed at 6-month intervals. By actuarial analysis, at 6 years, 34±6% of patients in the digoxin group underwent valve replacement versus 15±3% of those in the nifedipine group [60]. In the digoxin group, aortic valve replacement (AVR) was performed in 20 patients because of LV systolic dysfunction (ejection fraction less than 0.50) in 75%, LV systolic dysfunction plus symptoms in 10%, and symptoms in 15%. In the nifedipine group, all six patients underwent AVR because of development of LV dysfunction. In addition, all 26 patients who underwent AVR also had an increase in LV end-diastolic volume index of at least 15%.

This randomized trial demonstrates that long-term vasodilator therapy with nifedipine reduces or delays the need for AVR in asymptomatic patients with severe AR and normal LV systolic pump function. Slow-release nifedipine therapy should be used in all such patients unless there is a specific contraindication to such therapy. (*Adapted from* Scognamiglio *et al.* [60].)

Aortic Valve Replacement

INDICATIONS FOR VALVE REPLACEMENT/VALVE REPAIR IN CHRONIC SEVERE AR

SYMPTOMATIC PATIENTS

LV function normal: as soon as possible

LV dysfunction: urgent

Heart failure: emergent

Individualize if:

  Very severe LV dysfunction (LVEF ≤ 0.20)

  Severe LV dilatation (LVEDD ≥ 80 mm; LVEDVI ≥ 300 mL/m^2)

  Small R$_g$V (R$_g$V/EDV ≤ 0.14)

ASYMPTOMATIC PATIENTS

LV dysfunction (LVEF ≤ 0.50)

Normal LV function

  Associated severe obstructive coronary artery disease

  Other valve disease needing cardiac surgery

  Any of the following (additional testing needed):

    LVEDD ≥ 70 mm

    LVESD ≥ 50 mm

    LVEDVI ≥ 150 mL/m^2 *plus* PAWP on exercise ≥ 20 mm Hg

FIGURE 8-47. Indications for valve repair or replacement. Symptomatic patients with chronic severe aortic regurgitation (AR) are candidates for valve replacement. At the present time, various forms of valve repair appear to have encouraging early results. Symptomatic patients with severe AR should have valve surgery unless there is a specific contraindication to its performance. The urgency of surgery depends on the state of left ventricular (LV) function and severity of symptoms. For example, if there is LV dysfunction, the procedure is urgent; and in selected patients with heart failure, surgery is a relatively emergent procedure. In aortic stenosis there is no lower level of LV ejection fraction (LVEF) at which the patient becomes inoperable; the lower the LVEF, the more urgent the need for valve surgery. However, in AR there comes a time when valve surgery is associated with a much higher operative mortality and the postoperative results are not very satisfactory. The precise level at which this occurs has not been well defined. General guidelines are that one should individualize the performance of surgery in the presence of very severe LV dysfunction (LVEF 0.20 or less), in the presence of severe LV dilatation (probably LV end-diastolic dimension [LVEDD] 80 mm or more, or LV end-diastolic volume index [LVEDVI] 300 mL/m^2 or more) [61], and in patients who have a large LV with a small regurgitant volume (R$_g$V) (the ratio of R$_g$V to end-diastolic volume [EDV] probably 0.14 or less) [62].

Asymptomatic patients with severe chronic AR should undergo valve surgery in the presence of LV dysfunction (LVEF less than 0.50). In those with normal LV function, surgery is recommended in the presence of associated severe obstructive coronary artery disease that needs to be bypassed or if the patient is undergoing cardiac surgery for any other valve disease. In others, it is prudent to follow patients with changes in LV size and function. LVEDD on M-mode echocardiography of 70 mm or more, LV end-systolic dimension (LVESD) of 50 mm or greater, or LVEDVI of at least 150 mL/m^2 are markers of subsequent higher incidence of an adverse event, *ie*, these patients are at significant risk of developing symptoms or developing LV systolic dysfunction over the next 5-year period. Therefore, it is recommended that such patients should have an exercise study with a right heart balloon flotation catheter; if the pulmonary artery wedge pressure (PAWP) on exercise is 20 mm Hg or more, serious consideration should be given to undertaking valve surgery provided there is experience and skill in performing valve surgery at an acceptable and low risk at the institution where the procedure is to be performed. (© Copyright SH Rahimtoola, MB, FRCP, MACP, MACC.)

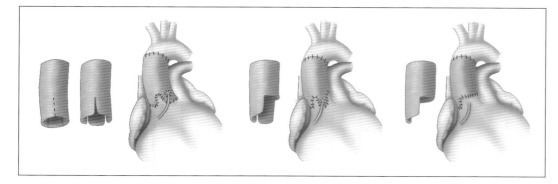

FIGURE 8-48. Aortic valve repair in patients with severe aortic regurgitation secondary to aneurysmal dilation of the aortic root. The aortic valve is spared and the aortic aneurysm is replaced. The conduit is fashioned to replace three (*left*), two (*middle*), or one (*right*) individual sinus. (*Adapted from* David *et al.* [63].)

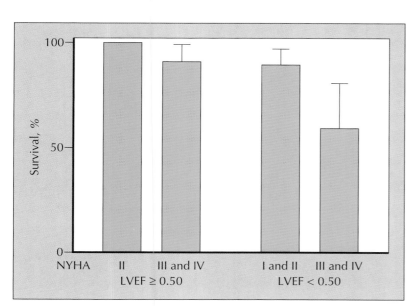

FIGURE 8-49. Five-year survival rates after aortic valve replacement (AVR). The 5-year survival after AVR for chronic severe aortic regurgitation is determined by the state of left ventricular (LV) systolic pump function and the New York Heart Association (NYHA) functional class of the patient [64]. The 5-year survival rates in patients with normal LV systolic pump function (LV ejection fraction [LVEF] 0.50 or greater) who were in NYHA functional class II or III/IV were 100% and 90%, respectively. In those with abnormal LV systolic pump function (LVEF less than 0.50) who are either asymptomatic or minimally symptomatic (NYHA classes I and II), the 5-year survival rate was 88%. The 5-year survival rates in these three subgroups were not statistically significantly different. Only patients who had reduced LVEF and were moderately or severely symptomatic (NYHA classes III and IV) had a lower 5-year survival of 63%. (*Adapted from* Greves *et al.* [64].)

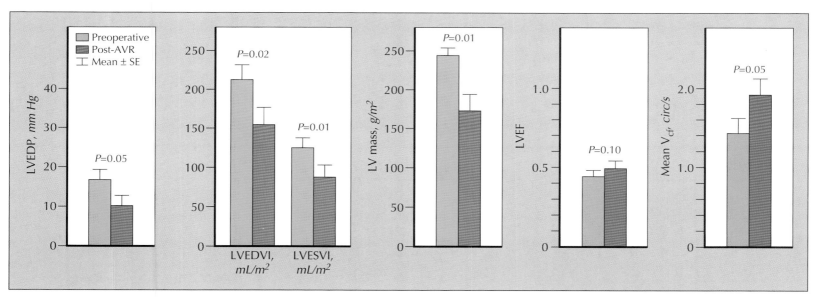

FIGURE 8-50. Effects of aortic valve replacement (AVR) on severe aortic regurgitation and left ventricular (LV) dysfunction. Patients who have abnormal LV systolic pump function undergo important changes in LV size and function over a 2-year period [65]. These patients had significant reductions in LV end-diastolic pressure (LVEDP), LV end-diastolic and end-systolic volume indices (LVEDVI and LVESVI) and LV hypertrophy (mass). LV systolic pump function was improved as demonstrated by increases in mean velocity of circumferential fiber (V_{cf}) shortening; however, LV ejection fraction (LVEF) in this study increased mildly and this change was not statistically significant.

However, it appears that these patients have no further changes in LV size, hypertrophy [66], or LVEF, which is different from those who have normal LV systolic function preoperatively. circ—circumferences. (*Adapted from* Clark *et al.* [65].)

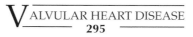

TRICUSPID AND PULMONIC VALVE DISEASE

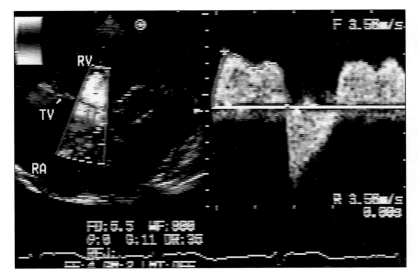

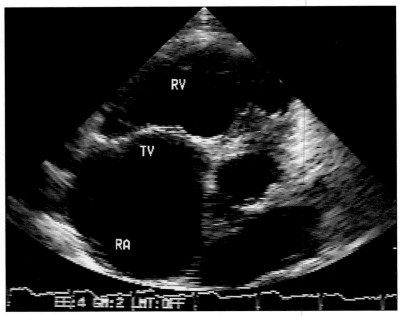

FIGURE 8-51. Doppler signal across the tricuspid valve (TV). This echocardiogram in a patient with tricuspid stenosis demonstrates the increased velocity in diastole across the tricuspid valve, calculating to a 17.8-mm Hg peak gradient with a 10-mm Hg mean gradient.

In systole there is a peak gradient of 30 mm Hg that rapidly decays in a manner consistent with severe tricuspid regurgitation. The hemodynamics of combined tricuspid stenosis and insufficiency are worse than with either lesion alone. The mean right atrial (RA) pressure is increased in tricuspid stenosis by the increase in RA volume in systole caused by the regurgitant volume due to the tricuspid insufficiency. With tricuspid regurgitation the mean RA pressure is increased by the presence of some degree of tricuspid stenosis because of the increase in RA pressure during diastole. Because the regurgitant volume increases the diastolic blood flow in the combined tricuspid stenosis and insufficiency lesion, the diastolic rumble of tricuspid stenosis is frequently very loud [67]. RV—right ventricle.

FIGURE 8-52. Two-dimensional echocardiogram in diastole in a 40-year-old patient with carcinoid tumor of the testes without metastases. He presented with a testicular mass and was found to have a grade III/VI pansystolic murmur and grade III/VI diastolic murmur; both increased with respiration. Note the thickened tricuspid valve (TV) and the lack of excursion of the TV from diastole to systole. This washer-like thickened TV is characteristic of carcinoid heart disease. It is common for a carcinoid TV to be both stenotic and insufficient. With carcinoid TV disease the valve becomes thickened and its mobility and flexibility are reduced [68]. RA—right atrium; RV—right ventricle.

PROSTHETIC VALVE

MECHANICAL VALVES

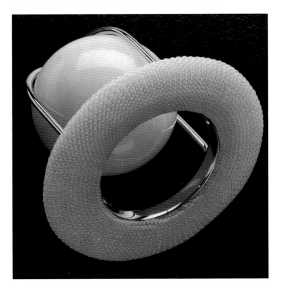

FIGURE 8-53. Starr-Edwards valve. The one-piece cage consists of a circular orifice and three (aortic) or four (mitral) thin struts joined at the apex. The poppet is molded from silicone rubber and impregnated with barium sulfate for radiopacity. The sewing ring is thickly upholstered to improve coaption with irregular tissue beds.

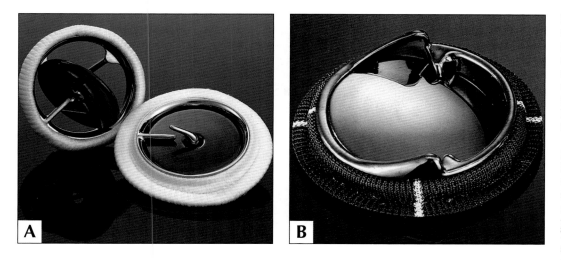

FIGURE 8-54. Medtronic Hall and Omnicarbon tilting disk valves. The Medtronic Hall valve (**A**) (Medtronic, Inc, Minneapolis, MN) has a Teflon sewing ring, a titanium housing machined from a solid cylinder, and a carbon-coated disk with flat parallel sides. The disk, which opens to 75° in the aortic model and 70° in the mitral, is retained by an S-shaped guide strut that protrudes through a hole in the center of the disk.

The Omniscience valve (not shown) (Medical, Inc), a successor of the discontinued Lillehei-Kaster Pivoting Disk valve, has a smoothly curved pyrolitic carbon disk, a one-piece titanium cage, and a polyester knit sewing ring. The disk opens to 80° and closes at an angle of 12° to the plane of the orifice, resulting in a 68° travel arc. The Omnicarbon valve (**B**) (Medical, Inc) is similar to the Omniscience valve, but is completely coated with pyrolitic carbon.

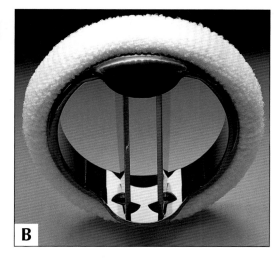

FIGURE 8-55. St. Jude bileaflet valve. The St. Jude valve (St. Jude Medical, St. Paul, MN) was the first clinically successful bileaflet valve and has been used over half a million times since its first implant in 1977. Previous bileaflet valves had been tried but were unsatisfactory; this design, with pyrolitic carbon coating and named after the patron saint of hopeless causes, led to unprecedented success and the beginning of a new family of heart valve designs.

The occluding mechanism consists of two semicircular leaflets that swing apart during opening, resulting in three separate flow areas. The housing of the valve is a cylindrically shaped piece of pyrolitic carbon with two rounded tabs, called pivot guards, which project up from the inflow side (**A**). The inside surfaces of these tabs are flat and contain two butterfly-shaped indentations that retain the leaflets (**B**). Small "ears" at the end of each diameter of the thin hemispherical leaflets fit into these indentations, which secure the leaflets in the housing and define their limits of travel.

BIOPROSTHETIC VALVES

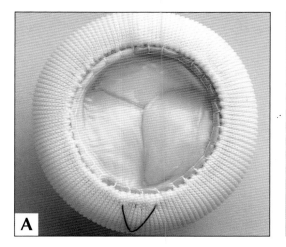

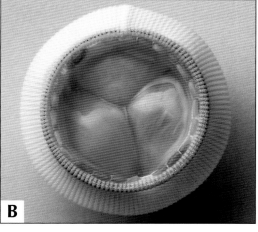

FIGURE 8-56. Hancock stented porcine valves: Standard, Modified Orifice, Hancock II, and MO II. Hancock Laboratories introduced the first commercial porcine heterograft valve in 1970, based on the glutaraldehyde treatment method developed by Carpentier *et al.* [69]. The stent is comprised of a flexible polypropylene cylinder with a radiopaque ring of Stellite 21 added for rigidity (**A**). The stent and silicone rubber sewing ring insert are covered with Dacron cloth.

The Hancock Modified Orifice (MO) valve (Medtronic, Inc, Minneapolis, MN) (**B**) was designed to overcome flow restrictions caused by the muscular shelf of the porcine right coronary cusp. The MO valve is produced by replacing its right coronary leaflet with the noncoronary cusp from a second porcine valve, creating a composite leaflet valve.

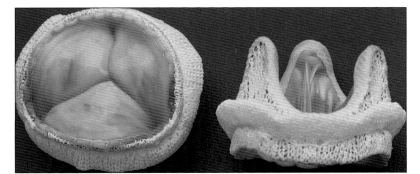

FIGURE 8-57. Carpentier-Edwards stented porcine valves: Standard, SAV, and Duraflex. The Carpentier-Edwards (Standard) (Baxter Healthcare Corporation, Irvine, CA) porcine bioprosthesis was released for general marketing shortly after the Hancock valve. The frame of the valve is a flexible wire stent made of Elgiloy, intended to reduce stresses on the leaflets and orifice. A flexible Mylar cylinder surrounds and supports the Elgiloy frame. The annulus is asymmetrically shaped, to obliterate the septal ridge of the porcine right coronary cusp.

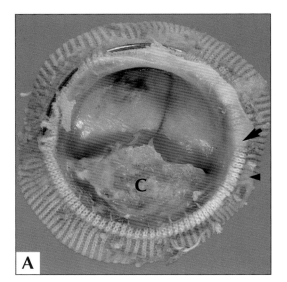

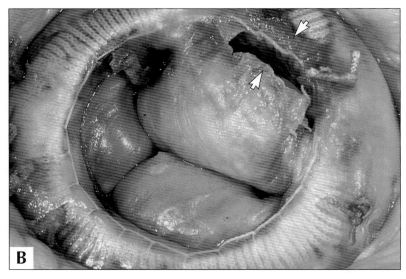

FIGURE 8-58. Bioprosthetic valves, degenerative changes. **A,** Mineralization occurs in virtually all bioprosthetic valves, especially in children and young adults. In this case calcification (C) was limited primarily to one cusp. The porcine AV is asymmetric, the right coronary cusp being larger, with a muscle shelf that results in less complete opening and accelerated calcification after xenotransplantation. The stent and sewing ring are denoted by the *arrow* and *arrowhead*, respectively. **B,** Perforation, bioprosthetic valve. This Hancock valve had been in the mitral position for 5 years. The patient died soon after hospitalization for sudden-onset congestive heart failure. There is a linear type II perforation (*arrows*) at the base of the cusp that does not involve the free edge.

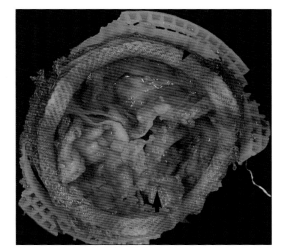

FIGURE 8-59. Bioprosthetic valve, endocarditis. Porcine valve viewed from aortic aspect is shown in this figure. Note destruction of valve leaflets by infectious vegetation (*arrow*). The infectious agent was *Staphylococcus epidermidis*; the valve was moved 1 month after insertion. Endocarditis occurs at a rate of about 5% at 5 years, and up to five times this rate in patients originally operated for endocarditis. Early infections are usually secondary to perioperative contaminants, whereas infections after 60 days result from bacteremic seeding. *Arrowhead* denotes cloth-covered stent.

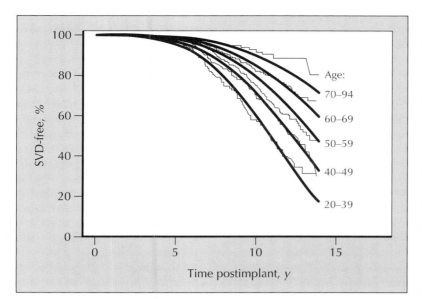

FIGURE 8-60. Actual versus actuarial freedom from structural valve deterioration (SVD). Time-related curves are required for the comparisons of biologic valves to incorporate the nonconstant risk of structural failure. It is important to understand that the usual actuarial curve gives the percentage free of an event at a given time, provided that the patients do not die (*ie*, that the risk of death has been eliminated). But many patients will die before their valve would have failed, so that the percent of patients who *actually* experience tissue failure will be lower than the usual *actuarial* estimates [70].

Shown here are the usual *actuarial* failure-free curves for 4910 operative survivors of isolated aortic or mitral replacement with Hancock or Carpentier-Edwards porcine valves from two centers (Stanford and Vancouver), followed up to 15 years, for a total of almost 30,000 valve-years [71]. The curves are stratified by age group, and a Weibull regression model based on patient age and valve position (*smooth lines*) was used to fit the actuarial Kaplan-Meier curves (*jagged lines*). Older patients have a much lower risk than younger patients.

An additional 164 patients with double valves from these same institutions were not used in the modeling above, but their risk of valve failure was as predicted based on the model for isolated valves only. Thus, the risk for a valve to fail does not seem to be influenced by the existence of a comparison valve in the same patient. (*Adapted from* Grunkemeier *et al.* [71].)

VALVE SELECTION FOR INDIVIDUAL PATIENTS

RECOMMENDATIONS FOR VALVE REPLACEMENT WITH A MECHANICAL PROSTHESIS

INDICATION	CLASS
Patients with expected long life spans	I
Patients with a mechanical prosthetic valve already in place in a different position than the valve to be replaced	I
Patients in renal failure, on hemodialysis, or with hypercalcemia	II
Patients requiring warfarin therapy because of risk factors* for thromboembolism	IIa
Patients age ≤ 65 years for AVR and age ≤ 70 years for MVR[†]	IIa
Valve re-replacement for thrombosed biologic valve	IIb
Patients who cannot or will not take warfarin	III

RECOMMENDATIONS FOR VALVE REPLACEMENT WITH A BIOPROSTHESIS

INDICATION	CLASS
Patients who cannot or will not take warfarin	I
Patients ages ≥ 65 years* needing AVR who do not have risk factors for thromboembolism[†]	I
Patients considered to have possible compliance problems with warfarin therapy	IIa
Patients ages > 70 years[‡] needing MVR who do not have risk factors for thromboembolism	IIa
Valve re-replacement for thrombosed mechanical valve	IIb
Patients ages < 65 years[‡]	IIb
Patients in renal failure, on hemodialysis, or with hypercalcemia	III
Adolescent patients who are still growing	III

*Risk factors: AF, severe LV dysfunction, previous thromboembolism, and hypercoagulable conditions.

[†]The age at which patients may be considered for biosprosthetic valves is based on the major reduction in the rate of structural valve deterioration after age 65 years and the increased risk of bleeding in this age group.

[‡]The age at which patients should be considered for biosprosthetic valves is based on the major reduction in the rate of structural valve deterioration after age 65 years and the increased risk of bleeding in this age group.

FIGURE 8-61. Selection of prosthesis for individual patients. The general principles in valve selection derive from the fundamental difference between the mechanical and biologic valves. Mechanical valves are extremely durable yet require lifetime anticoagulation to mitigate thromboembolic complications. Biologic valves have not eliminated thromboembolism, but they achieve rates comparable to those of mechanical valves without anticoagulation; however, they have limited lifetimes. Beyond this fundamental difference between types of valves, patient-specific factors influence the results as much as valve-specific factors.

Valve repair (not covered in this review) should be considered preferable to replacement for the mitral position [72,73]. Repair can also be considered for the aortic position [74]. Homografts or the Ross procedure may also be considered, especially for very young patients. However, the vast majority of patients requiring replacement will be served by one of the commercially available prostheses.

When prosthetic replacement is necessary, some general recommendations can be made with regard to valve selection, based on the above fundamental difference between valve types. A biologic valve would be preferred for a patient who cannot, or does not want to take, anticoagulants, who desires pregnancy, or who has a short life expectancy. A mechanical valve would be preferred for a patient who will be receiving anticoagulants for another reason (*eg*, previous stroke or infarction, atrial fibrillation, mechanical valve in another position), who is in renal failure or on dialysis, or who has a long life expectancy. AF—atrial fibrillation; AVR—aortic valve replacement; LV—left ventricle; MVR—mitral valve replacement. (*Adapted from* Bonow *et al.* [75].)

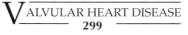

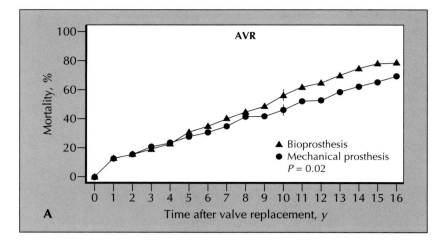

A

PROBABILITY OF AN OUTCOME EVENT AT 15 YEARS AFTER VALVE REPLACEMENT

B

	AORTIC VALVE REPLACEMENT			MITRAL VALVE REPLACEMENT		
	MECHANICAL	BIOPROSTHESIS	P VALUE	MECHANICAL	BIOPROSTHESIS	P VALUE
	n = 198	n = 196		n = 88	n = 93	
Death from any cause	66% ± 3%	79% ± 3%	0.02	81% ± 4%	79% ± 4%	0.30
Any valve related complication	65% ± 4%	66% ± 5%	0.26	73% ± 6%	81% ± 5%	0.56
Systemic embolism	18% ± 4%	18% ± 4%	0.66	18% ± 5%	22% ± 5%	0.96
Bleeding	51% ± 4%	30% ± 4%	0.0001	53% ± 7%	31% ± 6%	0.01
Endocarditis	7% ± 2%	15% ± 5%	0.45	11% ± 4%	17% ± 5%	0.37
Valve thrombosis	2% ± 1%	1% ± 1%	0.33	1% ± 1%	1% ± 1%	0.95
Perivalvular regurgitation	8% ± 2%	2% ± 1%	0.09	17% ± 5%	7% ± 4%	0.05
Re-operation	10% ± 3%	29% ± 5%	0.004	25% ± 6%	50% ± 8%	0.15
Primary valve failure	0% ± 0%	23% ± 5%	0.0001	5% ± 4%	44% ± 8%	0.0002

FIGURE 8-62. Data from the Department of Veterans Affairs randomized trial of a mechanical valve (Bjork-Shiley) versus a porcine bioprosthesis (Hancock). Maximum follow-up was 18 years, and average follow-up was 15 years. **A**, After aortic valve replacement (AVR), mortality was higher with a bioprosthesis than with a bioprosthesis; the difference started at 10 years, and at 15 years was 79% ± 3% versus 66% ± 3%, *P* = 0.02. **B**, All the complications at 15 years. Bleeding was higher with the mechanical valve; primary valve failure (structural valve deterioration) was higher with the bioprosthesis. There was no significant difference between the two valve types with regard to systemic embolism, endocarditits, valve thrombosis, or re-operation. (*Adapted from* Hammermeister *et al.* [76].)

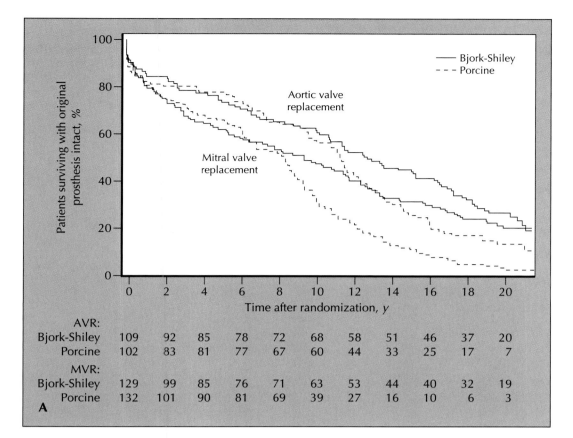

	AVR			MVR		
	MECHANICAL	PORCINE	*P* VALUE	MECHANICAL	PORCINE	*P* VALUE
Survival						
All survivors	28.4 (4.4)	31.3 (4.7)	0.57	22.4 (3.8)	18.4 (3.6)	0.41
With original prosthesis	27.5 (4.3)	13.7 (3.6)	0.025	20.7 (7.5)	3.1 (3.1)	0.002
Without major event	15.2 (3.5)	8.1 (3.0)	0.34	17.2 (7.0)	3.1 (3.1)	0.018
Valve-related events						
Re-operation	7.4 (3.0)	56.2 (8.4)	< 0.0001	13.4 (3.9)	77.6 (6.7)	< 0.0001
All bleeding	1.1 (7.6)	42.4 (12.1)	0.001	53.1 (8.2)	37.2 (0.9)	0.39
Major bleeding	37.8 (7.1)	32.0 (12.6)	0.021	47.3 (8.5)	9.5 (4.1)	0.044

TWENTY-YEAR OUTCOME DATA FROM THE EDINBURGH HEART VALVE TRIAL

B

FIGURE 8-63. Data from the Edinburgh Heart Valve Trial, a randomized trial of a mechanical valve (Bjork-Shiley) versus a bioprosthesis (Hancock or Carpentier-Edwards). Findings at 20 years are shown (**A** and **B**).

AVR—aortic valve replacement; MVR—mitral valve replacement. (*Adapted from* Oxenham *et al.* [77].)

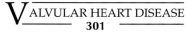

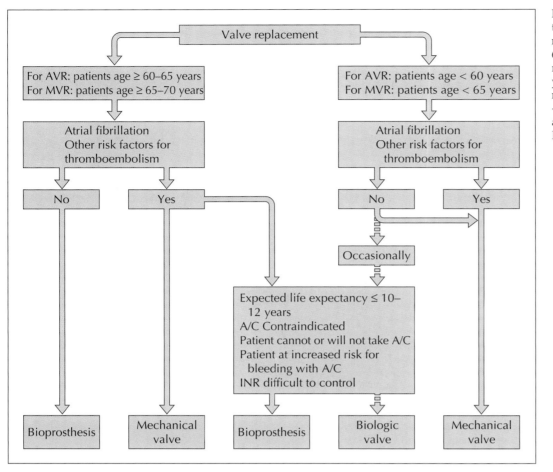

FIGURE 8-64. An algorithm for choice of a prosthetic heart valve for adult patients. Patients needing aortic valve replacement (AVR) at ages 60 to 65 years or older and patients needing mitral valve replacement (MVR) at ages 65 to 70 years or older are shown to the left. Patients needing AVR at age < 60 years and MVR at age < 65 years are shown to the right. A/C—anticoagulation; INR—International Normalized Ratio. (*Adapted from* Rahimtoola [78].)

REFERENCES

1. Dare AJ, Harrity PJ, Tazelaar HD, *et al.*: Evaluation of surgically excised mitral valves: revised recommendations based on changing operative procedures in the 1990s. *Hum Pathol* 1993, 24:1286–1293.

2. Wood P: An appreciation of mitral stenosis: Part 1. Clinical features. *BMJ* 1954, 1:1051–1063; Part 2. Investigations and results. *BMJ* 1954, 1:1113–1124.

3. Braunwald E: Valvular heart disease. In *Heart Disease*, 4th ed. Edited by Braunwald E. Philadelphia: WB Saunders; 1992:1007–1018.

4. Rahimtoola SH: Valvular heart disease. In *Internal Medicine*, 4th ed. Edited by Stein JH. St. Louis: Mosby–Year Book; 1994:214–215.

5. Ross RS: Right ventricular hypertension as a cause of precordial pain. *Am Heart J* 1961, 61:134–135.

6. Holen J, Aaslid R, Landmark K, *et al.*: Determination of pressure gradient in mitral stenosis with a noninvasive ultrasound Doppler technique. *Acta Med Scand* 1976, 199:455–460.

7. Nishimura RA, Tajik AJ: Quanititative hemodynamics by Doppler echocardiography: a noninvasive alternative to cardiac catheterization. *Prog Cardiovasc Dis* 1994, 36:309–342.

8. Inoue K, Owaki T, Nakamura T, *et al.*: Clinical application of transvenous mitral commissurotomy by a new balloon catheter. *J Thorac Cardiovasc Surg* 1984, 87:394–402.

9. Orrange SE, Kawanishi DT, Lopez BM, *et al.*: Actuarial outcome after balloon commissurotomy in patients with mitral stenosis. *Circulation* 1997, 95:382–389.

10. Iung B, Garbaz E, Michand P, *et al.*: Late results of percutaneous mitral commissurotomy in a series of 1024 patients. Analysis of late clinical deterioration: frequency, anatomic findings, and predictive factors. *Circulation* 1999, 99:3272–3278.

11. Rahimtoola SH, Durairaj A, Mehra A, *et al.*: Current evaluation and management of patients with mitral stenosis. *Circulation* 2002, 106:1183–1188.

12. Farb A, Tang AL, Atkinson JB, *et al.*: Comparison of cardiac findings in patients with mitral valve prolapse who die suddenly to those who have congestive heart failure from mitral regurgitation and to those with fatal noncardiac conditions. *Am J Cardiol* 1992, 70:234–239.

13. Carabello BA: Mitral regurgitation: basic pathophysiologic principles. Part 1. *Mod Concepts Cardiovasc Dis* 1988, 57:53–58.

14. Sonnenblick EH, Ross J Jr, Covell JW, *et al.*: Ultrastructure of the heart in systole and diastole: changes in sarcomere length. *Circ Res* 1967, 21:423–431.

15. Urschel CW, Covell JW, Sonnenblick EH, *et al.*: Myocardial mechanics in aortic and mitral valvular regurgitation: the concept of instantaneous impedance as a determinant of the performance of the intact heart. *J Clin Invest* 1968, 47:867–883.

16. Grossman W, Jones D, McLaurin LP: Wall stress and patterns of hypertrophy in the human left ventricle. *J Clin Invest* 1975, 56:56–64.

17. Wisenbaugh T, Skudicky D, Sareli P: Prediction of outcome after valve replacement for rheumatic mitral regurgitation in the era of chordal preservation. *Circulation* 1994, 89(1):191–197.

18. Helmcke F, Nanda N, Ming H, *et al.*: Color Doppler assessment of mitral regurgitation with orthogonal planes. *Circulation* 1987, 75:175–183.

19. Spain M, Smith M, Grayburn P, *et al.*: Quantitative assessment of mitral regurgitation by Doppler color-flow imaging: angiographic and hemodynamic correlations. *J Am Coll Cardiol* 1989, 13:585–590.

20. Cape E, Yoganathan P, Weyman A, *et al.*: Adjacent solid boundaries alter the size of regurgitant jets on Doppler color-flow maps. *J Am Coll Cardiol* 1991, 17:1094–1102.

21. Enriquez-Sarano M, Bailey KR, Seward JB, *et al.*: Quantitative Doppler assessment of valvular regurgitation. *Circulation* 1993, 87:841–848.

22. Jenni R, Ritter M, Eberli F, *et al.*: Quantification of mitral regurgitation with amplitude-weighted mean velocity. *Circulation* 1989, 79:1294–1299.

23. Bargiggia G, Tronconi L, Sahn D, *et al.*: A new method for quantification of mitral regurgitation based on color- flow Doppler imaging of flow convergence proximal to regurgitant orifice. *Circulation* 1991, 84:1481–1489.

24. Straub U, Feindt P, Huwer H, *et al.*: Mitral valve replacement with preservation of the subvalvular structures where possible: an echocardiographic and clinical comparison with cases where preservation was not possible. *Thorac Cardiovasc Surg* 1994, 42:2–8.

25. Goldman ME, Mora F, Guarino T, *et al.*: Mitral valvuloplasty is superior to valve replacement for preservation of left ventricular function. An intraoperative two-dimensional echocardiographic study. *J Am Coll Cardiol* 1987, 10:568–575.

26. Bonchek LI, Olinger GN, Siegel R, *et al.*: Left ventricular performance after mitral reconstruction for mitral regurgitation. *J Thorac Cardiovasc Surg* 1984, 88:122–127.

27. Lessana A, Herreman F, Boffety C, *et al.*: Hemodynamic and cineangiographic study before and after mitral valvuloplasty (Carpentier's technique). *Circulation* 1981, 64(suppl II):II-195–II-202.

28. Freeman WK, Schaff HV, Khandheria BK, *et al.*: Intraoperative evaluation of mitral valve regurgitation and repair by transesophageal echocardiography: incidence and significance of systolic anterior motion. *J Am Coll Cardiol* 1992, 20:599–609.

29. Grossi EA, Galloway AC, Parish MA, *et al.*: Experience with twenty-eight cases of systolic anterior motion after mitral valve reconstruction by the Carpentier technique. *J Thorac Cardiovasc Surg* 1992, 103:466–470.

30. Lucas RV Jr, Edwards JB: The floppy mitral valve. *Curr Probl Cardiol* 1982, 7:1–48.

31. King BD, Clark MA, Baba N, *et al.*: "Myxomatous" mitral valves: collagen dissolution as the primary defect. *Circulation* 1982, 66:288–296.

32. Stein PD, Wang CH, Riddle JM, *et al.*: Scanning electron microscopy of operatively excised severely regurgitant floppy mitral valves. *Am J Cardiol* 1989, 64:392–394.

33. O'Rourke RA, Carwford MH: The systolic click-murmur syndrome: clinical recognition and management. *Curr Probl Cardiol* 1976, 1:9–60.

34. Alpert MA, Cardney RJ, Flaker GC, *et al.*: Sensitivity and specificity of two-dimensional echocardiographic signs of mitral valve prolapse. *Am J Cardiol* 1984, 54:792–796.

35. Fontana ME, Sparks EA, Boudoulas H, *et al.*: Mitral valve prolapse and the mitral valve prolapse syndrome. *Curr Probl Cardiol* 1991, 16:315–375.

36. Devereux RB, Kramer-Fox R, Kligfield P: Mitral valve prolapse: causes, clinical manifestations, and management. *Ann Intern Med* 1989, 111:305–317.

37. Cosgrove DM, Altagracia M, Chavez MD, *et al.*: Results of mitral valve reconstruction. *Circulation* 1986, 74(suppl 1):82–87.

38. Salati M, Scrofani R, Fundaro P, *et al.*: Correction of anterior mitral prolapse: results of chordal transposition. *J Thorac Cardiovasc Surg* 1992, 104:1268–1273.

39. Cohn LH, Couper GS, Aranki SF, *et al.*: Long-term results of mitral valve reconstruction for regurgitation of the myxomatous mitral valve. *J Thorac Cardiovasc Surg* 1994, 107:143–151.

40. Passik CS, Ackermann DM, Pluth JR, Edwards WD: Temporal changes in the causes of aortic stenosis: a surgical pathologic study of 646 cases. *Mayo Clin Proc* 1987, 62(2):119–123.

41. Plantely G, Morton MJ, Rahimtoola SH: Effects of successful, uncomplicated valve replacement on ventricular hypertrophy, volume, and performance in aortic stenosis and aortic incompetence. *J Thorac Cardiovasc Surg* 1978, 75:383–391.

42. Braunwald E, Frahm CJ: Studies on the Starling's law of the heart. IV. Observations on the hemodynamic functions of the left atrium in man. *Circulation* 1961, 24:633–642.

43. Stott DK, Marpole DGF, Bristow JD, *et al.*: The role of left atrial transport in aortic and mitral stenosis. *Circulation* 1970, 41:1031–1041.

44. Ross J Jr: Afterload mismatch and preload reserve: a conceptual framework for the analysis of ventricular function. *Prog Cardiovasc Dis* 1976, 18:255–264.

45. Currie PJ, Seward JB, Reeder GS, *et al.*: Continuous-wave Doppler echocardiographic assessment of severity of calcific aortic stenosis: a simultaneous Doppler-catheter correlative study in 100 adult patients. *Circulation* 1985, 711:1162–1169.

46. Nishimura RA, Miller FA, Callahan MJ, *et al.*: Doppler echocardiography: theory, instrumentation, technique, and applications. *Mayo Clin Proc* 1985, 60:321–343.

47. Rahimtoola SH, Starr A: Valvular surgery. In *Congestive Heart Failure: Current Research and Clinical Applications*. Edited by Brunwald E, Mock M, Watson J. New York: Grune & Stratton; 1982:303–316.

48. Smith N, McAnulty JH, Rahimtoola SH: Severe aortic stenosis with impaired left ventricular function and clinical heart failure: results of valve replacement. *Circulation* 1978, 58:255–264.

49. Rahimtoola SH: Catheter balloon valvuloplasty for severe calcific aortic stenosis: a limited role. *J Am Coll Cardiol* 1994, 23:1076–1078.

50. DeMots H, Rahimtoola SH, McAnulty JH, Murphy ES: Pulmonary edema. In *Cardiac Emergencies*. Edited by Mason DT. Baltimore: Williams & Wilkins; 1978:173–223.

51. Kostuk W, Barr JW, Simon AL, Ross J Jr: Correlations between the chest film and hemodynamics in acute myocardial infarction. *Circulation* 1973, 48:624–632.

52. Kiely J, Kelly DT, Taylor DR, Pitt B: The role of furosemide in the treatment of left ventricular dysfunction associated with acute myocardial infarction. *Circulation* 1973, 48:581–587.

53. Rahimtoola SH: Management of heart failure in valve regurgitation. *Clin Cardiol* 1992, 15(suppl I):22–27.

54. Richardson JV, Karp RB, Kirklin JW, Dismukes WE: Treatment of infective endocarditis: a 10-year comparative analysis. *Circulation* 1978, 58:589–597.

55. Rahimtoola SH: Valvular heart disease: a prospective. *J Am Coll Cardiol* 1983, 1:199–215.

56. Nishimura RA, Vonk GD, Rumberger JA, *et al.*: Semiquantitation of aortic regurgitation by different Doppler echocardiographic techniques and comparison with ultrafast-computed tomography. *Am Heart J* 1992, 124:995–1001.

57. Perry G, Helmcke F, Nanda N, *et al.*: Evaluation of aortic insufficiency by Doppler color-flow mapping. *J Am Coll Cardiol* 1987, 9:952–959.

58. Pantely G, Morton MJ, Rahimtoola SH: Effects of successful, uncomplicated valve replacement on ventricular hypertrophy, volume, and performance in aortic stenosis and aortic incompetence. *J Thorac Cardiovasc Surg* 1978, 75:383–391.

59. Bonow RO, Lakatos E, Maron BJ, Epstein SE: Serial long-term assessment of the natural history of asymptomatic patients with chronic aortic regurgitation and normal left ventricular systolic function. *Circulation* 1991, 84:1625–1635.

60. Scognamiglio R, Rahimtoola SH, Fasoli G, *et al.*: Nifedipine in asymptomatic patients with severe aortic regurgitation and normal left ventricular function. *N Engl J Med* 1994, 331:689–694.

61. Taniguchi K, Nakano S, Hirose H, *et al.*: Preoperative left ventricular function: minimal requirement for successful late results of valve replacement for aortic regurgitation. *J Am Coll Cardiol* 1987, 10:510–518.

62. Levine HJ, Gaasch WH: Ratio of regurgitant volume to end-diastolic volume: a major determinant of ventricular response to surgical correction of chronic volume overload. *Am J Cardiol* 1983, 52:406–410.

63. David TE, Feindel CM, Bos J: Repair of the aortic valve in patients with aortic insufficiency and aortic root aneurysm. *J Thorac Cardiovasc Surg* 1995, 109(2):345–351.

64. Greves J, Rahimtoola SH, McAnulty JH, *et al.*: Preoperative criteria predictive of late survival following valve replacement for severe aortic regurgitation. *Am Heart J* 1981, 101:300–308.

65. Clark DG, McAnulty JH, Rahimtoola SH: Valve replacement in aortic insufficiency with left ventricular dysfunction. *Circulation* 1980, 61:411–421.

66. Bonow RO, Dodd JT, Maron BJ, *et al.*: Long-term serial changes in left ventricular function and reversal of ventricular dilatation after valve replacement for chronic aortic regurgitation. *Circulation* 1988, 78:1108–1120.

67. Pellikka PA, Tajik AJ, Khandheria BK, *et al.*: Carcinoid heart disease. Clinical and echocardiographic spectrum in 74 patients. *Circulation* 1993, 87:1188–1196.

68. Himelman RB, Schiller NB: Clinical and echocardiographic comparison of patients with the carcinoid syndrome with and without carcinoid heart disease. *Am J Cardiol* 1989, 63:347–352.

69. Carpentier A, Lemaigre G, Robert L, *et al.*: Biological factors affecting long-term results of valvular heterografts. *J Thorac Cardiovasc Surg* 1995, 58:467–483.

70. Starr A, Grunkemeier GL: The expected lifetime of porcine valves. *Ann Throac Surg* 1989, 48:317–318.

71. Grunkemeier GL, Jamieson WRE, Miller DC, Starr A: Actual vs. actuarial risk of structural valve deterioration. *J Thorac Cardiovasc Surg* 1994, 108:709–718.

72. Duran C: Mitral reconstruction in predominant mitral stenosis. In *Recent Progress in Mitral Valve Disease*. Edited by Duran C, Angell WW, Johnson AD, Oury JH. London: Butterworths; 1984:255–264.

73. Carpentier A: Mitral reconstruction in predominant mitral incompetence. In *Recent Progress in Mitral Valve Disease*. Edited by Duran C, Angell WW, Johnson AD, Oury JH. London: Butterworths; 1984:265–276.

74. Cosgrove DM, Rosenkranz ER, Hendren WG, *et al.*: Valvuloplasty for aortic insufficiency. *J Thorac Cardiovasc Surg* 1991, 102:571–576.

75. Bonow RO, Carabello B, de Leon AC Jr, *et al.*: ACC/AHA guidelines for the management of patients with valvular heart disease: a report of the American College of Cardiology/American Heart Association Task Force on Practice Guidelines (Committee on Management of Patients With Valvular Heart Disease.) *J Am Coll Cardiol* 1998; 32:1486–1588.

76. Hammermeister KE, Sethi GK, Henderson WG, *et al.*: Outcomes 15 years after valve replacement with mechanical versus bioprosthetic valve: final report of the Veterans Administration randomized trial. *J Am Coll Cardiol* 2000, 36:1152–1158.

77. Oxenham H, Bloomfield P, Wheatley DJ, *et al.*: Twenty-year comparison of a Bjork-Shiley mechanical heart valve with porcine bioprosthesis. *HEART* 2003, 89:715–721.

78. Rahimtoola SH: Choice of prosthetic heart valve for adult patients. *J Am Coll Cardiol* 2003, 41:893–904.

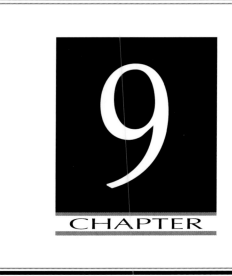

9 CHAPTER

CONGENITAL HEART DISEASE

Edited by Robert M. Freedom

Leland N. Benson, Christine Boutin, Scott D. Flamm,
Michael D. Freed, Charles B. Higgins, Paul R. Julsrud,
Luc C. Jutras, Ira A. Parness, P. Syamasundar Rao,
Stephen P. Sanders, Jeong-Wook Seo, Norman H. Silverman,
Gil Wernovsky, Shi-Joon Yoo

Congenital heart disease occurs in approximately one percent of live births. In this chapter, the pathophysiology, diagnosis, and treatment of many important congenital malformations of the heart are illustrated.

ATRIAL SEPTAL DEFECT

Atrial septal defect is a very common anomaly that occurs more frequently in females than males. There are three principal forms of atrial septal defect. Defects of the sinus venosus type occur in the superior portion of the atrial septum. They are usually associated with anomalous connection of the pul- monary veins of the right lung to the right atrium near the entry of the superior vena cava. Ostium secundum defects occur in the region of the foramen ovale, whereas ostium primum defects occur in the lower portion of the septum.

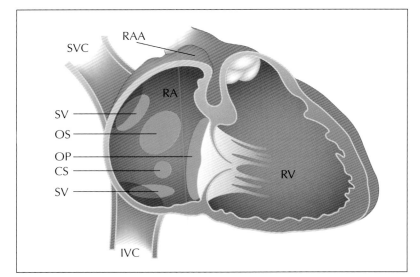

FIGURE 9-1. Diagrammatic representation of the sites of communication between the atria, shown from the perspective of the right atrium (RA). The RA, right ventricle (RV), superior vena cava (SVC), and inferior vena cava (IVC) are shown. The tricuspid valve apparatus lies between the RA and RV. The classic site of an ostium secundum (OS) atrial septal defect is shown in the confines of the fossa ovalis, the commonest site for intera- trial communications. The defects result from a deficiency of septum primum. The ostium primum (OP) defect lies adjacent to the atrioventric- ular valve. The upper sinus venosus (SV) defect occurs adjacent to SVC, while the lower SV defect occurs adjacent to the IVC. Interatrial commu- nications also occur through the coronary sinus (CS), related to a defi- ciency of the CS septum and entering through the mouth of the CS. In most patients with this defect, ultrasound is the primary mode of diag- nosis. This can be confirmed by a variety of techniques, including magnetic resonance imaging [1]. There is increasing experience with catheter-based strategies to close the secundum atrial septal defect using any number of catheter-deployed devices [2]. The relationship between cryptogenic stroke and patent foramen ovale continues to be explored [3–5]. Also, there is emerging information between migraine and patent foramen ovale [6–8]. RAA—right atrial appendage.

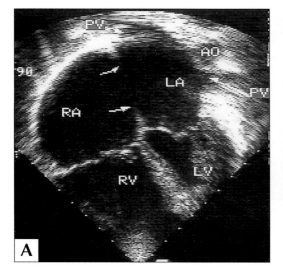

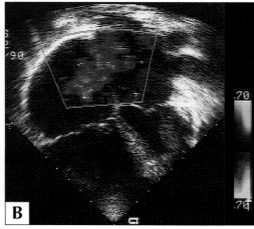

FIGURE 9-2. **A,** Apical four-chamber view of the left and right heart structures in a patient with a large ostium secundum atrial septal defect is shown (*arrows*). The pulmonary vein (PV) can be seen to enter the corners of the left atrium (LA), while the descending aorta (AO) is straddled by these two venous entry sites. **B,** During the Doppler color flow study, the diastolic frame shows transatrial flow across this large defect. The color scale on the lower left-hand part of the frame demonstrates the color assignment toward the transducer in yellow-orange, and flow away from the transducer in blue hues. The Nyquist limit, the velocity range defined by the map, is indicated at 0.70 m/s. LV—left ventricle; RA—right atrium; RV—right ventricle.

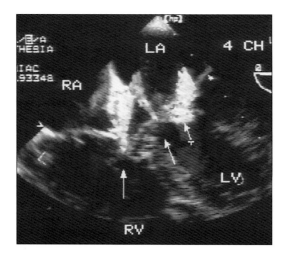

FIGURE 9-3. In this transesophageal frame of the four chambers of the heart in a patient with an ostium primum atrial septal defect taken in late systole, three regurgitation jets can be identified arising through the atrioventricular (AV) valve (*arrows*). There is lateral regurgitation between the left ventricle (LV) and left atrium (LA), probably arising from the junction between the mural leaflets and the opposed anlagen of the anterosuperior and posteroinferior bridging leaflets. There is a central jet adjacent to the atrial septum probably arising through the "cleft" between the bridging leaflets, and a separate jet between the right ventricle (RV) and right atrium (RA). Color flow Doppler study has revolutionized the definition of the shunting patterns in this group of lesions by allowing one to observe the pattern of shunt flow through the AV valve, the atrial and ventricular communication. The detection of shunting patterns is important surgically as well as prognostically [9–11]. Atrial and ventricular shunting patterns can be observed and the magnitude of the shunt size at the atrial or ventricular level estimated.

It is remarkable that there is so vast a degree of variability in the regurgitant patterns in valves that appear morphologically similar but have such a wide degree of functional impairment. Color flow is now the primary mode for Doppler ultrasound study in this condition. The AV valve regurgitation through the left side of the commissure most frequently is directed centrally and is part of the so-called LV-to-RA shunt. Less frequently the jet is directed more leftward and then becomes an LV-to-LA shunt. Ebels *et al.* [12] have suggested that this is related to the relative hypoplasia of the mural leaflet of the left component of the AV valve [9,11,12]. The regurgitation from the RA to the RV may be substantial as well.

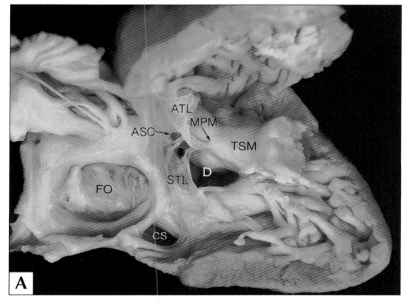

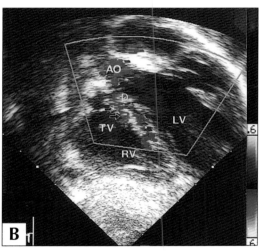

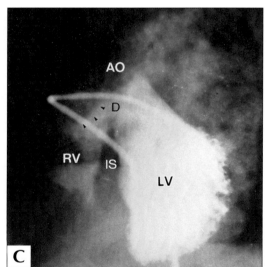

FIGURE 9-4. Perimembranous ventricular septal defects extending toward the inlet of the right ventricle (RV). Ventricular septal defect may occur as an isolated defect or as one component of a more complex congenital anomaly. Single defects usually occur in the membranous septum (perimembranous ventricular septal defect). Small defects at birth commonly close in early childhood. Large isolated defects may produce left ventricular failure in infancy and severe pulmonary hypertension in childhood leading to Eisenmenger's syndrome. **A,** RV aspect of a specimen. The defect (D) involves the inlet ventricular septum (IS) along the septal leaflet of the tricuspid valve (STL). It abuts on the anteroseptal commissure (ASC) superiorly. The medial papillary muscle (MPM) is seen at the anterosuperior aspect of the defect. **B,** Color Doppler echocardiogram in the subxyphoid long-axis plane from a different patient. The defect is located immediately below the aortic valve. The color-coded shunt flow (*arrows*) can be seen between the septal leaflet of the tricuspid valve (TV) and the IS. **C,** Left ventriculogram in long-axial oblique projection from another patient. The defect is seen immediately below the aortic valve. The initial shunt flow opacifies the inlet part of the RV between the septal leaflet (*arrowheads*) of the TV and the IS. There is increasing experience with catheter-based strategies to close the perimembranous and muscular ventricular septal defects, as well as the residual ventricular septal defect and the defect occurring after a myocardial infarction [13–16]. (Part C *from* Yoo and Choi [17]; with permission.) AO—aorta; ATL—anterior leaflet of the TV; CS—coronary sinus; FO—fossa ovalis; LV—left ventricle; TSM—trabecula septomarginalis.

Atrioventricular septal defects (AVSDs) are malformations characterized by varying degrees of incomplete development of the inferior portion of the atrial septum, the superior portion of the ventricular septum, and the mitral or tricuspid valve. The lesions include atrial septal defect of the ostium primum type, high ventricular septal defects, mitral regurgitation, and tricuspid regurgitation. These may occur singly or in any combination.

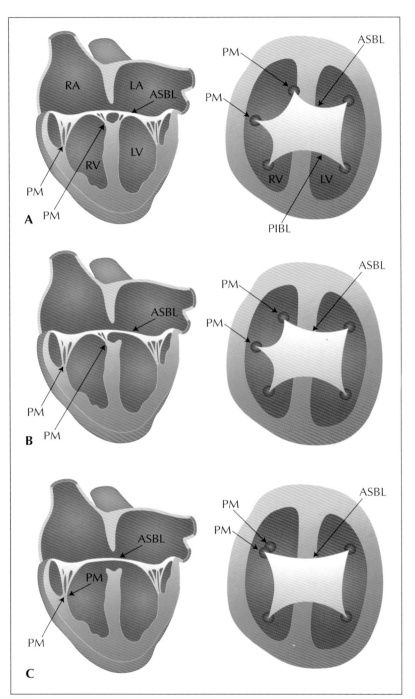

A

B

C

FIGURE 9-5. The classification of complete atrioventricular septal defects (AVSDs), popularized by Rastelli *et al.* [18], is based on the morphology of the anterosuperior bridging leaflet (ASBL), which can be displayed exquisitely echocardiographically. This diagram of a complete AVSD depicts the types of atrioventricular valve attachments of the ASBL that are identifiable echocardiographically and fit the surgical description of Rastelli. The *left-hand panels* are four-chamber views, while the *right-hand panels* are equivalent to subcostal short-axis or parasternal short-axis views.

A, Rastelli type A defect. Here the ASBL can be seen to be attached to the papillary muscle (PM) lying on the crest of the septum between the left (LV) and right (RV) ventricles. In the subcostal view, the posteroinferior bridging leaflet (PIBL) is depicted to be attached to the crest of the septum. **B,** Rastelli type B defect. The ASBL is not attached to the septum, but to PM arising from the RV. **C,** Rastelli type C defect. The ASBL is attached to PM, which also supports the other leaflet of the tricuspid valve yielding a free-floating nonattached leaflet. The *arrows* in the *right-hand panels* indicate how the PM attachment is from a septally attached (type A) to RV-originating PM (type B), and PM fused with the anterior PM within the RV (type C).

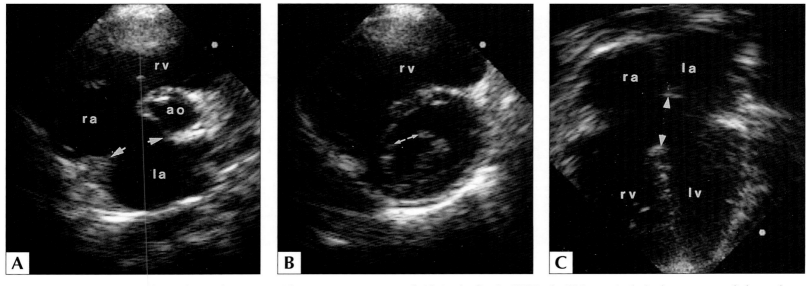

FIGURE 9-6. Transthoracic echocardiography can provide an accurate preoperative hemodynamic and morphologic evaluation of the wide spectrum of atrioventricular septal defects (AVSDs) [12,19–21]. Subcostal, parasternal short- and long-axis, and apical four-chamber views are complementary in assessing the extent of the atrial and ventricular communications, as well as the morphology, competency, and chordal attachments of the atrioventricular valves. The degree of septal malalignment, ventricular size, and outflow tract obstruction are also well defined by echocardiography. All of these different aspects of AVSDs, in addition to associated anomalies, must be addressed before surgical repair. **A,** Parasternal short-axis view illustrating the large primum defect component (*arrows*). In this patient, no ventricular septal defect was present. **B,** Parasternal short-axis view at the level of the papillary muscles (PMs). This view is ideal to evaluate the number of PMs, the distance separating them, and the cleft in the anterior bridging leaflet. In AVSDs the PMs, particularly the posteromedial muscle, are rotated counterclockwise from their normal position. This patient has two distinct PMs and the cleft is typically oriented toward the right ventricular (rv) outflow tract (*arrows*). **C,** Apical four-chamber view of a patient with a complete AVSD with the common atrioventricular valve open in diastole. Large atrial and ventricular communications are present (*arrowheads*), and there is no atrioventricular septal malalignment. Both ventricles are well developed. Because of the well-documented association with Down syndrome and the precocity for pulmonary vascular disease in this setting, most recommend early primary repair of the complete form of the atrial septal defect, preferably before 6 months of age [22.23]. Surgical results are excellent and intraoperative echocardiography has substantially improved the functional repair of the left atrioventricular valve. ao—aorta; la—left atrium; lv—left ventricular; ra—right atrium.

SUBAORTIC STENOSIS

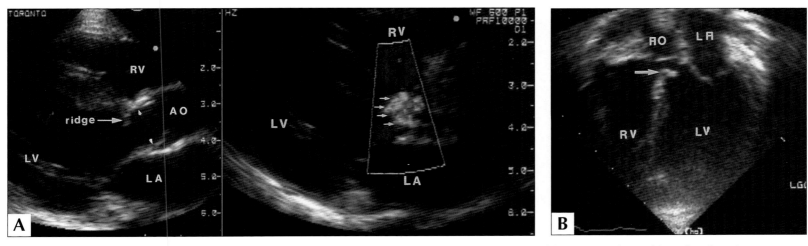

FIGURE 9-7. Although obstruction at the level of the aortic valve (congenital valvular aortic stenosis) is the most common form of congenital obstruction to left ventricular outflow, congenital subaortic stenosis due to a subaortic membrane or ridge is important to recognize since it can be readily corrected surgically. Subvalvular aortic stenosis can be the result of a discrete fibrous membrane, a thicker fibromuscular circumferential ridge, or a long tubular subaortic stenosis. This type of left ventricular (LV) outflow tract obstruction is frequently associated with ventricular septal defect, coarctation of the aorta (AO), and tubular hypoplasia of the aortic transverse arch. Optimal visualization of the subvalvular aortic stenosis can be achieved in parasternal long-axis and apical five-chamber views.
A, Parasternal long-axis view of a patient with subaortic stenosis caused by a fibrous ridge in close proximity to the aortic valve (*arrowheads*). Because of the parallel orientation of the membrane with the ultrasound beam part of the ridge (*arrow*) may not be fully imaged in this view (*left*). Color Doppler mapping is useful in confirming the LV outflow tract obstruction created by this ridge (*arrows* on *right*). **B,** The apical five-chamber view allows good delineation of the circumferential nature of the fibrous membrane beneath the aortic valve inserting at the mitral aortic junction (*arrow*). (*continued*)

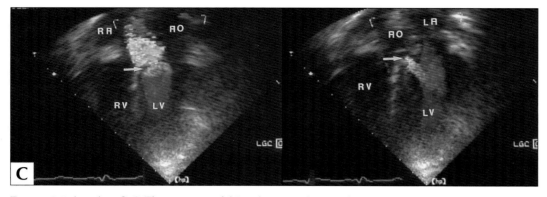

FIGURE 9-7. (*continued*) **C,** The presence of this subaortic ridge, its close proximity to the aortic valve, and the jet through the stenosis are responsible for progressive damage to the aortic valve. Color Doppler

interrogation in apical five-chamber view in the same patient illustrates the systolic flow turbulence created by the stenotic subaortic membrane (*left*), and the red diastolic aortic valve regurgitation jet directed toward the LV apex as a result of jet lesion of the aortic valve (*right*) [24,25]. *Arrows* indicate the level of the subaortic membrane. Subaortic stenosis is a peculiar disorder with features of a congenital and acquired disorder [26–28]. Subaortic stenosis seems progressive in childhood, while perhaps less so in the adult [29–31]. A sequela of this disorder is aortic regurgitation, and infective endocarditis is well known. There is ongoing debate as to the criteria for and timing of intervention [32,33]. LA—left atrium; RA—right atrium; RV—right ventricle.

COARCTATION OF THE AORTA

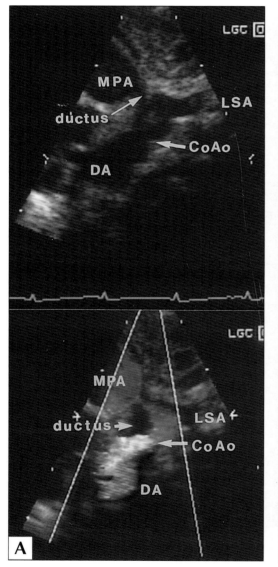

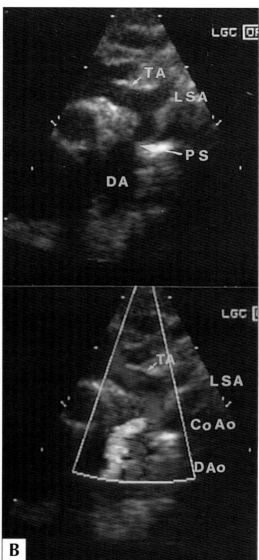

FIGURE 9-8. Coarctation of the aorta (CoAo). In this anomaly, which occurs twice as commonly in males as in females, there is constriction of the aorta, most commonly distal to the origin of the left subclavian artery. It is an important form of secondary hypertension. **A,** The ductal cut view with the transducer in the left subclavicular region is the best to show the relation between the site of coarctation created by the posterior shelf and the ductus arteriosus (*arrow*) and the origin of the left subclavian artery (LSA) (*top*). Color Doppler reveals turbulent flow beginning at the level of coarctation. In this patient, the ductus arteriosus (*arrow*) was closed as demonstrated by the absence of color signal in it (*bottom*). **B,** Coarctation of the aorta is also very well imaged from the suprasternal long-axis view. In this view the relation of the coarctation with ductus arteriosus is not well defined but the diameter of the transverse arch (*arrow*), which is often hypoplastic, can be well evaluated (*top*). As mentioned previously, color Doppler revealed the exact site of obstruction (*bottom*). (*continued*)

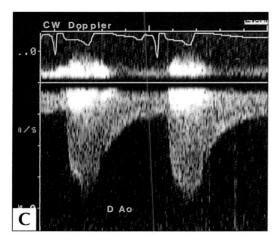

FIGURE 9-8. (continued) C, Continuous-wave Doppler examination of the descending aorta (DA/DAo) from the suprasternal notch of a patient with severe coarctation of the aorta. This negative signal represents flow away from the transducer. This is a typical flow signal observed in patients with coarctation of the aorta, with high-velocity systolic flow (3.7 m/s) continuing in diastole, representing the persistent gradient across the site of obstruction [34]. There is increasing experience with balloon angioplasty to treat native coarctation of the aorta, even in the young infant [35]. In the adult with coarctation of the aorta, endovascular stenting is being used with increasing frequency [36–39]. MPA—main pulmonary artery; PS—posterior shelf; TA—transverse arch.

EBSTEIN'S ANOMALY

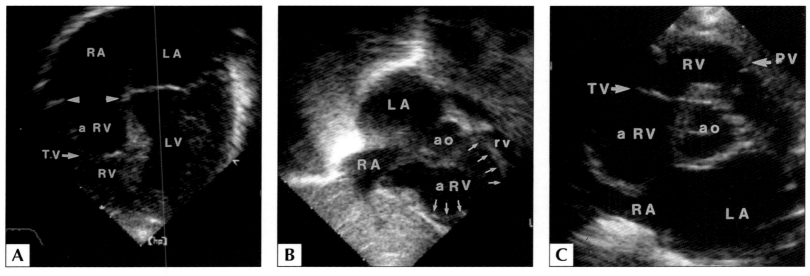

FIGURE 9-9. Patients with Ebstein's anomaly often are cyanotic due to right-to-left atrial shunting, and they frequently develop symptoms secondary to tricuspid regurgitation and right ventricular dysfunction due to hypoplasia of this chamber; paroxysmal atrial tachycardia is common as well. Surgical treatment includes prosthetic replacement of the tricuspid valve or creation of a competent unicuspid tricuspid valve by insertion of an anterior leaflet into the tricuspid annulus. Ebstein's anomaly of the tricuspid valve (TV) is characterized by dysplasia of the leaflets with downward displacement of the septal and posterior leaflets from the annulus. This results in atrialization of a portion of the right ventricle (aRV). Although the superoanterior leaflet is not displaced, its distal attachments are abnormal and may promote significant hemodynamic abnormalities. **A,** Apical four-chamber view of a patient with Ebstein's anomaly with severe inferior displacement of the TV septal leaflet (*arrow*). This view is the best to diagnose Ebstein's malformation. The anterosuperior and septal leaflets can be seen, and the degree of aRV can be evaluated as well as the severity of TV stenosis and/or regurgitation. *Arrowheads* indicate the right atrioventricular groove. **B,** Subcostal sagittal view, where inferior leaflets and the saillike anterior leaflet with its abnormal attachments can be visualized. Size and patency of the RV outflow tract can also be assessed in this plane. *Arrows* indicate the extent of the "atrialized" portion of the RV. **C,** Parasternal short-axis view showing the septal leaflet plastered down to the septal surface resulting in a displacement of the TV (*arrow*) and partial aRV. The anterior leaflet is also visualized in this view [40,41]. The outlook for the neonate presenting with Ebstein's

anomaly of the TV is far worse than those recognized later in childhood or adolescence [42–46]. Danielson *et al.* [47] have reported on the surgical results from the Mayo Clinic for this condition, analyzing the results in 189 patients operated on from 1972 to 1991. Closure of an atrial septal defect was performed on 169 patients, ablation of an accessory pathway(s) on 28 patients, and repair of ventricular septal defect in 7 patients. The perioperative mortality included 12 patients (6.3%). TV replacement was required in 69 patients, with four early deaths; eight early deaths were reported in the 110 patients undergoing placation and valvuloplasty. They were able to provide follow-up on 151 (85.3%) of the operative survivors. Ten late deaths occurred. In those who survived longer than 1-year after surgery, 92.9% were in New York Heart Association class I or II. Re-operations were required in four of the 110 patients who had undergone primary valve repair. This represented 3.6% in a follow-up extending to 19 years. This group has reviewed the late results of the bioprosthetic tricuspid valve replacement in 158 patients with Ebstein's anomaly, extending their observations from 1972 to 1997 (121). They had follow-up information on 149 patients (94.3%) who survived 30 days ranging up to 17.8 years (mean 4.5 years). The 10-year survival was 92.5% ± 2.5% (standard error). One hundred and twenty-nine late survivors (92.1%) were New York Heart Association class I or II, and 93.6% were free of anticoagulation. Freedom from bioprosthesis replacement was 97.5% ± 1.9% at 5 years and 80.6% ± 7.6% at 10 and 15 years. ao—aorta; LA—left atrium; LV—left ventricle; PV—pulmonary valve; RA—right atrium.

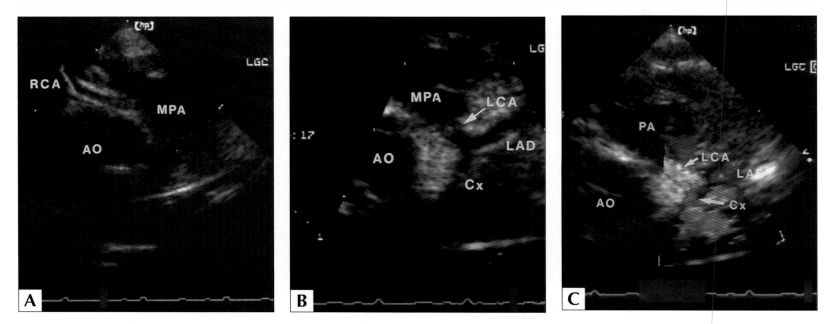

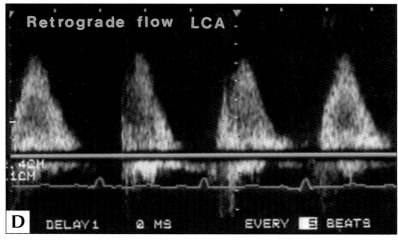

FIGURE 9-10. Infants with anomalous origin of the left coronary artery present with myocardial infarction and congestive heart failure as well as angina-like symptoms that may be misinterpreted as colic. The electrocardiogram shows deep Q waves and ST- and T-wave alterations in leads 1, aVL, V5, and V6. The chest roentgenogram usually demonstrates enlargement of the left atrium and left ventricle. Medical treatment consists of the management of heart failure, and surgical treatment involves reimplanting the left coronary artery into the aortic root. Echocardiography is critical to the diagnosis. The anomalous origin of the left main coronary artery (LCA) from the main pulmonary artery (MPA) results in progressive steal of the myocardial blood supply by retrograde flow from the coronary arteries into the pulmonary trunk as the pulmonary vascular bed resistance decreases. It is mandatory to eliminate a diagnosis of anomalous origin of the LCA when echocardiographic signs such as poorly contractile and dilated left ventricle with evidence of endocardial fibroelastosis and mitral valve regurgitation are present. **A,** One of the most pathognomonic echocardiographic signs is the diffuse dilation of the right coronary artery (RCA). **B,** Parasternal short-axis view with clockwise rotation of the transducer illustrating the LCA originating from the MPA trunk usually from the posterior surface. In some cases, the coronary ostium is difficult to visualize properly, and Doppler interrogation has proven to be very helpful in defining the origin and direction of the coronary blood supply. **C,** In the parasternal short-axis view, color Doppler examination reveals retrograde flow in the left anterior descending (LAD; *blue*) and the circumflex (Cx; *red*) coronary arteries going toward the MPA. **D,** In the same position, pulsed Doppler interrogation confirmed the retrograde diastolic flow in the LCA [48]. The results of re-implantation of the anomalous LCA in infancy are excellent, including those requiring left ventricular mechanical support [49–52]. Post-repair data reveal normalization of left ventricular function, or nearly so [49–52]. AO—aorta; PA—pulmonary artery.

TETRALOGY OF FALLOT

PATHOPHYSIOLOGY

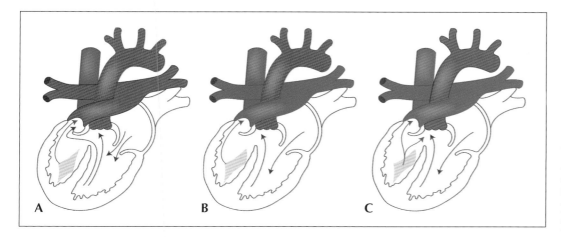

FIGURE 9-11. Pathophysiology of Tetralogy of Fallot (ToF). The physiology of ToF serves as the paradigm of VSD in association with pulmonary stenosis (PS). Because the VSD is usually nonrestrictive, the degree of PS determines the amount of pulmonary blood flow. Perhaps surprisingly in ToF, PS may be mild enough to allow a net left-to-right shunt (**A**), even to the extent of causing symptoms and signs of pulmonary overcirculation [53]. If the degree of PS is moderate (**B**), the circulation may be balanced with minimal shunting in either direction. As PS becomes more severe (**C**), right-to-left shunting at the level of the VSD increases, causing increasing cyanosis. With critical stenosis or atresia, pulmonary blood flow becomes dependent on alternate sources of supply. Patients may present with moderate, severe, or critical PS in infancy; others may present "pink" and then undergo "transformation" into the cyanotic form of ToF as the degree of stenosis progresses [54].

IMAGING

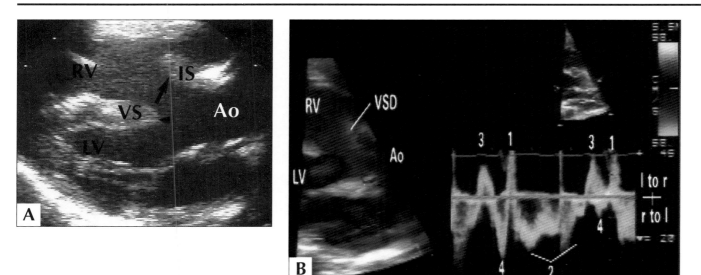

FIGURE 9-12. Parasternal long-axis views of the ventricular septal defect (VSD) in Tetralogy of Fallot (ToF). **A,** In ToF, the aorta (Ao) overrides the large defect left between the crest of the ventricular septum (VS) (*arrowhead*) and the anteriorly deviated infundibular septum (IS) (*arrow*). The latter "squeezes" the pulmonary infundibulum causing subpulmonary stenosis.

B, Although color flow mapping of the VSD in ToF demonstrates predominantly RV to LV shunting, this pulsed wave spectral display reveals complex phasic bidirectional shunting (phases 1 and 3, left to right; phases 2 and 4, right to left). Additional muscular VSDs occasionally may complicate ToF or TAC. LA—left atrium; LV—left ventricle; RV—right ventricle.

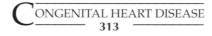

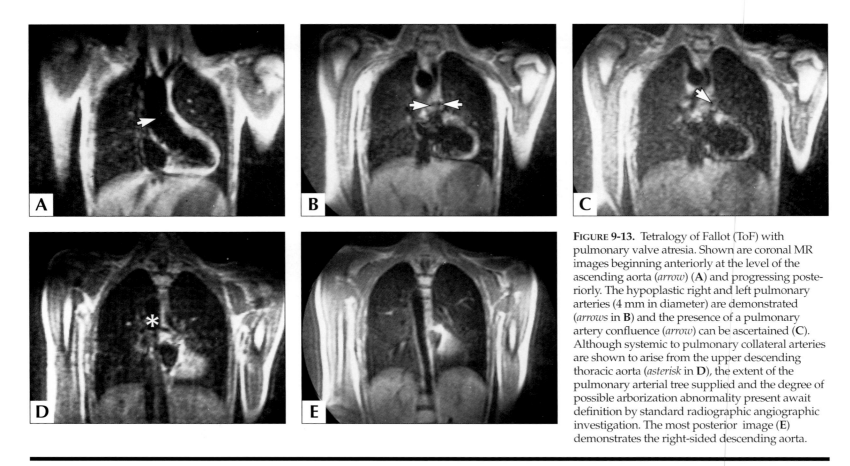

FIGURE 9-13. Tetralogy of Fallot (ToF) with pulmonary valve atresia. Shown are coronal MR images beginning anteriorly at the level of the ascending aorta (*arrow*) (**A**) and progressing posteriorly. The hypoplastic right and left pulmonary arteries (4 mm in diameter) are demonstrated (*arrows* in **B**) and the presence of a pulmonary artery confluence (*arrow*) can be ascertained (**C**). Although systemic to pulmonary collateral arteries are shown to arise from the upper descending thoracic aorta (*asterisk* in **D**), the extent of the pulmonary arterial tree supplied and the degree of possible arborization abnormality present await definition by standard radiographic angiographic investigation. The most posterior image (**E**) demonstrates the right-sided descending aorta.

CLINICAL PRESENTATION

CLINICAL PRESENTATION OF TOF					
DIAGNOSIS	AGE AT PRESENTATION	CLINICAL FINDINGS	CHEST RADIOGRAPHY	ECG	HYPEROXIA TEST (PASS: PO$_2$ ≥150 TORR WHEN FiO$_2$ = 1.0)
ToF with moderate sub-PS	Day 1 of life	Loud SEM; cyanosis proportional to degree of PS	"Boot-shaped" cardiac silhouette with scooped-out MPA segment; normal or decreased PBF	RV hypertrophy (upright T waves in V$_1$ after 3–5 d of age)	Pass or fail depending on degree of PS
ToF pulmonary atresia	1st day to months depending on source(s) and amount of PBF	Cyanosis, if too little PBF, classically with closing ductus arteriosus; CHF and continuous murmurs if too much PBF from collaterals	"Boot-shaped" cardiac silhouette with absent MPA segment; usually decreased PBF; may have abnormal PBF pattern if aortopulmonary collaterals are present	Same as ToF; may also develop LV hypertrophy if there are excessive aortopulmonary collaterals and PBF	Fail
ToF with AV canal defect	Day 1 of life	Often, trisomy 21; loud SEM; cyanosis proportional to the degree of PS	Similar to ToF; ± RA enlargement if AV valve incompetence	RV hypertrophy + superior frontal plane axis with counterclockwise looping	Pass or fail depending on degree of PS
ToF with absent pulmonary valve syndrome	Day 1 of life	Air trapping + CO$_2$ retention improved in prone position; classic loud to-and-fro murmur of PS and PR	Cardiac enlargement, bilateral hyperinflation, aneurysmal hilar PAs	Same as ToF	Fail, but picture confused by associated hypoventilation

FIGURE 9-14. Clinical presentation of Tetralogy of Fallot (ToF). This table presents the salient clinical features, common signs, symptoms, and initial laboratory evaluation of ToF, TAC, and their major variations. The "hyperoxia" test [55] involves evaluating the arterial partial pressure of oxygen (PO$_2$) of the patient 20 minutes after administration of 100% fraction of inspired oxygen (FiO$_2$), and requires normal ventilation for meaningful interpretation. AV—atrioventricular; CHF—congestive heart failure; LV—left ventricular; MPA—main pulmonary artery; PA—pulmonary artery; PBF—pulmonary blood flow; PR—pulmonary regurgitation; PS—pulmonary stenosis; RA—right atrium; RV—right ventricular; SEM—systolic ejection murmur.

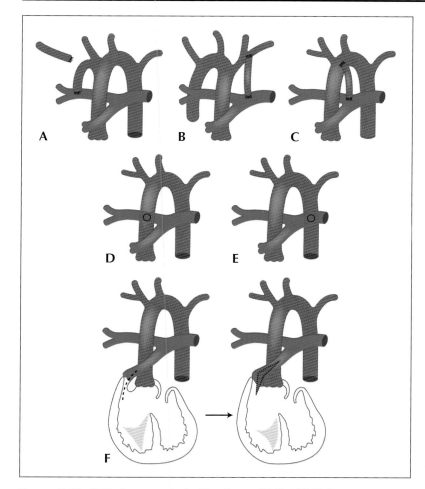

FIGURE 9-15. Palliative surgery for Tetralogy of Fallot (ToF). In most cases, complete surgical correction is the treatment of choice for ToF. However, a number of palliative procedures are also possible. **A–E,** Various palliative shunt procedures that do not require cardiopulmonary bypass. These shunts are designed to increase pulmonary blood flow and allow growth of the branch pulmonary arteries (PAs), but must be small enough to restrict transmission of aortic pressure to the PAs. The classic Blalock-Taussig (B-T) shunt (**A**) devised by dividing the subclavian artery and anastomosing it to the ipsilateral branch PA, usually on the side opposite the arch. The modified (*left*) B-T shunt (**B**) involves interposition of a prosthetic tube graft between the ipsilateral subclavian artery and branch PAs. The "central shunt" (**C**) has many variations and is usually created by placing a prosthetic tube graft between the ascending aorta and the area of the PA bifurcation. The Waterston (**D**) and Potts (**E**) shunts involve creation of direct "window" anastomoses between the right PA and the overlying ascending aorta or the left PA and the underlying descending aorta, respectively. The Waterston and Potts shunts have largely been abandoned because they were associated with a high incidence of complications such as pulmonary vascular disease and/or severe branch PA distortion. **F,** In patients with severe branch PA hypoplasia, which is associated more frequently with ToF and pulmonary atresia, a transannular outflow patch can be performed without closure of the ventricular septal defect, improving pulmonary blood flow, and allowing access for subsequent transcatheter balloon angioplasty of branch PA stenoses.

Patients with ToF are undergoing repair with excellent results in infancy, and in the majority of patients, a preoperative cardiac catheterization is not required. Pulmonary regurgitation is inevitable for most post-repair patients, with its impact on the form and function of the right ventricle [56]. In this regard, late sudden death remains a tragic event for some patients. Silka *et al.* [57] wrote that the risk of late sudden death for patients surviving operation for common congenital heart defects is 25 to

100 times greater than an age-matched control population. In their review, they found the incidence of sudden cardiac death in ToF to be approximately 1.5 per 1000 patient-years [57]. For comparison, the incidence of sudden cardiac death in complete transposition was 4.9 per 100 patient-years, and for aortic stenosis 5.4 per 1000 patient-years. Deanfield *et al.* [58] found that 12% of a cohort of unoperated patients had ventricular arrhythmia, with 0% in patients < 8 years to 58% in those > 8 years. In the corrected group of Fallot patients, 44% had a ventricular arrhythmia. This group found that the incidence of ventricular arrhythmia was associated with older age at repair, but not with era of surgery, duration of follow-up or postoperative hemodynamic status [58]. Gatzoulis *et al.* [59] studied the late follow-up of 178 adult survivors of ToF repair. These patients were observed for a mean duration since repair of 21.4 years. In this study of mechanoelectrical interaction, they found that chronic right ventricular volume overload was related to diastolic function and this correlated with QRS prolongation [60]. They found that the risk of symptomatic arrhythmia was high in patients with marked right ventricular enlargement and QRS prolongation. Their data indicate that a QRS duration on the resting electrocardiogram of 180 milliseconds or longer was the most sensitive predictor of life-threatening ventricular arrhythmia [60]. This issue is not as simple as it seems. Sarubbi *et al.* [61] have studied the accuracy and reproducibility of the measurement of QRS duration in right bundle branch block. Their findings led them to conclude that the measurement of QRS duration is difficult, can be operator-dependent, and influenced by the presence of conduction abnormalities, which reduce its accuracy and reproducibility. Kugler [62] also urges caution in using QRS duration as a marker for predicting sudden death. However, others have found that QRS prolongation is associated with inducible ventricular tachycardia after repair of ToF [63]. In the study published by Balaji *et al.* [63], induced sustained monomorphic ventricular tachycardia was related to QRS duration, right ventricular dimension, and H-V interval and symptoms. Via multivariate analysis, QRS duration was related to induced sustained monomorphic ventricular tachycardia. Furthermore, QRS duration of 180 milliseconds or longer was 35% sensitive and 97% specific for induced sustained monomorphic ventricular tachycardia [63]. Extending their original observations that QRS prolongation is a risk marker for sustained ventricular tachycardia, Gatzoulis *et al.* [64] studied depolarization-repolarization inhomogeniety after repair of ToF. They found that depolarization and repolarization abnormalities were associated with post-repair ventricular tachycardia, and that increased QT, QRS, and JT dispersion combined with a QRS of 180 milliseconds or longer refined risk stratification in these patients [64]. Berul *et al.* [65] found that the combination of QRS prolongation and increased JT dispersion had very good positive and negative predictive values for sudden death. These observations support the findings of Gatzoulis *et al.* [64] that arrhythmogenesis in post-repair ToF patients involves depolarization as well as repolarization abnormalities. Hokanson and Moller [66] studied the incidence of late sudden death in a large cohort of patients with ToF operated at the University of Minnesota between 1954 and 1974. The operative mortality during this period was 30%, and they defined an incidence of sudden death of 9%. Of the 288 patients observed for this report, no patient with sudden death had documented QRS duration of > 180 milliseconds. Ten patients had at least one electrocardiogram with QRS duration of > 180 milliseconds, but none died suddenly [66]. Rather than QRS prolongation as a marker for late sudden death, Hokanson and Moller found that transient complete heart block persisting beyond the third postoperative day most strongly correlated with sudden death [66].

In those patients with ToF, pulmonary atresia, with multiple aortopulmonary collateral arteries, there remains discussion as to the best approach. The group from the University of California at San Francisco [67–69] advocated primary repair including unifocalization with encouraging results. This group also provided guidelines as to when the ventricular septal defect should be closed, often a thorny problem [69]. Murthy *et al.* [70,71] and Cherian and Murthy [72] also have had excellent results with this approach.

TRUNCUS ARTERIOSUS COMMUNIS

In truncus arteriosus communis, a single vessel forms the outlet for both ventricles and gives rise to both the systemic and pulmonary arteries.

CLASSIFICATION OF TRUNCUS ARTERIOSUS

	Collett-Edwards	VanPraagh
	Type 1	Type A1
	Type 2	Type A2
	Type 3	Type A2
	Type 4	Tetralogy of Fallot with pulmonary atresia
	Subtype of type 3	Type A3
	Subtype of types 1 or 2	Types A4
	Type "5" (incomplete form of TAC)	Type B2
	Not encountered	Type B3

FIGURE 9-16. The classification schemes of persistent truncus arteriosus communis (TAC) as devised by Collett and Edwards [73] and VanPraagh and VanPraagh [74]. The existence of two different popular classification schemes that employ similar numerical labeling is a recipe for confusion. This figure contrasts the classification schemes of the variants of TAC encountered by these two groups of investigators. A basic disagreement over the embryologic origin of the two defects partly underlies the differing approaches to nomenclature and categorization [75–77].

Collett and Edwards [73] call the defect "persistent truncus arteriosus" and classify the anomaly according to the origin of the branch pulmonary arteries (PAs). In type 1 TAC, the branches arise from a main pulmonary artery (MPA) component; in type 2, the branches arise adjacent to one another without a distinct MPA component; and in type 3, the branches arise remotely from one another. Collett and Edwards claim that each stage, in ascending numerical order, represents persistence of an even earlier embryonic phase of development. Type 4, in which true mediastinal branch PAs are absent and "collateral" arteries from the descending aorta supply the lungs, probably does not fulfill the criteria for TAC. Calder et al. [78] have argued that Collett-Edwards type 4 TAC is really tetralogy of Fallot with pulmonary atresia, a view with which Edwards [77] later agreed.

VanPraagh and VanPraagh [74] omit "persistent" from the name TAC, believing that the defect is not the consequence of *persistence* of the embryonic truncus, but rather is a variant of pulmonary infundibular and (often) valvar atresia associated with solitary aortic trunk, and completely absent aorticopulmonary septum. They first divide TAC according to whether a ventricular septal defect (VSD) is present (type A) or absent (type B). Type B TAC in their scheme has separate semilunar valves and an intact ventricular septum, a defect that other authorities classify as the complete form of aorticopulmonary septal defect [79]. Types A1 and A2 are identical to types 1 and 2 of Collett-Edwards. The VanPraagh scheme assigns a separate category, type A3, to highlight the rare but important group of TAC with absence or discontinuity of either branch PA. In this situation, the involved lung derives its supply from a ductus or an aorticopulmonary collateral vessel. Type A4 of VanPraagh comprises the uncommon but serious group in which there is associated aortic arch interruption or coarctation. Other rare but important variants not covered in either classification include TAC with atrioventricular canal defect [80], TAC with restrictive aorticopulmonary or VSD components [81], or a common truncal valve with intact ventricular septum [82], among others [83].

PATHOPHYSIOLOGY

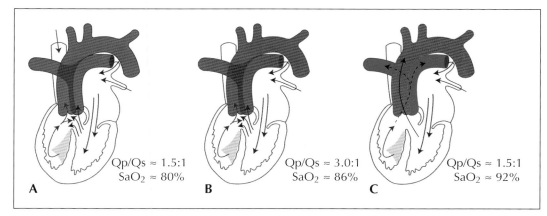

FIGURE 9-17. Pathophysiology of truncus arteriosus communis (TAC). The physiology of TAC depends in part on the presence or absence of *streaming*, separating oxygenated from deoxygenated blood despite the absence of anatomic aortopulmonary septation. Such streaming, when it occurs, is presumably related to favorable spatial orientation of the branch pulmonary arteries relative to the ventricular septal defect (VSD) and results in unexpectedly high arterial oxygen saturation (SaO$_2$). More typically, however, physiology in TAC is analogous to single ventricle in which there is common mixing of oxygenated and deoxygenated blood (at the level of the VSD in TAC). The SaO$_2$ is wholly dependent on the ratio of pulmonary-to-systemic blood flow (Qp/Qs), which in turn is inversely proportional to the pulmonary:systemic resistance ratio (Rp/Rs). As the elevated pulmonary vascular resistance (PVR) of the newborn falls, pulmonary blood flow increases associated with parallel increases in SaO$_2$ and symptoms of congestive heart failure.

A, Mixing of oxygenated with deoxygenated blood at the level of the VSD. With only mildly reduced PVR, symptoms of congestive heart failure are absent or mild. **B,** As pulmonary flow increases, consequent to a falling Rp/Rs ratio in the first weeks of life, more oxygenated blood mixes with the deoxygenated blood, resulting in a more highly oxygen-saturated systemic mixture. Unfortunately, this improved SaO$_2$ is at the expense of pulmonary overcirculation and consequent heart failure. **C,** The less common situation in which the oxygenated and deoxygenated blood streams cross each other with little mixing, allowing excellent systemic oxygen saturation irrespective of the amount of pulmonary blood flow. This situation may allow the patient to pass a "hyperoxia" test and to have a high SaO$_2$ without the expected signs and symptoms of pulmonary overcirculation.

IMAGING

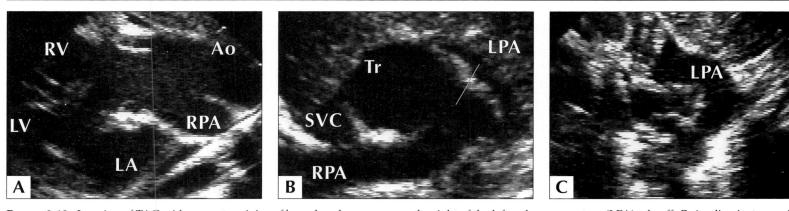

FIGURE 9-18. Imaging of TAC with separate origins of branch pulmonary arteries from the truncus (type A2 of the VanPraagh classification). **A,** A parasternal long-axis view shows excellent systolic excursion of the thin truncal valve overriding the crest of the ventricular septum. **B,** The course of the right pulmonary artery (RPA) posterior to the truncus (Tr) is best displayed in a high parasternal transverse plane. The right pulmonary artery (RPA) arises from the posterior aspect of the truncus, immediately to the right of the left pulmonary artery (LPA) takeoff. **C,** Angling just superior to the RPA orifice and rotating counterclockwise displays the course of the LPA. Not infrequently, it is difficult by any imaging modality to distinguish between adjacent separate branch pulmonary artery origins from the truncus versus a very short MPA component, a situation somewhat facetiously referred to as type A "1 and 1/2." Ao—aorta; LA—left atrium; LV—left ventricle; RV—right ventricle.

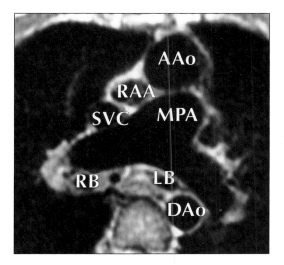

FIGURE 9-19. Axial spin-echo image showing a patient with d-transposed great arteries. The ascending aorta (AAo) is clearly seen anterior to the main pulmonary artery (MPA). Caudal images allow us to follow the AAo to the right ventricle and the MPA to the left ventricle. Although the coronary arteries are often seen in thin axial images, in many cases, their small size compared with the image thickness makes it difficult to define their precise anatomy and course. Surgical results for repair of truncus ateriosus continue to improve, including those patients with interrupted aortic arch or severe truncal valve regurgitation [84–88]. Long-term follow-up issues are related primarily for the requirement for conduit replacement and re-repair/replacement of the dysfunctional truncal valve [89,90]. DAo—descending aorta; LB—left mainstem bronchus; RAA—right atrial appendage; RB—right mainstream bronchus; SVC—superior vena cava.

COMPLETE TRANSPOSITION OF THE GREAT ARTERIES

In complete transposition of the great arteries, the aorta arises from the right ventricle, and the pulmonary artery arises from the left ventricle to the left and posterior to the aorta. In most cases there is an interatrial septal defect and a patent ductus arteriosus. Patients are characterized by severe cyanosis, congestive heart failure, and in the absence of aortic stenosis, the development of pulmonary vascular changes.

SURGICAL TREATMENT

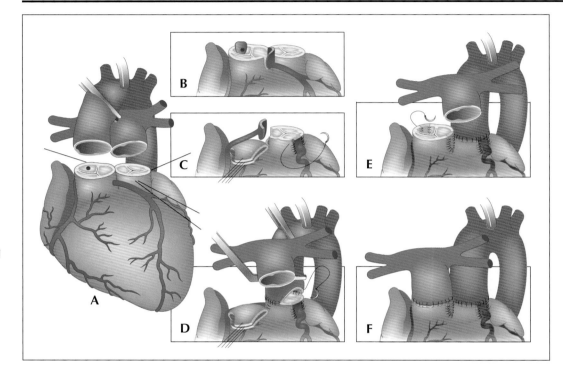

FIGURE 9-20. Technique of the arterial switch operation (ASO). The anatomic challenges of arterial switching have been met by the application of novel surgical techniques [91–95] with many individual modifications. **A,** The great arteries are transected in a manner that allows eventual reanastomosis of the distal aortic segment to the proximal pulmonary artery (PA) (neoaortic root). **B,** Transfer of the coronary arteries to this pulmonary segment is facilitated by their excision from the aortic sinus with a cuff of adjacent aortic wall. **C,** Posterior translocation of the coronary "buttons" with incorporation into the neoaortic root. **D,** The proximal neoaortic root is connected to the distal aorta by an end-to-end anastomosis; Lecompte's innovative maneuver [92] passes the previously anterior aorta behind the bifurcation of the PA. **E,** The coronary artery "donor sites" are patched with glutaraldehyde-treated pericardium. **F,** The distal PA is directly anastomosed to the neopulmonary root. Alternatively, the right ventricular–PA connections can be established by using an interposed prosthetic tubular conduit [93]. (*Adapted from* Castañeda [96].)

FIGURE 9-21. Operative mortality and risk factors for death. This graph shows survival after the arterial switch operation in patients with transposition of the great arteries (TGA) with intact ventricular septum (simple TGA) or TGA with ventricular septal defect (VSD). The *circles* and *squares* and the *t-bars* represent actuarial estimates based on reported experience from a multi-institutional study of outcomes after surgery for TGA conducted by the Congenital Heart Surgeons Society [97]. "Life table" refers to the actual Kaplan-Meier depiction; "parametric" refers to the average risk-adjusted survival obtained in the 513 patients repaired at 22 separate institutions from January 1, 1985 through March 1, 1989. Recent surgical results have improved significantly [98,99]. It is now approximately 20 years since the arterial switch procedure for neonates with transposition of the great arteries ± VSD was introduced. Mortality for coronary-uncomplicated TGA is less than 2% and long-term follow-up shows improving freedom from re-intervention. Aortic regurgitation is a well-known occurrence of follow-up, but relatively few patients require valve replacement. There are ongoing concerns about neurodevelopmental issues for these patient repaired as neonates. (*Adapted from* Kirklin *et al.* [97].)

The graph shows:

Simple TGA (*n* = 384)
TGA with VS (*n* = 129)

P (Gehan-Wilcoxon) = 0.3
P (Parametric) = 0.4

Interval, mo	Simple TGA, %		TGA with VSD, %	
	Life table	Parametric	Life table	Parametric
1	87	85	81	80
12	84	84	79	78
24	83	83	(79)	78
60	(83)	83	(79)	77

TRICUSPID ATRESIA

Tricuspid atresia is accompanied by an obligatory interatrial septal defect and usually by hypoplasia of the right ventricle and pulmonary artery. The patients are usually severely cyan-otic. The electrocardiogram shows right atrial hypertrophy, left axis deviation, and left ventricular hypertrophy.

IMAGING

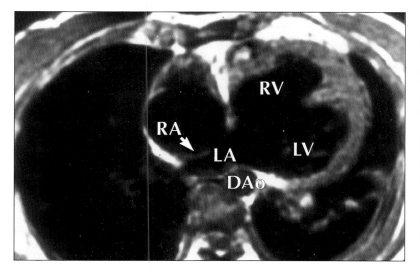

FIGURE 9-22. Axial spin-echo image from a patient with tricuspid atresia. The atrial septum (*arrow*) bulges leftward and an atrial septal defect allows systemic venous blood to drain into the left atrium (LA) and through the mitral valve. Note the bright signal intensity of the fat found in the right-sided atrioventricular (AV) groove where the tricuspid valve is expected. This entity can be differentiated from the common AV valve of an endocardial cushion defect by the preserved alignment between the right atrium (RA) and the underdeveloped right ventricle (RV) and the presence of atrial septal tissue at the crux interposed between the mitral valve and the bright signal intensity area where one expects the tricuspid valve. Note the large-inlet ventricular septal defect allowing blood from the smooth-walled morphologic left ventricle (LV) to the underdeveloped RV, and ultimately to the pulmonary artery. The four-chamber view is useful in assessing AV valve morphology and function. Cine sequences allow qualitative assessment of AV valve function in terms of valve motion and identification of stenotic or regurgitant jets. Quantitative assessment of the flow velocity and volume across the valve can be achieved using velocity-encoded cine sequences. DAo—descending aorta.

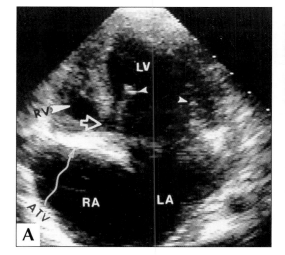
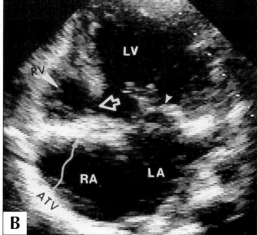

FIGURE 9-23. Apical four-chamber two-dimensional echocardiographic views (with open [**A**] and closed [**B**] mitral valve) of an infant with tricuspid atresia showing an enlarged left ventricle (LV), a small right ventricle (RV; *large arrowheads*), and a dense band of echoes at the site where the tricuspid valve should be. The ventricular septal defect (*open arrows*) and the mitral valve (*small arrowheads*) are also visible. ATV—atretic tricuspid valve; LA—left atrium; RA—right atrium.

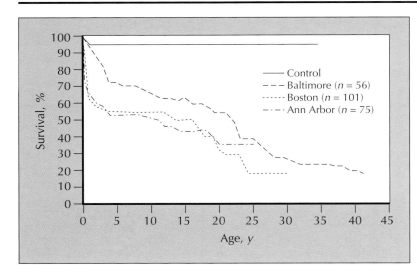

FIGURE 9-24. Actuarial survival curves from three reported clinical series of patients with tricuspid atresia [100–102] showing 1) high initial mortality in the first year of life; 2) a plateau between the first year and the middle of the second decade of life; and 3) a second bout of mortality from the middle of the second decade onward, presumably related to impaired left ventricular function [101]. The slightly higher survival rate in the Baltimore group appears to be related to the inclusion of a number of self-selected early survivors.

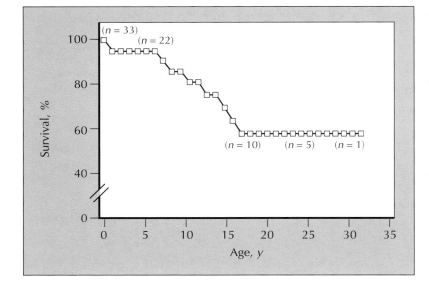

FIGURE 9-25. Actuarial survival curve of patients with tricuspid atresia who eventually underwent the Fontan operation (atrio-pulmonary artery connection) at C.S. Mott Children's Hospital in Ann Arbor, Michigan. Note that survival is slightly better in this subgroup when compared with the entire group [103]. From data published by Tam *et al.* [104] and Franklin *et al.* [105] some years ago, the outlooks for patients with tricuspid atresia, especially those with concordant ventriculoarterial connections, continue to improve. Ashburn *et al.* [106] have studied the outcomes of 112 infants with tricuspid atresia and concordant ventriculoarterial connections seen at the participating institutions within the first 3 months of age. The mean birth-weight was 3.1 kg and 15% had noncardiac anomalies. Twenty percent had pulmonary atresia; 50% had restricted pulmonary blood flow, and 20% excessive pulmonary blood flow. An arterial shunt was performed as the initial shunt in 67%, cavopulmonary shunt as the initial shunt in 24%, and pulmonary artery banding in 9%. By the conclusion of the study, 11 patients died, 10 before the Fontan. With a variety of strategies to reach a Fontan, current survival was estimated to 92% and 88% at 1 and 3 years, respectively. Thus, results for patients with the "ideal" form of tricuspid atresia continue to improve.

CATHETER-BASED INTERVENTIONS IN CONGENITAL HEART DISEASE

CATHETER THERAPEUTICS

LESIONS AMENABLE TO REPAIR

Pulmonary stenosis

Recurrent or native coarctation of the aorta

Persistent arterial duct

Atrial septal defect

Muscular ventricular septal defect

Perimembranous ventricular septal defect

LESIONS AMENABLE TO PALLIATION

Aortic valve stenosis

Postoperative systemic or venous obstruction

Prosthetic tissue valve obstruction

Pulmonary arteriovenous fistula

LESIONS AMENABLE TO PALLIATION OR AS AN ADJUNCT TO SURGERY

Occlusion of systemic to pulmonary collaterals/shunts

Venous obstructions (systemic/pulmonary)

Interarterial communications (fenestrated Fontan)

Peripheral pulmonary artery stenosis (angioplasty, stent)

FIGURE 9-26. Therapeutic catheter interventions may be corrective, reparative or palliative. As with cardiac surgery, there are three principal objectives: to improve and/or preserve cardiac function, to improve longevity, and to maintain or improve quality of life. When these ends are met, interventional catheterization obviates surgical morbidity and mortality. Unsuccessful outcomes, including complications and nondefinitive outcomes, may in part yield to experience and improvements in technique. The ingenuity of the interventional cardiologist continues to grow. Perhaps the most exciting frontier that is now being breached is fetal cardiac intervention, extending the collaboration between the pediatric cardiologist and obstetrician. There is now increasing experience with fetal intervention for critical pulmonary stenosis or aortic stenosis. Another area that warrants close observation is percuatneous implantation of the pulmonary or aortic valve. Percutaneous insertion of a pulmonary valve may dramatically alter the management of the postrepair patient with tetralogy of Fallot and free pulmonary regurgitation. In such patients, there is ongoing debate as to the indications for and timing of pulmonary valve replacement.

BALLOON ATRIAL SEPTOSTOMY

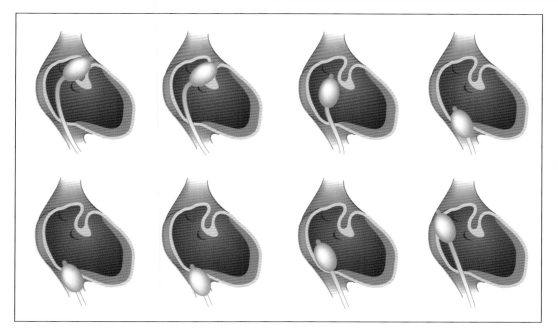

FIGURE 9-27. Sequential diagrams of a balloon atrial septostomy. The indications for this procedure include anatomic situations that have mandated a parallel pulmonary and systemic circulation or cases in which there is no egress for venous return to the concordant ventricle. Whereas these patients initially were destined for an atrial switch repair (Mustard or Senning procedure), today an anatomic correction is performed in the newborn period. Balloon septostomy is still performed frequently at diagnosis to ensure adequate arterial oxygen saturation while awaiting surgery.

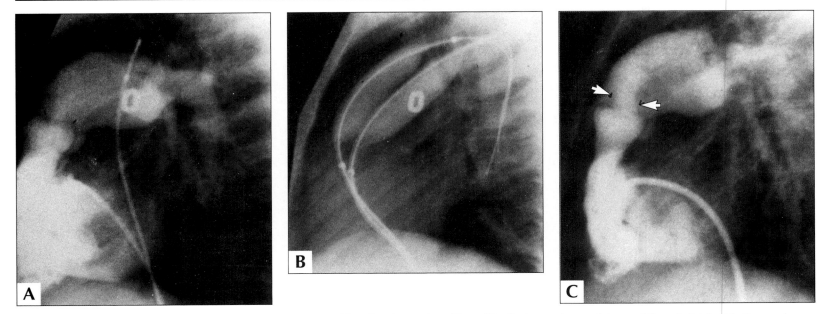

FIGURE 9-28. Typical pulmonary valve stenosis in a teenager. **A,** Thin doming valve leaflets. **B,** Two balloons inflated across the valve. **C,** Disrupted valve leaflets (*arrowheads*). Indications for pulmonary valve balloon dilation include a peak systolic right ventricular–to–main pulmonary artery gradient greater than 40 mmHg. Owing to the persistence of the arterial duct in the newborn, tricuspid regurgitation, and pulmonary hypertension, the gradient may be low (<40 mmHg). Such cases require intervention based on clinical and echocardiographic findings.

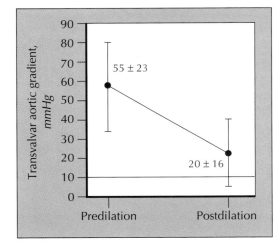

FIGURE 9-29. Results of balloon dilation of the aortic valve in 125 patients (newborns [$n = 20$] through 18 years of age). Although considered a palliative procedure, the recurrence rate requiring reintervention has been surprisingly low over the 8 years of follow-up. Surgical intervention has only been required in cases in which the hemodynamic results were not satisfactory, although a second dilation is attempted first. More often surgery is required to repair the aortic valve in those few patients ($n = 4$) with balloon-induced severe aortic regurgitation. No replacements have yet been required in our patient group due to this complication. Gradient reduction of 60% of predilation values can be achieved. An increase in angiographic grade of aortic regurgitation is frequent, but generally mild.

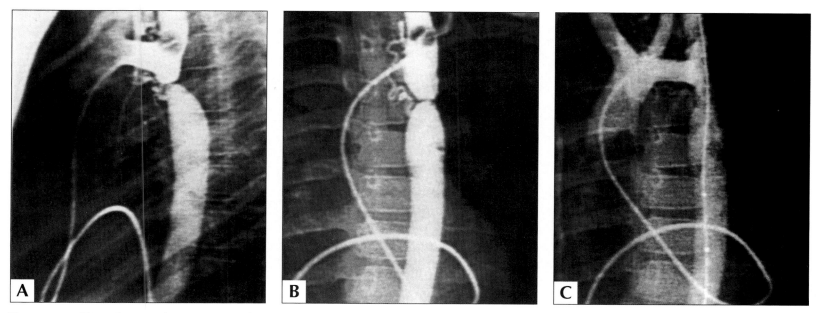

FIGURE 9-30. The indications for intervention for unoperated lesions are the same as those for recurrent coarctation. Early experience has suggested that the response to dilation in the neonatal expression of the disease is transient, and few centers routinely apply this technique in that age group. At the Hospital for Sick Children in Toronto, the technique is offered as initial therapy to all patients older than 1 year of age. **A** and **B**, Ascending aortograms from a 5-year-old showing the typical weblike coarctation of the aorta, with the catheter placed from the venous circulation. **C**, After angioplasty, the stabilizing wire was placed into the left subclavian artery, which guided the balloon catheter to the site of dilation.

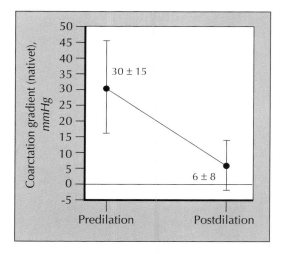

FIGURE 9-31. Results of native coarctation angioplasty at the Hospital for Sick Children, Toronto. A significant reduction in gradient was achieved. Follow-up from this patient group found a persistence of gradient reduction to 11 ± 12 mmHg [107] over a 2-year period.

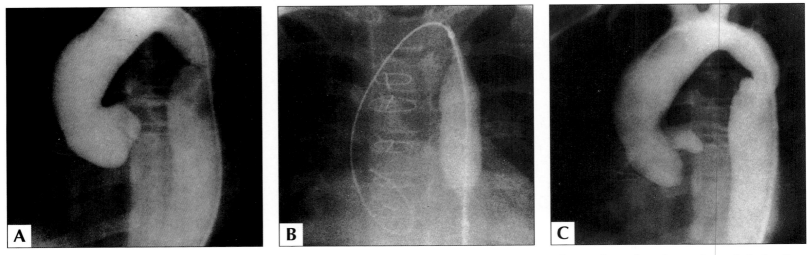

FIGURE 9-32. Recurrent coarctation after subclavian flap aortoplasty.
A, Retrograde aortogram localizing the level and extent of the coarctation.
B, Balloon dilation (usually inflated for 30 seconds) with guidewires in place
in the ascending aorta. **C,** Postdilation aortogram showing marked
improvement in stenotic segment. Balloon dilation is the primary treatment
choice for postsurgical repair of a recurrent obstruction. Its effectiveness is
not influenced by the type of repair, *ie*, patch, end-to-end, or subclavian flap.
Patients generally have systemic hypertension or an arm-leg blood pressure
difference of more than 20 mmHg at rest. As in all angioplasty procedures,
catheters should not be maneuvered past dilated segments unless guided
over a wire to prevent inadvertent transmural catheter passage.

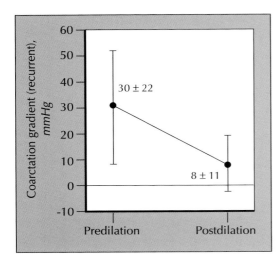

FIGURE 9-33. Results of angioplasty procedures in 89 patients with recurrent coarctation at the Hospital
for Sick Children, Toronto, over an 8-year period (1987–1995). These results are similar to those reported
by the multicenter Valvuloplasty and Angioplasty of Congenital Anomalies (VACA) Registry [108].
Follow-up data from this population (mean, 3 years) would suggest long-term gradient relief, although
surgical reintervention was required when there was an associated hypoplastic transverse arch.

REFERENCES

1. Higgins CB, Silverman NH, Kersting-Sommerhoff BA, *et al.*: Congenital
   Heart Disease: Echocardiography and Magnetic Resonance Imaging. New
   York: Raven Press; 1990.

2. Freedom RM, Yoo S-J, Mikailian H, Williams WG: *The Natural and Modified
   History of Congenital Heart Disease*. Oxford: Blackwell-Futura; 2003.

3. Lamy C, Giannesini C, Zuber M, *et al.*: Clinical and imaging findings in
   cryptogenic stroke patients with and without patent foramen ovale: the
   PFO-ASA Study. Atrial Septal Aneurysm. *Stroke* 2002, 33:706–711.

4. Schuchlenz HW, Saurer G, Weihs W: Patent foramen ovale, atrial septal
   aneurysm, and recurrent stroke. *N Engl J Med* 2002, 346:1331–1332.

5. Meier B, Lock JE: Contemporary management of patent foramen ovale.
   Circulation 2003, 107:5–9.

6. Sztajzel R, Genoud D, Roth S, *et al.*: Patent foramen ovale, a possible cause
   of symptomatic migraine: a study of 74 patients with acute ischemic stroke.
   Cerebrovasc Dis 2002, 13:102–106.

7. Morandi E, Anzola GP, Angeli S, *et al.*: Transcatheter closure of patent
   foramen ovale: a new migraine treatment? *J Interv Cardiol* 2003, 16:39–42.

8. Wilmshurst PT; Nightingale S; Walsh KP; Morrison WL: Effect on migraine
   of closure of cardiac right-to-left shunts to prevent recurrence of decom-
   pression illness or stroke or for hemodynamic reasons. *Lancet* 2000,
   356:1648-1651.

9. Ebels T: Surgery of the left atrioventricular valve and of the left atrioventricular outflow tract in atrioventricular septal defect. *Cardiol Young* 1991,
   1:344–355.

10. Silverman NH, Anderson RH, Zuberbuhler JR: Atrioventricular septal
    defects: cross-sectional echocardiographic and morphologic comparisons.
    Int J Cardiol 1986, 13:309–331.

11. Meijboom EJ, Wyse RK, Ebels T, *et al.*: Doppler mapping of postoperative
    left atrioventricular valve regurgitation. *Circulation* 1988, 77:311–315.

12. Ebels T, Meijboom EJ, Anderson RH, *et al.*: Anatomic and functional
    "obstruction" of the outflow tract in atrioventricular septal defects with
    septal valve orifices ("ostium primum atrial septal defect"): an echocardio-
    graphic study. *Am J Cardiol* 1984, 54:843–847.

13. Marshalland AC, Lang P: Closing ventricular septal defects in the cardiac catheterization laboratory. *Heart Dis* 2002, 4:51–53.

14. Hijazi ZM, Hakim F, Haweleh AA, *et al.*: Catheter closure of perimembranous ventricular septal defects using the new Amplatzer membranous VSD occluder: initial clinical experience. *Catheter Cardiovasc Interv* 2002, 56:508–515.

15. Arora R, Trehan V, Kumar A, *et al.*: Transcatheter closure of congenital ventricular septal defects: experience with various devices. *J Interv Cardiol* 2003, 16:83–91.

16. Chessa M, Carminati M, Cao QL, *et al.*: Transcatheter closure of congenital and acquired muscular ventricular septal defects using the Amplatzer device. *J Invasive Cardiol* 2002, 14:322–327.

17. Yoo S-J, Choi Y-H: Ventricular septal defect. In *Angiograms in Congenital Heart Disease*. Edited by Yoo S-J, Choi Y-H. Oxford: Oxford University Press; 1991:29–54.

18. Rastelli GC, Kirklin JW, Titus JL: Anatomic observations on complete form of persistent common atrioventricular canal with septal reference to atrioventricular valves. *Mayo Clin Proc* 1996, 41:296–308.

19. Lipshultz SE, Sanders SP, Mayer JE, *et al.*: Are routine preoperative cardiac catheterization and angiography necessary before repair of ostium primum atrial septal defect? *J Am Coll Cardiol* 1988, 11:373–378.

20. Cabrera A, Pastor E, Galdeano JM, *et al.*: Cross-sectional echocardiography in the diagnosis of atrioventricular septal defect. *Int J Cardiol* 1990, 28:19–23.

21. Sreeram N, Stumper OFW, Kaulitz R, *et al.*: Comparative value of transthoracic and transesophageal echocardiography in the assessment of congenital abnormalities of the atrioventricular junction. *J Am Coll Cardiol* 1990, 16:1205–1214.

22. Hanley FL, Fenton KN, Jonas RA, *et al.*: Surgical repair of complete atrioventricular canal defects in infancy: twenty-year trends. *J Thorac Cardiovasc Surg* 1993, 106:387–397.

23. Najm HK, Coles JG, Endo M, *et al.*: Complete atrioventricular septal defects: results of repair, risk factors, and freedom from reoperation. *Circulation* 1997, 96:311–315.

24. Davidson WR Jr, Pasqual MJ, Fanelli C: A Doppler echocardiographic examination of the aortic valve and left ventricular outflow tract. *Am J Cardiol* 1991, 67:547–549.

25. Kleinert S, Geva T: Echocardiographic morphometry and geometry of the left ventricular outflow tract in fixed subaortic stenosis. *J Am Coll Cardiol* 1993, 22:1501–1508.

26. Freedom RM: The long and the short of it: some thoughts about the fixed forms of left ventricular outflow tract obstruction. *JACC* 1997, 30:1843–1846.

27. Cape EG, Vanauker MD, Sigfusson G, *et al.*: Potential role of mechanical stress in the etiology of pediatric heart disease: septal shear stress in subaortic stenosis. *J Am Coll Cardiol* 1997, 30:247–254.

28. Cilliers AM, Gewillig M: Rheology of discrete subaortic stenosis. *Heart* 2002, 88:335–336.

29. Bezold LI, Smith EO, Kelly K, *et al.*: Development and validation of an echocardiographic model for predicting progression of discrete subaortic stenosis in children. *Am J Cardiol* 1998, 81:314–320.

30. Rohlicek CV, del Pino SF, Hosking M, *et al.*: Natural history and surgical outcomes for isolated discrete subaortic stenosis in children. *Heart* 1999, 82:708–713.

31. Oliver JM, Gonzalez A, Gallego P, *et al.*: Discrete subaortic stenosis in adults: increased prevalence and slow rate of progression of the obstruction and aortic regurgitation. *J Am Coll Cardiol* 2001, 38:835–842.

32. Brauner R, Laks H, Drinkwater DC, *et al.*: Benefits of early surgical repair in fixed subaortic stenosis. *J Am Coll Cardiol* 1997, 30:1835–1842.

33. Gersony WM: Natural history of discrete subvalvar aortic stenosis: management implications. *J Am Coll Cardiol* 2001, 38:843–845.

34. Snider AR, Serwer GA: *Echocardiography in Pediatric Heart Disease*, ed 1. Littleton, MA: Year Book Medical Publishers; 1990.

35. McCrindle BW, Jones TK, Morrow WR, *et al.*: Acute results of balloon angioplasty of native coarctation versus recurrent aortic obstruction are equivalent. For the Valvuloplasty and Angioplasty of Congenital Anomalies (VACA) Registry Investigators. *J Am Coll Cardiol* 1996, 28:1810–1817.

36. Ledesma M, Alva C, Gomez FD, *et al.*: Results of stenting for aortic coarctation. *Am J Cardiol* 2001, 88:460–462.

37. Rosenthal E: Stent implantation for aortic coarctation: the treatment of choice in adults? *J Am Coll Cardiol* 2001, 38:1524–1527.

38. Hamdan MA, Maheshwari S, Fahey JT, Hellenbrand WE: Endovascular stents for coarctation of the aorta: initial results and intermediate-term follow-up. *J Am Coll Cardiol* 2001, 38:1518–1523.

39. Harrison DA, McLaughlin PR, Lazzam C, *et al.*: Endovascular stents in the management of coarctation of the aorta in the adolescent and adult: one-year follow-up. *Heart* 2001, 85:561–566.

40. Roberson DA, Silverman NH: Ebstein's anomaly: echocardiographic and clinical features in the fetus and neonate. *J Am Coll Cardiol* 1989, 14:1300–1307.

41. Quaegebeur JM, Sreeram N, Fraser AG, *et al.*: Surgery for Ebstein's anomaly: the clinical and echocardiographic evaluation of a new technique. *J Am Coll Cardiol* 1991, 17:722–728.

42. Celermajer DS, Cullen S, Sullivan ID, *et al.*: Outcome in neonates with Ebstein's anomaly. *JACC* 1992, 19:1041–1046.

43. Celermajer DS, Dodd SM, Greenwald SE, *et al.*: Morbid anatomy in neonates with with Ebstein's anomaly of the tricuspid valve: pathophysiologic and clinical implications. *JACC* 1992, 19:1049–1053.

44. Yetman AT, Freedom RM, McCrindle BW: Outcome in cyanotic neonates with Ebstein's anomaly. *Am J Cardiol* 1998, 81:749–754.

45. Hong YM, Moller JH: Ebstein's anomaly: a long-term study of survival. *Am Heart J* 1993, 125:1419–1424.

46. Attie F, Rosas M, Rijlaarsdam M, *et al.*: The adult patient with Ebstein anomaly: outcome in 72 unoperated patients. *Medicine* 2000, 79:27–36.

47. Danielson GK, Driscoll DJ, Mair DD, *et al.*: Operative treatment of Ebstein's anomaly. *J Thorac Cardiovasc Surg* 1992, 104:1195–1202.

48. Koike K, Musewe NN, Smallhorn JF, Freedom RM: Distinguishing between anomalous origin of the left coronary artery from the pulmonary trunk and dilated cardiomyopathy: role of echocardiographic measurement of the right coronary artery diameter. *Br Heart J* 1989, 61:192–197.

49. Azakie A, Russell JL, McCrindle BW, *et al.*: Anatomic repair of anomalous left coronary artery from the pulmonary artery by aortic reimplantation: early survival, patterns of ventricular recovery and late outcome. *Ann Thorac Surg* 2003, 75:1535–1541.

50. Cochrane AD, Coleman DM, Davis AM, *et al.*: Excellent long-term functional outcome after an operation for anomalous left coronary artery from the pulmonary artery. *J Thorac Cardiovasc Surg* 1999, 117:332–342.

51. Schwartz ML; Jonas RA; Colan SD: Anomalous origin of left coronary artery from pulmonary artery: recovery of left ventricular function after dual coronary repair. *J Am Coll Cardiol* 1997, 30:547–553.

52. del Nido PJ, Duncan BW, Mayer JE, *et al.*: Left ventricular assist device improves survival in children with left ventricular dysfunction after repair of anomalous origin of the left coronary artery from the pulmonary artery. *Ann Thorac Surg* 1999, 67:169–172.

53. Rowe RD, Vlad P, Keith JD: Atypical tetralogy of Fallot: noncyanotic form with increased lung vascularity. Report of four cases. *Circulation* 1955, 12:230–238.

54. Gasul BM, Dillon RF, Urla V, Hait G: Ventricular septal defects: their natural transformation into those with infundibular stenosis or into the cyanotic or noncyanotic types of tetralogy of Fallot. *JAMA* 1957, 164:847–853.

55. Nadas AS: Hypoxemia. In *Nadas' Pediatric Cardiology*. Edited by Fyler DC. Philadelphia: Hanley & Belfus; 1992:73–82.

56. Kirklin JW, Barratt-Boyes BG: *Cardiac Surgery*, edn 2. New York: Churchill Livingstone; 1993:861–1012.

57. Silka MJ, Hardy BG, Menashe VD, *et al.*: A population-based prospective evaluation of risk of sudden cardiac death after operation for common congenital heart defects. *J Am Coll Cardiol* 1998, 32:245–251.

58. Deanfield JE, McKenna WJ, Presbitero P, *et al.*: Ventricular arrhythmia in unrepaired and repaired tetralogy of Fallot: relation to age, timing of repair, and haemodynamic status. *Br Heart J* 1984, 52:77–81.

59. Gatzoulis MA, Balaji S, Webber SA, *et al.*: Risk factors for arrhythmia and sudden cardiac death late after repair of tetralogy of Fallot: a multicenter study. *Lancet* 2000, 356:975–981.

60. Gatzoulis MA, Till JA, Somerville J, Redington AN: Mechanoelectrical interaction in tetralogy of Fallot: QRS prolongation relates to right ventricular size and predicts malignant ventricular arrhythmias and sudden death. *Circulation* 1995, 92:231–237.

61. Sarubbi B, Li W, Somerville J: QRS width in right bundle branch block: accuracy and reproducibility of manual measurement. *Int J Cardiol* 2000, 75:71–74.

62. Kugler JD: Predicting sudden death in patients who have undergone tetralogy of Fallot repair: is it really as simple as measuring ECG intervals? *J Cardiovasc Electrophysiol* 1998, 9:103–106.

63. Balaji S, Lau YR, Case CL, Gillette PC: QRS prolongation is associated with inducible ventricular tachycardia after repair of tetralogy of Fallot. *Am J Cardiol* 1997, 80:160–163.

64. Gatzoulis MA, Till JA, Redington AN: Depolarization-repolarization inhomogeneity after repair of tetralogy of Fallot: the substrate for malignant ventricular tachycardia? *Circulation* 1997, 95:401–404.

65. Berul CI, Hill SL, Geggel RL, *et al.*: Electrocardiographic markers of late sudden death risk in postoperative tetralogy of Fallot children. *J Cardiovasc Electrophysiol* 1997, 8:1349–1356.

66. Hokanson JS, Moller JH: Significance of early transient complete heart block as a predictor of sudden death late after operative correction of tetralogy of Fallot. *Am J Cardiol* 2001, 87:1271–1277.

67. McElhinney DB, Reddy VM, Hanley FL: Tetralogy of Fallot with major aortopulmonary collaterals: early total repair. *Pediatr Cardiol* 1998, 19:289–296.

68. Reddy VM, McElhinney DB, Amin Z, *et al.*: Early and intermediate outcomes after repair of pulmonary atresia with ventricular septal defect and major aortopulmonary collateral arteries: experience with 85 patients. *Circulation* 2000, 101:1826–1832.

69. Reddy VM, Petrossian E, McElhinney DB, *et al.*: One-stage complete unifocalization in infants: when should the ventricular septal defect be closed? *J Thorac Cardiovasc Surg* 1997, 113:858–868.

70. Murthy KS, Krishnanaik S, Coelho R, *et al.*: Median sternotomy single stage complete unifocalization for pulmonary atresia, major aorto-pulmonary collateral arteries and VSD-early experience. *Eur J Cardiothorac Surg* 1999, 16:21–25.

71. Murthy KS, Rao SG, Naik SK, *et al.*: Evolving surgical management for ventricular septal defect, pulmonary atresia, and major aortopulmonary collateral arteries. *Ann Thorac Surg* 1999, 67:760–764.

72. Cherian KM, Murthy KS: Single-stage complete unifocal-ization and repair for tetralogy of Fallot, pulmonary atresia, and major aortopulmonary collateral arteries. *Adv Card Surg* 2001, 13:89–106.

73. Collett RW, Edwards JE: Persistent truncus arteriosus: a classification according to anatomic types. *Surg Clin North Am* 1949, 29:1245–1270.

74. VanPraagh R, VanPraagh S: The anatomy of common aorticopulmonary trunk (truncus arteriosus communis) and its embryologic implications: a study of 57 necropsy cases. *Am J Cardiol* 1965, 406–425.

75. Van Mierop LHS, Patterson DF, Schnarr WR: Pathogenesis of persistent truncus arteriosus in light of observations made in a dog embryo with the anomaly. *Am J Cardiol* 1978, 41:755–762.

76. Anderson RH, Thiene G: Categorization and description of hearts with a common arterial trunk. *Eur J Cardiothorac Surg* 1989, 3:481–487.

77. Edwards JE: Persistent truncus arteriosus: a comment [editorial]. *Am Heart J* 1976, 92:1–2.

78. Calder AL, Brandt PWT, Barratt-Boyes BG, Neutze JM: Variant of tetralogy of Fallot with absent pulmonary valve leaflets and origin of one pulmonary artery from the ascending aorta. *Am J Cardiol* 1980, 46:106–116.

79. Kutsche LM, Van Mierop LHS: Anatomy and pathogenesis of aorticopulmonary septal defect. *Am J Cardiol* 1987, 59:443–447.

80. Butto F, Lucas RV, Edwards JE: Persistent truncus arteriosus: pathologic anatomy in 54 cases. *Pediatr Cardiol* 1986, 7:95–101.

81. Rosenquist GC, Bharati S, McAllister HA, Lev M: Truncus arteriosus communis: truncal valve anomalies associated with small conal or truncal septal defects. *Am J Cardiol* 1976, 37:410–412.

82. Carr I, Bharati S, Kusnoor VS, Lev M: Truncus arteriosus communis with intact ventricular septum. *Br Heart J* 1979, 42:97–102.

83. Gatzoulis MA, Shore D, Yacoub M, Shinebourne EA: Complete atrioventricular septal defect with tetralogy of Fallot: diagnosis and management. *Br Heart J* 1994, 71:579–583.

84. Thompson LD, McElhinney DB, Reddy M, *et al.*: Neonatal repair of truncus arteriosus: continuing improvement in outcomes. *Ann Thorac Surg* 2001, 72:391–395.

85. Williams JM, de Leeuw M, Black MD, *et al.*: Factors associated with outcomes of persistent truncus arteriosus. *J Am Coll Cardiol* 1999, 34:545-53

86. McElhinney DB, Reddy VM, Rajasinghe HA, *et al.*: Trends in the management of truncal valve insufficiency. *Ann Thorac Surg* 1998, 65:517–524.

87. Jahangiri M, Zurakowski D, Mayer JE, et al.: Repair of the truncal valve and associated interrupted arch in neonates with truncus arteriosus. J Thorac Cardiovasc Surg 2000, 119:508–514.

88. Black MD: Truncal valve repair in common arterial trunk. *Prog Pediatr Cardiol* 2002, 15:59–63.

89. Rajasinghe HA, McElhinney DB, Reddy VM, *et al.*: Long-term follow-up of truncus arteriosus repaired in infancy: a twenty-year experience. *J Thorac Cardiovasc Surg* 1997, 113:869–879.

90. McElhinney DB, Rajasinghe HA, Mora BN, *et al.*: Reinterventions after repair of common arterial trunk in neonates and young infants. *J Am Coll Cardiol* 2000, 35:1317–1322.

91. Jatene AD, Fontes VF, Paulista PP, *et al.*: Anatomic correction of transposition of the great vessels. *J Thorac Cardiovasc Surg* 1976, 72:364–370.

92. Lecompte Y, Zannini L, Hazan E, *et al.*: Anatomic correction of transposition of the great arteries: new technique without use of a prosthetic conduit. *J Thorac Cardiovasc Surg* 1981, 82:629–631.

93. Piccoli GP, Hamilton DI: Interposition of a modified aortic homograft conduit as main pulmonary trunk in anatomic correction of transposition of the great arteries. *J Thorac Cardiovasc Surg* 1981, 82:429–435.

94. Yacoub MH, Radley-Smith R, Hilton CJ: Anatomical correction of complete transposition of the great arteries and ventricular septal defect in infancy. *BMJ* 1976, May:1112–1114.

95. Yacoub MH, Radley-Smith R, Maclaurin R: Two-stage operation for anatomical correction of transposition of the great arteries with intact interventricular septum. *Lancet* 1977, 1:1275–1278.

96. Castañeda AR: Anatomic correction of transposition of the great arteries at the arterial level. Edited by Sabiston Jr DC, Spencer FC. In *Surgery of the Chest*, ed 5. Philadelphia: W.B. Saunders; 1990:1435–1446.

97. Kirklin JW, Blackstone EH, Tchervenkov CI, Castañeda AR, and the Congenital Heart Surgeons Society: Clinical outcomes after the arterial switch operation for transposition: patient, support, procedural and institutional risk factors. *Circulation* 1992, 86:1501–1515.

98. Wernovsky G, Mayer Jr JE, Jonas RA, *et al.*: Factors influencing early and late outcome of the arterial switch operation for transposition of the great arteries. *J Thorac Cardiovasc Surg* 1995, 109:289–302.

99. Planche C, Bruniaux J, Lacour-Gayet F, *et al.*: Switch operation for transposition of the great arteries in neonates: a study of 120 patients. *J Thorac Cardiovasc Surg* 1988, 96:354–363.

100. Dick M, Fyler DC, Nadas AS: Tricuspid atresia: clinical course in 101 patients. *Am J Cardiol* 1975, 36:327–337.

101. Dick M, Rosenthal A: The clinical profile of tricuspid atresia. In *Tricuspid Atresia*. Edited by Rao PS. Mt Kisco, NY: Futura Publishing Co; 1982:83–111.

102. Taussig HB, Keinonen R, Momberger N, *et al.*: Long-term observations in the Blalock-Taussig operation IV: tricuspid atresia. *Johns Hopkins Med J* 1973, 132:135–142.

103. Dick M II, Rosenthal A: The clinical profile of tricuspid atresia. In *Tricuspid Atresia*, ed 2. Edited by Rao PS. Mt Kisco, NY: Futura Publishing Co; 1992:117–140.

104. Tam CKH, Lightfoot NE, Finlay CD, *et al.*: Course of tricuspid atresia in the Fontan era. *Am J Cardiol* 1989, 63:589–593.

105. Franklin RCG, Spiegalhalter DJ, Sullivan ID, *et al.*: Tricuspid atresia presenting in infancy: survival and suitability for the Fontan operation. *Circulation* 1993, 87:427–439.

106. Ashburn D, Van Arsdell GVS, Willliams WG: Management and outcomes for tricuspid atresia. Paper presented at the 83rd Annual Meeting of the American Association for Thoracic Surgery. Boston, MA; May 4-7, 2003.

107. Houde C, Zahn EM, Burrows PE, *et al.*: Native coarctation angioplasty, medium-term results. *J Am Coll Cardiol* 1992, 19:25A.

108. Hellenbrand WE, Allen HD, Golinko RJ, *et al.*: Balloon angioplasty for aortic recoarctation: results of valvuloplasty and angioplasty of congenital anomalies registry. *Am J Cardiol* 1990, 117:1157–1158.

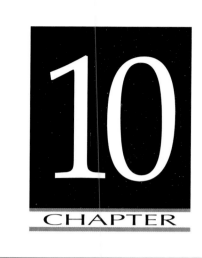

PULMONARY EMBOLISM, PULMONARY HYPERTENSION, AND CARDIAC TUMORS

Edited by Samuel Z. Goldhaber

Michael F. Allard, Richard N. Channick, Evan Loh,
Bruce M. McManus, Glenn P. Taylor, Janet E. Wilson

COR PULMONALE

The term *cor pulmonale* describes a spectrum of cardiopulmonary syndromes that are characterized by pulmonary hypertension, right ventricular hypertrophy, and right ventricular dilatation. Cor pulmonale includes a diverse range of etiologies, pathophysiologic mechanisms, and clinical characteristics. The common denominator of all these syndromes is pulmonary hypertension [1,2].

DEFINITION AND NATURAL HISTORY

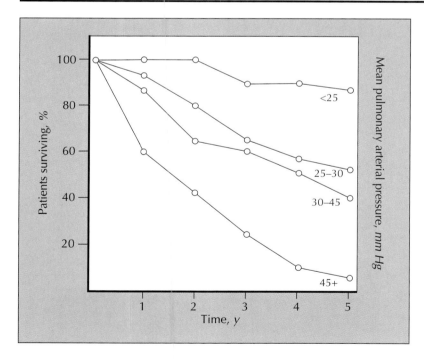

FIGURE 10-1. Correlation between survival (in years) and base-line mean pulmonary arterial pressure in patients with pulmonary hypertension secondary to parenchymal lung disease. A higher initial presenting mean pulmonary artery pressure was associated with significantly higher mortality. These findings suggest that regardless of the etiology of pulmonary hypertension, mean pulmonary artery pressure remains the single best determinant of long-term survival. (*Adapted from* Bishop [3].)

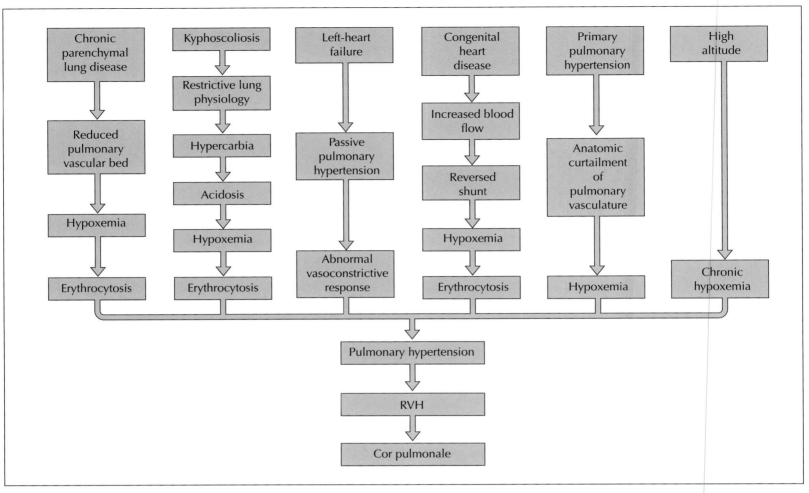

Figure 10-2. Flow diagram demonstrating the etiology and pathophysiology of cor pulmonale. General categories of disease states and the various pathophysiologic mechanisms that lead to development of the disorder are shown. Acute and chronic thromboembolic disease constitute a major cause of cor pulmonale. Note that the final common pathway for the group of diseases that comprises cor pulmonale is advanced, long-standing pulmonary hypertension. RVH—right ventricular hypertrophy.

PATHOPHYSIOLOGY

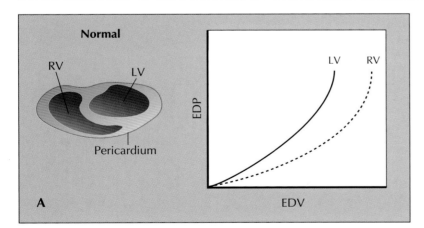

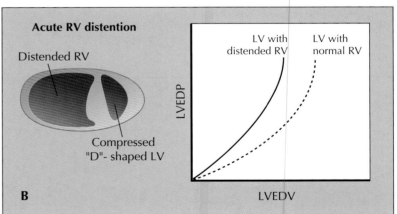

Figure 10-3. Interdependence of the right (RV) and left (LV) ventricles. **A,** Under normal conditions, the RV is much more distensible than the LV. **B,** In patients who develop acute cor pulmonale, there is a sudden and large increase in RV volume. Because of space limitations imposed by the pericardium, the distended RV impinges upon and compresses the LV cavity. The increase in RV volume causes the interventricular septum to shift toward the LV, thus causing a decrease in the dimension of the septum to free wall of the LV. The distention of the RV decreases the overall LV end-diastolic volume (LVEDV), even though the LV end-diastolic pressure (LVEDP) remains the same (*arrow*). As the LV becomes progressively less compliant, increases in LVEDP do not normally augment LVEDV. Therefore, the LV is unable to compensate for its loss of volume. Eventually, the LV cavity is obliterated, resulting in low forward cardiac output and hemodynamic collapse. (*Adapted from* Weber *et al.* [4].)

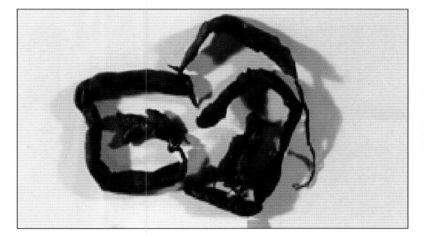

FIGURE 10-4. Acute massive pulmonary embolism (PE). This 64-year-old woman was hospitalized with "atypical chest pain." Her electrocardiogram showed sinus tachycardia, incomplete right bundle branch block, and an "S1Q3TIII pattern" with an S wave in lead I, Q wave in lead III, and inverted T wave in lead III, findings indicative of right ventricular strain. A 3- by 4-cm round mass was observed in the right ventricle, just below the tricuspid valve. This mass turned out to be a giant, curled-up venous thrombus, which embolized to the pulmonary arteries and caused massive acute PE. She was referred for emergency open surgical pulmonary embolectomy. The surgical specimen, demonstrating acute massive PE, is shown in this figure. She had an uncomplicated post-operative course [5].

PATHOPHYSIOLOGY OF PULMONARY HYPERTENSION

A — INCREASED RESISTANCE TO PULMONARY VENOUS DRAINAGE

Elevated left ventricular diastolic pressure
  Left ventricular systolic failure
  Left ventricular diastolic dysfunction
  Constrictive pericarditis
Left atrial hypertension
  Mitral valve disease
  Cor triatriatum
  Left atrial myxoma or thrombus
Pulmonary venous obstruction
  Congenital stenosis of pulmonary veins
  Anomalous pulmonary venous connection with obstruction
  Pulmonary veno-occlusive disease
  Mediastinal fibrosis

C — INCREASED RESISTANCE TO FLOW THROUGH LARGE PULMONARY ARTERIES

Pulmonary thromboembolism
Peripheral pulmonic stenosis
Unilateral absence or stenosis of the pulmonary artery

B — INCREASED RESISTANCE TO FLOW THROUGH PULMONARY VASCULAR BED

Decreased cross-sectional area of pulmonary vascular bed secondary to parenchymal diseases
  Chronic obstructive pulmonary disease
  Restrictive lung disease
  Collagen-vascular diseases (scleroderma, systemic lupus erythematosus, rheumatoid arthritis)
  Fibrotic reactions (Hamman-Rich syndrome, desquamative interstitial pneumonitis, pulmonary hemosiderosis)
  Sarcoidosis
  Neoplasm
  Pneumonia
  Status after pulmonary resection
  Congenital pulmonary hypoplasia
Decreased cross-sectional area of pulmonary vascular bed secondary to Eisenmenger's syndrome
Other conditions associated with decreased cross-sectional area of the pulmonary vascular bed
  Primary pulmonary hypertension
  Hepatic cirrhosis and/or portal thrombosis
  Chemically induced aminorex fumarate, *Crotalaria* alkaloids
  Persistent fetal circulation in the newborn

FIGURE 10-5. Clinical causes of pulmonary hypertension that either result in or are associated with cor pulmonale, including (**A**) increased resistance to pulmonary venous drainage; (**B**) increased resistance to flow through pulmonary vascular bed; (**C**) increased resistance to flow through large pulmonary arteries;

Continued on next page

FIGURE 10-5. *(Continued)* **(D)** hypoventilation; and **(E)** miscellaneous causes.

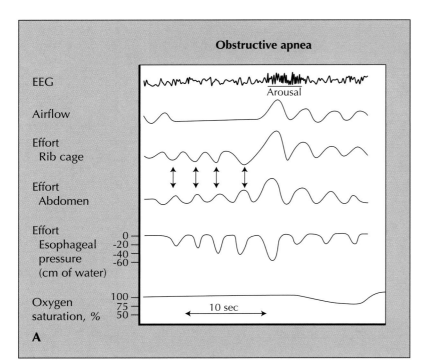

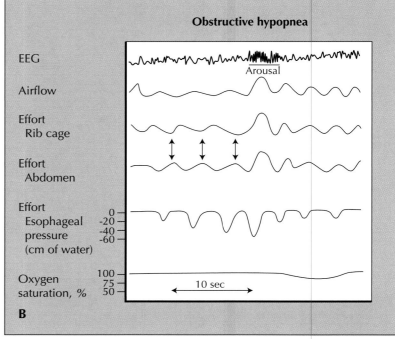

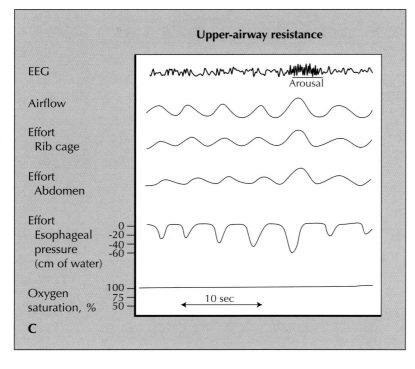

FIGURE 10-6. A–C, The sleep apnea syndrome should be suspected after eliciting a history of both daytime sleepiness and snoring while sleeping. Sleep apnea is underdiagnosed even though most patients can be effectively treated with continuous positive airway pressure. Cardiac complications include nocturnal sudden death caused by cardiac arrhythmia (especially bradyarrhythmia), myocardial ischemia, cardiomyopathy, and pulmonary and systemic arterial hypertension [6]. The major societal complication is an increased risk of traffic accidents [7] caused, in part, by lax governmental regulation of affected patients [8]. (*Adapted from* Strollo and Rogers [6].)

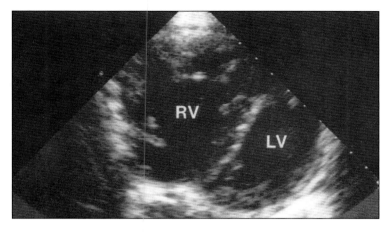

FIGURE 10-7. Echocardiographic features of the heart in a patient with cor pulmonale. Shown here is a short-axis view demonstrating a markedly enlarged right ventricle (RV) with RV hypertrophy. Abnormal bowing of the interventricular septum into the left ventricle (LV) gives a characteristic *D* configuration of the LV, consistent with volume and pressure overload of the RV.

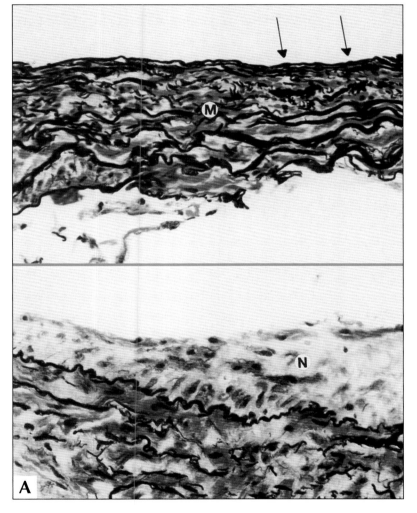

FIGURE 10-8. A–C, Assessing the etiology of pulmonary hypertension has been difficult, in part because of the inaccessibility of pulmonary vascular tissue for analysis. A novel endoarterial biopsy catheter appears successful in obtaining endovascular biopsy samples from distal canine pulmonary arteries that are 2 to 3 mm in luminal diameter [9]. (*From* Rothman *et al.* [9]; with permission.)

Continued on next page

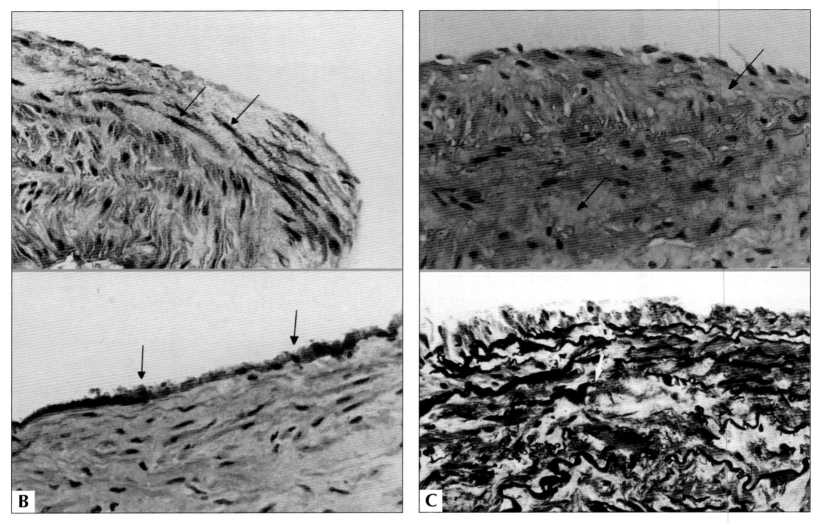

FIGURE 10-8. *(Continued)*

TREATMENT

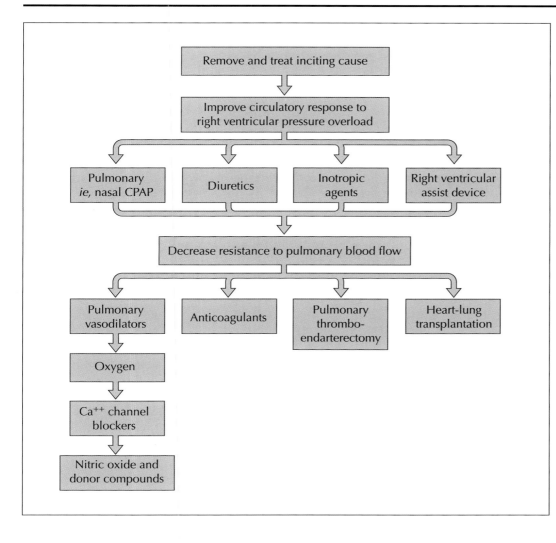

```
┌─────────────────────────────────────┐
│  Remove and treat inciting cause     │
└─────────────────────────────────────┘
                 │
                 ▼
┌─────────────────────────────────────┐
│  Improve circulatory response to     │
│  right ventricular pressure overload │
└─────────────────────────────────────┘
```

| Pulmonary *ie*, nasal CPAP | Diuretics | Inotropic agents | Right ventricular assist device |

Decrease resistance to pulmonary blood flow

| Pulmonary vasodilators | Anticoagulants | Pulmonary thrombo-endarterectomy | Heart-lung transplantation |

Oxygen

Ca++ channel blockers

Nitric oxide and donor compounds

FIGURE 10-9. Therapy for patients with advanced cor pulmonale. It is important to establish the underlying cause of the disease in order to direct therapy appropriately. General goals of therapy include improving the circulatory response to right ventricular overload and/or decreasing resistance to pulmonary blood flow by various means, such as the administration of pulmonary vasodilators, anticoagulation therapy, pulmonary thromboendarterectomy, and also heart-lung transplantation as indicated. CPAP—continuous positive airway pressure.

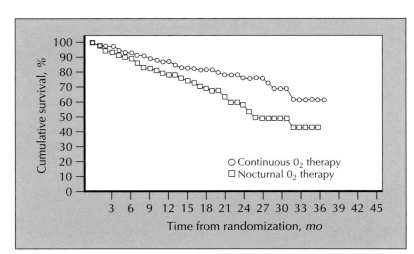

FIGURE 10-10. Oxygen therapy for hypoxemic chronic obstructive lung disease. When chronic bronchitis or emphysema is complicated by hypoxic cor pulmonale, the prognosis for surviving several years is poor. Therefore, the Medical Research Council sponsored a controlled clinical trial of administering nocturnal oxygen at home (15 hours per night of nasal prong oxygen; usually 2 L/min) versus no oxygen to determine whether oxygen

therapy reduced the 3-year mortality rate [10]. The annual mortality rate was 29% among controls compared with 12% among those who received oxygen ($P = 0.04$). Interestingly, no difference in the survival curves appeared until after approximately 500 days of oxygen therapy. It was not apparent whether continuous oxygen therapy would be superior to nocturnal oxygen. Therefore, the National Heart, Lung and Blood Institute initiated a trial at six centers in which 203 patients with hypoxemic chronic obstructive lung disease were allocated randomly either to continuous oxygen therapy or 12-hour nocturnal oxygen therapy and followed up for an average of 19 months [11]. The mortality rate was almost halved among patients who received continuous oxygen. The mechanism for this beneficial effect is not clear. Continuous oxygen reduced pulmonary vascular resistance more than nocturnal oxygen at 6 months after entry into the study; however, patients with larger decreases in pulmonary vascular resistance (> 20 dynes/s × cm^5) paradoxically tended to have a greater mortality rate than patients with smaller decreases. Patients receiving continuous oxygen therapy had an average decrement of 11% in pulmonary vascular resistance, whereas patients receiving nocturnal oxygen therapy had an average increase of 6% in pulmonary vascular resistance ($P = 0.04$). Thus, these data suggest that although continuous O$_2$ therapy reduced both mortality and pulmonary vascular resistance, the two phenomena appeared unrelated. (*Adapted from* Nocturnal Oxygen Therapy Trial Group [11].)

PRIMARY PULMONARY HYPERTENSION

Primary pulmonary hypertension (PPH) is defined clinically as a mean pulmonary arterial pressure of more than 25 mm Hg at rest or 30 mm Hg during exercise when all known causes of pulmonary hypertension have been excluded [12]. Primary pulmonary hypertension is a condition characterized by marked, chronic elevations of pulmonary vascular resistance in the absence of underlying cardiac or pulmonary disease. It occurs more often in women than in men and is observed most commonly in the third or fourth decade of life. Without treatment, the median survival is 2.8 years, with survival rates of 68%, 48%, and 34% at 1, 3, and 5 years, respectively. During the past decade, there has been a surge of interest and progress in understanding the genetics, pathophysiology, and management of this illness [13].

EPIDEMIOLOGY

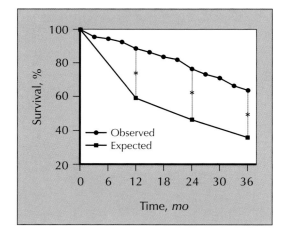

FIGURE 10-11. Three-year survival observed and predicted by the National Institutes of Health equation using baseline hemodynamics. Intravenous epoprostenol was the first Food and Drug Administration–approved therapy for primary pulmonary hypertension (PPH). It has changed the epidemiology of PPH by improving long-term survival. In this study of 162 consecutive patients, observed survival with epoprostenol therapy at 1, 2, and 3 years was 88%, 76%, and 63%, significantly greater than the expected survival of 59%, 46%, and 35% based upon historical data [14]. Baseline predictors of survival included exercise tolerance, functional class, right atrial pressure, and vasodilator response to adenosine. Predictors of survival after the first year of therapy included functional class and improvement in exercise tolerance, cardiac index, and mean pulmonary artery pressure.

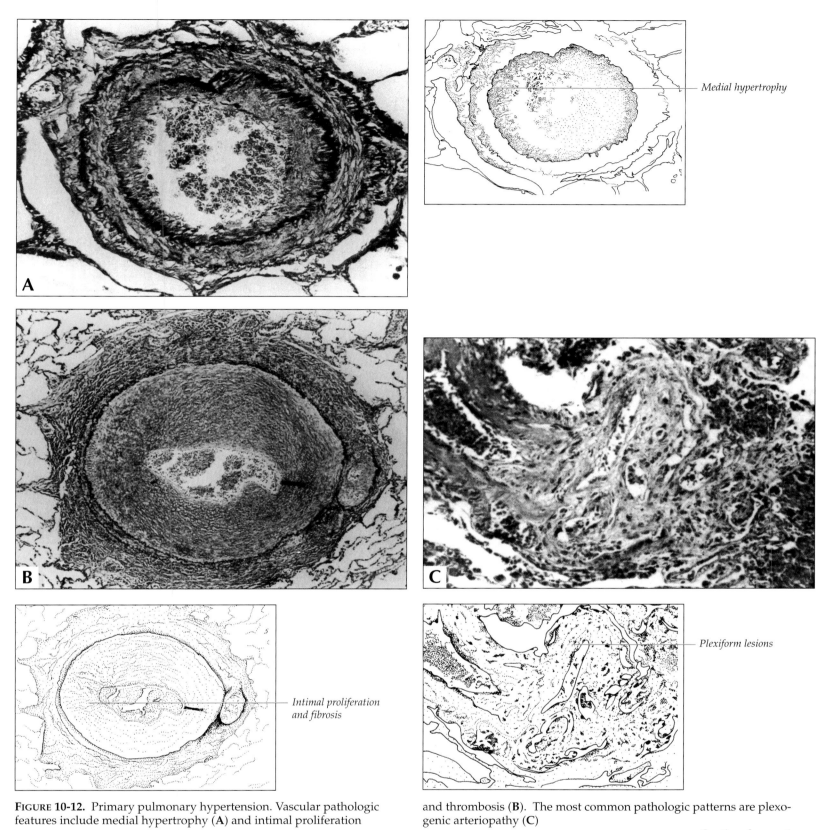

FIGURE 10-12. Primary pulmonary hypertension. Vascular pathologic features include medial hypertrophy (**A**) and intimal proliferation and thrombosis (**B**). The most common pathologic patterns are plexogenic arteriopathy (**C**)

Continued on next page

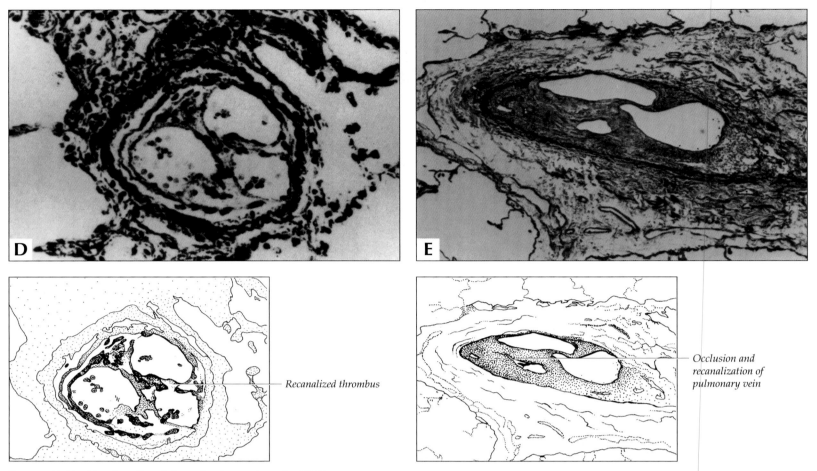

FIGURE 10-12. *(Continued)* and thrombotic arteriopathy (**D,E**).

Recanalized thrombus

Occlusion and recanalization of pulmonary vein

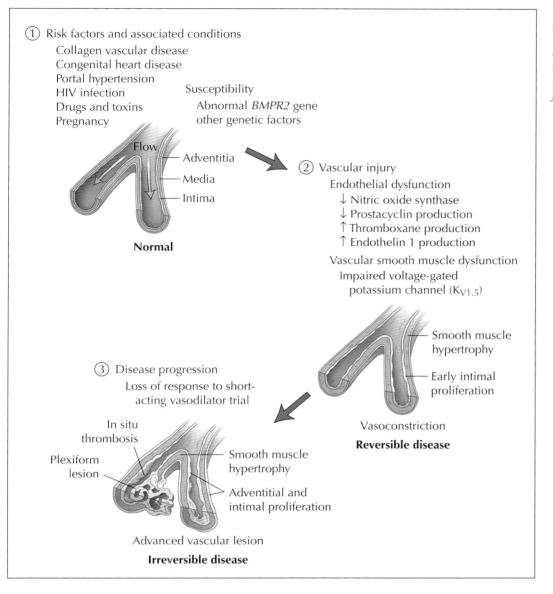

1. Risk factors and associated conditions
   Collagen vascular disease
   Congenital heart disease
   Portal hypertension
   HIV infection
   Drugs and toxins
   Pregnancy

   Susceptibility
      Abnormal *BMPR2* gene
      other genetic factors

   Flow
     — Adventitia
     — Media
     — Intima

   Normal

2. Vascular injury
   Endothelial dysfunction
     ↓ Nitric oxide synthase
     ↓ Prostacyclin production
     ↑ Thromboxane production
     ↑ Endothelin 1 production

   Vascular smooth muscle dysfunction
   Impaired voltage-gated
     potassium channel ($K_{V1.5}$)

   — Smooth muscle
     hypertrophy

   — Early intimal
     proliferation

   Vasoconstriction
   Reversible disease

3. Disease progression
   Loss of response to short-
     acting vasodilator trial

   In situ
   thrombosis

   Plexiform
   lesion

   Smooth muscle
   hypertrophy

   Adventitial and
   intimal proliferation

   Advanced vascular lesion
   Irreversible disease

FIGURE 10-13. Pathogenesis of pulmonary arterial hypertension. Pulmonary arterial hypertension occurs in susceptible patients as a result of an insult to the pulmonary vascular bed resulting in an injury that progresses to produce the characteristic pathologic features. (*Adapted from* Gaine [15].)

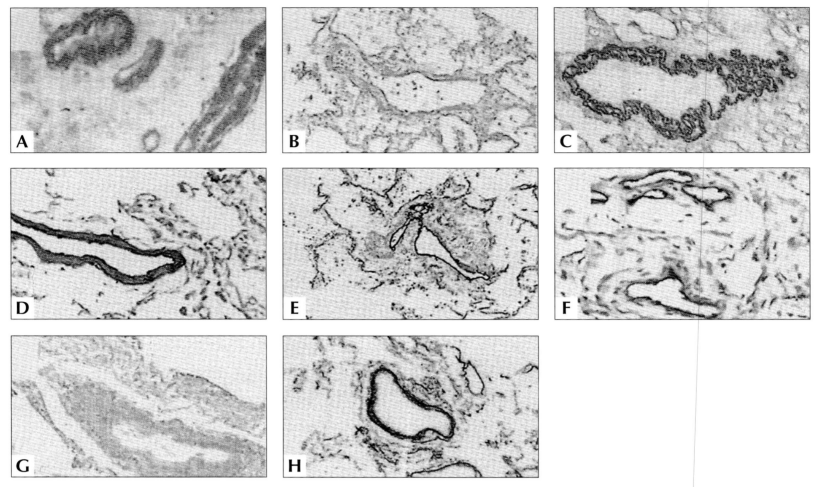

Figure 10-14. Immunohistochemical analysis of representative lung samples from patients with pulmonary hypertension (**A**, **C**, **E**, and **G**) and normotensive control patients (**B**, **D**, **F**, and **H**). Smooth muscle proliferation around small pulmonary vessels is an essential part of the pathogenesis. Mutations in the bone morphogenetic protein receptor type 2 (BMPR2) have been linked to familial cases of pulmonary hypertension. A signaling pathway involved in smooth muscle proliferation has been found to be altered in both familial and nonfamilial forms of pulmonary hypertension [16]. The pathway includes angiopoietin-l (Ang-1), a molecule that signals the recruitment of smooth muscle cells; its receptor, (called TIE2); and BMPR2.

Ang-1 is present in vascular smooth muscle cells in arterioles from a patient with pulmonary hypertension (**A**) but not in lung tissue from a control (**B**). Angiopoietin-2 (Ang-2) is present in vascular smooth muscle cells in vessels of all sizes in a patient with pulmonary hypertension (**C**) and in a control (**D**). TIE2 is present in endothelial cells lining vessels of all sizes in a patient with pulmonary hypertension (**E**) and in a control (**F**). Bone morphogenetic protein receptor type 1A (BMPR1A) is absent in endothelial cells in vessels less than 800 microns in diameter in lung tissue from a patient with pulmonary hypertension (**G**) but is present in a control (**H**). (*From* Du *et al.* [16]; with permission.)

DIAGNOSTIC APPROACH

DIAGNOSTIC EVALUATION OF PRIMARY PULMONARY HYPERTENSION

Blood tests: antinuclear antibodies, HIV, thryroid function
Electrocardiogram
Chest radiograph
Spiral chest CT
Echocardiogram
Exercise treadmill test
Pulmonary function tests
Cardiac catheterization

Figure 10-15. Diagnostic evaluation of primary pulmonary hypertension (PPH). (*Adapted from* McLaughlin [17].)

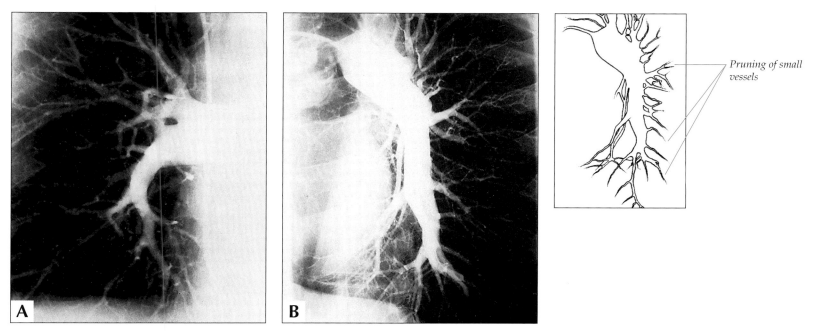

FIGURE 10-16. Pulmonary angiograms. **A**, The normal angiogram demonstrates a diffuse branching pattern with smoothly tapering vessels and branches leading to the periphery of the lung. **B**, In PPH, pulmonary angiography demonstrates marked "pruning" of small vessels with absent peripheral flow. No segmental or larger vascular abnormalities are noted.

Pruning of small vessels

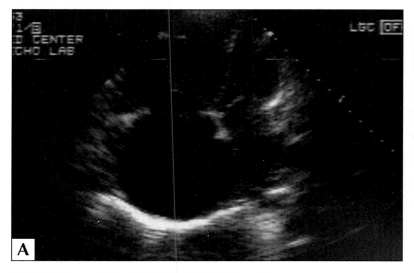

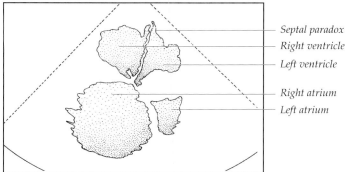

Septal paradox
Right ventricle
Left ventricle
Right atrium
Left atrium

FIGURE 10-17. This echocardiogram in a patient with primary pulmonary hypertension (PPH) demonstrates an enlarged right atrium and right ventricle, and a reduced size of the left ventricle (**A**). Doppler ultrasound of the tricuspid regurgitant jet is 4.7 meters per second (**B**), yielding an estimated pulmonary artery systolic pressure of at least 90 mm Hg. Echocardiographic predictors of adverse outcomes in PPH include pericardial effusion, right atrial enlargement, and interventricular septal displacement toward the left ventricle [18].

TREATMENT OPTIONS IN PRIMARY PULMONARY HYPERTENSION

Anticoagulation

Round-the-clock oxygen, if necessary

Calcium channel blockers (effective in 10% to 20% of patients)

Continuous infusion prostacyclin (improves survival and may heal endothelium)

Oral bosentan

Oral sildenafil (investigational)

Inhaled prostacyclin or nitric oxide (both investigational)

FIGURE 10-18. Treatment options in primary pulmonary hypertension (PPH). Continuous intravenous infusion of epoprostenol (prostacyclin) is the most effective treatment available for the management of PPH. New therapies include the recently US Food and Drug Administration--approved oral antagonist of endothelin receptors, bosentan [19]. Investigational therapies include an aerosolized prostacyclin analogue [20], iloprost, as well as inhaled nitric oxide [21] and combined therapy with aerosolized iloprost plus oral sildenafil [22].

Therapeutic interventions may be supportive if aimed at symptomatic relief, or "definitive" if significant survival prolongation is possible; no treatment in PPH is truly curative. Limitation of activity is strongly recommended. Pregnancy is contraindicated. Some patients will demonstrate significant oxygen desaturation upon exercising, due to impaired cardiac reserve. In this group, supplemental oxygen is indicated. Diuretics are useful in relieving symptoms of right-sided heart failure, such as hepatic congestion, ascites, and peripheral edema. These agents, however, must be used with extreme caution, as the right ventricle is quite preload-dependent in these patients and precipitous reductions in intravascular volume can be hazardous. Continuous intravenous prostacyclin infusion (PGI_2) improves exercise tolerance and survival in patients with PPH [23]. It also appears to be effective for patients with pulmonary hypotension caused by the scleroderma spectrum of disease [24]. More recently, inhaled nitric oxide [25] and aerosolized iloprost (an analogue of prostacyclin) [26] have been used in patients with PPH.

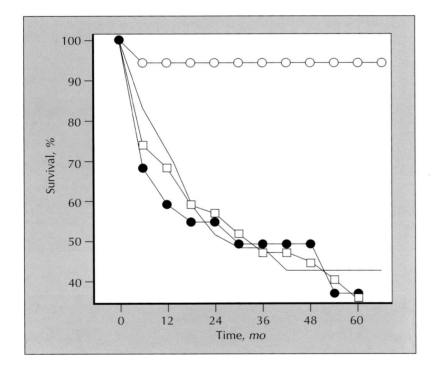

FIGURE 10-19. Survival curves in patients who responded acutely to calcium channel blockers (nifedipine or diltiazem) and were continued on treatment with one of these agents (*open circles*), compared with patients in the same study who did not respond favorably to calcium channel blockers (*solid line*), patients from the NIH Registry treated at the study institution (*solid circles*), and patients in the NIH Registry Cohort (*open squares*). This is the first evidence of improved survival with long-term pharmacologic therapy for PPH. The group that responded to calcium channel blockers also had a sustained reduction in pulmonary arterial pressure, pulmonary vascular resistance, and right ventricular chamber size diameter; symptoms were significantly alleviated. (*Adapted from* Rich *et al.* [27].)

CARDIAC TUMORS

As cardiac imaging becomes more common, with increasing resolution and tissue definition provided by echocardiography, computed tomography, and magnetic resonance imaging, cardiac tumors are being diagnosed with increasing frequency. Among adults, myxomas account for about half of the primary tumors; among children, rhabdomyomas and fibromas account for more than half of the primary tumors.

Of those tumors that are resected, myxomas account for about 75%. The most common malignant primary cardiac tumor is sarcoma, specifically angiosarcoma. With regard to metastatic tumors, hematologic malignancies are especially likely to involve the heart. As many as 25% of patients dying of lymphoma and 30% dying with leukemia have metastases to the heart.

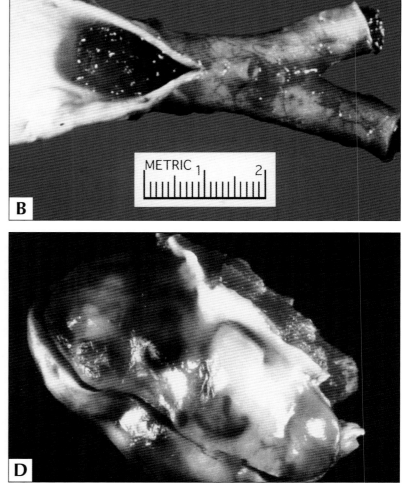

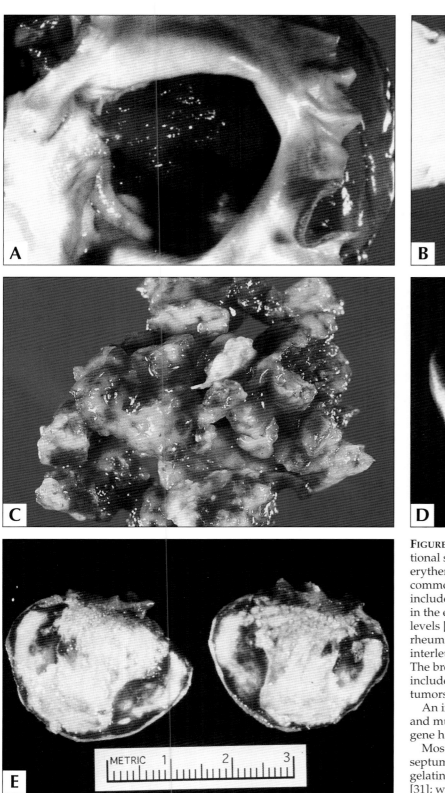

FIGURE 10-20. Myxomas. Patients with myxomas present with constitutional symptoms, embolism, or intracardiac obstruction. Fatigue, fever, erythematous rash, arthralgia, myalgia, and weight loss are the most common constitutional symptoms. Common laboratory abnormalities include anemia (usually normochromic and hypochromic) and elevation in the erythrocyte sedimentation rate, C-reactive protein, and globulin levels [28]. Constitutional symptoms mimicking autoimmune and rheumatologic diseases may be caused by the myxoma's production of interleukin 6 [29]. The skin has lentiginosis, blue nevi, and myxomas. The breast has myxoid fibroadenomas. The endocrine abnormalities include adrenal cortical hyperplasia, acromegaly, and Sertoli cell tumors of the testes.

An inherited syndrome with cardiac myxomas that are often recurrent and multiple is called the Carney complex. The Carney complex disease gene had been identified at the human chromosome 17q2 locus [30].

Most myxomas develop in the left atrium and arise from the interatrial septum. As shown in the gross specimens (**A** to **E**), they may appear gelatinous, irregular, smooth, or calcified [31]. (*From* Burke and Virmani [31]; with permission.)

Left Atrial Myxoma

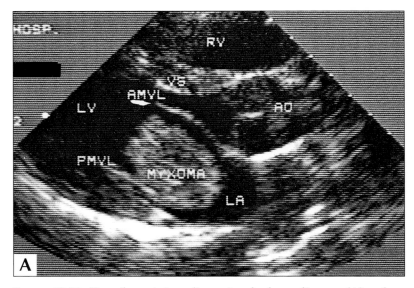

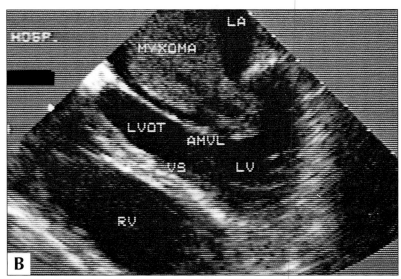

FIGURE 10-21. Transthoracic two-dimensional echocardiogram (**A**) and transesophageal two-dimensional echocardiogram (**B**) showing a left atrial (LA) mass prolapsing into and obstructing the mitral valve orifice. Note the superior resolution of the transesophageal echocardiogram. Although not visible here, the myxoma was attached to the mid-portion of the atrial septum.

Typically, LA myxomas attach to the fossa ovalis; although myxomas are rarely located posteriorly, a mass in this location should arouse suspicion of malignancy. During diastole, an atrial myxoma is visualized on M-mode echocardiography as multiple echoes behind the AMVL on the left and the tricuspid valve on the right. M-mode echocardiography is most useful for intracavitary, pedunculated masses of the LA;

however, it is less effective for visualizing tumors during systole and immobile tumors. Although ventricular myxomas can be seen as multiple intracavitary echoes, they are less frequently detected by this method. Two-dimensional echocardiography provides sufficient information (*ie*, size, attachment, and mobility) for surgical treatment. This imaging modality reveals intracavitary masses with alternating areas of echodensity and lucency and is useful for visualizing small, ventricular, and nonprolapsed tumors. Two-dimensional echocardiography also allows recognition of multiple masses. LV—left ventricle; LVOT—left ventricular outflow tract; PMVL—posterior leaflet of mitral valve; RV—right ventricle; VS—ventricular septum. (*Courtesy of* C.R. Thompson, MD, St. Paul's Hospital, Vancouver, BC.)

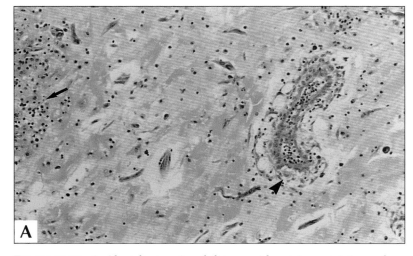

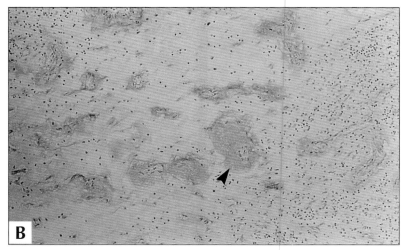

FIGURE 10-22. **A**, Abundant eosinophilic myxoid matrix containing polygonal to stellate myxoma cells distributed singly, in small groups, and around thin-walled vascular channels (*arrowhead*). Focal collections of mononuclear cells (macrophages, lymphocytes, plasma cells) are also seen (*arrow*). Myxomas may also contain glands, areas of recent and old

hemorrhage, as well as calcification and metaplastic bone formation (hematoxylin and eosin, × 200).

B, Large quantities of acid mucopolysaccharide are present in the myxoma matrix, primarily in the vicinity of vascular channels (*arrowhead*) (Alcian blue, × 100).

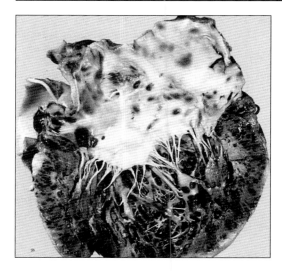

FIGURE 10-23. Malignant melanoma. Tumor metastases to the heart are hundreds of times more common than primary cardiac tumors. They are seen in about 15% of autopsies of patients with disseminated cancer. Some uncommon tumors, such as malignant melanoma [27], involve the heart almost half the time. Lung and breast carcinoma involve the heart and pericardium about 20% to 25% of the time. (*From* Burke and Virmani [31]; with permission.)

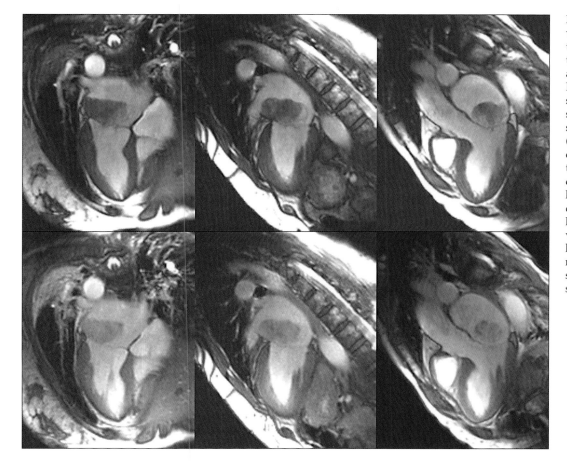

FIGURE 10-24. Mesothelioma. A 55-year-old woman with a remote history of mesothelioma treated with surgery and combined chemotherapy and radiation therapy presented with atypical chest pain and was found to have a large left atrial mass. Steady-state free precession gradient echo MRI revealed a 4x2x3-cm solid mobile mass, which attached to the atrial surface of the tricuspid annulus. Pre-contrast (gadolinium-DTPA) images on the *top row* indicated signal intensity of the cardiac mass similar to the left ventricular myocardium. Post-contrast images on the *bottom row* indicated heterogeneous enhancement of the mass. The degree of enhancement of the atrial mass was higher than the myocardium due to the larger volume of contrast distribution as a result of higher tissue vascularity, cellular edema, or necrosis. Histopathology of this resected mass showed high-grade poorly differentiated sarcoma with areas of necrosis.

REFERENCES

1. Farber HW, Loscalzo J: Pulmonary arterial hypertension. *N Engl J Med* 2004, 351:1655–1665.

2. Humbert M, Sitbon O, Simonneau G: Treatment of pulmonary arterial hypertension. *N Engl J Med* 2004, 351:1425–1436.

3. Bishop JM: Hypoxia and pulmonary hypertension in chronic bronchitis. *Prog Respir Res* 1975, 9:10.

4. Weber KT, Janicki JS, Shroff S, Fishman AP: Contractile mechanisms and interaction of the right and left ventricles. *Am J Cardiol* 1981, 47:686–695.

5. Aklog L, Williams CS, Bryne JG, Goldhaber SZ: Acute pulmonary embolectomy: a contemporary approach. *Circulation* 2002, 105:1416–1419.

6. Strollo PJ Jr, Rogers RM: Obstructive sleep apnea. *N Engl J Med* 1996, 334:99–104.

7. Teran-Santos J, Jimenez-Gomez A, Cordero-Guevara J: The association between sleep apnea and the risk of traffic accidents. *N Engl J Med* 1999, 340:847–851.

8. Suratt PM, Findley LJ: Driving with sleep apnea. *N Engl J Med* 1999, 340:881–883.

9. Rothman A, Mann DM, House MT, *et al.*: Transvenous procurement of pulmonary artery smooth muscle and endothelial cells using a novel endoarterial biopsy catheter in a canine model. *J Am Coll Cardiol* 1996, 27:218–224.

10. Report of the Medical Research Council Working Party: Long term domiciliary oxygen therapy in chronic hypoxic cor pulmonale complicating chronic bronchitis and emphysema. *Lancet* 1981, 1:681–686.

11. Nocturnal Oxygen Therapy Trial Group: Continuous or nocturnal oxygen therapy in hypoxemic chronic obstructive lung disease: a clinical trial. *Ann Intern Med* 1980, 93:391–398.

12 Gaine SP, Rubin LJ: Primary pulmonary hypertension. *Lancet* 1998, 352:719–725.

13. Cool CD, Rai PR, Yeager ME, *et al.*: Expression of human herpesvirus 8 in primary pulmonary hypertension. *N Engl J Med* 2003, 349:1113–1122.

14. McLaughlin VV, Shillington A, Rich S: Survival in primary pulmonary hypertension: the impact of epoprostenol therapy. *Circulation* 2002,106:1477–1482.

15. Gaine S: Pulmonary hypertension. *JAMA* 2000, 284:3160–3168.

16. Du L, Sullivan CC, Chu D, *et al.*: Signaling molecules in nonfamilial pulmonary hypertension. *N Engl J Med* 2003, 348:500–509.

17. McLaughlin VV: Pulmonary arterial hypertension: current diagnosis and management. *ACC Curr J Rev* 2002, 17–21.

18. Raymond RJ, Hinderliter AL, Willis PW, *et al.*: Echocardiographic predictors of adverse outcomes in primary pulmonary hypertension. *J Am Coll Cardiol* 2002, 39:1214–1219.

19. Rubin LJ, Badesch DB, Barst RJ, *et al.*: Bosentan therapy for pulmonary arterial hypertension. *N Engl J Med* 2002, 346:896–903.

20. Hoeper MM, Schwarze M, Ehlerding S, *et al.*: Long-term treatment of primary pulmonary hypertension with aerosolized iloprost, a prostacyclin analogue. *N Engl J Med* 2000, 342:1866–1870.

21. Rimensberger PC, Spahr-Schopfer I, Berner M, et al.: Inhaled nitric oxide versus aerosolized iloprost in secondary pulmonary hypertension in children with congenital heart disease: vasodilator capacity and cellular mechanisms. *Circulation* 2001, 103:544–548.

22. Ghofrani HA, Wiedemann R, Rose F, *et al.*: Combination therapy with oral sildenafil and inhaled iloprost for severe pulmonary hypertension. *Ann Intern Med* 2002, 136:515–522.

23. Barst RJ, Rubin LJ, Long WA, *et al.*: A comparison of continuous intravenous epoprostenol (prostacyclin) with conventional therapy for primary pulmonary hypertension. *N Engl J Med* 1996, 334:296–301.

24. Badesch DB, Tapson VF, McGoon MD, *et al.*: Continuous intravenous epoprostenol for pulmonary hypertension due to the scleroderma spectrum of disease: a randomized, controlled trial. *Ann Intern Med* 2000, 132:425–434.

25. Hoeper MM, Olschewski J, Ghofrani HA, *et al.*, and the German PPH Study Group: A comparison of the acute hemodynamic effects of inhaled nitric oxide and aerosolized iloprost in primary pulmnonary hypertension. *J Am Coll Cardiol* 2000, 35:176–182.22.

26. Olschewski H, Ghofrani A, Schemehl T, *et al.*, for the German PPH Study Group: Inhaled iloprost to treat severe pulmonary hypertension: an uncontrolled trial. *Ann Intern Med* 2000, 132:435–443.

27. Rich S, Kaufman E, Levy PS: The effect of high doses of calcium-channel blockers on survival in primary pulmonary hypertension. *N Engl J Med* 1992, 327:76–81.

28. Reynen K: Cardiac myxomas. *N Engl J Med* 1995, 333:1610–1617.

29. Seguin JR, Beigbeder JY, Hvass U, *et al.*: Interleukin 6 production by cardiac myxomas may explain constitutional symptoms. *J Thorac Cardiovasc Surg* 1992, 103:599–600.

30. Casey M, Mah C, Merliss AD, *et al.*: Identification of a novel genetic locus for familial cardiac myxomas and Carney complex. *Circulation* 1998, 98:2560–2566.

31. Burke A, Virmani R: *Tumors of the Heart and Great Vessels: Atlas of Tumor Pathology*, 3rd series, fascicle 16. Washington, DC: Armed Forces Institute of Pathology; 1996.

NUCLEAR CARDIOLOGY

Vasken Dilsizian and Jagat Narula

Daniel S. Berman, Jeffrey S. Borer, Guido Germano,
Rory Hachamovitch, Leo Hofstra, Diwakar Jain, D. Douglas Miller,
Maria Angela Oxilia-Estigarribia, Heinrich R. Schelbert,
Markus Schwaiger, H. William Strauss, James E. Udelson,
Renu Virmani, Frans J. Th. Wackers, Barry L. Zarat

CHAPTER 11

SPECT MYOCARDIAL PERFUSION IMAGING

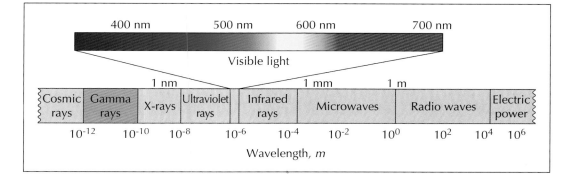

FIGURE 11-1. The spectrum of electromagnetic waves. Radioisotopes commonly used with single-photon emission computed tomography (SPECT) emit gamma rays of varying energies and have relatively long physical half-lives. Gamma rays are part of the spectrum of the electromagnetic waves. All of these waves travel at the speed of light (3×10^{10} cm/s, or 186,000 mile/s in a vacuum). Localization of gamma rays emitted by single photon–emitting radiotracers in the heart is accomplished by an Anger scintillation camera (gamma camera), which converts the gamma rays to light photons via sodium iodide scintillation detectors. The gamma camera limits the direction of photons entering the detector by a collimator and then positions each event electronically. Thus, the radioisotopes used for optimal scintigraphic registration with SPECT are limited to those that emit gamma rays with an energy range that is suitable for the gamma camera and related single-photon devices, such as ^{201}Tl, ^{99m}Tc, and iodine-123. The spatial resolution of SPECT system is in the range of 12 to 15mm. Although clinically useful, estimates of relative myocardial blood flow by SPECT are significantly affected by attenuation artifacts. The development and validation of attenuation correction devices is extremely important for the further advancement of clinical myocardial perfusion SPECT. (*Courtesy of* Thinkquest, http://library.thinkquest.org.)

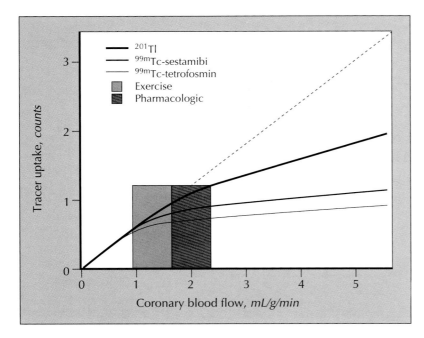

FIGURE 11-2. Radionuclide myocardial perfusion imaging. Two classes of radiotracers are used for stress myocardial perfusion single-photon emission computed tomography imaging: [201]Tl, used since the mid-1970s, and ^{99m}Tc-labeled perfusion tracers, used since the early 1990s. These two classes of radiotracers have different physical half-lives, energy of photons emitted, and dosage allowances. Both ^{201}Tl and ^{99m}Tc-labeled perfusion tracers distribute within the myocardium proportional to regional blood flow. This schematic illustrates radiotracer uptake and regional myocardial blood flow. An ideal myocardial perfusion tracer would be expected to show a perfect linear relationship (line of identity: *dotted line*) to myocardial blood flow over a wide range of flow rates in mL/g/min. Under resting conditions, myocardial blood flow is approximately 1 mL/g/min. During physical exercise, myocardial blood flow may increase to 2 mL/g/min; with pharmacologic vasodilation (adenosine or dipyridamole), flow may exceed 2 mL/g/min. All three radiotracers demonstrate "roll-off" at high flow levels (ie, the relationship between tracer uptake and flow deviates more and more from the line of identity). Although this is true for ^{201}Tl, it is particularly marked for ^{99m}Tc-sestamibi and ^{99m}Tc-tetrofosmin. The practical implication of this is that at higher flow levels, relative myocardial uptake of these radiotracers may underestimate regional myocardial blood flow deficits. Clinical studies have shown that this "roll-off" phenomenon does not significantly affect the detection of significant (> 80%) coronary artery stenoses. However, mild coronary artery stenoses (50%–70%) may go undetected, especially with ^{99m}Tc-sestamibi and ^{99m}Tc-tetrofosmin.

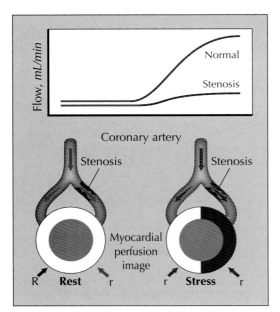

FIGURE 11-3. Pathophysiology underlying radionuclide myocardial perfusion imaging. Coronary blood flow in each of the coronary artery branches at rest and during stress is shown in the graph. At rest, regional myocardial blood flow is similar in both coronary artery branches. When a myocardial perfusion radiotracer is injected at rest, myocardial uptake of radiotracer is homogeneous; consequently, the short-axis image is normal. During stress, coronary blood flow increases 2.0 to 2.5 times in the normal branch but not to the same extent in the stenotic branch, resulting in heterogeneous distribution of regional myocardial blood flow. This heterogeneity of blood flow can be visualized with ^{201}Tl, ^{99m}Tc-sestamibi, or ^{99m}Tc-tetrofosmin as an area with relatively decreased myocardial accumulation (ie, an image with a myocardial perfusion defect; *bottom right*). Anatomic delineation of a normal (left branch) and an abnormal (right branch) coronary artery is shown. R—normal resistance; r—low resistance.

SPECT TECHNIQUES: [201]TI

Monovalent cation with biologic properties similar to potassium

80 keV mercury radiograph emission, 74-h physical half-life

High first-pass extraction fraction (~ 85%)

Transported across myocyte sarcolemmal membrane via the Na-K ATPase transport system and by facilitative diffusion

Peak myocardial concentration within 5 min of intravenous injection

Rapid clearance from the intravascular compartment

Redistribution begins 10 to 15 min after injection

FIGURE 11-4. Single-photon emission computed tomography (SPECT) techniques: [201]Tl. Myocardial extraction of ^{201}Tl is dependent on energy utilization, membrane adenosine triphosphate (ATPase), and active transport. [201]Tl does not actively concentrate in regions of infarcted or scarred myocardium. Thus, decreased myocardial ^{201}Tl uptake early after injection may be caused either by reduced regional blood flow or by infarction. Experimental studies with ^{201}Tl have shown that the cellular extraction of ^{201}Tl across the cell membrane is unaffected by hypoxia unless irreversible injury is present. Similarly, pathophysiologic conditions of chronic hypoperfusion (hibernation) and postischemic dysfunction (stunning), in which regional contractile function is impaired in the presence of myocardial viability do not adversely alter extraction of [201]Tl.

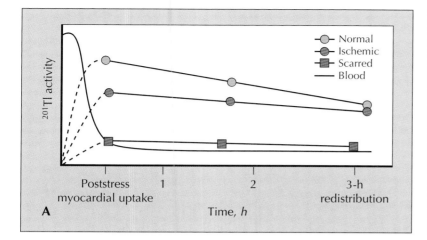

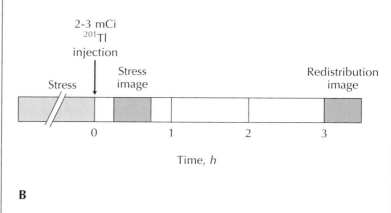

FIGURE 11-5. Stress-redistribution ^{201}Tl protocol. Schematic diagrams of ^{201}Tl uptake and redistribution in normal and ischemic myocardium (**A**) and a stress-redistribution protocol (**B**) are shown. Although the initial distribution of ^{201}Tl (early after intravenous injection) is proportional to regional blood flow, the later distribution of ^{201}Tl over a 3- to 4-hour period, the redistribution phase, is a function of regional blood volume and is unrelated to flow. During the redistribution phase, there is a continuous exchange of ^{201}Tl between the myocardium and the extracardiac compartments, driven by the concentration gradient of tracer and myocyte viability. Thus, the extent to defect resolution, from the initial to

delayed redistribution images over time (a reversible defect), reflects one index of myocardial viability. When only nonviable, scarred myocardium is present, the initial ^{201}Tl defect (an irreversible defect) persists over time without redistribution. When both viable and scarred myocardium are present, ^{201}Tl redistribution is incomplete, giving the appearance of partial reversibility. Thus, whereas the initial phase of ^{201}Tl studies reflect reductions in flow caused by coronary artery narrowing, the delayed, redistribution phase of ^{201}Tl studies reflect myocardial potassium space, differentiating viable from scarred myocardium.

A. SPECT TECHNIQUES: ^{99m}Tc-LABELED SESTAMIBI AND TETROFOSMIN

Lipid-soluble cationic compounds

140 keV photopeak energy, 6-h physical half-life

First-pass extraction fraction ~ 60%

Uptake is passive across mitochondrial membranes

At equilibrium, they are retained within the mito-chondria because of a large negative trans-membrane potential

Clearance from the intravascular compartment via hepatobiliary excretion

Minimal redistribution when compared with ^{201}Tl

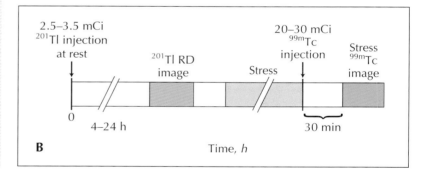

FIGURE 11-6. Single-photon emission computed tomography (SPECT) techniques: ^{99m}Tc-labeled sestamibi and tetrofosmin. **A,** ^{99m}Tc-sestamibi (isonitrile) (MIBI) and ^{99m}Tc-tetrofosmin (diphosphine) are both lipophilic cationic complexes with similar myocardial uptake and blood clearance kinetics. However, the clearance of tetrofosmin from the lungs and the liver is faster than that of ^{99m}Tc-sestamibi, which may improve the resolution of cardiac images and reduce the overall radiation burden. Both ^{99m}Tc-sestamibi and tetrofosmin are taken up across sarcolemmal and mito-chondrial membranes of myocytes by passive distribution and are retained within the mitochondria at equilibrium because of a large negative trans-membrane potential. Experimental studies with ^{99m}Tc-sestamibi have shown that myocardial uptake and clearance of ^{99m}Tc-sestamibi are related to the mitochondrial transmembrane potential and do not differ from ischemic to nonischemic regions. In addition, experimental studies of myocardial infarction, with and without reperfusion, have fueled optimism

in the use of ^{99m}Tc-sestamibi clinically for myocardial viability assessment.

In the clinical setting, however, with the exception of a few studies, both ^{99m}Tc-sestamibi and tetrofosmin appear to underestimate myocardial viability. Compared with ^{201}Tl and positron emission tomography (PET) tracers, factors that may contribute to the impaired ^{99m}Tc-sestamibi or tetrofosmin accumulation in viable regions at rest include differences in extraction fraction, blood clearance, redistribution (RD), and response to altered metabolic states. Perhaps a likely improvement in viability assessment with ^{99m}Tc-sestamibi and tetrofosmin could be achieved through nitrate administration before rest ^{99m}Tc injection and quantitation of regional radiotracer uptake. **B,** Alternatively, dual-isotope gated SPECT imaging could be performed, which combines rest–redistribution ^{201}Tl (for viability) with stress ^{99m}Tc—sestamibi or tetrofosmin (for perfusion), thereby taking advantage of the favorable properties of each of the two tracers.

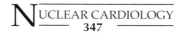

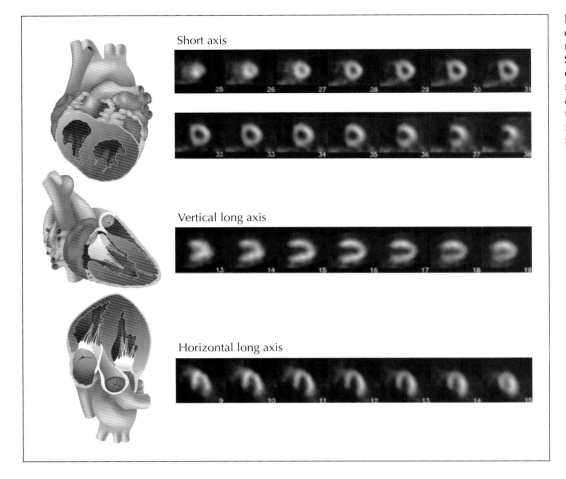

FIGURE 11-7. Normal exercise single-photon emission computed tomography (SPECT) myocardial perfusion images. The display of SPECT myocardial perfusion imaging is standardized. The short-axis slices are presented from apex to base, the vertical long-axis slices are displayed from septum to lateral wall, and the horizontal long-axis slices are displayed from inferior to anterior. The radiotracer uptake is homogeneous in each of the slices.

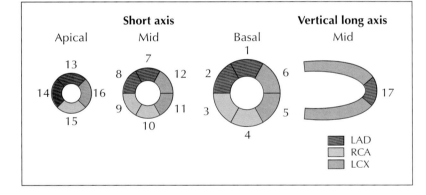

FIGURE 11-8. Coronary artery territories. Although the anatomy of coronary arteries may vary substantially in individual patients, the location of myocardial perfusion abnormalities on single-photon emission computed tomography imaging allows for a general prediction of which coronary artery is likely to be diseased. The diagram shown represents the standardized assignment of coronary artery territories of the left anterior descending coronary artery (LAD), right coronary artery (RCA), and left circumflex coronary artery (LCX). The prediction of disease in the LAD is often quite accurate. The prediction of disease in the RCA and LCX is often less accurate because of substantial variation in extent of myocardial territories supplied by these arteries. (*Adapted from* Port [1].)

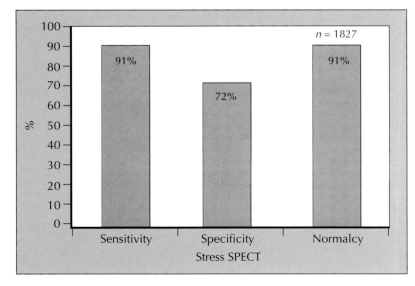

FIGURE 11-9. Detection of angiographic coronary artery disease with radiotracers. Extensive literature exists on the diagnostic yield of stress single-photon emission computed tomography (SPECT) myocardial perfusion imaging [2–13]. Among 1827 patients referred for evaluation of chest discomfort (pooled data from 12 studies performed between 1989 and 1999), the overall sensitivity of myocardial perfusion SPECT for the detection of angiographic coronary artery disease was 91%, the specificity was 72%, and the normalcy rate (in subjects with low likelihood for coronary artery disease who did not undergo coronary angiography) was 91%.

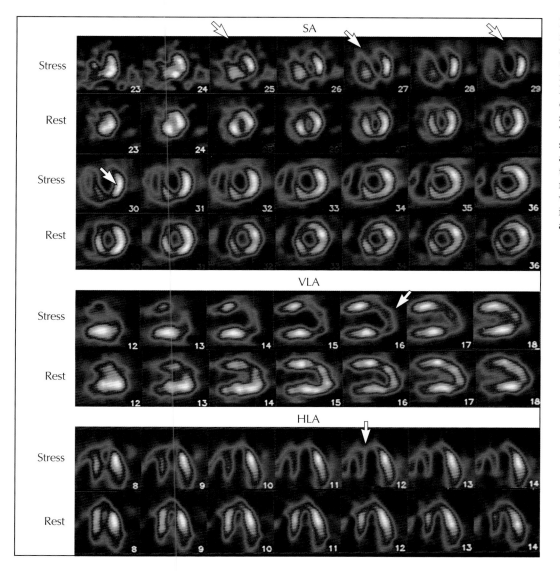

FIGURE 11-10. Example of a patient with a large, reversible myocardial perfusion defect. Large, severely reduced anteroseptal and apical defects (*arrows*) are present on stress images but not on rest images, suggestive of myocardial ischemia. In addition, mild transient ischemic cavity dilatation of the left ventricle is present on the stress images compared with the rest images. The rest images are almost normal except for a small residual defect in the anterior wall on the apical short-axis (SA) slices. These images are typical for a large reversible stress-induced myocardial perfusion defect. The transient left ventricular cavity dilation suggests severe ischemia during stress. HLA—horizontal long axis; VLA—vertical long axis.

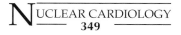

FIGURE 11-11. Example of a patient with a large, fixed (irreversible) myocardial perfusion defect. Both on the stress and rest images, large, severely reduced, anteroseptal and apical defects are evident (*arrows*). HLA—horizontal long axis; SA—short axis; VLA—vertical long axis.

HIGH- AND LOW-RISK SPECT IMAGES

HIGH RISK

Large perfusion defect on stress imaging
Multiple coronary artery territories
Large reversibility
Increaed lung uptake
Transient LV dilation

LOW RISK

Normal stress images
Small stress defect
Small reversibility

FIGURE 11-12. High- and low-risk single-photon emission computed tomography (SPECT) images. SPECT images should not be interpreted as either normal or abnormal. The prognosis of a patient is related to the degree of myocardial perfusion abnormality. Quantification or semiquan-

tification provides that important prognostic information. High-risk SPECT images are characterized by large perfusion defects on the stress images that involve multiple coronary artery territories (if two or more coronary territories are involved, the study should be considered to indicate high risk for the patient). Large stress-induced reversible defects represent extensive myocardial ischemia, which may be associated with increased lung uptake, transient ischemic left ventricular (LV) cavity dilatation, and transient increased right ventricular myocardial visualization. One of the strongest features of stress myocardial perfusion SPECT imaging is its ability to identify low-risk patients. Patients with unequivocal normal exercise or pharmacologic stress myocardial perfusion SPECT images exhibit less than a 1% future cardiac event rate, the same as the general population. For those undergoing an exercise study, this presumes that the patient achieved greater than 85% predicted maximum heart rate for a man or woman of his or her age. Similarly, presuming that adequate exercise was performed, patients with small myocardial perfusion defects on stress and small regions of defect reversibility have low risk for future cardiac events. These patients should be treated aggressively with medical therapy because of the presence of coronary artery disease. It is important to emphasize that stress myocardial perfusion SPECT images should always be interpreted in conjunction with clinical and electrocardiographic data. For example, a rare patient may have a markedly abnormal exercise portion of the test but normal or near-normal SPECT images. It is the responsibility of the nuclear cardiologist to determine the significance of such disparate data.

POSITRON EMISSION TOMOGRAPHY TRACERS AND PROTOCOLS

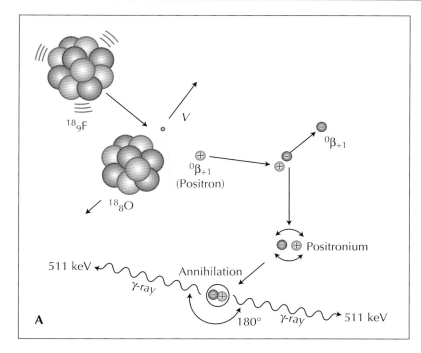

A

FIGURE 11-13. Cardiac positron emission tomography (PET) applications and positron-emitting radiotracers. **A**, Positron-emitting radioisotopes commonly used with PET emit two gamma rays, 511 keV each, and have relatively short physical half-lives. When the high-energy positron is emitted from a nucleus, it travels a short distance and collides with an electron. The result is complete annihilation of both the positron and the electron and conversion of the combined mass to energy in the form of electromagnetic radiation (two gamma rays, 511 keV energy each). Because the gamma rays are perfectly collinear (discharged at 180° to each other) and travel in opposite directions, the PET detectors can be programmed to register only events with temporal coincidence of photons that strike directly at opposing detectors. This results in improved spatial (4 to 6 mm) and temporal resolution. Moreover, the PET system is more sensitive than a single-photon emission computed tomography system (which has a higher count rate) and provides the possibility of attenuation correction. The consequence of these advantages with PET is the possibility for quantitation of tracer concentration in absolute units. **B,** Clinically available cardiac PET radiotracers fall within two broad categories: those that evaluate myocardial blood flow and those that evaluate specific metabolic pathways. By labeling various compounds of physiologic interest, valuable insights into biochemical pathways and tissue metabolism can be obtained in functional and dysfunctional myocardium. Because estimates of both myocardial blood flow and metabolism can be obtained in absolute terms beyond the diagnosis of ischemic left ventricular dysfunction, PET may allow monitoring of both the progression of disease and the effect of various treatments in such patients.

B. CARDIAC PET APPLICATIONS AND POSITRON-EMITTING RADIOTRACERS

MYOCARDIAL BLOOD FLOW

Rubidium-82	75 s half-life; produced from strontium-82 generator
^{15}O-water	2 min half-life; cyclotron-produced
^{13}N-ammonia	10 min half-life; cyclotron-produced

MYOCARDIAL METABOLISM

^{11}C-palmitate	20 min half-life; cyclotron-produced
^{11}C-acetate	20 min half-life; cyclotron-produced
[^{18}F]-fluorodeoxyglucose	110 min half-life; cyclotron-produced

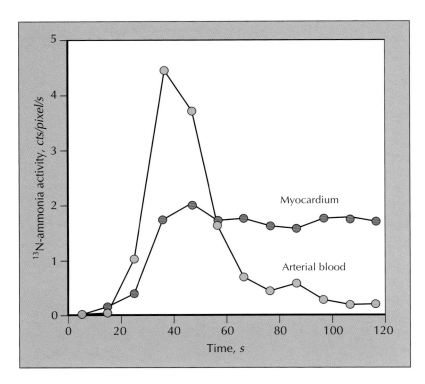

Time, s

FIGURE 11-14. Arterial radiotracer input function and myocardial tissue response. From regions of interest assigned to the left ventricular blood pool and the left ventricular myocardium on the serially acquired images, time–activity curves are derived that describe the changes in radiotracer activity in arterial blood and in myocardium as a function of time. Through fitting of the time–activity curves with the operational equation formulated from the tracer kinetic model, estimates of myocardial blood flow in units of milliliters of blood per minute per gram myocardium are obtained.

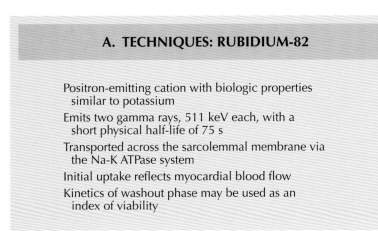

A. TECHNIQUES: RUBIDIUM-82

Positron-emitting cation with biologic properties similar to potassium

Emits two gamma rays, 511 keV each, with a short physical half-life of 75 s

Transported across the sarcolemmal membrane via the Na-K ATPase system

Initial uptake reflects myocardial blood flow

Kinetics of washout phase may be used as an index of viability

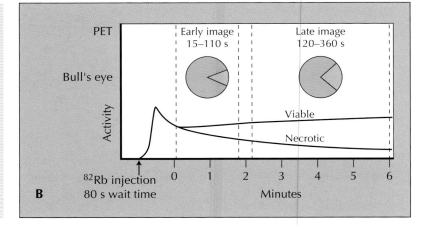

FIGURE 11-15. Positron emission tomography (PET) technique: rubidium-82. **A,** ^{82}Rb is a generator-produced, short-lived, positron-emitting cation with biologic properties that are similar to potassium and ^{201}Tl. As with potassium and ^{201}Tl, intracellular uptake of ^{82}Rb across the sarcolemmal membrane reflects active cation transport via the Na-K ATPase transport system. In patients with chronic coronary artery disease, myocardial uptake of ^{82}Rb is preserved in viable regions and severely reduced in scarred regions. In the setting of acute myocardial injury and reperfusion, initial uptake of ^{82}Rb reflects blood flow. **B,** Because necrotic myocardium cannot retain ^{82}Rb, the kinetics of ^{82}Rb washout may be used as an index of myocardial viability. This is demonstrated in the schematic bull's-eye diagram of ^{82}Rb on early and late image. Such application of ^{82}Rb washout kinetics provides myocardial viability information comparable to metabolic imaging with PET. In the clinical setting, 40 to 60 mCi of ^{82}Rb is administered intravenously. (*Panel B adapted from* Gould *et al.* [14].)

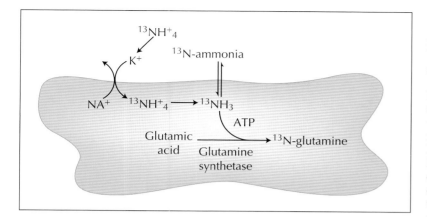

FIGURE 11-16. Positron emission tomography (PET) technique: ^{13}N-ammonia. ^{13}N-ammonia is the extractable perfusion tracer most commonly used with PET. At physiologic pH, ammonia is in its cationic form with a

physical half-life of 10 minutes. Myocardial distribution of ammonia is related inversely and nonlinearly to blood flow. Although the exact mechanism of ^{13}N-ammonia transport across the myocardial membrane has not been conclusively established, it has been suggested that ^{13}N-ammonia may cross cell membranes by passive diffusion or as ammonium ion (^{13}NH$^+_4$) by the active sodium–potassium transport mechanism influenced by the concentration gradient across the cell membrane. Once in the myocyte, myocardial retention of ^{13}N-ammonia involves predominantly the conversion of ^{13}N-ammonia and glutamic acid to ^{13}N-labeled glutamine mediated by adenosine triphosphate and glutamine synthetase. Hence, absolute quantification requires two- and three-compartment kinetic models that incorporate both extraction and retention rate constants. Quantification of ammonia is further complicated by the rapid degradation of ammonia, which occurs within 5 minutes after administration, producing metabolic intermediates such as urea and glutamine that are also extracted by the heart. Experimental studies suggest that myocardial uptake of ammonia reflects absolute blood flows up to 2.0 to 2.5 mL/g/min and plateaus at flows in the hyperemic range. In the clinical setting, 10 to 20 mCi of ^{13}N-ammonia is administered intravenously.

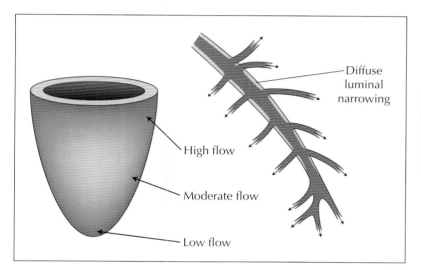

FIGURE 11-17. Diffuse coronary artery luminal narrowing and myocardial blood flow. Diffuse luminal narrowing of the epicardial conduit vessels can cause a longitudinal base to apex myocardial perfusion gradient [15,16]. Because resistance to flow through the conduit vessel relates according to the Hagen-Poiseuille equation to the fourth power of the radius, the intracoronary pressure may decline progressively along the epicardial vessels from proximal to distal so that the perfusion pressure significantly declines in myocardium in the distal distribution of the coronary arteries. Such longitudinal perfusion can be especially prominent during hyperemic blood flows when resistance to coronary flow is especially high and accentuated if the conduit vessel does not dilate. (*Adapted from* Gould *et al.* [16].)

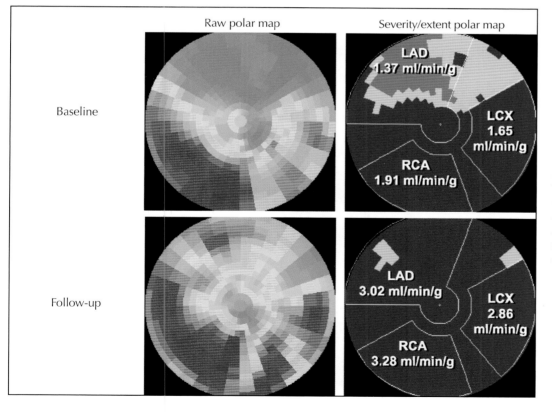

FIGURE 11-18. HMG CoA–reductase inhibitors and regional myocardial blood flow. Polar maps of the distribution of myocardial blood flow during adenosine-stimulated hyperemia in a patient with coronary artery disease at baseline and after 1 year of treatment with pravastatin. The extent of the stress-induced defect declined from 51% of the left anterior descending coronary artery (LAD) territory to only 3%. Myocardial blood flow in each of the three coronary artery territories increased and normalized in the region with a prior stress-induced defect. Only measurements of myocardial blood flow but not the evaluation of the relative distribution of the radiotracer uptake in the myocardium demonstrate the improvement in the flow reserve in remote or normal-appearing myocardium. LCX—left circumflex coronary artery; RCA—right coronary artery.

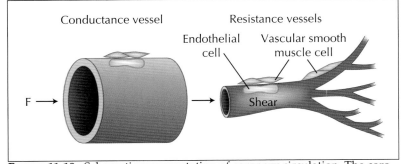

FIGURE 11-19. Schematic representation of coronary circulation. The coronary circulation has been viewed as a two-compartment system consisting of the large epicardial conductance and resistance vessels. In normal coronary circulation, the intraluminal pressure in the conductance vessels equals that in the aortic root (or the coronary driving pressure), but the pressure steeply declines within the resistance vessels to values moderately higher than those in the right atrium, so that a pressure gradient between the coronary circulation and the right atrium is maintained. Direct vascular smooth muscle dilatation, as affected through adenosine or dipyridamole, lowers the resistance to flow. Acceleration of coronary flow (F) prompts a flow-dependent, endothelium-mediated additional dilation of the resistance vessels but also an approximately 15% to 25% flow-dependent increase in the diameter of the conductance vessels. This flow-dependent dilatation of the conductance vessels offsets an increase in resistance to higher flow velocities. The total adenosine- or dipyridamole-stimulated hyperemic flows, therefore, reflect the total integrated vasodilator capacity of the coronary circulation. Factors that modify hyperemic myocardial blood flow in the normal heart include gender; age; cardiac work; the coronary driving pressure; heart rate; left ventricular diastolic and systolic pressures; effects of insulin, norepinephrine, and epinephrine; and nitric oxide bioactivity.

FIGURE 11-20. Patient protocol selection algorithm. The decision analysis for pharmacologic stress imaging illustrates the clinical issues that should be addressed: whether the patient can perform dynamic exercise, whether there are contraindications for drug stress, the type of drug stress (*ie*, hyperemic or inotropic), and the resulting physiologic and pathophysiologic endpoints. ETT—exercise treadmill testing.

Testing indication

Diagnosis → Prognosis

Dynamic exercise capacity?

Maximal → ETT

Submaximal → Isometric exercise → Low-level exercise

Incapable of any exercise → Contraindication(s) to drug stress?

Yes →

No → Hyperemic therapy / Inotropic therapy

Hyperemic therapy → Dipyridamole (indirect) ← Adenosine (direct)

Inotropic therapy → Dobutamine

Dipyridamole (indirect) → (-) Dromotropic

Dobutamine → (+/-) Atropine

(-) Dromotropic → Coronary vasodilation

(+/-) Atropine → Increased cardiac work

Coronary vasodilation → Coronary "steal" → Myocardial ischemia

Increased cardiac work → Myocardial ischemia

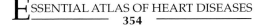

INDICATIONS FOR PHARMACOLOGIC IMAGING

Inability to exercise
   Physical limitations (amputation, etc.)
   Recent operation
   Comorbidity
Limited exercise capacity
   Deconditioning
   Limiting physical conditions (COPD, claudication)
   Medications (β-blockers)
   Poor motivation
Contraindications to exercise
   Early post–myocardial infarction
   Unstable angina
   Aortic aneurysm (coexisting medical conditions)
   LBBB

FIGURE 11-21. Indications for pharmacologic stress imaging. These indications include inability to exercise, limited exercise capacity, and relative or absolute contraindications to exercise. Although exercise remains the preferred modality of stress testing in the majority of cases, a significant number of patients cannot complete a maximum stress test. Some patient populations are well suited for vasodilator stress imaging, such as patients with aortic stenosis, with which excellent diagnostic accuracy and safety have been shown [17]. Patients with electrocardiographic left bundle branch block (LBBB) have a high false-positive rate with exercise or dobutamine stress testing attributable to abnormal patterns of septal perfusion and contraction [18,19]. The diagnostic accuracy in patients with LBBB is 86% to 90% with adenosine or dipyridamole compared with 50% or less with exercise perfusion imaging. Supplemental exercise is not advised for patients with LBBB. COPD—chronic obstructive pulmonary disease.

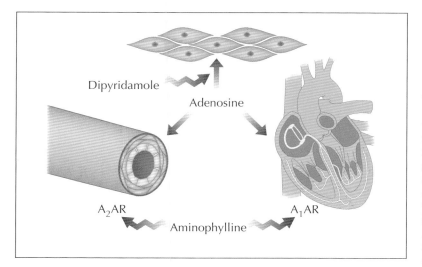

FIGURE 11-22. The direct and indirect action of adenosine and dipyridamole on vascular smooth muscle cells (A2 receptors [A2AR]) and on cardiac conduction cells (A1 receptors [A1AR]). The "antidote" that reverses the effects of dipyridamole or adenosine is aminophylline. Patient preparation for pharmacologic stress testing is similar to that for 12 to 24 hours for exercise stress, although all methylxanthines must be withheld before adenosine or dipyridamole testing [20]. ß-Blockers should be withheld for 24 hours before dobutamine stress testing. With vasodilator single-photon emission computed tomography imaging, the increased splanchnic activity mandates a delay in image acquisition for 30 to 60 minutes after the injection of a ^{99m}Tc agent [21,22]. Adenosine is a small, heterocyclic, endogenous compound produced by the endothelial cell. It activates A2 receptors, causing vasodilatation via the production of adenyl cyclase and the subsequent local increase in cylic AMP. Theophylline and other methylxanthines, including caffeine, are competitive antagonists of adenosine, blocking their effects at the A2 receptor. Adenosine enters endothelial and red blood cells by a facilitated transport mechanism. Intracellular adenosine is then deaminated or converted to other inactive metabolites. Selective A2 receptor agonists, such as MRI-0470, CVT-3146, ATL-146e, and CGS-21680, induce coronary hyperemia with less systemic vasodilation and fewer side effects, including chest pain and atrioventricular block [23,24]. Stress testing with intravenous adenine triphosphate has also been successful.

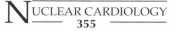

CHARACTERISTICS OF METHODS OF STRESS TESTING

	EXERCISE	DOBUTAMINE	DIPYRIDAMOLE	ADENOSINE
CBF increase	2–3X	2X	3–4X	3–5X
Ischemia provocation	Frequent	Common	Rare	Uncommon
Onset of effect	3–5 min	2–4 min	4–6 min	1–2 min
Duration after stopping	2–5 min	4–6 min	10–30 min	0.5–1 min
AV block occurrence	No	No	Rare	Common (transient)
Ventricular ectopy	Uncommon	Common	Rare	Rare

FIGURE 11-23. Characteristics of stress testing with regard to responses from exercise, dobutamine, dipyridamole, and adenosine. AV—atrioventricular; CBF—coronary blood flow.

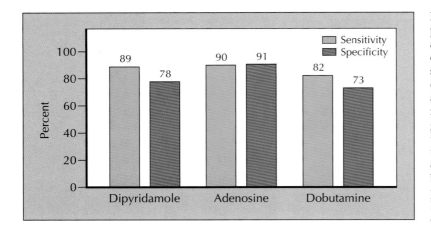

FIGURE 11-24. Cumulative test accuracy data from multiple studies of pharmacologic stress imaging using dipyridamole, adenosine, or dobutamine in combination with myocardial perfusion single-photon emission computed tomography. Average sensitivity ranges from 82% to 90%, and specificity ranges from 73% to 91%. Drug stress provides comparable diagnostic value to exercise for the detection of coronary artery disease as well as superior accuracy to submaximal exercise testing. The diagnostic accuracy of drug stress imaging is high, regardless of age or gender. Transient left ventricular cavity dilatation and increased lung ^{201}Tl activity are markers of more severe or extensive coronary disease; these markers of disease burden also portend an increased risk for cardiac events. Adenosine, dipyridamole, and dobutamine have each been successfully used in conjunction with all available myocardial perfusion tracers (*ie*, ^{201}Tl, ^{99m}Tc-sestamibi, ^{99m}Tc-tetrofosmin) [20]. Diagnostic accuracy may be slightly reduced with certain protocol combinations, such as dobutamine–[99m]Tc-sestamibi [21] and dipyridamole–[99m]Tc-tetrofosmin [22].

DIPYRIDAMOLE-²⁰¹TI IMAGING FOR PEROPERATIVE ASSESSMENT OF CARDIAC RISK*

| | | | | PERIOPERATIVE EVENTS | |
STUDY VASCULAR SURGERY	N	PATIENTS WITH ISCHEMIA BY ²⁰¹TL-RD, N (%)	MI/DEATH, N (%)	RD SCAN POSITIVE PREDICTIVE VALUE, % (N)†	NORMAL SCAN NEGATIVE PREDICTIVE VALUE, % (N)†
Boucher *et al.*	48	16 (33)	3 (6)	19 (3/160)	100 (32/32)
Cutler and Leppo	116	54 (47)	11 (10)	20 (11/54)	100 (60/60)
Fletcher *et al.*	67	15 (22)	3 (4)	20 (3/15)	100 (56/56)
Sachs *et al.*	46	14 (31)	2 (4)	14 (2/14)	100 (24/24)
Eagle *et al.*	200	82 (41)	15 (8)	16 (13/82)	98 (61/62)
McEnroe *et al.*	95	34 (36)	7 (7)	9 (3/34)	96 (44/46)
Younis *et al.*	111	40 (36)	8 (7)	15 (6/40)	100 (51/51)
Mangano *et al.*	60	22 (37)	3 (5)	5 (1/22)	95 (19/20)
Strawn and Guernsey	68	NA	4 (6)	NA	100 (21/21)
Watters *et al.*	26	15 (58)	3 (12)	20 (3/15)	100 (11/11)
Hendel *et al.*	327	167 (51)	28 (9)	14 (23/167)	99 (97/98)
Lette *et al.*	355	161 (45)	30 (8)	17 (28/161)	99 (160/162)
Madsen *et al.*	65	45 (69)	5 (8)	11 (5/45)	100 (20/20)
Brown and Rowen	231	77 (33)	12 (5)	13 (10/77)	99 (120/121)
Kresowik *et al.*	170	67 (39)	5 (3)	4 (3/67)	98 (64/64)
Baron *et al.*	457	160 (35)	22 (5)	4 (7/160)	96 (195/203)‡
Bry *et al.*	237	110 (46)	17 (7)	11 (12/110)	100 (97/97)
Total	2679	107 (41)	178 (6.6)	12 (33/1079)	99 (1132/1149)
NONVASCULAR SURGERY					
Camp *et al.*	40	9 (23)	6 (15)	67 (6/9)	100 (23/23)
Iqbal *et al.*	31	11 (41)	3 (11)	27 (3/11)	100 (20/20)
Coley *et al.*	100	36 (36)	4 (4)	8 (3/36)	98 (63/64)
Shaw *et al.*	60	28 (47)	6 (10)	21 (6/28)	100 (19/19)
Takase *et al.*	53	15 (28)	6 (11)	27 (4/15)	100 (32/32)
Younis *et al.*	161	50 (31)	15 (9)	18 (9/50)	98 (87/89)
Total	445	149 (33)	40 (9)	21 (31/149)	99 (244/247)

*All studies except those by Coley *et al.* acquired patient information prospectively. Only in reports by Mangano *et al.* and Baron *et al.* were scan results blinded from attending physicians.

†Patients with fixed defects were omitted from calculation of positive and negative predictive value.

‡Nonfatal MI only.

FIGURE 11-25. Dipyridamole-²⁰¹Tl imaging for preoperative assessment of cardiac risk. Dipyridamole-²⁰¹Tl myocardial scintigraphy has been used extensively as a noninvasive approach to assess perioperative cardiac risk in patients before vascular and nonvascular surgery [25–30]. Dipyridamole–⁹⁹ᵐTc-sestamibi scintigraphy for preoperative risk stratification has also been evaluated [31,32]. Patients with a normal ²⁰¹Tl or sestamibi myocardial perfusion study are at very low likelihood for perior postoperative cardiac events. Events (including death and nonfatal myocardial infarction [MI]) occur in approximately 20% of patients with scintigraphic evidence of ischemia. Patients with fixed perfusion defects are at lower risk for perioperative cardiac events, but their long-term prognosis is similar to that in patients with chronic coronary artery disease with myocardial ischemia. Although drug-induced myocardial hypoperfusion or ischemia predicts a high risk for cardiac events, approximately 80% of patients survive the surgical procedure without complications (*ie*, low positive predictive value). Risk stratification may be improved by identifying not only the presence but also the extent of myocardial ischemia. Patients with multiple ischemic defects in several vascular beds are at higher risk than those with a single ischemic segment. Quantitative single-photon emission computed tomography (SPECT) imaging permits the determination of the percent and location of ischemic myocardium.

Continued on next page

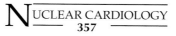

FIGURE 11-25. *(Continued)* Of 231 patients undergoing noncardiac surgery who had dipyridamole studies with 1 month of operation [33], the number of segments with ^{201}Tl redistribution (RD) was the best predictor of perioperative cardiac death or nonfatal MI (*P* = 0.0001), although a history of diabetes mellitus was also predictive in this study (*P* = 0.006). When dipyridamole perfusion scintigraphy was performed in 66 consecutive patients undergoing predominantly vascular surgeries, only 9% of patients with a "small" ischemic defect had a cardiac event compared with 80% of patients with more extensive ischemia. Levinson *et al.* [34] reported a significantly higher cardiac event rate in patients with ^{201}Tl redistribution in four or more segments (38%) compared with those with less extensive ischemia (12%). The optimal approach for identifying risk in surgical candidates should integrate clinical and imaging variables. In 200 patients undergoing major vascular surgery [35], clinical and imaging parameters were evaluated to optimize risk stratification in patient subsets. Logistic regression analysis identified five clinical predictors of cardiac event risk: electrocardiographic Q waves, ventricular ectopic activity, diabetes, age over 70 years, and a history of angina. The presence of ^{201}Tl redistribution was also found to be a significant risk predictor. In the 64 patients who had no clinical predictors, only 3.1% had ischemic events, with no deaths. Most of these patients also had no scintigraphic evidence of ischemia and, therefore, would have been classified as low risk by imaging. Conversely, 50% of patients with more than three clinical risk factors had cardiac events, and scintigraphic ischemia involving multiple vascular territories was frequent in this subgroup. The majority of patients had one or two clinical variables (68%); of these, 15.5% had a postoperative event, defining a large group at intermediate clinical risk. Without dipyridamole-^{201}Tl redistribution, 3.2% had a subsequent cardiac event compared with 30% with defect redistribution. Among younger patients without a prior cardiovascular history, clinical criteria can effec-tively define a low-risk group, and stress imaging is generally not warranted [36]. In patients with multiple cardiac risk factors, imaging is useful as a guide to coronary revascularization before surgery. In heterogeneous clinical populations with variable risk, drug stress perfusion imaging is valuable for defining patients most likely to have cardiac events based on the presence and extent of myocardial ischemia.

Despite the increased use of adenosine and dobutamine as pharmacologic stressors [30–41], less data are available for these agents in preoperative risk stratification than for dipyridamole. When adenosine-^{201}Tl tomography was used as a preoperative screening test in patients referred for vascular orthopedic or general surgery, patients with defect redistribution had a 25% event rate, but no events occurred in patients without myocardial ischemia [40].

Adenosine-^{201}Tl tomography, when performed in 106 patients undergoing vascular surgery, was abnormal in 54% of patients, of whom 82% demonstrated defect ischemia [39]. Eleven percent of the patients with scintigraphic ischemia had an event, but none of the patients without ischemia had an event. By quantitative analysis, the size of the total and reversible perfusion defects was larger in patients with events compared with those without perfusion defects. In 126 patients awaiting vascular surgery, dobutamine was administered in doses up to 20 μg/kg/min, with atropine given to 47 patients to further increase heart rate [30]. Sixty-seven percent had either a normal ^{201}Tl SPECT or only a fixed defect, with cardiac event rates of 1.8% and 11%, respectively. In the 42 patients who demonstrated ^{201}Tl defect redistribution, 15 operations were canceled, nine patients underwent coronary revascularization, and 18 patients proceeded with their vascular procedures. Nine of the 18 patients who did not undergo revascularization with scintigraphic ischemia (50%) had a postoperative cardiac event.

MYOCARDIAL VIABILITY

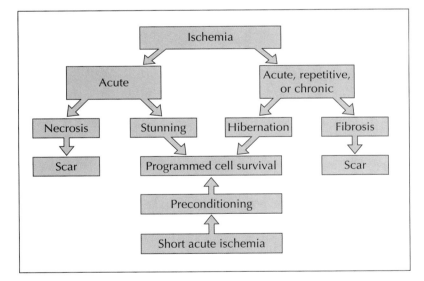

FIGURE 11-26. Imbalance between oxygen supply, usually caused by reduced myocardial perfusion, and oxygen demand, determined primarily by the rate and force of myocardial contraction, is termed *ischemic myocardium*. If the oxygen supply–demand imbalance is transient (*ie*, triggered by exertion), it represents reversible ischemia. On the other hand, if the regional oxygen supply–demand imbalance is prolonged, high-energy phosphates become depleted, regional contractile function progressively deteriorates, and cell membrane rupture with cell death follows (*ie*, myocardial necrosis and fibrosis). The phenomena of stunning, hibernation, and ischemic preconditioning represent different mechanisms of acute and chronic adaptation to a temporary or sustained reduction in coronary blood flow. Such modulated responses to ischemia are regulated to preserve sufficient energy to protect the structural and functional integrity of the cardiac myocyte. In contrast to programmed cell death, or apoptosis, Taegtmeyer [42] has coined the term *programmed cell survival* to describe the commonality between myocardial stunning, hibernation, and ischemic preconditioning independent from their disparate myocardial responses to acute and chronic ischemia. (*Adapted from* Taegtmeyer [42].)

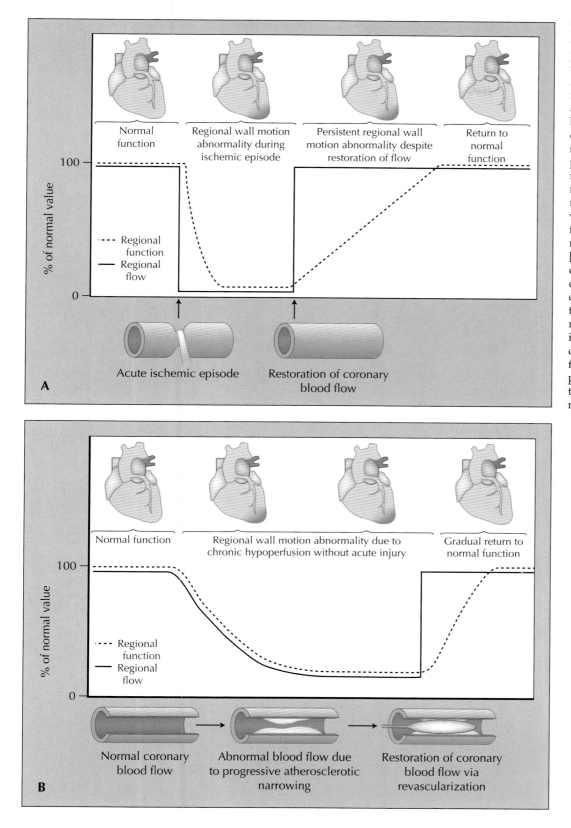

Figure 11-27. Pathophysiologic paradigms concerning the relationship between myocardial perfusion and left ventricular function in stunned and hibernating myocardium. **A,** Stunned myocardium is the state of delayed recovery of regional left ventricular dysfunction after a transient period of ischemia that has been followed by reperfusion [43]. The ischemic episodes that ultimately lead to myocardial stunning can be single or multiple, brief or prolonged, but never severe enough to result in myocardial necrosis. **B,** Hibernating myocardium is an adaptive rather than injurious response of the myocardium in which viable but dysfunctional myocardium arises from prolonged myocardial hypoperfusion at rest in the absence of clinically evident ischemia [44]. In stunning, interventions aimed at decreasing the frequency, severity, or duration of ischemic episodes result in improved contractile function. In hibernation, interventions that favorably alter the supply–demand relationship of the myocardium, either improvement in blood flow or reduction in demand, are expected to improve contractile function. It is very likely, however, that in patients with chronic coronary artery disease, the adaptive responses of hibernation and injurious responses of stunning coexist.

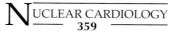

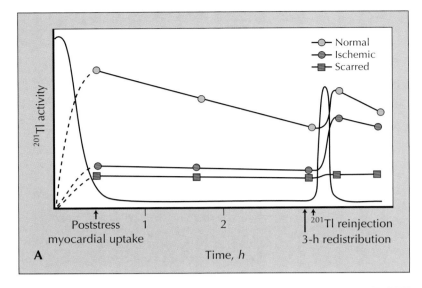

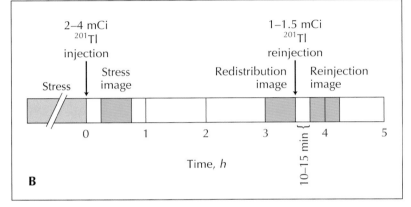

FIGURE 11-28. Thallium reinjection. **A,** ^{201}Tl reinjection differentiates ischemic but viable myocardium from scarred myocardium by augmenting the blood levels of ^{201}Tl at rest. A viable segment may be asynergic on the basis of repetitive stunning and hibernation. Thus, an asynergic but viable region may have reduced (but not absent) blood flow at rest (hibernation) or transient reduction in blood flow after a period of ischemia (stunning). Although standard stress–3- to 4-hour redistribution ^{201}Tl scintigraphy may underestimate the presence of ischemic but viable myocardium in many patients with coronary artery disease, reinjection of ^{201}Tl at rest after stress–3- to 4-hour redistribution imaging substantially improves the assessment of myocardial ischemia and viability in up to 49% of patients with apparently irreversible defects [45]. The theory that myocardial regions identified by ^{201}Tl uptake after ^{201}Tl reinjection represent viable myocardium is supported by improved regional function after revascularization and preserved metabolic activity by [18F]-fluorodeoxyglucose positron emission tomography (PET). In addition, a significant inverse correlation between the magnitude of ^{201}Tl activity after reinjection and regional volume fraction of interstitial fibrosis has been demonstrated in comparative clinicopathologic studies [46]. It is possible that whereas the initial myocardial uptake of ^{201}Tl (postinjection) reflects regional blood flow, redistribution of ^{201}Tl in a given defect depends not only on the severity of the initial defect but also on the presence of viable myocytes, the concentration of the tracer in the blood, and the rate of decline of ^{201}Tl levels in the blood. Thus, the heterogeneity of regional blood flow observed on the initial stress-induced ^{201}Tl defects may be independent of the subsequent extent of ^{201}Tl redistribution. If the blood level of ^{201}Tl remains the same (or increases) during the period between stress and 3- to 4-hour redistribution imaging, then an apparent defect in a region with viable myocytes that can retain ^{201}Tl should improve. On the other hand, if the serum ^{201}Tl concentration decreases during the imaging interval, the delivery of ^{201}Tl may be insufficient and the ^{201}Tl defect may remain irreversible even though the underlying myocardium is viable. This suggests that some ischemic but viable regions may never redistribute, even with late (24-hour) imaging, unless serum levels of ^{201}Tl are increased.

B, This hypothesis is supported by a study in which ^{201}Tl reinjection was performed immediately after 24-hour redistribution images were obtained [47]. Improved ^{201}Tl uptake after reinjection occurred in 40% of defects that appeared irreversible on late (24-hour) redistribution images. Thus, reinjection of 1 mCi of ^{201}Tl at rest immediately after either stress–3- to 4-hour redistribution or stress–24-hour redistribution studies, followed by image acquisition 10 to 15 minutes later, improves significantly the assessment of myocardial ischemia and viability. (*Adapted from* Dilsizian [48].)

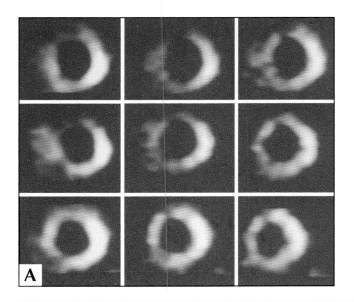

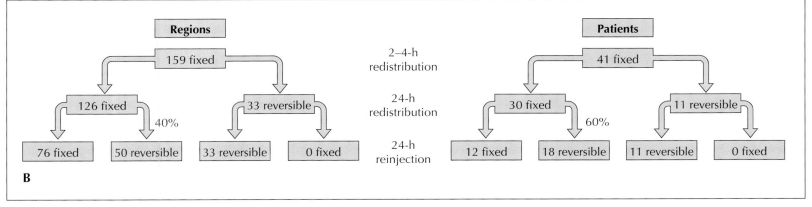

FIGURE 11-29. The beneficial effect of ^{201}Tl reinjection in the clinical setting. **A,** Short-axis tomograms demonstrate extensive ^{201}Tl defects in the anterior and septal regions on stress images (*top row*) that persist on redistribution images (*center row*) but improve markedly on reinjection images (*bottom row*). Among patients who underwent coronary artery revascularization, 87% of myocardial regions identified as viable by reinjection studies had normal ^{201}Tl uptake and improved regional wall motion after revascularization. In contrast, all regions with irreversible defects on reinjection imaging before revascularization had persistent wall motion abnormality after revascularization [5]. **B,** Similar results were obtained when ^{201}Tl reinjection was performed immediately after late (24-hour) redistribution imaging. Improved ^{201}Tl uptake after reinjection occurred in 40% of regions (involving 60% of patients) that appeared fixed on late redistribution imaging. (*Panel A* courtesy of Vasken Dilsizian, National Institutes of Health, Bethesda, MD; *Panel B adapted from* Kayden *et al.* [47].)

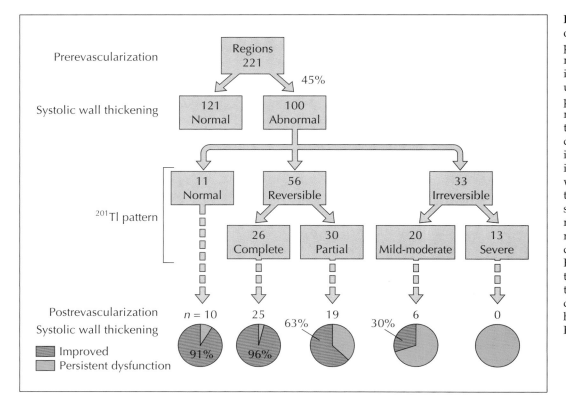

Prerevascularization

Systolic wall thickening

^{201}Tl pattern

Postrevascularization
Systolic wall thickening

- ▨ Improved
- ▥ Persistent dysfunction

FIGURE 11-30. Post-revascularization functional outcome of asynergic regions in relation to prerevascularization ^{201}Tl patterns of normal, reversible, partially reversible, mild to moderate irreversible, and severe irreversible defects using a stress–redistribution–reinjection ^{201}Tl protocol. The probabilities of functional recovery after revascularization were greater than 90% in normal or completely reversible defects, 63% in partially reversible defects, 30% in mild to moderate irreversible defects, and 0% in severe irreversible defects. Asynergic regions with reversible defects (complete or partial) on the prerevascularization ^{201}Tl study were shown more likely to improve function after revascularization compared with asynergic regions with mild to moderate irreversible defects (79% vs 30%, respectively; $P < 0.001$). Even at a similar mass of viable myocardial tissue (as reflected by the final ^{201}Tl content), the presence of inducible ischemia (reversible defect) was associated with an increased likelihood of functional recovery. (*Adapted from* Kitsiou *et al.* [49].)

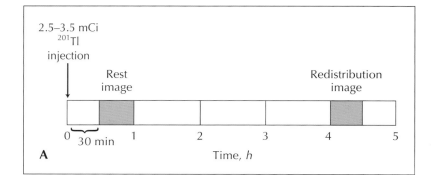

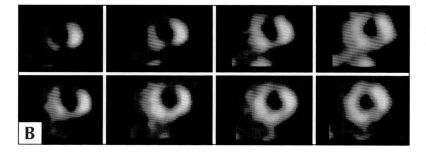

FIGURE 11-31. Rest–redistribution ^{201}Tl protocol. **A,** The stress–redistribution–reinjection ^{201}Tl protocol provides important diagnostic information regarding both inducible ischemia and myocardial viability. In most cases, the identification of myocardial ischemia is much more important clinically in terms of patient management and risk stratification than knowledge of myocardial viability. However, if the clinical question is one of the presence and extent of viable myocardium within a dysfunctional region and not inducible ischemia, then it is reasonable to perform rest–redistribution ^{201}Tl imaging only. **B,** Rest–redistribution short-axis ^{201}Tl tomograms are shown from a patient with chronic coronary artery disease. There are extensive ^{201}Tl perfusion defects in the anteroapical, anteroseptal, and inferior regions on the initial rest images (*top row*). On the delayed (3- to 4-hour) redistribution images (*bottom row*), whereas the inferior region remains fixed (scarred myocardium), the anteroapical and anteroseptal regions show significant reversibility, suggestive of viable myocardium [50]. (*Panel B courtesy of* Vasken Dilsizian, National Institutes of Health, Bethesda, MD.)

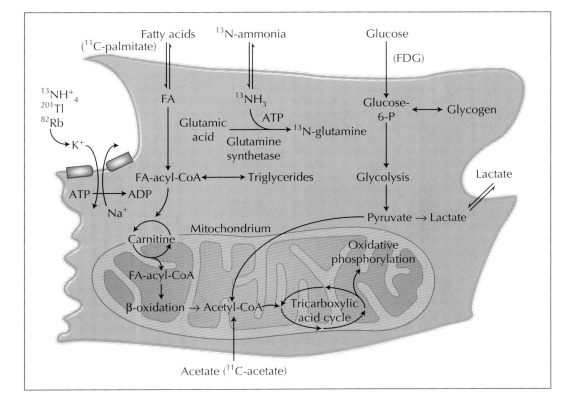

FIGURE 11-32. Major metabolic pathways and regulatory steps of a myocyte. Breakdown of fatty acids in the mitochondria via ß-oxidation is exquisitely sensitive to oxygen deprivation. Therefore, in the setting of reduced oxygen supply, the myocytes compensate for the loss of oxidative potential by shifting toward greater utilization of glucose to generate high-energy phosphates. Glycolysis occurs in the cytoplasm under anaerobic conditions and leads to the formation of pyruvate. For every mol of glucose metabolized through glycolysis, 2 mol of ATP are generated (anaerobic condition), and 36 mol of ATP are generated from pyruvate entering the citric acid cycle in the mitochondria (aerobic oxidative phosphorylation). Because glycolysis can generate ATP under anaerobic conditions, glycolysis becomes an attractive alternate metabolic pathway for ATP generation in hypoperfused myocardium with a limited supply of oxygen. Although the amount of energy produced by glycolysis may be adequate to maintain myocyte viability and preserve the electrochemical gradient across the cell membrane, it may not be sufficient to sustain contractile function. In hibernation, the adaptive response of the myocardium in the setting of prolonged resting hypoperfusion (reduced oxygen supply) is a reduction in myocardial contractile function (reduced oxygen demand), thereby preserving myocardial viability in the absence of clinically evident ischemia. FDG—[18F]-fluorodeoxyglucose. (*Adapted from* Dilsizian [51].)

PET TECHNIQUES: FDG

Glucose analogue that competes with glucose for hexokinase

Phosphorylated by hexokinase to FDG-6-phosphate

Trapped within myocytes

Impermeable to the sarcolemma

Poor substrate for further metabolism

Slow dephosphorylation

Myocardial uptake is influenced by metabolic and hormonal milieu

FIGURE 11-33. Positron emission tomography (PET) technique: [18F]-fluorodeoxyglucose (FDG). FDG is a glucose analogue used to image myocardial glucose utilization with PET. After intravenous injection of 5 to 10 mCi FDG, FDG rapidly exchanges across the capillary and cellular membranes and is phosphorylated by hexokinase to FDG-6-phosphate. After it is phosphorylated, FDG is not metabolized further in the glycolytic pathway, fructose–pentose shunt, or glycogen synthesis. Because the dephosphorylation rate of FDG is slow, it essentially becomes trapped in the myocardium, allowing adequate time to image regional glucose uptake by PET or single-photon emission computed tomography. In the fasting and aerobic conditions, fatty acids are the preferred source of myocardial energy production, with glucose accounting for some 15% to 20% of the total energy supply. However, in the fed state, plasma insulin levels increase, glucose metabolism is stimulated, and tissue lipolysis is inhibited, resulting in reduced fatty acid delivery to the myocardium. The combined effects of insulin on these processes and the increased arterial glucose concentration associated with the fed state result in preferred glucose utilization by the myocardium.

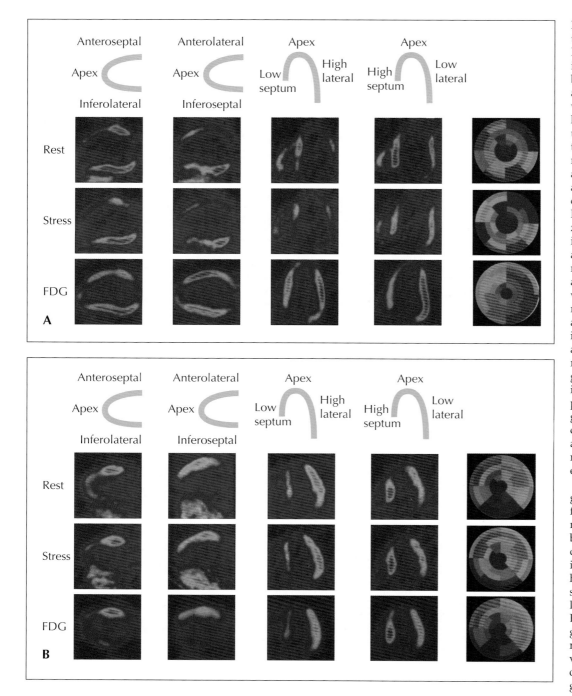

FIGURE 11-34. Examples of positron emission tomography (PET) mismatch and match patterns. Increased [18F]-fluorodeoxyglucose (FDG) uptake in asynergic myocardial regions with reduced blood flow at rest (mismatch pattern) has become a scintigraphic marker of hibernation. **A,** A patient with severely dilated left ventricle, diffuse hypotension, and apical dyskinesis (left ventricular ejection fraction [LVEF], 12%) had severe triple vessel disease. The coronary angiogram revealed 100% occlusion of the proximal left anterior descending coronary artery (LAD), D1, and D2; subtotal occlusion of the proximal right coronary artery (RCA); and 90% OM1 occlusion. In this patient, four long-axis slices (two horizontal long-axis and two vertical long-axis images) encompassing the entire left ventricle along with corresponding bull's-eye images for rest and stress ^{13}N-ammonia and FDG uptake are shown. Rest ^{13}N-ammonia images show irreversible defects in the apical and anterolateral regions with partial reversibility in the anterior and inferoseptal regions. Stress ^{13}N-ammonia images show markedly decreased perfusion in the apical, anterior, anterolateral, and inferoseptal regions. However, FDG images acquired under glucose-loaded conditions show preserved or increased glucose utilization in all abnormally perfused myocardial regions at rest, the scintigraphic hallmark of hibernation. In patients with chronic ischemic left ventricular dysfunction, rest and stress myocardial perfusion images alone may significantly underestimate the presence and extent of hibernating but viable myocardium.

B, Decreased or absent FDG uptake in asynergistic myocardial regions with reduced blood flow at rest (match pattern) represents scarred myocardium. A patient with previous coronary bypass surgery presented with significantly dilated left ventricle, apical dyskinesis, septal and inferior akinesis (LVEF, 36%), and congestive heart failure. The coronary angiogram revealed severe native disease of all three vessels, patent left and right internal mammary grafts to the LAD and RCA, critical stenoses of the OM1 vein graft, and a patent OM2 vein graft. In this patient, rest and stress ^{13}N-ammonia images show irreversible defects in the inferior, apical, and inferoseptal regions. FDG images acquired under glucose-loaded condition show absence of glucose utilization in all abnormally perfused myocardial regions at rest. Such asynergic myocardial regions demonstrating matched reduction in perfusion and metabolism represent scarred myocardium and are unlikely to recover function after revacularization.

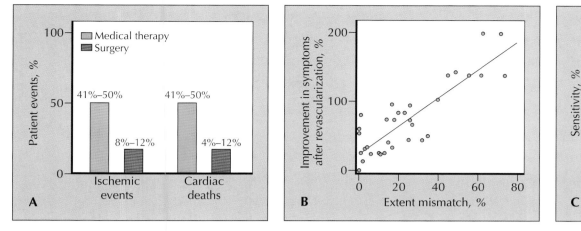

FIGURE 11-35. Positron emission tomography (PET) mismatch and prognosis. The prognostic significance of perfusion–metabolism mismatch pattern in ischemic cardiomyopathy has been shown in a number of nonrandomized, retrospective studies with PET [52,53]. **A,** Patients with perfusion–metabolism mismatch pattern who were treated surgically had lower ischemic event rates and fewer deaths compared with those treated with medical therapy. In contrast, patients with perfusion–metabolism match pattern displayed no such difference in outcomes between surgical and medical management. Moreover, the patients with myocardial viability (mismatch pattern) who underwent revascularization manifested a significant improvement in heart failure symptoms and exercise tolerance [54,55].

B, The relationship between the anatomic extent of perfusion–metabolism PET mismatch pattern (expressed as percent of the left ventricle)

and the change in functional status after revascularization (expressed as percent improvement from baseline) is shown. The scatterplot shows that the greatest improvement in heart failure symptoms occurs in patients with the largest mismatch defects on quantitative analysis of PET images.

C, Receiver-operating characteristic curve for different anatomic extent of perfusion–metabolism mismatch to predict a change (at least 1 grade) in functional status after revascularization is shown. When the extent of PET mismatch involves 18% or more of the left ventricular mass, the sensitivity for predicting a change in functional status after revascularization is 76% and the specificity is 78% (area under the fitted curve = 0.82). (*Panel A adapted from* Eitzman *et al.* [52] *and* Di Carli *et al.* [53]; *panels B and C adapted from* Di Carli *et al.* [54].)

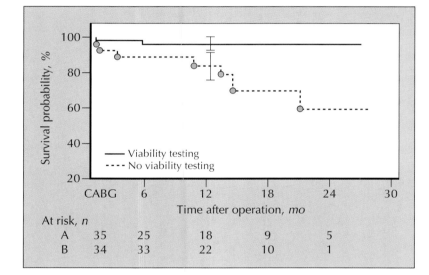

FIGURE 11-36. Assessment of myocardial viability before surgery and clinical outcome. Because patients with chronic ischemic left ventricular dysfunction are at higher risk for perioperative complications associated with coronary artery bypass surgery (CABG), one might question whether assessment of myocardial viability by means of positron emission tomography (PET) before surgery affects the clinical outcome with respect to perioperative and postoperative survival. In this retrospective study, the actuarial survival curve, which includes in-hospital mortality after surgery and mortality during follow-up, shows significant different survival between patients who were selected for surgery on the basis of clinical presentation and angiographic data (group A, no viability testing) compared with those who were selected for surgery according to extent of viable myocardium determined by PET (group B, viability testing). One year after surgery, whereas the survival rate of patients with viability testing was 97% ± 3%, the survival rate of patients with no viability testing was 79% ± 8% (*P* < 0.01). These data suggest that beyond providing prognostic information with regard to recovery of function after revascularization, myocardial viability studies with PET also allow selection of patients who are at low risk for serious perioperative and postoperative complications. (*Adapted from* Haas *et al.* [55].)

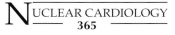

DIAGNOSIS OF ACUTE CORONARY SYNDROMES

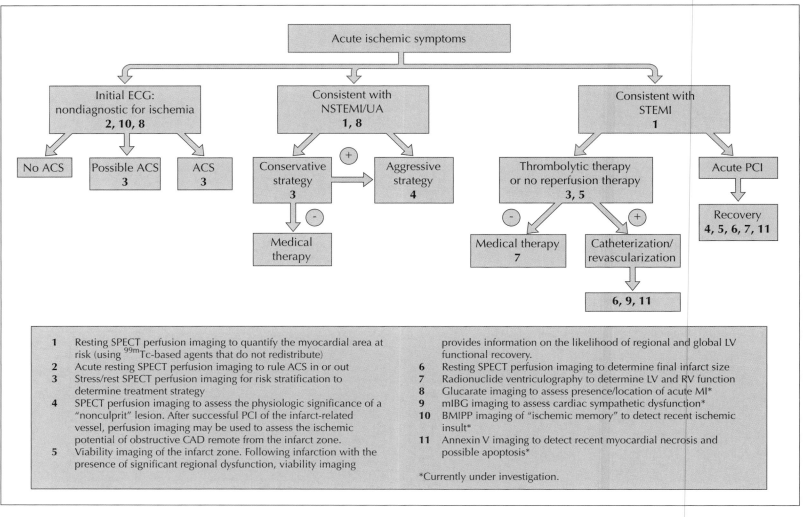

FIGURE 11-37. Diagnostic and therapeutic decision points in three categories of acute ischemic coronary syndromes (ACS). This schematic demonstrates the role of radionuclide techniques in patients seen in the emergency department with suspected ACS who have nondiagnostic ECG changes, patients with non–ST segment elevation myocardial infarction/unstable angina (NSTEMI/UA), and patients with ST segment elevation myocardial infarction (STEMI). Radionuclide imaging techniques that have been applied in either a research or clinical setting are listed, keyed to the appropriate clinical time points where they would be most useful. BMIPP—15-(p-[iodine-123] iodophenyl)-3-(R,S) methylpentadecanoic acid; CAD—coronary artery disease; LV—left ventricle; mIBG—metaiodobenzylguanidine; PCI—percutaneous coronary intervention; RV—right ventricle.

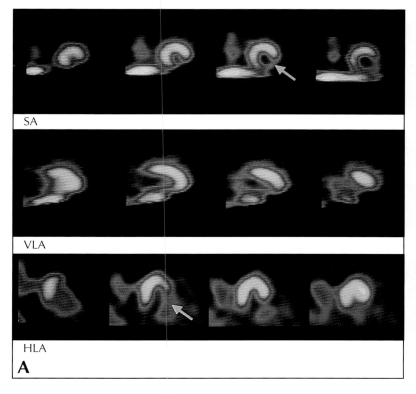

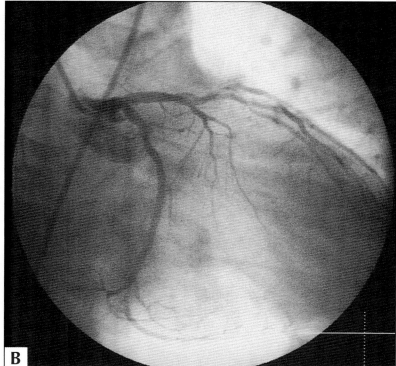

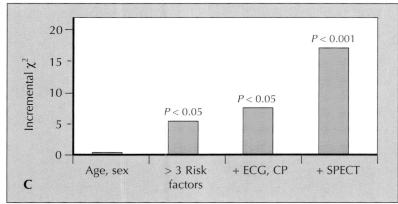

C

FIGURE 11-38. Significant myocardial perfusion abnormalities in patients with chest pain but nondiagnostic electrocardiographic alterations. **A,** Short-axis (SA), vertical long-axis (VLA), and horizontal long-axis (HLA) resting single-photon emission computed tomography (SPECT) myocardial perfusion images (MPIs) of a 39-year-old man who presented to the emergency room (ER) with chest pain atypical for angina and a normal initial electrocardiogram (ECG). The patient was injected with ^{99m}Tc-sestamibi at rest in the ER and underwent SPECT imaging soon thereafter.

The images show a dense inferolateral resting perfusion defect (*arrows*), which, in the setting of ongoing symptoms, was most suggestive of resting ischemia and acute coronary syndrome (ACS). He was immediately triaged to the catheterization laboratory.

B, Right anterior oblique view of the left coronary artery injection showing an acutely occluded left circumflex artery in the patient in *A.* Left circumflex occlusions are not always well seen on the standard 12-lead ECG. The patient subsequently underwent successful percutaneous coronary intervention of the left circumflex artery, with an excellent anatomic result. Had MPI not been performed, he may have been admitted for observation, and serial enzyme analysis may have been positive for a myocardial infarction. The use of MPI likely allowed significantly earlier intervention in this case.

C, Analysis of the incremental value of resting MPI data to predict cardiac events in patients presenting to the ER with suspected ischemia. The incremental χ^2 value measures the strength of the association between individual factors added to a clinician's knowledge base in incremental fashion and unfavorable cardiac events. Addition of resting SPECT MPI data (+ SPECT) in the ER setting adds highly statistically significant value on detection of ACS and events even given knowledge of age, gender, multiple (> three) risk factors for coronary artery disease, and ECG changes and the presence or absence of chest pain (CP). (*Panel C adapted from* Heller *et al.* [56].)

MYOCARDIAL FUNCTION: RADIONUCLIDE ANGIOGRAPHY AND GATED SINGLE-PHOTON EMISSION COMPUTED TOMOGRAPHY

LEFT VENTRICULAR EJECTION FRACTION DURING DOXORUBICIN THERAPY

BASELINE EF	PERFORM EQUILIBRIUM RADIONUCLIDE ANGIOGRAPHY	AT RISK FOR CHF
Normal (~ 50%)	At baseline	≥ 10% EF fall from baseline to < 50%
	At ~ 450 mg/m²	
	At 250–300 mg/m²	
≥ 30% to < 50 %	At baseline	≥ 10% EF fall from baseline or EF < 30%
< 30 %	Prior to each subsequent dose	
	Avoid doxorubicin	

FIGURE 11-39. Directing doxorubicin therapy. Radionuclide angiography (RNA) is the most widely accepted method for serial evaluation of cardiac function in patients undergoing doxorubicin therapy. Left ventricular ejection fraction (LVEF) is an important and universally accepted index of cardiac function. Overt congestive heart failure caused by doxorubicin cardiotoxicity is preceded by a progressive decrease in LVEF. Serial studies can detect a change in cardiac function over time, and doxorubicin administration can be stopped when a predetermined decrease in LVEF is observed. Both the absolute LVEF and the magnitude of the decrease are important strategic determinants. The guidelines for using serial RNA at rest during the course of doxorubicin therapy are standardized and are based on experience with nearly 1500 patients over a

7-year period. A greater than fourfold reduction in the incidence of overt cardiac failure was observed when these guidelines were followed. Moreover, if congestive heart failure (CHF) develops, it was mild and rapidly responsive to medical therapy. A recent study [57] has reestablished the clinical relevance and cost effectiveness of serial LVEF monitoring with equilibrium RNA for the prevention of congestive heart failure during the course of doxorubicin therapy. Exercise RNA has also been used in patients undergoing treatment with doxorubicin. However, patients with malignancies are often unable to undergo exercise testing because of generalized debility, fever, anemia, or musculoskeletal problems. Moreover, exercise testing does not appear to provide additional information compared with resting RNA. Some caution may be required in interpreting changes in LVEF during the course of chemotherapy because these values are also affected by several noncardiac conditions such as anemia, fever, and sepsis. Resting RNA continues to be the most practical and effective way of monitoring doxorubicin cardiotoxicity. EF—ejection fraction (*Adapted from* Schwartz *et al.* [58].)

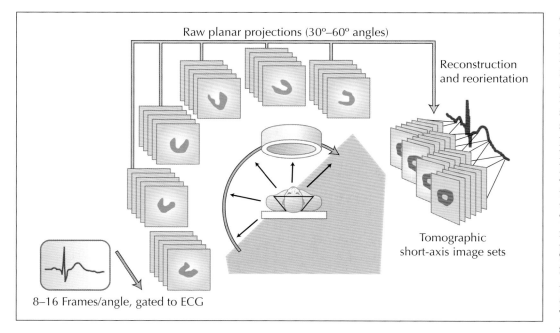

FIGURE 11-40. Gated myocardial perfusion single-photon emission computed tomography (SPECT): acquisition. A gated cardiac SPECT acquisition proceeds almost exactly like an ungated one: the camera detector (or detectors) rotate around the patient, collecting projection images at

equally spaced angles along a 180° or 360° arc, and these projections are then filtered and reconstructed into tomographic short- and long-axis images [59,60]. The distinguishing feature of gated SPECT imaging is that at each angle, several (eight, 16, or even 32) projection images are acquired, each corresponding to a specific phase of the cardiac cycle. Reconstruction of all same-phase projections produces a 3-dimensional "snapshot" of the patient's heart, frozen in time at that particular phase. Doing so for all phases results in 4-dimensional image volumes (x, y, z, and time, tomographic short-axis image sets) from which cardiac function can be readily assessed. Typical parameters used are low-energy, high-resolution collimator (or collimators), patient weight–based injection of 25 to 40 mCi of ^{99m}Tc-sestamibi/tetrofosmin or 3 to 4.5 mCi of ^{201}Tl, 3° of spacing between adjacent projections, and 25 seconds (^{99m}Tc) or 35 seconds (^{201}Tl) acquisition time per projection [61]. The resulting total acquisition time can be as short as 12.5 minutes (^{99m}Tc) or 17.5 minutes (^{201}Tl), if a dual detector camera with the detectors at a 90° angle is used. (*Adapted from* Germano and Berman [62].)

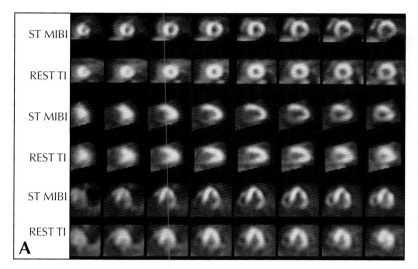

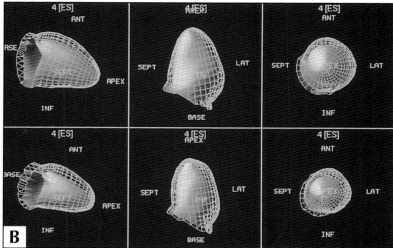

FIGURE 11-41. Assessment of risk using gated myocardial perfusion single-photon emission computed tomography (SPECT). **A,** Perfusion results from a 73-year-old patient with atypical chest pain who had undergone coronary artery bypass surgery at a remote time and angioplasty 5 years before this SPECT study. The patient had hypertension and hypercholesterolemia but no history of prior myocardial infarction. Adenosine stress testing demonstrated ST segment depression (-1.5 mm downsloping in lead V5), and there was no ST segment depression at rest. Exercise stress ^{99m}Tc-sestamibi (ST MIBI) and rest ^{201}Tl (REST Tl) images are interlaced in the alternate rows, which show short-axis images (*top two rows*), vertical long-axis images (*middle two rows*), and horizontal long-axis images (*bottom two rows*). The stress and rest images demonstrate extensive ischemia in the right coronary territory and evidence of ischemia in the diagonal coronary

territory. The stress perfusion defects alone indicate a high-risk state. There is also evidence of transient ischemic dilation in the left ventricle, further adding to the proof that ischemia is severe in this patient.

B, Stress (*top row*) and rest (*bottom row*) of the gated SPECT study. Shown are the vertical long-axis (*left column*), horizontal long-axis (*middle column*), and short-axis (*right column*) views. The *white grid* is the computer-defined endocardial surface from the gated SPECT study at end-diastole, and the *shaded gray surface* represents the computer-defined endocardial surface at end-systole. This patient demonstrates septal wall motion abnormality at rest (with normal thickening not shown) consistent with prior bypass surgery. After stress, there is the development of a new wall motion abnormality in the anterior apical and inferior left ventricular walls.

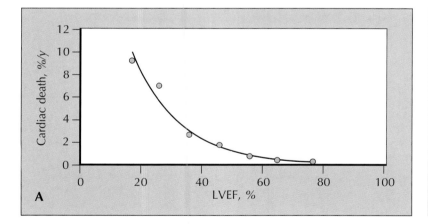

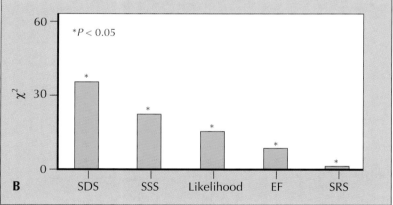

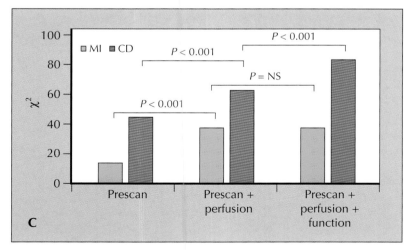

FIGURE 11-42. Relationship between left ventricular ejection fraction (LVEF) measured by gated single-photon emission computed tomography (SPECT) and mortality rate and nonfatal myocardial infarction (MI). **A,** In 2686 consecutive patients undergoing stress ^{99m}Tc myocardial perfusion gated SPECT, there is a curvilinear inverse relationship between LVEF at rest and cardiac death [63]. The LVEF was the strongest predictor of mortality in this group. The findings are similar to those reported for LVEF acquired with radionuclide angiography in patients after MI. **B,** When the predictors of nonfatal MI are considered, although LVEF remains a significant predictor, the extent of reversible ischemia, as measured by the summed difference score (SDS), is the strongest univariate predictor. Previous studies have also shown that the extent of reversible ischemia is more predictive for cardiac events than the extent of coronary artery disease, as assessed by coronary angiography [64]. **C,** When considered from the standpoint of incremental information, stress SPECT perfusion data add significantly to clinical information for predicting nonfatal MI, and there is no further information gained from other variables provided by gated SPECT (*orange bars*). However, when the risk of cardiac death is considered (*green bars*), incremental information is provided over clinical data not only by the stress perfusion findings but also by LVEF assessed by gated SPECT. EF—ejection fraction; SRS—summed rest score; SSS—summed stress score. (*Adapted from* Sharir *et al.* [63].)

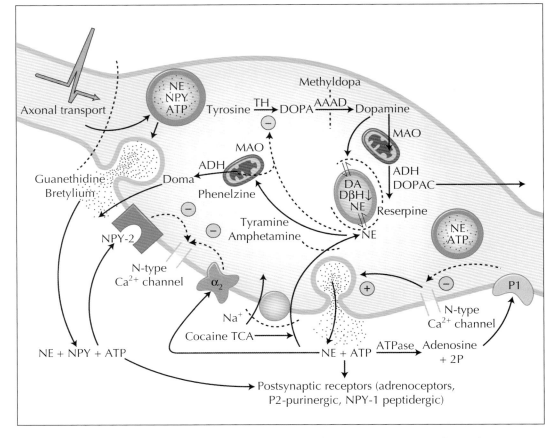

FIGURE 11-43. Neurotransmitter synthesis and release at adrenergic nerve terminals: mechanisms controlling transmitter synthesis and release at adrenergic nerve terminals. Transmitters are stored in two types of synaptic vesicles, small vesicles containing only the principal transmitter norepinephrine (NE) and cotransmitter adenosine triphosphate (ATP) (each synthesized within the nerve terminal itself), and larger dense-core vesicles containing the polypeptide cotransmitter neuropeptide Y (NPY) and chromogranin (both of which are exclusively synthesized in the cell soma) as well as NE and ATP. The rate-limiting step for NE synthesis in the nerve terminal is tyrosine hydroxylase (TH) enzyme activity, which is negatively controlled by the cytoplasmic concentration of NE. The TH enzymatic product dopa is decarboxylated to dopamine by (unspecific) aromatic L-amino acid decarboxylase (AAAD) in a step subject to therapeutic interference by provision of the "false" substrate methyldopa (resulting in the eventual formation of the "false transmitter" -methyl-NE). Dopamine is to equal proportions either deaminated and excreted as DOPAC (3,4-dihydroxyphenylacetic acid) or

taken up into storage vesicles containing dopamine–hydroxylase (DH) via a reserpine-sensitive active uptake process and hydroxylated to NE. The cytoplasmic concentration of NE is determined by a dynamic equilibrium established between diffusion (leakage) out of storage vesicles; reserpine-sensitive (active) reuptake into storage vesicles; cytoplasmic displacement and extrusion by indirect sympathomimetics such as tyramine and amphetamine; reuptake from the extracellular space via a Na^+-dependent cotransport mechanism sensitive to inhibition by cocaine or tricyclic antidepressants; and elimination after metabolizing to 3,4-dihydroxymandelic acid (DOMA) by mitochondrial monoamine oxidase (MAO) and aldehyde dehydrogenase (ADH), a pathway sensitive to inhibition by MAO inhibitors such as phenelzine. In adrenal medullary neurons, 80% of cytoplasmic NE is methylized by N-methyl transferase into epinephrine before being packaged into storage vesicles. Nerve stimulation–evoked physiologic transmitter release occurs via fusion of synaptic storage vesicles with the cell membrane after the invasion of the nerve terminal by propagated action potentials (sensitive to blockade by guanethidine or bretylium) and the resulting increase in cytoplasmic Ca^{2+} through activation of voltage-sensitive (predominantly N-type) Ca^{2+} channels. Upon release, ATP, NE, and NPY produce neuroeffector responses through actions on postsynaptic membrane receptors. In addition, all three transmitters inhibit further release through action on presynaptic (P1, 2-adrenergic, NPY-2) receptors [65,66]. Transmitter actions are terminated by hydrolysis (ATP), reuptake into nerve terminals (NE), uptake into nonneuronal tissue and metabolism by catechol-O-methyl transferase (COMT) (NE), and diffusion away from the terminal and into the bloodstream (NE, NPY). ADH—aldehyde dehydrogenase; TCA—tricyclic antidepressant; TH—tyrosine hydroxylase. (*Adapted from* Nicholls *et al.* [67].)

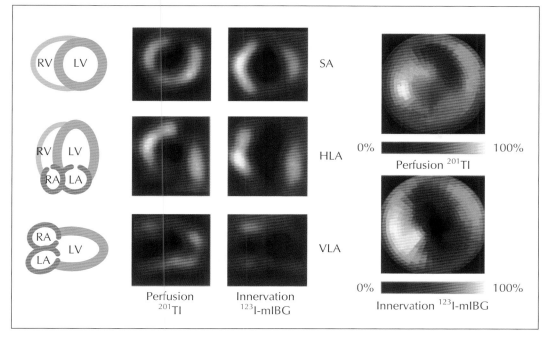
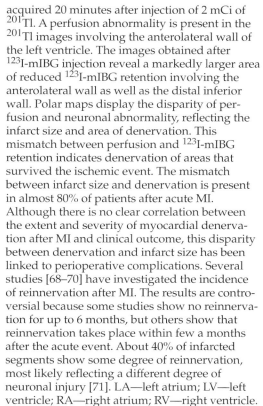

SA

HLA

0% [   ] 100%
Perfusion ²⁰¹Tl

VLA

0% [   ] 100%
Innervation ¹²³I-mIBG

Perfusion ²⁰¹Tl   Innervation ¹²³I-mIBG

FIGURE 11-44. Assessment of neuronal function in the infarct zone. Single-photon emission computed tomography (SPECT) images were obtained in a patient within 14 days of an anterior myocardial infarction (MI). The tomographic slices are displayed in short-axis (SA), horizontal long-axis (HLA), and vertical long-axis views (VLA). Regional retention of 10 mCi I-123 metaiodobenzylguanidine (¹²³I-mIBG) after 4 hours was compared with the myocardial perfusion as assessed from images acquired 20 minutes after injection of 2 mCi of ²⁰¹Tl. A perfusion abnormality is present in the ²⁰¹Tl images involving the anterolateral wall of the left ventricle. The images obtained after ¹²³I-mIBG injection reveal a markedly larger area of reduced ¹²³I-mIBG retention involving the anterolateral wall as well as the distal inferior wall. Polar maps display the disparity of perfusion and neuronal abnormality, reflecting the infarct size and area of denervation. This mismatch between perfusion and ¹²³I-mIBG retention indicates denervation of areas that survived the ischemic event. The mismatch between infarct size and denervation is present in almost 80% of patients after acute MI. Although there is no clear correlation between the extent and severity of myocardial denervation after MI and clinical outcome, this disparity between denervation and infarct size has been linked to perioperative complications. Several studies [68–70] have investigated the incidence of reinnervation after MI. The results are controversial because some studies show no reinnervation for up to 6 months, but others show that reinnervation takes place within few a months after the acute event. About 40% of infarcted segments show some degree of reinnervation, most likely reflecting a different degree of neuronal injury [71]. LA—left atrium; LV—left ventricle; RA—right atrium; RV—right ventricle.

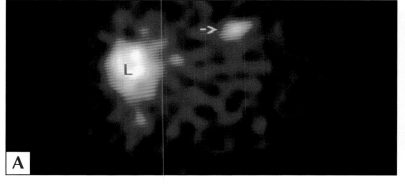

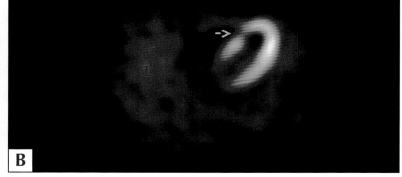

FIGURE 11-45. Noninvasive detection of apoptosis in acute myocardial infarction (MI). Postmortem studies in patients with acute MI have shown high frequency of apoptotic cell death program in the infarct area. The apoptotic cells are predominantly seen in the infarct periphery, where the severity of ischemic insult is milder. However, upon reperfusion, the infarct center shows an extensive admixture of apoptotic and necrotic cells as the doomed cells are rescued from necrosis but die by apoptosis. Furthermore, reperfusion injury may accelerate apoptosis in the cells in the center of the infarct. Accordingly, annexin V studies have been performed in patients with acute MI [72].

A, Patient with acute anteroapical infarction was injected with annexin V labeled with ⁹⁹ᵐTc immediately after reperfusion; the transverse single-photon emission computed tomography (SPECT) image shows enhanced uptake of annexin V in the apical region of the heart (*arrow*). **B,** The sestamibi perfusion scan obtained 48 hours later shows a perfusion defect that corresponds to the region of annexin uptake. The defect on the sestamibi SPECT indicates that cells that bound annexin V on day 1 must have undergone cell death. One intriguing possibility is that the binding of annexin V in the infarct area may indicate that cell death in this region may be preventable through intervention in the cell death program. (*From* Hofstra *et al.* [72]; with permission.)

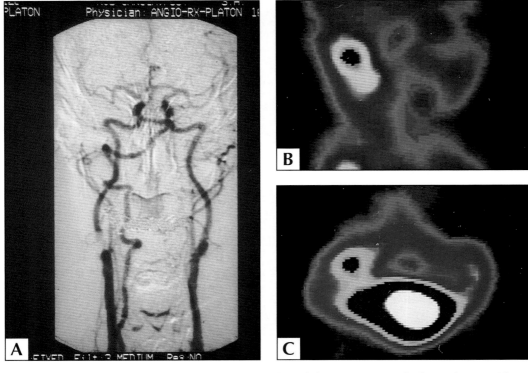

FIGURE 11-46. Clinical imaging of smooth muscle cell proliferation in carotid atherosclerosis. After the successful demonstration of the feasibility of imaging of proliferating smooth muscle cells (SMCs), the safety, biodistribution, accumulation, and elimination of Z2D3 were assessed in 11 patients who were candidates for carotid endarterectomy [73]. Arteriographic and Doppler echographic studies demonstrated significant stenosis in one carotid bed of all 11 patients; nine patients had bilateral disease. The arteriographic degree of stenosis ranged from 70% to 90% in the vessel on which endarterectomy was going to be performed, and from 10% to 70% in the contralateral sides of patients with bilateral disease. Z2D3 (250 µg) labeled with 5 mCi of ^{111}In was administered by slow intravenous injection. Planar and single-photon emission computed tomography (SPECT) images were obtained 4, 24, 48, and 72 hours later. Positive antibody uptake was observed in all of the 11 carotid arteries that underwent endarterectomy. Positive uptake also was seen in five contralateral sites with minimal evidence of stenosis in the arteriograms.

A, Significant obstructive lesion is observed in the carotid angiogram (*arrow*). Uptake of ^{111}In-Z2D3 at the site of the carotid plaques was seen in the planar and SPECT views at 4 hours (**B**, sagittal; **C**, transverse). The antibody uptake was localized discretely in the stenotic artery and corresponded with the angiographic location of the disease. The antibody uptake in planar images occasionally resulted in diffuse increase in radioactivity on the affected side compared with the contralateral normal carotid artery. SPECT images demonstrated the atherosclerotic plaques with more intense focal uptake in the majority of lesions, providing better delineation of the lesion sites. The intensity of uptake at the site of the plaques reached a maximum at 4 hours and decreased at subsequent time intervals. The target-to-control ratios were 2.20 ± 0.3, 1.98 ± 0.3, 1.60 ± 0.2, and 1.45 ± 0.2 at 4, 24, 48, and 72 hours, respectively. Comparison of the pattern of antibody uptake with the appearance of the plaques on arteriography revealed that the region with severe stenosis did not always correspond precisely with the site of more intense antibody uptake. In addition, the pattern of uptake was frequently more extended than the stenotic regions as delineated by the angiograms. Pathologic examination of the specimens by direct avidin––biotin–peroxidase immunocytochemistry revealed staining of neointimal SMC in scan-positive plaques (data not shown). Endarterectomy specimens were intensely radioactive, and the mean percent of the injected dose per gram localization in the specimens was 0.0475 ± 0.007. (*From* Carrio *et al.* [73]; with permission.)

FUTURE DIRECTIONS

The future of nuclear imaging depends on two factors: new radioligand development and new imaging and detection technology. It is clear that the explosion of information in cardiovascular molecular biology and atherosclerosis research will be ultimately translated into effective imaging strategies. Initial approaches to molecular imaging have already yielded exciting results. However, detection of radioligand uptake with superior resolution is a significant technologic undertaking. Whether this challenge will be best met by higher resolution imaging cameras or by intravascular radiation detectors comparable to intravascular ultrasound remains to be determined. In any event, the future appears extremely promising as imaging moves toward molecular paradigms in defining its next phase.

1. Port SC: Imaging guidelines for nuclear cardiology procedures: Part 2. *J Nucl Cardiol* 1999, 6:G49–G84.

2. Maddahi J, Van Train K, Prigent F, *et al.*: Quantitative single photon emission computed thallium-201 tomography for detection and localization of coronary artery disease: optimization and prospective validation of a new technique. *J Am Coll Cardiol* 1989, 14:1689.

3. Fintel DJ, Links JM, Brinker JA, *et al.*: Improved diagnostic performance of exercise thallium-201 single photon emission computed tomography over planar imaging in the diagnosis of coronary artery disease: a receiver operating characteristic analysis. *J Am Coll Cardiol* 1989, 13:600.

4. Iskandrian AS, Heo J, Kong B, *et al.*: Effect of exercise level on the ability of thallium-201 tomographic imaging in detecting coronary artery disease: analysis of 461 patients. *J Am Coll Cardiol* 1989, 14:1477.

5. Go RT, Marwick TH, MacIntyre WJ, *et al.*: A prospective comparison of rubidium-82 PET and thallium-201 SPECT myocardial perfusion imaging utilizing a single dipyridamole stress in the diagnosis of coronary artery disease. *J Nucl Med* 1990, 31:1899.

6. Mahmarian JJ, Boyce, Goldberg RK, *et al.*: Quantitative exercise thallium-201 single photon emission computed tomography for the enhanced diagnosis of ischemic heart disease. *J Am Coll Cardiol* 1990, 15:318.

7. van Train KF, Maddahi J, Berman DS, *et al.*: Quantitative analysis of tomographic stress thallium-201 myocardial scintigrams: a multicenter trial. *J Nucl Med* 1990, 31:1168.

8. Kiat H, Maddahi J, Roy L, *et al.*: Comparison of technetium 99m methoxy isobutyl isonitrile and thallium-201 for evaluation of coronary artery disease by planar and tomographic methods. *Am Heart J* 1989, 117:111.

9. Iskandrian AS, Heo J, Long B, *et al.*: Use of technetium-99m isonitrile (RP-30A) in assessing left ventricular perfusion and function at rest and during exercise in coronary artery disease, and comparison with coronary arteriography and exercise thallium-201 SPECT imaging. *Am J Cardiol* 1989, 64:270.

10. Kahn JK, McGhie I, Akers MS, *et al.*: Quantitative rotational tomography ^{201}Tl and ^{99m}Tc 2-methoxly-isobutyl-isonitrile. *Circulation* 1989, 79:1282.

11. Solot G, Hermans J, Merlo P, *et al*: Correlation of 99Tcm-sestamibi SPECT with coronary angiography in general hospital practice. *Nucl Med Commun* 1993, 14:23.

12. Van Train KF, Garcia EV, Maddahi J, *et al.*: Multicenter trial validation for quantitative analysis of same-day rest-stress technetium-99m-sestamibi myocardial tomograms. *J Nucl Med* 1994, 35:609.

13. Azzarelli S, Galassi AR, Foti R, *et al.*: Accuracy of 99m-tetrofosmin myocardial tomography in the evaluation of coronary artery disease. *J Nucl Cardiol* 1999, 6:183.

14. Gould KL, Yoshida K, Hess MJ, *et al.*: Myocardial metabolism of fluorodeoxyglucose compared to cell membrane integrity for the potassium analogue rubidium-82 for assessing infarct size in man by PET. *J Nucl Med* 1991, 32:1–9.

15. Bruyne B, Hersbach F, Pijls NH, *et al.*: Abnormal epicardial coronary resistance in patients with diffuse atherosclerosis but "normal" coronary angiography. *Circulation* 2001, 104:2401–2406.

16. Gould KL, Nakagawa Y, Nakagawa K, *et al.*: Frequency and clinical implications of fluid dynamically significant diffuse coronary artery disease manifest as graded, longitudinal, base-to-apex myocardial perfusion abnormalities by noninvasive positron emission tomography. *Circulation* 2000, 101:1931–1939.

17. Samuels B, Kiat H, Friedman JD, Berman DS: Adenosine pharmacologic stress myocardial perfusion tomographic imaging in patients with significant aortic stenosis. Diagnostic efficacy and comparison of clinical, hemodynamic and electrocardiographic variables with 100 age-matched control subjects. *J Am Coll Cardiol* 1995, 25:99–106.

18. O'Keefe JH Jr, Bateman TM, Barnhart CS: Adenosine thallium-201 is superior to exercise thallium-201 for detecting coronary artery disease in patients with left bundle branch block. *J Am Coll Cardiol* 1993, 21:1332–1338.

19. Wagdy HM, Hodge D, Christian TF, *et al.*: Prognostic value of vasodilator perfusion imaging in patients with left bundle-branch block. *Circulation* 1998, 97:1563–1570.

20. Pennell DJ, Ell PJ: Whole-body imaging of thallium-201 after six different stress regimens. *J Nucl Med* 1994, 35:425–428.

21. Wu JC, Yuyn JJ, Heller EN, *et al.*: Limitations of dobutamine for enhancing flow heterogeneity in the presence of single coronary artery stenosis: implications for technetium-99m-sestamibi imaging. *J Nucl Med* 1998, 39:417–425.

22. Levine MG, Ahlberg A, Mann A, *et al.*: Comparison of exercise, dipyridamole, adenosine, and dobutamine stress with the use of Tc-99m tetrofosmin tomographic imaging. *J Nucl Cardiol* 1999, 6:389–396.

23. Homma S, Gilliland Y, Guiney TE, *et al.*: Safety of intravenous dipyridamole for stress testing with thallium imaging. *Am J Cardiol* 1987, 59:152–154.

24. Verani MS, Mahmarian JJ, Hixson JB, *et al.*: Diagnosis of coronary artery disease by controlled coronary vasodilation with adenosine and thallium-201 scintigraphy in patients unable to exercise. *Circulation* 1990, 82:80–87.

25. Watters TA, Botvinick EH, Dae MW, *et al.*: Comparison of the findings on preoperative dipyridamole perfusion scintigraphy and intraoperative transesophageal echocardiography: implications regarding the identification of myocardium at ischemic risk. *J Am Coll Cardiol* 1991, 18:93–100.

26. Fletcher JP, Antico JF, Gruenewald S, *et al.*: Dipyridamole-thallium scan for screening of coronary artery disease prior to vascular surgery. *J Cardiovasc Surg (Torino)* 1988, 29:666–669.

27. Younis LT, Aguirre F, Byers SL, *et al.*: Perioperative and long-term prognostic value of intravenous dipyridamole thallium scintigraphy in patients with peripheral vascular disease. *Am Heart J* 1990, 119:1287–1292.

28. Strawn DJ, Guernsey JM: Dipyridamole thallium scanning in the evaluation of coronary artery disease in elective abdominal aortic surgery. *Arch Surg* 1991, 126:880–884.

29. Younis LT, Stratmann HG, Takase B, *et al.*: Preoperative clinical assessment and dipyridamole thallium-201 scintigraphy for prediction and prevention of cardiac events in patients having major noncardiovascular surgery and known or suspected coronary artery disease. *Am J Cardiol* 1994, 74:311–317.

30. Elliott BM, Robison JG, Zellner JL, *et al.*: Dobutamine-thallium-201 imaging: assessing cardiac risks associated with vascular surgery. *Circulation* 1991; 84(suppl III):54–60.

31. Stratmann HG, Younis LT, Wittry MD, *et al.*: Dipyridamole technetium-99m sestamibi myocardial tomography for preoperative cardiac risk stratification before major or minor nonvascular surgery. *Am Heart J* 1996, 132:536–541.

32. Amanullah AM, Berman DS, Erel J, *et al.*: Incremental prognostic value of adenosine myocardial perfusion single-photon emission computed tomography in women with suspected coronary artery disease. *Am J Cardiol* 1998, 15:725–730.

33. Brown KA, Rowen M: Extent of jeopardized viable myocardium determined by myocardial perfusion imaging best predicts perioperative cardiac events in patients undergoing noncardiac surgery. *J Am Coll Cardiol* 1993, 21:325–330.

34. Levinson JR, Boucher CA, Coley CM, *et al.*: Usefulness of semiquantitative analysis of dipyridamole-thallium-201 redistribution for improving risk stratification before vascular surgery. *Am J Cardiol* 1990, 66:406–410.

35. Eagle KA, Singer DE, Brewster DC, *et al.*: Dipyridamole-thallium scanning in patients undergoing vascular surgery: optimizing preoperative evaluation of cardiac risk. *JAMA* 1987, 257:2185–2189.

36. Eagle KA, Brundage BH, Chaitman BR, *et al.*: Report of the American College of Cardiology/American Heart Association Task Force on Practice Guidelines (Committee on Perioperative Cardiovascular Evaluation for Noncardiac Surgery). *J Am Coll Cardiol* 1996, 27:910–948.

37. Hachamovitch R, Berman DS, Kiat H, *et al.*: Incremental prognostic value of adenosine stress myocardial perfusion single-photon emission computed tomography and impact on subsequent management in patients with or suspect of having myocardial ischemia. *Am J Cardiol* 1997, 80:426–433.

38. Shaw LJ, Eagle KA, Gersh BJ, Miller DD: Meta-analysis of intravenous dipyridamole-thallium-201 imaging (1985 to 1994) and dobutamine echocardiography (1991 to 1994) for risk stratification before vascular surgery. *J Am Coll Cardiol* 1996, 27:787–798.

39. Koutelou MG, Asimacopoulos PJ, Mahmarian JJ, *et al.*: Preoperative risk stratification by adenosine thallium-201 single-photon emission computed tomography in patients undergoing vascular surgery. *J Nucl Cardiol* 1995, 2:389–394.

40. Shaw LJ, Miller DD, Kong BA, *et al.*: Determination of perioperative cardiac risk by adenosine thallium-201 myocardial imaging. *Am J Heart J* 1992, 124:861–869.

41. Stratmann HG, Younis LT, Wittry MD, *et al.*: Dipyridamole technetium-99m sestamibi myocardial tomography in patients evaluated for elective vascular surgery: prognostic value for perioperative and late cardiac events. *Am Heart J* 1996, 131:923–929.

42. Taegtmeyer H: Modulation of responses to myocardial ischemia: metabolic features of myocardial stunning, hibernation, and ischemic preconditioning. In *Myocardial Viability: A Clinical and Scientific Treatise.* Edited by Dilsizian V. Armonk, NY: Futura; 2000:25–36.

43. Braunwald E, Kloner RA: The stunned myocardium: prolonged, postischemic ventricular dysfunction. *Circulation* 1982, 66:1146–1149.

44. Rahimtoola SH: A perspective on the three large multicenter randomized clinical trials of coronary bypass surgery for chronic stable angina. *Circulation* 1985, 72(suppl V):123–135.

45. Dilsizian V, Rocco TP, Freedman NM, *et al.*: Enhanced detection of ischemic but viable myocardium by the reinjection of thallium after stress-redistribution imaging. *N Engl J Med* 1990, 323:141–146.

46. Zimmermann R, Mall G, Rauch B, *et al.*: Residual Tl-201 activity in irreversible defects as a marker of myocardial viability: clinicopathological study. *Circulation* 1995, 91:1016–1021.

47. Kayden DS, Sigal S, Soufer R, *et al.*: Thallium-201 for assessment of myocardial viability: Quantitative comparison of 24-hour redistribution imaging with imaging after reinjection at rest. *J Am Coll Cardiol* 1991, 18:1480–1486.

48. Dilsizian V: Thallium-201 Scintigraphy: experience of two decades. In *Myocardial Viability: A Clinical and Scientific Treatise.* Edited by Dilsizian V. Armonk, NY: Futura; 2000:265–313.

49. Kitsiou AN, Srinivasan G, Quyyumi AA, *et al.*: Stress-induced reversible and mild-to-moderate irreversible thallium defects: are they equally accurate for predicting recovery of regional left ventricular function after revascularization? *Circulation* 1998, 98:501–508.

50. Arrighi JA, Dilsizian V: Identification of viable, nonfunctioning myocardium. In *Cardiac Intensive Care.* Edited by Brown DL. Philadelphia: W.B. Saunders; 1998:307–327.

51. Dilsizian V: Perspectives on the study of human myocardium: viability. In *Myocardial Viability: A Clinical and Scientific Treatise.* Edited by Dilsizian V. Armonk, NY: Futura; 2000:3–22.

52. Eitzman D, Al-Aouar Z, Kanter HL, *et al.*: Clinical outcome of patients with advanced coronary artery disease after viability studies with positron emission tomography. *J Am Coll Cardiol* 1992, 20:559–565.

53. Di Carli MF, Davidson M, Little R, *et al.*: Value of metabolic imaging with positron emission tomography for evaluating prognosis in patients with coronary artery disease and left ventricular dysfunction. *Am J Cardiol* 1994, 73:527–533.

54. Di Carli MF, Asgarzadie F, Schelbert HR, *et al.*: Quantitative relation between myocardial viability and improvement in heart failure symptoms after revascularization in patients with ischemic cardiomyopathy. *Circulation* 1995, 92:3436–3444.

55. Haas F, Haehnel CJ, Picker W, *et al.*: Preoperative positron emission tomography viability assessment and perioperative and postoperative risk in patients with advanced ischemic heart disease. *J Am Coll Cardiol* 1997, 30:1693–1700.

56. Heller GV, Stowers SA, Hendel RC, *et al.*: Clinical value of acute rest technetium-99m tetrofosmin tomographic myocardial perfusion imaging in patients with acute chest pain and nondiagnostic electrocardiograms. *J Am Coll Cardiol* 1998, 31:1011–1017.

57. Mitani I, Jain D, Joska TM, Burtness B, Zaret BL: Doxorubicin cardiotoxicity: prevention of congestive heart failure with serial cardiac function monitoring with equilibrium radionuclide angiocardiography in the current era. *J Nucl Cardiol* 2003, 10:132–139.

58. Schwartz RG, McKenzie WB, Alexander J, *et al.*: Congestive heart failure and left ventricular dysfunction complicating doxorubicin therapy. Seven-year experience using serial radionuclide angiocardiography. *Am J Med* 1987, 82:1109–1118.

59. Germano G: Technical aspects of myocardial SPECT imaging. *J Nucl Med* 2001, 42:1499–1507.

60. The Cardiovascular Imaging Committee, American College of Cardiology, The Committee on Advanced Cardiac Imaging and Technology, *et al.*: Standardization of cardiac tomographic imaging. *J Am Coll Cardiol* 1992, 20:255–256.

61. Sharir T, Germano G, Kavanagh PB, *et al.*: Incremental prognostic value of post-stress left ventricular ejection fraction and volume by gated myocardial perfusion single photon emission computed tomography. *Circulation* 1999, 100:1035–1042.

62. Germano G, Berman D, eds: Acquisition and processing for gated perfusion SPECT: technical aspects. In *Clinical Gated Cardiac SPECT.* Armonk, NY: Futura; 1999:93–113.

63. Sharir T, Germano G, Kang X, *et al.*: Prediction of myocardial infarction versus cardiac death by gated myocardial perfusion SPECT: risk stratification by the amount of stress-induced ischemia and the poststress ejection fraction. *J Nucl Med* 2001, 42:831–837.

64. Berman DS, Hayes SW, Shaw LJ, *et al.*: Recent advances in myocardial perfusion imaging. *Curr Probl Cardiol* 2001, 26:1–140.

65. Lipscombe D, Kongsamut S, Tsien RW, *et al.*: Adrenergic inhibition of sympathetic neurotransmitter release mediated by modulation of N-type calcium-channel gating. *Nature* 1989, 340:639–642.

66. Toth PT, Bindokas VP, Bleakman D, *et al.*: Mechanism of presynaptic inhibition by neuropeptide Y at sympathetic nerve terminals. *Nature* 1993, 364:635–639.

67. Nicholls JG, Martin AR, Wallace BG, *et al.*: *From Neuron to Brain.* Sunderland, MA: Sinauer Associates; 1992.

68. Allman KC, Wieland DM, Muzik O, *et al.*: Carbon-11 hydroxyephedrine with positron emission tomography for serial assessment of cardiac adrenergic neuronal function after acute myocardial infarction in humans. *J Am Coll Cardiol* 1993, 22:368–375.

69. Fallen EL, Coates G, Nahmias C, *et al.*: Recovery rates of regional sympathetic reinnervation and myocardial blood flow after acute myocardial infarction. *Am Heart J* 1999, 137:863–869.

70. Simula S, Lakka T, Kuikka J, *et al.*: Cardiac adrenergic innervation within the first 3 months after acute myocardial infarction. *Clin Physiol* 2000, 20:366–373.

71. Patel A, Iskandrian A: MIBG imaging. *J Nucl Cardiol* 2002, 9:75–94.

72. Hofstra L, Liem IH, Dumont E, *et al.*: Visualisation of cell death in vivo in patients with acute myocardial infarction. *Lancet* 2000, 356:209–212.

73. Carrio I, Pieri P, Narula J, *et al.*: Noninvasive localization of human atherosclerotic lesions with indium-111-labeled monoclonal Z2D3 antibody specific for proliferating smooth muscle cells. *J Nucl Cardiol* 1998, 5:551–557.

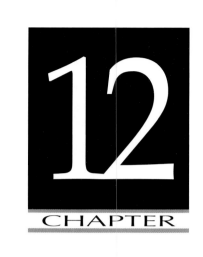

INTERVENTIONAL CARDIOLOGY

Verghese Mathew and David R. Holmes, Jr.

John D. Altman, Gregory W. Barsness, John F. Bresnahan,
Anoop Chauhan, Ali E. Denktas, Andrew Farb, Kirk N. Garratt,
Stuart T. Higano, Amir Lerman, Dieter F. Lubbe, Ranjit S. More,
Charanjit S. Rihal, Robert S. Schwartz, Mandeep Singh,
Farris K. Timimi, Renu Virmani

CHAPTER 12

CORONARY ARTERIAL RESPONSE TO INJURY

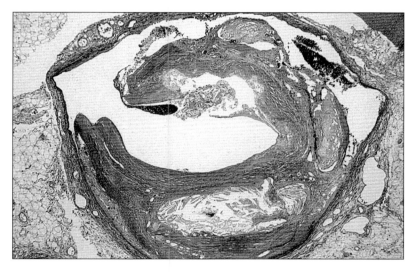

FIGURE 12-1. Acute pathology specimen of a patient who underwent balloon coronary angioplasty. Percutaneous coronary intervention induces significant injury in the coronary artery. The arterial response to injury, which is a critical determinant to the long-term success or failure of such procedures [1], results in neointimal hyperplasia and adventitial thickening (the latter may manifest as negative remodeling). The primary mechanism of lumen improvement after balloon angioplasty appears to be fracture of the atheromatous plaque or the media itself. In this figure, note the dissection across the superior border of the artery and laceration of the vessel at the plaque site. (Hematoxylin and eosin stain.)

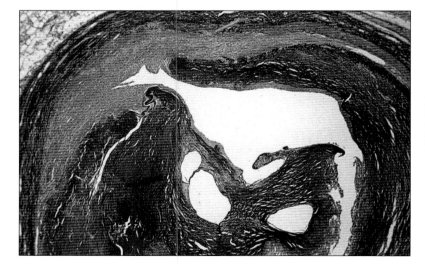

FIGURE 12-2. Pathology specimen of a coronary artery long after balloon angioplasty. The initial hemostatic event after deep arterial injury is a rapid activation and deposition of platelets with subsequent cellular recruitment and proliferation. This sequence of histopathologic events results in neointimal formation, which, in its most exuberant form, manifests clinically as restenosis. However, in addition to neointimal hyperplasia, negative vessel remodeling also factors importantly into the occurrence of restenosis. In the pathologic specimen shown here, representing a coronary artery long after balloon angioplasty, renarrowing of the vessel has occurred despite the presence of only a small amount of neointima, underscoring the important role of negative remodeling on restenosis. (Verhoeff–van Gieson elastic stain.)

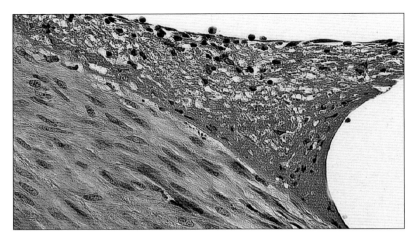

FIGURE 12-3. Normal porcine artery 4 days after stent placement. For all practical purposes, placement of a stent eliminates the possibility of negative vessel remodeling after coronary intervention. Therefore, neointimal hyperplasia is the prime determinant of in-stent restenosis. In this figure, a normal porcine coronary artery is shown 4 days after stent placement. Accumulation of mural thrombus along the stent strut is apparent. Macrophages and lymphocytes are colonizing the thrombus at this early stage; an inflammatory response is much more common when the stent strut has been embedded in a lipid core or injured media rather than in fibrous plaque. Endothelialization is present at this early stage in this porcine coronary injury model; in general, by 30 days after implantation in humans, stent endothelialization is present, although not necessarily complete.

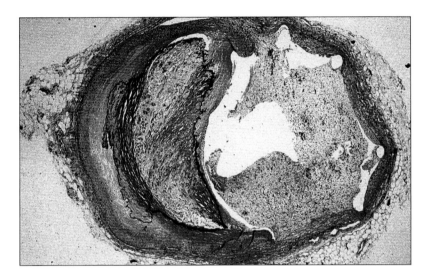

FIGURE 12-4. Pathology specimen of a coronary artery 30 days after stent placement. Inflammation is the clear source of neointimal thickening. In this pathologic specimen of a coronary artery 30 days after stent implantation, densely cellular neointimal proliferation has caused severe restenosis. In summary, coronary revascularization results in vessel injury (*ie*, disruption of the vascular endothelium and exposure of deep tissue components to blood). Potential repair mechanisms that are basic to survival of the species are triggered by these occurrences, which result in thrombus formation and acute inflammation with subsequent neointimal formation. A better understanding of these processes enables the development of more effective anti-restenosis strategies to complement the currently available technologies of brachytherapy and drug-eluting stents.

INVASIVE LESION ASSESSMENT: BEYOND CORONARY ANGIOGRAPHY

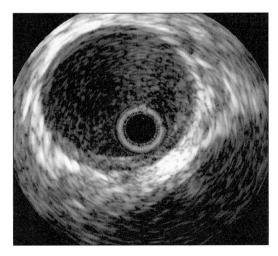

FIGURE 12-5. Intravascular ultrasound (IVUS) image of a normal left main coronary artery. IVUS complements coronary angiography in the qualitative and quantitative assessment of coronary anatomy. An IVUS image represents a tomographic cross-section of a vessel, although when using an automated pullback system and associated software, a three-dimensional reconstruction of the vessel is possible. A normal coronary artery was initially thought to have a trilayer appearance composed of an inner bright layer, a middle sonolucent area, and an outer dense layer. These layers were initially believed to correspond to the intima, media, and adventitia, respectively, although subsequent studies have shown that this three-layered appearance is not always present. For example, in young patients with completely normal coronary arteries on histopathologic examination, the inner bright layer is often absent; this layer is usually seen in older patients who have an intimal thickness of at least 178 μm. Shown is an intravascular ultrasound image of a normal left main coronary artery with a partial demonstration of the inner bright layer from approximately 4 o'clock to 8 o'clock. The catheter is the dark circle at 5 o'clock with a surrounding bright halo, also known as ring-down artifact.

QUANTITATIVE CORONARY ULTRASOUND (QCU)

DIRECT MEASUREMENTS

Lumen measurements
  Diameter (D_{Max}, D_{Min})
  Cross-sectional lumen area
EEM measurements
  EEM area
Atheroma measurements
  Plaque thickness (PT_{Max}, PT_{Min})
Calcium measurements
  Degrees
  Grade
    Grade 0, none
    Grade 1, $< 90°$
    Grade 2, $90–180°$
    Grade 3, $180–270°$
    Grade 4, $> 270°$
  Location
Stent measurements
  Stent diameter (SD_{Max}, SD_{Min})
  Cross-sectional stent area

DERIVED MEASUREMENTS

Lesion atheroma area = EEM area – lumen area
(Also termed "plaque + media area")

$$\text{Atheroma burden \%} = \frac{\text{Atheroma area} \times 100\%}{\text{EEM area}}$$

$$\text{Lumen area stenosis \%} = \frac{\text{MLA - reference LA}^* \times 100\%}{\text{Reference LA}}$$

$$\text{Remodeling index} = \frac{\text{Lesion EEM}}{\text{Averaged reference EEM}}$$

$$\text{Lesion lumen eccentricity index} = \frac{D_{Max} - D_{Min}}{D_{Max}}$$

$$\text{Atheroma eccentricity index} = \frac{PT_{Max} - PT_{Min}}{PT_{Max}}$$

Original lesion atheroma area = EEM area – stent area
Neointima (NI) lesion area = stent area – lumen area

$$\text{Atheroma + NI burden} = \frac{\text{EEM area - lumen area} \times 100\%}{\text{EEM area}}$$

$$\text{Lumen area stenosis} = \frac{\text{MLA - reference LA}^* \times 100\%}{\text{Reference LA}}$$

$$\text{Stent symmetry} = \frac{SD_{Max} - SD_{Min}}{SD_{Max}}$$

$$\text{Stent expansion} = \frac{\text{Stent area}}{\text{Reference LA}^*}$$

*Specify proximal, distal, largest, or average.

FIGURE 12-6. Quantitative coronary ultrasound. Quantitative assessment of intravascular ultrasound images includes direct and derived measurements. D_{Max}—maximum lumen diameter; D_{Min}—minimum lumen diameter; EEM—external elastic membrane; LA—lumen area; MLA—minimum lumen area; NI—neointima; PT_{Max}—maximum plaque thickness; PT_{Min}—minimum plaque thickness; SD_{Max}—maximum stent diameter; SD_{Min}—minimum stent diameter.

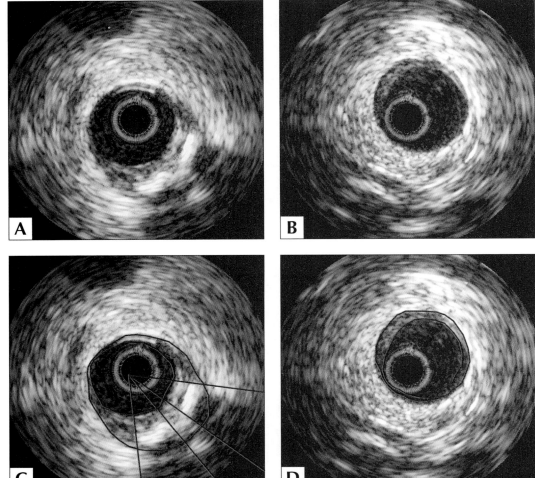

FIGURE 12-7. Intravascular ultrasound images from the left anterior descending artery demonstrating quantitative coronary ultrasound measurements. **A** shows remodeled plaque with associated quantitative measurements shown in **C**. **B** is the image from the proximal reference segment demonstrating mild intimal thickening between 9 o'clock and 12 o'clock with associated measurements shown in **D**. **E** demonstrates the quantitative measurements; note the large atheromatous burden with only a small lumen area stenosis primarily attributable to positive arterial remodeling.

E. QUANTITATIVE CORONARY ULTRASOUND

DIRECT MEASUREMENTS	REFERENCE (B, D)	LESION (A, C)
Lumen area, mm^2	9.0	8.0
EEM area, mm^2	11.1	18.0
Maximum thickness, mm	0.5	1.9
Minimum thickness, mm	0.2	0.3
Maximum diameter, mm	3.4	3.4
Minimum diameter, mm	3.2	3.1
Calcium arc, degrees	0	67
DERIVED MEASUREMENTS		
Lesion atheroma area (plaque plus media), mm^2	2.1	10.0
Atheroma burden, %	19	56
Lumen area stenosis, %	–	11
Remodeling index	–	1.62

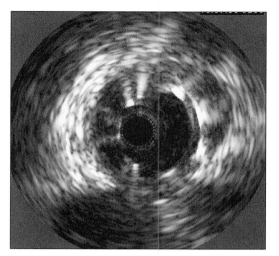

FIGURE 12-8. Intravascular ultrasound (IVUS) image during stent implantation demonstrating incomplete stent apposition. IVUS imaging is useful for guiding coronary intervention. This image demonstrates incomplete stent apposition from approximately 6 o'clock to 1 o'clock, which is not appreciated by coronary angiography. Although multiple IVUS criteria have been formulated to define optimal stent implantation, it has not been clearly demonstrated that IVUS improves clinical outcome during stent implantation, particularly in the era of high-pressure stent deployment during post-inflation.

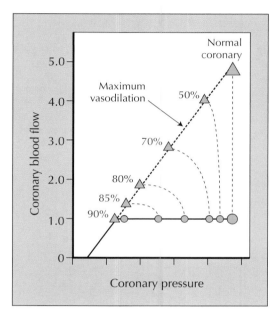

FIGURE 12-9. Coronary pressure–flow relationship at rest and during hyperemia. The addition of Doppler and pressure wire modalities have enabled us to offer invasive coronary physiologic assessments, although a basic understanding of coronary physiology is needed before one incorporates physiologic guidewires into clinical practice. Alterations in coronary blood flow (CBF) can be understood by considering a two-resistor model. Whereas coronary atherosclerosis typically occurs in the epicardial conduit vessel and contributes to the proximal resistance, the distal resistance represents the microcirculation. At rest, CBF is maintained at near constant levels over a wide range of perfusion pressures by the process of autoregulation. In the presence of an obstructive atherosclerotic stenosis in the epicardial conduit vessel, the distal coronary pressure is reduced and the microcirculation undergoes compensatory vasodilatation. With increasingly severe stenoses, the translesional pressure drop increases and autoregulation is eventually overcome because the resistance vessels are unable to further dilate. The figure illustrates that at rest, even with relatively high-grade stenoses, coronary blood flow is preserved over a wide range of pressures (circles). However, with increased demand or induced hyperemia, the ability to increase coronary blood flow becomes diminished with increasingly severe epicardial stenosis (triangles). It is this principle that aids in the assessment of lesion significance as well as distal microvascular function.

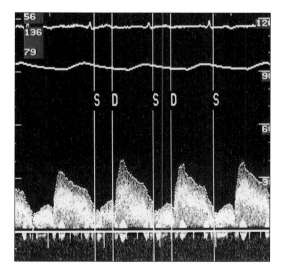

FIGURE 12-10. Normal phasic flow patterns in the left anterior descending and distal right coronary arteries. The limitations of coronary angiography are well recognized; however, even when the vessel lumen is well projected and imaged, the physiologic significance of the coronary stenosis cannot always be determined by the angiogram itself, particularly for what might be considered intermediate stenoses (50% to 70% diameter). In addition to ultrasound imaging, coronary flow reserve (CFR) and fractional flow reserve (FFR) may be useful adjunctive modalities to assess lesion significance. Additionally, CFR can be used to assess microvascular function. This figure demonstrates normal phasic flow patterns in the left anterior descending artery. Note the predominant diastolic flow. The numbers along the right ordinate indicate velocity in centimeters per second. D—onset of diastole; S—onset of systole.

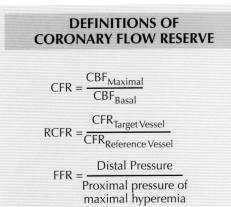

DEFINITIONS OF CORONARY FLOW RESERVE

$$CFR = \frac{CBF_{Maximal}}{CBF_{Basal}}$$

$$RCFR = \frac{CFR_{Target\ Vessel}}{CFR_{Reference\ Vessel}}$$

$$FFR = \frac{Distal\ Pressure}{Proximal\ pressure\ of\ maximal\ hyperemia}$$

FIGURE 12-11. The definitions of various types of coronary flow reserve (CFR) that are referenced. CBF—coronary blood flow; FFR—fractional flow reserve; RCFR—relative coronary flow reserve.

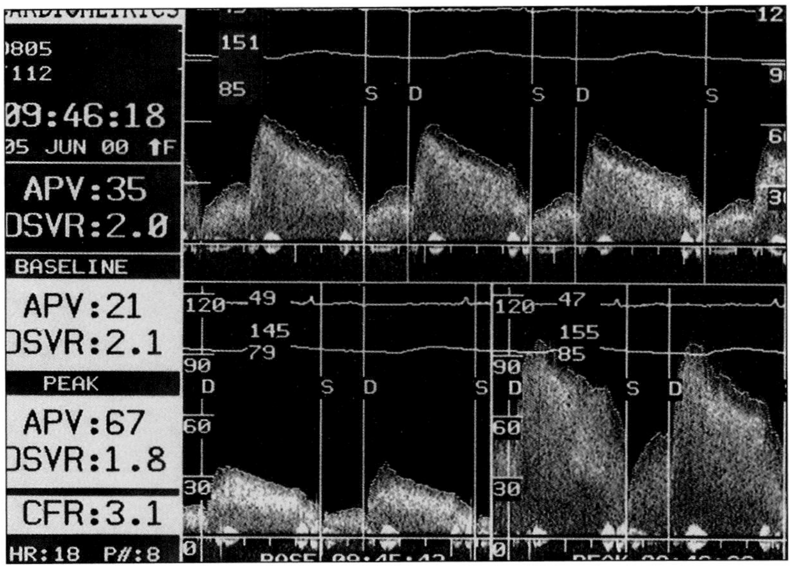

FIGURE 12-12. Intracoronary Doppler study demonstrating the measurement of coronary flow reserve (CFR). To assess coronary flow reserve, incremental doses of adenosine (18 μg to 54 μg in the authors' practice) are administered into the guiding catheter. The baseline or resting average peak velocity (APV) was 21 in this case, and the hyperemic APV after intracoronary adenosine administration was 67, signifying a coronary flow reserve of 3.1. A CFR of 2.5 or greater is generally considered to be consistent with intact microvasculature. With respect to lesion assessment, most clinicians would accept that a CFR greater than or equal to 2.0 would be consistent with a non–flow-limiting lesion. However, a potential problem arises when microvascular impairment may exist, in which case a low CFR may not differentiate between a significant epicardial lesion and impaired microcirculation. In such a case, a relative CFR can be measured, which involved the additional measurement of a CFR in a reference vessel. A relative CFR less than 0.8 suggests that the epicardial lesion is physiologically significant [2]. Of note, an abnormal CFR (< 2.0) has been shown to correspond with a lumen area of less than 4.0 mm^2, as measured by intravascular ultrasound [3]. It is safe to defer revascularization in patients with intermediate lesions and normal coronary flow physiology by Doppler guidewire because these patients have a low cardiac event rate [4,5].

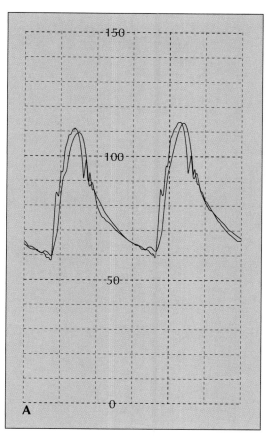

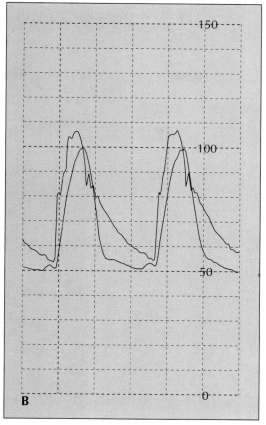

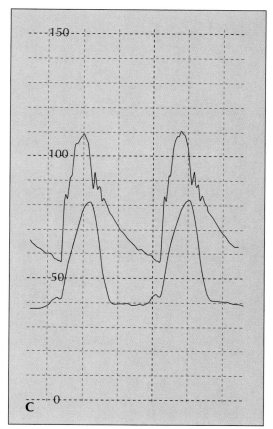

FIGURE 12-13. Translesional pressure gradients measured at rest. The pressure guidewire is also an angioplasty-style guidewire with a pressure sensor near its tip. The concept of myocardial fractional flow reserve (FFR) was developed to overcome the inherent inaccuracies of measuring a resting gradient. Myocardial FFR is defined as the ratio of hyperemic flow in a target vessel with a stenosis to the hyperemic flow in the same target vessel if the stenosis were not present. In relating flow to pressure, there should obviously be no pressure gradient in a vessel where a lesion does not exist, as demonstrated in **A**. However, with a stenosis of increasing severity, a pressure decrease in response to induced hyperemia may be observed, as demonstrated in **B** and **C**. Several studies have shown that an FFR less than 0.75 correlates with an abnormal noninvasive functional test for ischemia and is generally thought to be consistent with a flow-limiting lesion [6,7]. However, both technical and theoretical limitations should be considered when one assesses coronary lesions with pressure guidewire, including signal drift, guide catheter–induced pressure damping, ostial stenoses, tandem lesions or diffuse disease, and microvascular disease.

EQUIPMENT SELECTION AND TECHNIQUES OF VASCULAR ACCESS

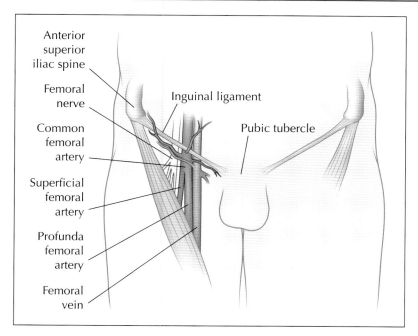

FIGURE 12-14. Anatomic relationship of vascular structures in the inguinal triangle. One of the most important—yet perhaps most overlooked—aspects of interventional procedures is vascular access. The majority of coronary interventional procedures are still performed from the femoral artery using the Seldinger technique. The arterial puncture should be in the common femoral artery below the inguinal ligament but above the bifurcation of the superficial and deep femoral arteries to ensure that adequate compression of the vessel against the femoral head will be possible when the sheath is removed.

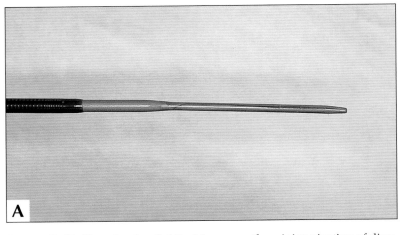

A

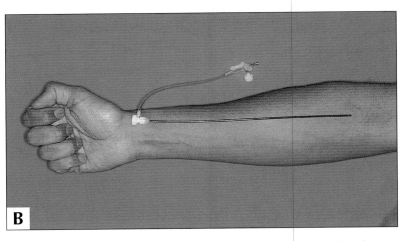

B

FIGURE 12-15. Vascular sheath kits. More recently, miniaturization of diagnostic and therapeutic catheters has enabled consideration of alternative arterial access sites such as the radial artery. Specially designed sheath kits using hydrophilic sheaths allow relatively easy passage into the radial artery (**A**). A 45-cm sheath allows one to get past the radial artery up toward the brachial artery, where spasm should be much less of an issue (**B**). Potential advantages to a radial approach include the fact that it is a superficial, easily evaluable, and compressible vessel that is not an end artery. As long as the ulnar artery is patent, no major complications have been reported as a result of radial artery occlusion. From a patient perspective, bed rest time can be substantially minimized. In the authors' practice, sublingual nitroglycerin is administered before accessing the radial artery and verapamil (1 to 5 mg) is administered into the radial artery upon cannulation. Use of systemic heparin (2500 to 5000 U) appears to be an important factor in reducing the likelihood of late radial artery occlusion.

GUIDE SELECTION

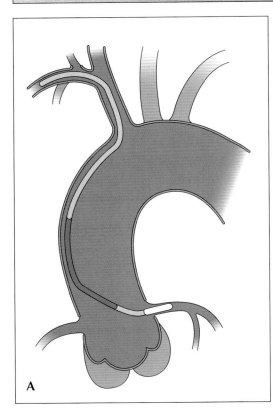

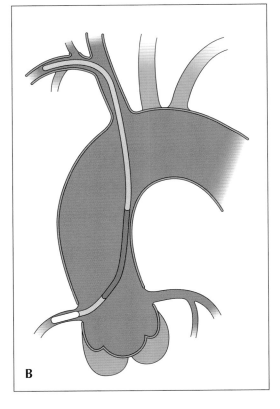

A

B

FIGURE 12-16. The Kimny guide. **A** and **B**, Specially designed catheters are available for diagnostic as well as interventional purposes. This multipurpose catheter provides sufficient fit and support for native left and right coronary arteries and vein grafts in the majority of patients.

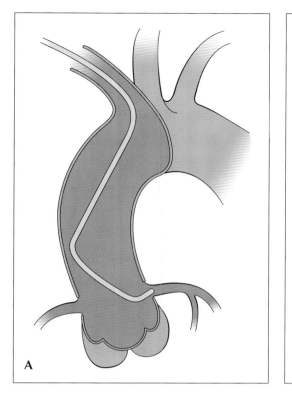

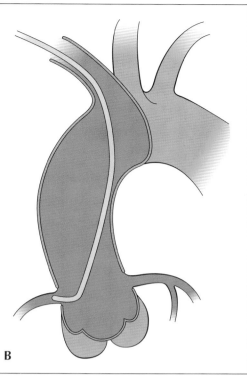

A

B

FIGURE 12-17. Judkins catheters. These catheters (**A** and **B**) can also be used from a radial approach. Using a Judkins catheter from the right transradial approach, a Judkins left catheter that is 0.5 cm smaller than would be used from the groin and a Judkins right catheter that is 1 cm larger than would be used from the groin are recommended for optimal engagement and support. If the left arm is used, the same size Judkins catheters as are used from the groin would be appropriate.

STENT DESIGNS

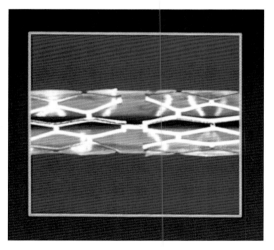

FIGURE 12-18. Evolution of Cordis (Miami Lakes, FL) stents. Stents can be classified according to their basic design (slotted tube, coil, ring, mesh, open cell), composition (stainless steel, tantalum, gold, nitinol), and mode of deployment (balloon expandable, self-expanding). An ideal stent would have the positive attributes of flexibility, trackability, adequate surface coverage, visibility, radial strength, side branch access, adequate adherence to deployment balloon to eliminate the possibility of stent loss, low crossing profile, and reliable expandability. Each stent design has relative advantages and disadvantages in each of these categories; no single stent design possesses all of these positive attributes to a sufficient degree; therefore, stent selection needs to take into account angiographic and procedural issues for a specific case. This photograph demonstrates the original Palmaz-Schatz stent, which was the first approved coronary stent that was widely used in the United States. This is the original slotted tube design, laser cut from a continuous cylinder of stainless steel. Although the stent and the associated delivery system were relatively difficult to deliver, the 1-mm articulation site shown in the middle of two 7-mm segments improved deliverability.

FIGURE 12-19. The Gianturco-Roubin (GR) (Cook, Bloomington, IN) stent. This stent was constructed from a single strand of 0.006-inch stainless steel wire, which made the stent very flexible and deliverable. The second-generation stent (GR-II) had the same basic design, with an added longitudinal spine to reduce deformability. Restenosis rates of GR-II stents were observed to be higher than those of the Palmaz-Schatz stents [8], although this may have been partly related to the use of smaller stents than would have been recommended based on the reference segment [9]. This stent is no longer on the market.

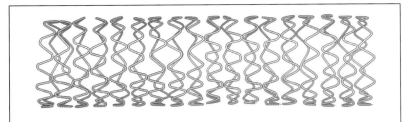

Figure 12-20. The Medtronic-Arterial Vascular Engineering (AVE) (Medtronic, Santa Rosa, CA) stent. These stents are based on a single sinusoidal element configured in a series of interconnected crowns and struts. Although the early generation of this stent focused on deliverability, the more recent generations have evolved to emphasize radial strength and vessel scaffolding with radiopacity. The S7 is the most recent version of Medtronic's coronary stent offerings.

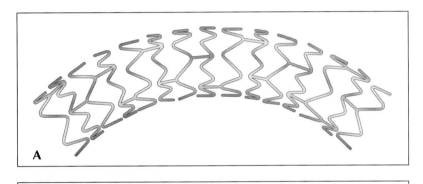

Figure 12-21. The ACS Guidant (Guidant, Indianapolis, IN) stents. These stents are originally based on a slotted tube design composed of multiple rings interconnected with small bridges. The Multi-Link Penta stent (shown), the fifth generation version of this stent, has recently been replaced by the Zeta stent.

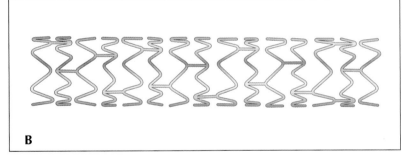

A

Figure 12-22. Previously, the NIR stent was the Boston Scientific (Natick, MA) offering in the coronary arena. The current generation of their stent is called the EXPRESS II stent, in which the stent design and delivery system have been modified substantially to allow for greater flexibility and trackability (**A**). The TAXUS stent (**B**) is a paclitaxel-eluting stent . The TAXUS stent is the same platform as the EXPRESS II stent; the only difference is the TAXUS stent's paclitaxel coating.

B

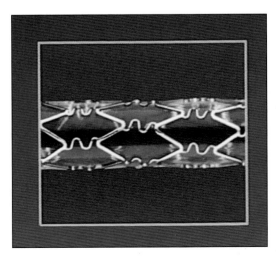

Figure 12-23. Cordis (Miami Lakes, FL) stent. The most recent generation of stents from Cordis include the Bx Velocity stent, which, similar to its predecessor, the Palmaz-Schatz stent, is laser cut from a single tube of stainless steel. It uses a closed-cell design to maintain flexibility while trying to preserve vessel coverage. The rapamycin-eluting version of this stent (CYPHER stent) possesses the same structural design.

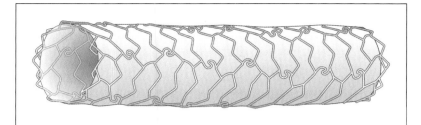

FIGURE 12-24. JOMED (Rancho Cordova, CA) stent. Approved for the indication of coronary perforation in the United States, although used in the treatment of saphenous vein graft disease elsewhere, is the JOMED JOSTENT, which possesses a polytetrafluoroethylene (PTFE) layer sandwiched between two stainless steel stents. There can be significant foreshortening of the stent, especially at the larger diameters. Nonetheless, this is an effective stent for the treatment of coronary perforations that are not responsive to conventional measures of prolonged balloon inflation and reversal of anticoagulation, and it prevents for emergent surgery in some proportion of patients experiencing this unusual complication of coronary intervention.

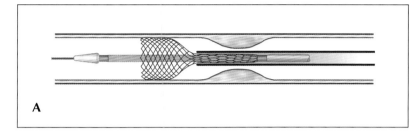

A

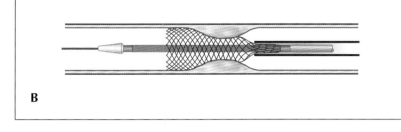

B

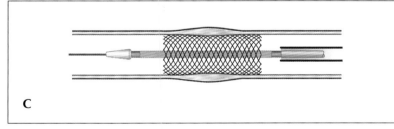

C

FIGURE 12-25. Magic Wallstent (Boston Scientific, Natick, MA). Although all the stents discussed thus far are balloon-expandable stents (*ie*, they are premounted on a balloon and deployed within the coronary artery), the Wallstent, which is a self-expandable stent, was one of the first stents to undergo clinical evaluation. A version of the stent was withdrawn in 1990 because of high rates of stent thrombosis, and the newer version, the Magic Wallstent, was reintroduced in 1994. This and other self-expanding stents are advanced across the target coronary lesion in a protective sheath, at which point the protective sheath is withdrawn, as shown in the figure, resulting in stent deployment. **A–C,** The stent shortens to a moderate extent and does not allow easy side branch access. Clinically important beneficial effects on restenosis have not been clearly demonstrated for self-expanding stent designs compared with balloon-expandable designs.

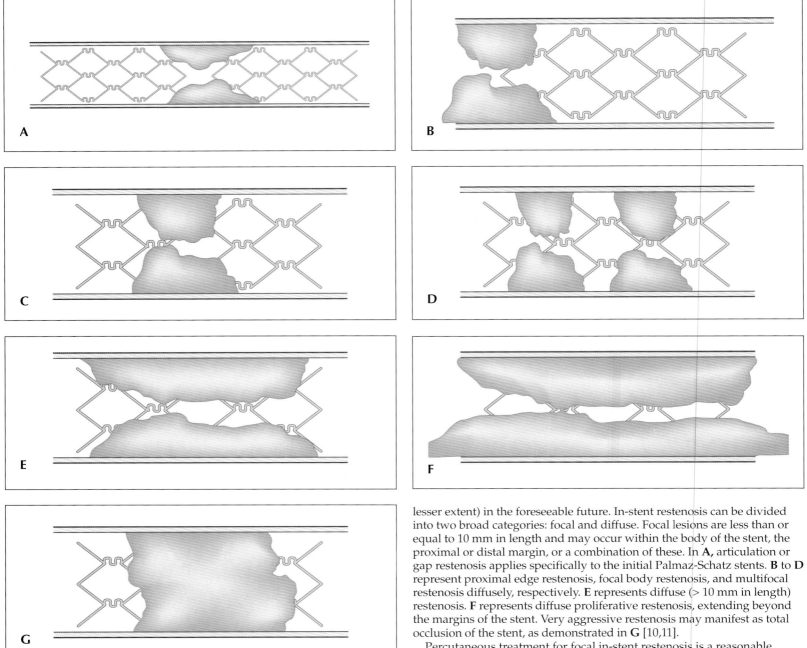

FIGURE 12-26. Classification of restenosis. Although the availability of coronary stents has largely reduced restenosis compared with conventional balloon angioplasty, the increasing number of stents used has resulted in an increasing absolute number of cases of in-stent restenosis. Although the availability of drug-eluting stents may reduce this likelihood, in-stent restenosis continues to be a therapeutic challenge in the current era of interventional cardiology and will likely continue to be a challenge (albeit to a lesser extent) in the foreseeable future. In-stent restenosis can be divided into two broad categories: focal and diffuse. Focal lesions are less than or equal to 10 mm in length and may occur within the body of the stent, the proximal or distal margin, or a combination of these. In **A,** articulation or gap restenosis applies specifically to the initial Palmaz-Schatz stents. **B** to **D** represent proximal edge restenosis, focal body restenosis, and multifocal restenosis diffusely, respectively. **E** represents diffuse (> 10 mm in length) restenosis. **F** represents diffuse proliferative restenosis, extending beyond the margins of the stent. Very aggressive restenosis may manifest as total occlusion of the stent, as demonstrated in **G** [10,11].

Percutaneous treatment for focal in-stent restenosis is a reasonable approach and is associated with acceptable rates of repeat in-stent restenosis. Diffuse proliferative or occlusive restenosis has a high rate of recurrence after conventional percutaneous interventional techniques (*ie*, percutaneous transluminal coronary angioplasty, repeat stenting, or ablative techniques). In such cases, intracoronary brachytherapy should be strongly considered because repeat percutaneous intervention without this modality is highly unlikely to afford a lasting benefit. The use of drug-eluting stents to treat in-stent restenosis is currently being investigated.

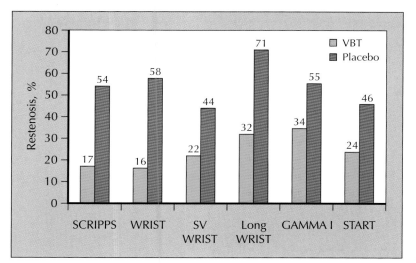

FIGURE 12-27. Angiographic restenosis rates in trials of vascular brachytherapy versus conventional percutaneous treatment of in-stent restenosis.

PREDICTORS OF IN-STENT RESTENOSIS AND RECURRENT IN-STENT RESTENOSIS

PATIENT/LESION-RELATED FACTORS

Diabetes

Age

Female gender

Hyperlipidemia

D/D genotype of the ACE gene

Shorter time interval between placement and
  restenosis episode (< 90 days)

Prior restenosis

Restenosis class/pattern

Previous CABG surgery

Multivessel disease; multivessel stenting not a factor

LAD

Vein graft

Ostial stenosis

Bifurcation

Lesion length

Smaller reference vessel size

Plaque burden by IVUS

ACC/AHA lesion classification

PROCEDURE-RELATED FACTORS

Stent length

Multiple contiguous stents

Postprocedure minimal stent diameter or
  percent stenosis

Postprocedure CSA

Stent type

No IVUS use (univariate)

FIGURE 12-28. Predictors of in-stent restenosis and recurrent in-stent restenosis. A number of angiographic and patient-related factors may predict the occurrence of restenosis. Among the angiographic predictors, length of the stented segment, multiple stents, nominal vessel size less than 3.0 mm, restenotic lesions, ostial lesions, smaller stent cross-sectional area, and stent design have all been implicated as factors that increase the likelihood of in-stent restenosis. Patient-related factors include diabetes, prior restenosis, and genetic phenotypes. ACC/AHA—American College of Cardiology/American Heart Association; ACE—angiotensin-converting enzyme; CABG—coronary artery bypass graft; CSA—cross-sectional area; IVUS—intravascular ultrasound; LAD—left anterior descending coronary artery.

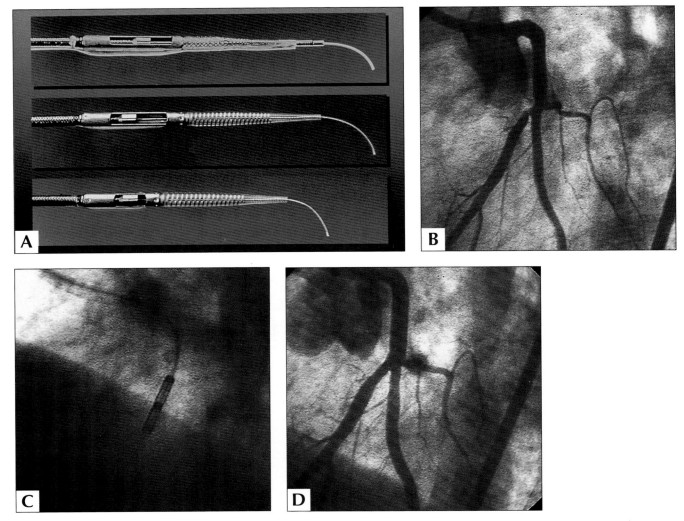

FIGURE 12-29. Three generations of Simpson atherocaths (Devices for Vascular Intervention, Redwood, CA) and proximal left anterior descending coronary artery (LAD) stenosis. A variety of ablative technologies have been developed and tested in registries and randomized clinical trials. These devices were developed based on the concept that removal or modification of the atheromatous plaque would improve the safety of the procedure, giving a more stable initial result and that this would translate into improved, longer-term outcome with a reduction in restenosis. Directional atherectomy (DCA) was the first of the devices to be introduced (**A**). This multilumen catheter terminates in a nose cone, which serves as collection chamber for tissue fragments that are shaved off by the cutting element. This device requires considerable expertise and skill to use but can result in excellent initial outcomes (**B** to **D**). In this patient, a severe ostial LAD stenosis was treated with DCA with an excellent initial result. Although the initial angiographic results with this device are often very favorable for bulky, eccentric, or selected ostial lesions, in most series and trials, restenosis rates have not been improved substantially compared with the control device tested. This device is currently used infrequently in interventional practice. Nevertheless, it is helpful for selected bulky, ostial, noncalcified lesions.

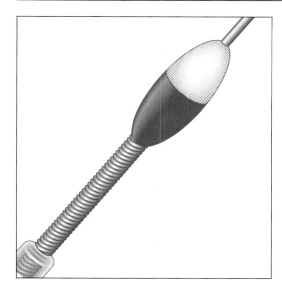

FIGURE 12-30. Burr, drive shaft, and sheath loaded onto a RotaWire (Boston Scientific, Natick, MA). Another ablative technique, rotational coronary atherectomy, has also been widely tested and used. This device is a nickel-plated brass elliptical burr coated on its leading edge with diamond chips. The device, which comes in a variety of sizes from 1.5 to 2.5 mm, is advanced through the atherosclerotic lesion while rotating at approximately 150,000 RPM. This results in selective ablation of diseased (*ie*, inelastic) tissue and sparing of more normal arterial wall. It has been studied as an adjunct to percutaneous transluminal coronary angioplasty (PTCA) or to stent placement and as a technique if PTCA cannot be performed because of dense calcification or rigidity of the lesion that does not respond to conventional balloon angioplasty. It has also been tested as a sole therapy. In general, it has not resulted in a decrease in restenosis rates (*see* Fig. 12-31). It is still very useful as a niche technique for lesions that are undilatable (*see* Figs. 12-32A–F).

FIGURE 12-31. Data from the SPORT trial (Stenting Post-Rotational Atherectomy Trial). NS—not significant; PTCA—percutaneous transluminal coronary angioplasty; QCA—quantitative coronary angiography.

THE SPORT TRIAL

BASELINE QCA	PTCA + STENT, N = 364	ROTABLATOR + STENT, N = 349	PVALUE
Lesion length, *mm*	16.0	17.0	NS
Reference visual diameter, *mm*	2.83 ± 0.48	2.87 ± 0.49	NS
Preprocedure minimum lumen diameter, *mm*	0.88 ±0.42	0.87 ± 0.38	NS
Diameter stenosis preprocedure, %	86.0 ± 9.3	85.8 ± 10.4	NS
Postprocedure minimum lumen diameter, *mm*	2.74	2.81	0.032
Acute gain, *mm*	1.86	1.94	0.041

SUCCESS RATES, %	PTCA + STENT, N = 375	ROTABLATOR + STENT, N = 360	PVALUE
Angiographic success*	100	100	NS
Procedural success	88.1	93.6	0.0114
Clinical success*	87.3	91.6	NS

*Procedure success with no major adverse cardiac events.

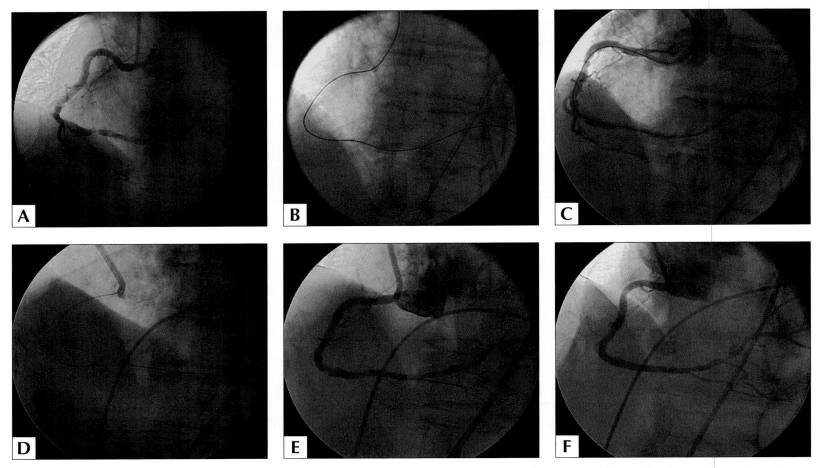

FIGURE 12-32. Treatment of nondilatable stenosis. **A,** Focal, high-grade stenosis in distal right coronary artery. **B,** Balloon angioplasty is attempted. Appropriately sized balloons will not pass; angioplasty is attempted with a 1.5-mm balloon. **C,** The 1.5-mm balloon fails to improve the lesion. **D,** After exchange of the 0.014-inch coronary guidewire for a rotational coronary atherectomy (RCA) guidewire, RCA is performed using serial burrs. **E,** After RCA, the lesion is improved and distal blood flow is enhanced. **F,** After RCA balloon angioplasty with an appropriately sized balloon and stent placement, excellent results are achieved.

CUTTING BALLOON ANGIOPLASTY

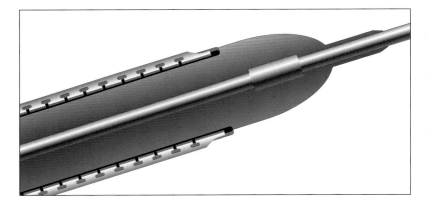

FIGURE 12-33. Cutting balloon. One of the most recent additions to the field of mechanical treatment to modify lesions has been the cutting balloon. This device has longitudinal steel atherotomes on the surface of the balloon. When the balloon is inflated, these atherotomes create controlled incisions in the atheromatous plaque. The cutting balloon has been used to treat rigid fibrotic lesions, ostial lesions, and in-stent restenotic lesions to optimize the initial result of therapy. In general, as has been true of both directional coronary atherectomy and rotational coronary atherectomy, although initial results are excellent, the cutting balloon has not been shown to dramatically reduce restenosis rates. It remains useful, however, for selected ostial lesions, in-stent restenosis, and fibrotic lesions (*see* Figs. 12-34A–C).

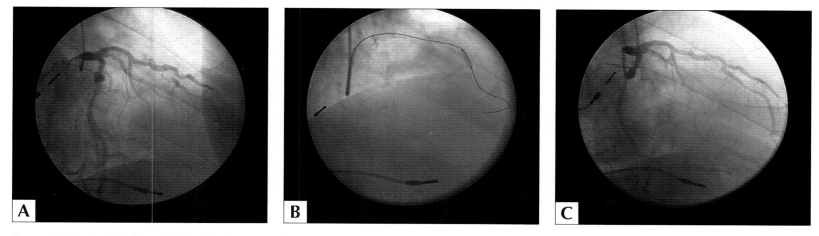

FIGURE 12-34. **A**, A high-grade distal left anterior descending artery stenosis at the take-off of a large second diagonal branch is noted. **B**, A 3 × 10 mm cutting balloon is advanced with only mild difficulty to the target lesion and inflated three times to a maximum of 8 atm of pressure. **C**, Final angiographic images reveals an excellent result in the target lesion and no compromise of the diagonal branch.

SPECIFIC LESION SUBSETS

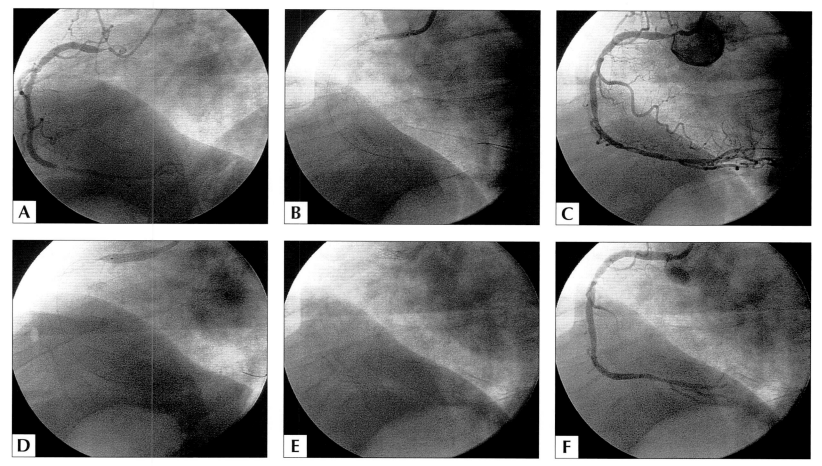

FIGURE 12-35. High-grade aorto-ostial stenosis of the right coronary artery. Coronary arterial stenosis exists in almost infinite variety because of the number of variables involved in each lesion. Some of these anatomic variables and features may have a major impact on procedural performance, selection of equipment, risks and complications of the procedure, and longer-term outcome. From the earliest days of interventional cardiology, there have been classification schemes; the most commonly used modified American College of Cardiology/American Heart Association system includes variables such as location and severity of stenosis, tortuosity, presence of major or minor branches, and presence or absence of calcification. Some lesion types are associated with decreased procedural success, and others are associated with higher complications. Ostial lesions remain a significant problem, particularly in placing the stent so that the lesion is adequately covered but that the stent does not protrude excessively into the aorta. In this patient, high-grade aorto-ostial stenosis of the right coronary artery was present (**A**). Because the stenosis was not calcified, the initial treatment was with balloon angioplasty (**B**), which was associated with significant recoil (**C**). A high-visibility NIRoyal stent (Boston Scientific, Natick, MA) was chosen to optimize positioning of the stent (**D** and **E**). The final result (**F**) reveals complete lesion coverage without significant stent protrusion into the ascending aorta.

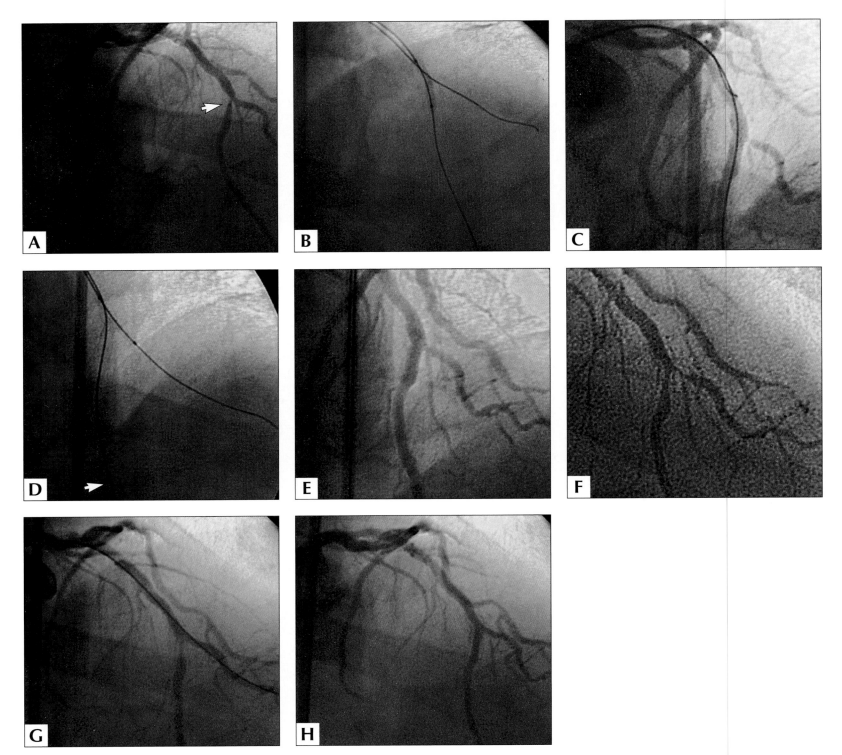

FIGURE 12-36. Pre- and posttreatment angiograms. Bifurcation lesions are also problematic. With these lesions, acute success rates are decreased, and restenosis rates are increased. The problem for this lesion subset is that either the major parent or the branch vessel may be compromised while treating the entire lesion. Pre- and post-treatment angiograms are shown here. A 65-year-old man presented with crescendo angina and demonstrable ischemia in the anterior, anteroseptal, anterolateral, and apical segments. Coronary angiography (**A**) demonstrates significant disease at the branch point of a moderate-sized second diagonal and the distal left anterior descending (LAD) coronary artery, primarily involving the parent vessel (*arrow*). After passing separate guidewires into each branch (**B**), the LAD was dilated with a 3.0-mm balloon. A suboptimal angiographic result led to placement of a 3 mm × 12 mm S7 stent with a relatively open geometry. The resulting lesion (**C**) at the ostium of the second diagonal was treated with a 2.5-mm balloon placed through the stent struts (**D**) while maintaining guidewire protection of the LAD (*arrow*), with good acute angiographic result (**E**). Five months later, the patient returned with restenosis in both limbs of the bifurcation (**F**). Balloon angioplasty using a 2.5-mm balloon produced a good angiographic result in the diagonal (**G**). After performing intracoronary ultrasound for optimal stent sizing, a 3.5 × 10 mm cutting balloon (Boston Scientific, Natick, MA) was used to dilate within the previously placed stent. Optimization of the angiographic result was followed by the intracoronary application of gamma radiation (**H**).

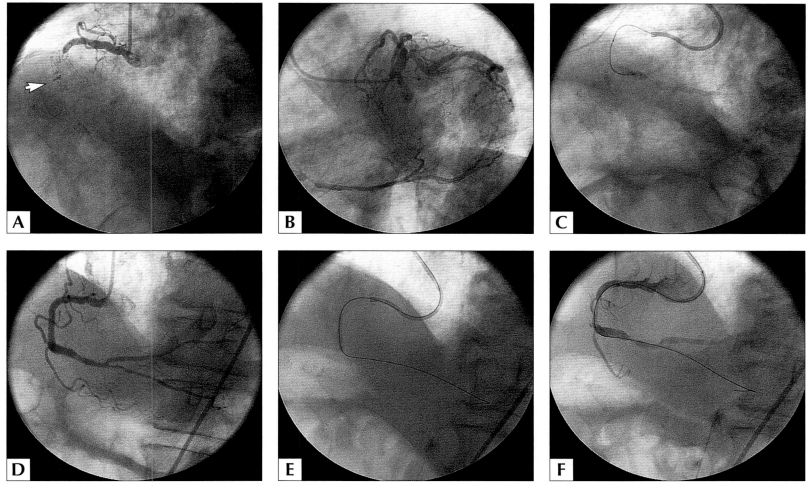

FIGURE 12-37. Recanalization of a chronic total occlusion estimated clinically to be between 3 and 6 months old. Chronic total occlusion supplying viable myocardium remains the most common reason for referral for coronary artery bypass graft surgery. Although a variety of new guidewires and devices are available, success rates in lesions that are attempted are still only approximately 70%. **A,** The proximal right coronary artery occlusion received collaterals from the left coronary artery (**B**). Note the presence of bridging collaterals (**A,** *arrow*). A left Amplatz guide catheter provided excellent support and, after failing with soft and intermediate wires, the occlusion was crossed with a Cross-It (Guidant, Indianapolis, IN), a relatively stiff-tipped guidewire. **C,** Because of uncertainty regarding the position of the guidewire distal to the point of occlusion, a 2.3-F Rapid Transit perfusion catheter (Cordis, Miami Lakes, FL) was advanced over the guidewire, the wire was removed, and contrast medium was injected to confirm an intraluminal location. **D,** Balloon angioplasty restored normal flow, and stenting optimized the final result (**E** and **F**).

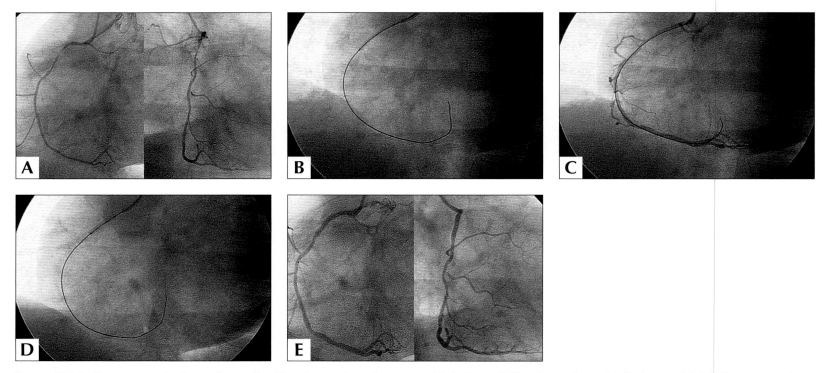

FIGURE 12-38. Coronary angioplasty of a small-caliber (approximately 2 mm) proximal right coronary artery lesion. Small vessels are another problem. In most patients, small size is related to diffuseness of disease. The use of drug-eluting stents may offer particular advantages in this setting. **A,** The stenosis was initially dilated with a 20-mm-long, 2.0-mm-wide balloon. **B,** Despite prolonged inflations and full balloon expansion, a significant lesion remained (**C**). **D,** This area was stented with a 2.5-mm stent inflated to nominal pressures (10 atm). **E,** A small stepdown is noted at the junction of the stented and dilated regions.

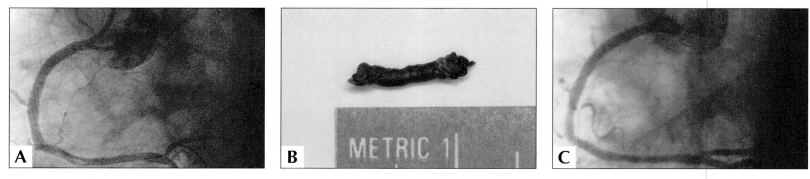

FIGURE 12-39. Thrombus progression. Lesions containing thrombus are associated with increased acute complications despite advances in adjunctive therapy. **A,** Despite reasonable anticoagulation with unfractionated heparin (activated clotting time, 305 seconds), thrombus formation was noted during elective right coronary artery (RCA) intervention. The thrombus (*arrow*) developed after stent placement in the proximal and mid-RCA and was noted to move with the guidewire. **B,** Under fluoroscopic guidance, the guidewire was carefully withdrawn into the guide catheter and the thrombus was aspirated as the entire guide catheter was extracted from the body. **C,** No distal embolization was found, and coronary flow remained brisk.

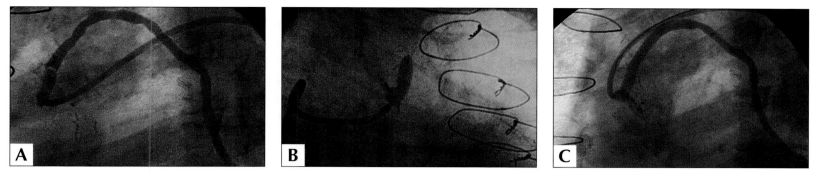

FIGURE 12-40. Adequate visualization and positioning in treating vein graft ostia. Treatment of vein graft disease is often complex and can be associated with distal embolization and slow flow or no reflow. Vein graft disease will become increasingly frequent because of the well-documented limited lifespan of vein grafts; it has been found that at 10 years, approximately 75% of vein grafts are either significantly diseased or occluded. **A,** After multiple angiographic views confirmed a significant proximal vein graft anastomotic lesion, an appropriate oblique view was identified to isolate the ostium for planned intervention. **B,** After backing the guiding catheter from the vein graft ostium to permit complete balloon expansion outside the catheter, a stent was deployed so the proximal struts extended just outside the ostium, confirmed by the injection of a small amount of contrast agent. **C,** The guide catheter was then carefully reapproximated to the vein graft ostium as the stent balloon and guidewire were removed for a final angiogram.

DRUG-ELUTING STENTS

CLASSES OF AGENTS THAT HAVE BEEN ASSESSED OR ARE BEING ASSESSED FOR LOCAL DRUG ELUTION FROM COATED STENTS

IMMUNOSUPPRESSANTS	ANTINEOPLASTIC AGENTS	ANTITHROMBOTICS	MIGRATION INHIBITORS	ENDOTHELIAL MODULATORS
Sirolimus (rapamycin)	Paclitaxel	Abciximab	Batimastat (metallopro-teinase inhibitor)	17β-Estradiol
Tacrolimus	Taxol derivative (PQ-2)	Heparin		HMG-CoA reductase inhibitors
Dexamethasone	Actinomycin D	Hirudin		VEGF
Leflunomide	Angiopeptin			
Tranilast	C-*myc* antisense			
Cyclosporine				

HMG-CoA—3-hydroxy-3-methylglutaryl coenzyme A; VEGF—vascular endothelial growth factor.

FIGURE 12-41. Classes of agents that have been assessed or are being assessed for local drug elution from coated stents. Drug eluting stents are revolutionary technology. Two devices have been approved—CYPHER utilizing sirolimus (Cordis, Miami Lakes, FL) and TAXUS utilizing pacli-taxel (Boston Scientific, Natick, MA). The results have been dramatic with marked decreases in angiographic and clinical restenosis (*see* Figs. 12-42 and 12-43). These drug-eluting stents have become predicate devices and are now used in the majority of procedures in the United States.

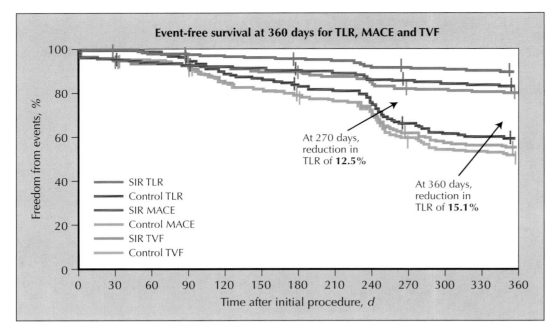

FIGURE 12-42. Event-free survival at 360 days from the SIRIUS trial. An increasing amount of information is available on the follow-up of patients in the multicenter SIRIUS trial, which randomized patients to either a sirolimus drug-eluting stent or a control bare metal Bx Velocity (Cordis, Miami Lakes, FL) stent. Irrespective of what measure of outcome was used (target lesion revascularization [TLR], major adverse cardiac events [MACE], or target vessel failure [TVF]), patients receiving the drug-eluting stent fared better. There was an absolute reduction in TLR or 12.5% at 270 days with the drug-eluting stent; this widened at 360 days to 15.1%.

TAXUS IV			
	9-MONTH EVENTS		
	TAXUS	CONTROL	*P*
Cardiac death	1.4	1.1	0.80
QMI	0.8	0.3	0.45
Non-QMI	2.7	3.4	0.52
TVR	4.7	12.0	< 0.0001
TLR	3.0	11.3	< 0.0001
TLR-CABG	0.6	3.1	0.008
Stent thrombosis	0.6	0.8	0.75
MACE	8.5	15.0	0.0002

FIGURE 12-43. The TAXUS IV trial. The paclitaxel-eluting stent TAXUS (Boston Scientific, Natick, MA) has been released and has been used extensively. The pivotal TAXUS IV trial, which randomized 1314 patients to the paclitaxel-eluting stent or a bare metal stent, found a striking reduction in angiographic and clinical restenosis. CABG—coronary artery bypass graft; MACE—major adverse cardiac event; QMI—Q-wave myocardial infarction; TLR—target lesion revascularization; TVF—target vessel failure.

DISTAL PROTECTION DEVICES—ADVANTAGES AND DISADVANTAGES

BALLOON OCCLUSION /ASPIRATION

ADVANTAGES	DISADVANTAGES
Effective	Ischemia during occlusion
Studied in randomized clinical trials	Blood stasis
Safe, deliverable	Visualization of complex anatomy is difficult after balloon inflation
Material aspirated	Failure of complete aspiration
Can trap all emboli	Failure of complete apposition
	Potential for systemic embolization during treatment of aorto-ostial lesions
	Potential for embolization into side branches proximal to the lesion being treated

FILTERS

ADVANTAGES	DISADVANTAGES
Effective	Larger crossing profile
Allow continued flow, minimizing ischemia	Pore size allows some particles and vasoactive substances to pass downstream
Material removed	Complete device apposition difficult to gauge
Allow visualization of anatomy during stent deployment	May fill with material, making removal difficult

FIGURE 12-44. Distal protection devices—advantages and disadvantages. The issue of distal embolization is receiving increased interest as patients with more complex lesions such as acute myocardial infarction (MI) and vein graft disease are being treated. In addition, recognition of the clinical significance of slow flow or no reflow has further heightened interest. A number of different approaches for distal protection have been developed, and each one has advantages and disadvantages. Two devices are now approved, and several others are under evaluation (*see* Figs. 12-45A and B). The approved devices, Percusurge Guardwire and FilterWire, have been tested in multicenter, randomized trials for vein graft disease (*see* Figs. 12-46 and 12-47). In each of these trials, the distal protection device has been found to decrease major adverse cardiac events compared with dilatation and stenting alone. These devices have become predicate devices for treatment of vein graft disease. They are currently being tested in the setting of acute MI to improve initial microvascular flow and prevent no reflow, thus improving outcome.

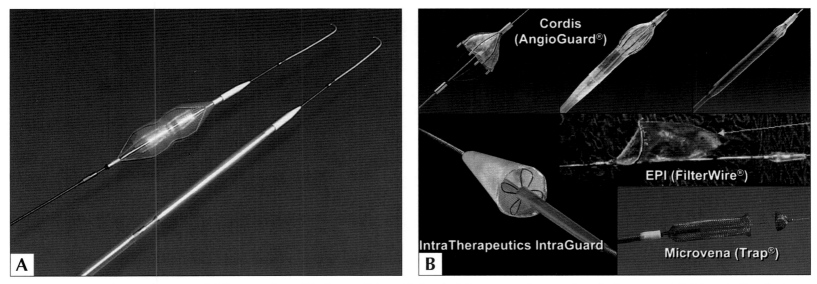

FIGURE 12-45. A, Filter guidewire and delivery catheter (Mednova, Galway, Ireland). **B,** Representative samples of other current distal protection devices.

SAFER TRIAL: 30-DAY ENDPOINTS

	GUARDWIRE	CONTROL	P
MACE, n (%)	39 (9.6)	65 (16.5)	0.004
MI, n (%)	35 (8.6)	58 (14.7)	0.008
Non–Q-wave MI, n (%)	30 (7.4)	54 (13.7)	
Any CK elevation above normal, n (%)	66 (16.3)	95 (24.1)	0.006
Death, n (%)	4 (1.0)	9 (2.3)	0.17
Emergency CABG, n (%)	0	2 (0.5)	0.24

FIGURE 12-46. Saphenous Vein Graft Angioplasty Free of Emboli Randomized (SAFER) trial: 30-day endpoints. CABG—coronary artery bypass graft; CK—creatine kinase; MACE—major adverse cardiac event; MI—myocardial infarction.

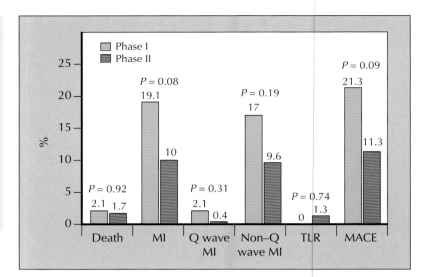

FIGURE 12-47. Results of a randomized trial of FilterWire: phase I versus phase II. MACE—major adverse cardiac event; MI—myocardial infarction; TLR—target lesion revascularization.

PERIPHERAL INTERVENTIONS

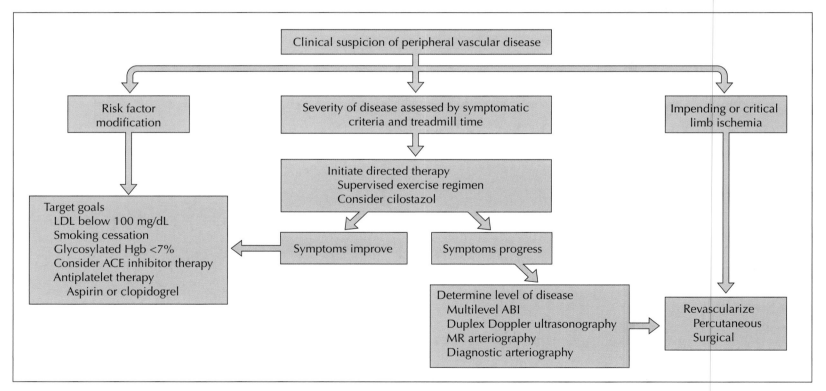

FIGURE 12-48. Clinical approach to and management of patients with suspected peripheral vascular disease. The incidence of peripheral arterial disease is increasing as the patient population becomes older. Some data suggest that peripheral arterial disease is often present but not diagnosed. This may relate to the fact that symptoms can be misinterpreted, the patient is not severely symptomatic, or there is limited expertise in exam-

ining the peripheral vascular tree. The clinical approach and management of patients with suspected peripheral arterial disease requires a heightened clinical suspicion of its presence. ABI—ankle/brachial index; ACE—angiotensin-converting enzyme; Hgb—hemoglobin; LDL—low-density lipoprotein. (*Adapted from* Hiat [12].)

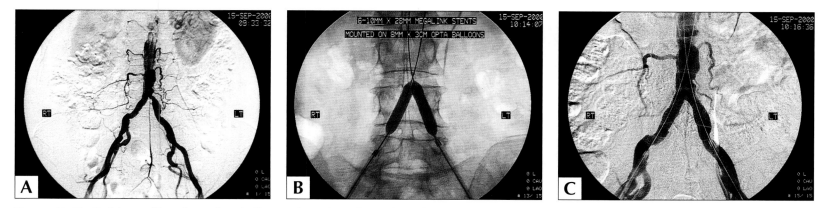

FIGURE 12-49. Ostial aortoiliac atherosclerotic disease. Aortoiliac atherosclerotic disease is well treated by interventional cardiovascular approaches. In this case, lifestyle-limiting left lower extremity claudication was present. Treatment of this type of anatomic stenosis may involve implantation of stents in both iliac arteries to prevent plaque shift or embolization. **A,** Diagnostic ateriography demonstrates high-grade left aortoiliac ostial stenosis in this patient with lifestyle-limiting left lower extremity claudication. Note a small infrarenal abdominal aortic aneurysm. **B,** Given the ostial location of the left iliac stenosis, a bilateral approach is chosen. Bilateral 8-F 24-cm Vista Brite Tip sheaths (Cordis Corporation, Miami, FL) were placed, and 0.035-inch Storq guidewires (Cordis) were used to cross the iliac vessels and were parked in the descending abdominal aorta. Two 28-mm Megalink stents (Guidant, Santa Clara, CA) were then handmounted on 8 × 3 cm OPTA balloons (Cordis) and deployed in a "kissing" fashion, with concomitant inflation and deflation. **C,** Final arteriography demonstrates no evidence of plaque burden transfer or embolization.

SVS/ICVS CLASSIFICATION OF ACUTE EXTEMITY ISCHEMIA

	VIABLE	THREATENED	NONVIABLE
Pain	Mild	Severe	Unpredictable
Capillary refill	Intact	Delayed	Absent
Motor deficit	None	Partial	Complete
Sensory deficit	None	Partial	Complete
Arterial Doppler	Audible	Inaudible	Inaudible
Venous Doppler	Audible	Audible	Inaudible
Treatment	Urgent evaluation	Emergent surgery	Amputation

FIGURE 12-50. Assessment of patients with peripheral vascular disease with acute extremity ischemia. This assessment can be classified according to clinical and noninvasive parameters. This has important implications in terms of subsequent procedures such as the need for amputation. ISCS—International Society of Cardiovascular Surgeons; SVS—Society of Vascular Surgeons.

RENAL ARTERY DUPLEX ULTRASOUND

DEGREE OF STENOSIS	PEAK SYSTOLIC VELOCITY	RENAL ARTERY/AORTIC RATIO
Normal	< 60 cm/s	< 3.5
Moderate	≥ 180 cm/s	< 3.5
Severe stenosis	≥ 180 cm/s	> 3.5
Occlusion	Unobtainable	Unobtainable

FIGURE 12-51. Renal artery duplex ultrasound. There is great interest in the relationship between renal artery stenosis and hypertension. Given the increased emphasis and interest in secondary causes of hypertension, the potential for renal artery restenosis as a cause must be at least entertained. This figure and Figure 12-50 document the clinical algorithm to facilitate the evaluation of patients with potential or probable renal artery stenosis. In patients with documented renal artery stenosis, there is increasing information on the effect of revascularization with stent implantation with or without distal protection.

FIGURE 12-52. Clinical algorithm to facilitate the evaluation of patients with probable renal artery stenosis. (*Adapted from* Saifan and Textor [13].)

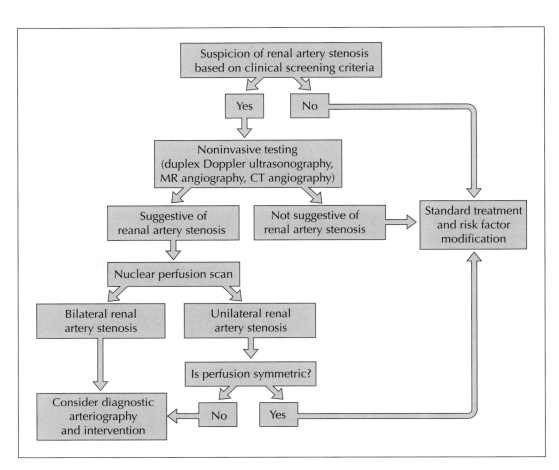

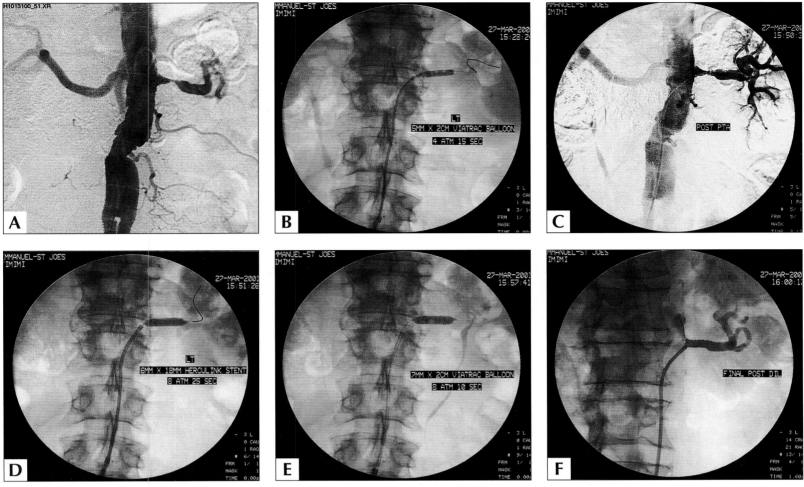

FIGURE 12-53. Proximal (nonostial) atherosclerotic renal artery stenosis. Detection of a proximal but not ostial atherosclerotic renal artery stenosis in this patient led to the selection of an interventional approach as therapy. When these patients are well selected, improvement and control of blood pressure often result. Complete abolition of the need for antihypertensive medications is relatively infrequent. However, in patients who have significant hypertension and impaired renal function, revascularization may substantially improve clinical outcome. The use of distal protection is being explored in these patients to try to prevent the acute decrease in renal function that may be seen after intervention. **A,** Diagnostic nonselective arteriography demonstrates a proximal high-grade atherosclerotic lesion in this patient with hypertension requiring multiple pharmacologic agents. **B,** A 6-F renal double curve catheter was used to engage the ostium of the right renal artery. A 0.014-inch Sparta Core wire (Guidant, Santa Clara, CA) was used to cross the lesion, and dilatation was conducted with a 5 × 2 cm Via Trac (Guidant) balloon. **C,** After balloon dilatation, significant residual stenosis is shown. **D** and **E,** Therefore, the 6-F renal double curve was exchanged for an 8-F 55-cm hockey stick guide, and a 6 × 18 mm Herculink stent (Guidant) was deployed. A 7 × 2 mm Via Trac balloon was used for postdilatation. **F,** Final arteriography demonstrates no significant residual stenosis or marginal dissection.

SEVERITY OF ICA STENOSIS BY CAROTID DUPLEX

SEVERITY, %	PEAK SYSTOLIC VELOCITY	INTERNAL CAROTID/COMMON CAROTID RATIO	END DIASTOLIC VELOCITY	SPECTRAL BROADENING
1–39	< 125 cm/s	< 1.6		Mild or none
40–69	125–230 cm/s	1.6–3.2		Moderate
70–99	≥ 230 cm/s	≥ 3.2	≥ 70 cm/s	Marked
100	None	NA	None	None

FIGURE 12-54. Severity of internal carotid artery (ICA) stenosis by carotid duplex. Given the high degree of expertise in stent implantation and the finding that patients with carotid arterial disease benefit from revascularization, a percutaneous approach has been used to treat patients with carotid arterial disease. The severity of intercranial stenosis is usually assessed by carotid duplex. This is combined with data on the expected perioperative stroke or death rate (*see* Fig. 12-53) in different groups of patients undergoing carotid surgical intervention. NA—not applicable.

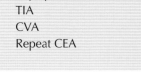

AHA STROKE COUNCIL GUIDELINES FOR CEA

CLINICAL GROUP	EXPECTED PERIOPERATIVE STROKE/DEATH RATE, %
Asymptomatic	< 3
TIA	< 5
CVA	< 7
Repeat CEA	< 10

FIGURE 12-55. American Heart Association (AHA) Stroke Council guidelines for carotid endarterectomy (CEA). CVA—cerebrovascular aneurysm; TIA—transient ischemic attack.

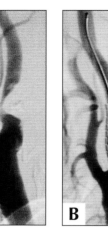 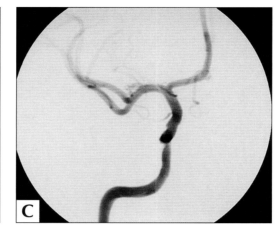

A **B** **C**

FIGURE 12-56. Symptomatic carotid artery stenosis. Increasing information is now available on the use of stent implantation with distal protection to improve outcomes in patients with significant carotid arterial stenosis (**A–C**). Recently, a randomized trial has documented improved outcome in patients who could either be treated with a surgical approach or an interventional approach who are at high risk for intervention. It is believed that in the future, a majority of patients in whom the carotid arterial lesion is suitable for stent implantation and distal protection will be treated in that fashion.

REFERENCES

1. Schwartz RS, Murphy JG, Edwards WD, *et al.*: Restenosis occurs with internal elastic lamina laceration and is proportional to severity of vessel injury in a porcine coronary artery model [abstract]. *Circulation* 1990, 82:III-656.

2. Kern MJ, Bach RG, Mechem CJ, *et al.*: Variations in normal coronary vasodilatory reserve stratified by artery, gender, heart transplantation and coronary artery disease. *J Am Coll Cardiol* 1996, 28:1154–1160.

3. Abizaid A, Mintz GS, Pichard AD, *et al.*: Clinical, intravascular ultrasound, and quantitative angiographic determinants of the coronary flow reserve before and after percutaneous transluminal coronary angioplasty. *Am J Cardiol* 1998, 82:423–428.

4. Kern MJ, Donohue TJ, Aguirre FV, *et al.*: Clinical outcome of deferring angioplasty in patients with normal translesional pressure-flow velocity measurements. *J Am Coll Cardiol* 1995, 25:178–187.

5. Ferrari M, Schnell B, Werner GS, Figulla HR: Safety of deferring angioplasty in patients with normal coronary flow velocity reserve. *J Am Coll Cardiol* 1999, 33:82–87.

6. Pijls NH, De Bruyne B, Peels K, *et al.*: Measurement of fractional flow reserve to assess the functional severity of coronary-artery stenoses. *N Engl J Med* 1996, 334:1703–1708.

7. De Bruyne B, Bartunek J, Sys SU, Heyndrickx GR: Relation between myocardial fractional flow reserve calculated from coronary pressure measurements and exercise-induced myocardial ischemia. *Circulation* 1995, 92:39–46.

8. Dean LS: The Gianturco-Roubin II (GR-II) intracoronary stent. In *Strategic Approaches in Coronary Intervention*. Edited by Ellis SG, Holmes DR Jr. Baltimore: Williams & Wilkins; 1996.

9. Dean LS, Holmes DR Jr, Roubin GS: One year follow-up: the effect of proper stent size on clinical outcome. *Am J Cardiol* 1998, 82:69S.

10. Kimura T, Tamura T, Yokoi H, *et al.*: Long-term clinical and angiographic follow-up after placement of Palmaz-Schatz coronary stent: a single center experience. *J Intervent Cardiol* 1994, 7:129–139.

11. Mehran R, Dangas G, Abizaid AS, *et al.*: Angiographic patterns of in-stent restenosis: classification and implications for long-term outcome. *Circulation* 1999,100:1872–1878.

12. Hiat R: Medical treatment of peripheral arterial disease and claudication. *N Engl J Med* 2001, 344:1608–1621.

13. Saifen R, Textor S: Renal artery stenosis. *N Engl J Med* 2001, 344:431–442.

INDEX

A

ABCA1 transporter, 16–17
Ablation
  alcohol septal, 157–158
  of arrhythmias, 225
ACS Guidant stent, 384
Acute aortic regurgitation, 289–291
Acute coronary syndromes
  drug therapy of, 55–61
  nomenclature of, 55
  nuclear cardiology in diagnosis of, 366–367
  overview of, 47
Acute heart failure
  treatment of, 143–145
Acute ischemic syndromes
  pathology of, 49–54
Acute myocardial infarction, 47–81
  cardiac rupture and, 54, 81
  cardiogenic shock in, 77–80
  coronary occlusion in, 53
    reperfusion and, 62–68
  drug therapy in, 55–61
    antiplatelet, 71–73
    thrombolytic, 65–68, 75–76
  mitral regurgitation and, 80
  pathophysiology of, 49–55
  percutaneous transluminal coronary
    angioplasty in, 74–77
  platelets in, 68–71
  SPECT assessment of, 369, 371
  triggering of, 48
  ventricular septal defect and, 80
Acute myocarditis, 174–175
Acute pericarditis, 180–181
Adenosine
  in pharmacologic stress imaging, 354–356
Adrenal tumor
  hypertension from, 244
Adrenergic nervous system
  in heart failure, 123–125
  in hypertension, 231–232
  neurotransmitter synthesis in, 370
Alcohol septal ablation
  in hypertrophic cardiomyopathy, 157–158
Aldosterone agents
  in heart failure, 137
Aldosteronism
  hypertension in, 243–245
Alpha blockers
  in hypertension, 251
Alteplase
  in acute myocardial infarction, 65
Ambulatory blood pressure monitoring, 258
Ammonia
  in positron emission tomography, 353
Amyloidosis
  cardiomyopathy in, 163–164
Angina
  in chronic ischemic heart disease,
    83–85, 105–106
  pathophysiology of, 83–85

therapy of
  stable, 105–106
  unstable, 60–61, 68
Angiography
  in ischemic heart disease, 99–100
Angioplasty
  cutting balloon, 390–395
  in ischemic heart disease, 99–104
  in myocardial infarction, 74–76
Angiotensin
  in hypertension, 235–237
Angiotensin receptor antagonists
  in heart failure, 138
Angiotensin-converting enzyme inhibitors
  in acute myocardial infarction, 58
  in chronic ischemic heart disease, 108
  in heart failure, 135–136
  in hypertension, 234, 251
Anistreplase
  in acute myocardial infarction, 65
Anomalous left coronary artery origin, 312
Antiarrhythmic agents
  class III, 206
  effect on reentry of, 192–193
  prophylactic, 58–59
Antibiotics
  in Lyme disease, 162
Antihypertensive agents
  clinical trials of, 252–255
  factors in selection of, 255
  principles of treatment with, 249–251
  in treatment algorithm, 256
Antiplatelet agents
  in acute myocardial infarction, 71–73
  heart disease prevention and, 42
Aorta
  coarctation of, 310–311, 323–324
Aortic regurgitation, 289–295
  acute, 289–291
  chronic, 291–294
  valve replacement in, 294–295
Aortic stenosis, 284–288
  echocardiography in, 286–287
  pathophysiology of, 284–285
  physical examination in, 286
  treatment of, 287–288
Apoptosis
  SPECT assessment in myocardial
    infarction of, 371
Arrhythmias, 187–225.
    See also specific arrhythmias
  antiarrhythmic drugs and, 192–193
  cardiac resynchronization therapy for, 224
  catheter ablation for, 225
  internal defibrillators in prevention of,
    222–223
  mechanisms of, 190–192
  normal conduction and excitation *versus,*
    187–189
  pacemaker therapy in, 216–221
  sinus node, 193–199
  sudden cardiac death and, 222

supraventricular tachycardias as, 199–206
triggered, 191
ventricular, 207–215
Arrhythmogenic right ventricular
  cardiomyopathy
  diagnosis of, 176
Aspirin
  in acute myocardial infarction, 71
  heart disease prevention and, 42
Atherectomy
  coronary, 388–390
Atherosclerosis, 1–42
  diabetes and risk of, 85
  dietary treatment of, 24–29
  drug therapy in, 29–42
    bile acid sequestrants in, 31–32
    combination, 37–42
    fibric acids in, 35–36
    lipoprotein metabolism and, 30–31
    nicotinic acid in, 34–35
    statins in, 32–33
  hyperlipoproteinemias in, 8–23
    chylomicrons and, 19
    high-density lipoproteins and, 14–17
    low-density lipoproteins and, 11–14
    triglyceride-rich lipoproteins and, 17–18
    very low-density lipoproteins and, 20
  plaque formation in, 1–7, 14
  SPECT assessment of, 372
Atrial fibrillation, 203–206
  in mitral stenosis, 271
Atrial flutter, 203
Atrial natriuretic factor
  in heart failure, 127
Atrial septal defect, 305–306
Atrial tachycardia, 199–200
Atrioventricular nodal reentry tachycardia,
  200–203
Atrioventricular septal defect, 308–309
Automatic implantable cardioverter/
  defibrillators, 222–223
  in advanced heart disease, 182–183
  drug therapy *versus,* 213–214
  in hypertrophic cardiomyopathy, 158
  indications for, 213
  in ventricular arrhythmias,
    211–214, 222–224
Automaticity
  in arrhythmogenesis, 190

B

Balloon angioplasty
  cutting, 390–395
Balloon atrial septostomy, 321
Balloon commissurotomy
  in mitral stenosis, 273–275
Balloon septostomy
  atrial, 321
Balloon valvuloplasty
  in aortic stenosis, 288
Becker muscular dystrophy
  cardiomyopathy in, 168

Beta blockers
 in acute myocardial infarction, 56
 in heart failure, 141–142
 in hypertension, 250
Bile acid sequestrants, 31–32
Bioprosthetic valves, 298
Blood pressure. *See also* Hypertension
 ambulatory monitoring of, 258
 classification of, 256–257, 266
Brachytherapy
 in chronic ischemic heart disease, 102–103
Brain natriuretic peptide
 in heart failure treatment, 143–144
Brugada's syndrome, 210
Bypass surgery
 in chronic ischemic heart disease, 109–110

C

Calcium
 in heart failure, 122
Calcium antagonists
 in acute myocardial infarction, 57
 in chronic ischemic heart disease, 108
Captopril test
 in renovascular hypertension, 240
Cardiac amyloidosis, 163–164
Cardiac arrhythmias. *See* Arrhythmias;
 specific arrhythmias
Cardiac murmurs
 in aortic stenosis, 286
 in mitral stenosis, 271–272
 in mitral valve prolapse, 281
Cardiac pacemaker therapy.
 See Pacemaker therapy
Cardiac resynchronization
 in advanced heart disease, 183–184, 224
Cardiac rupture
 acute myocardial infarction and, 54, 81
Cardiac sarcoidosis, 162–163
Cardiac tamponade, 178–180
Cardiac transplantation, 146–152.
 See also Heart transplantation
Cardiac tumors, 341–343
Cardiogenic shock
 diagnosis of, 78
 pathophysiology of, 77
 treatment of, 79–80
Cardiomyopathy, 155–170
 in amyloidosis, 163–164
 arrhythmogenic right ventricular, 176
 in Friedreich's ataxia, 169
 genetic causes of dilated, 170
 hypertrophic, 155–158
 idiopathic dilated, 159–161
 in Kearns-Sayre syndrome, 169–170
 in Lyme disease, 161–162
 in muscular dystrophy, 167–169
 restrictive, 164–165
 in sarcoidosis, 162–163
Cardiovascular disease
 aspirin in prevention of, 42
 risk factors for, 24
Carotid artery stenosis, 401–402
Carotid endarterectomy
 guidelines for, 402
Carpentier-Edwards prosthetic valve, 298
Carvedilol

in heart failure, 141–142
Catheter ablation
 of arrhythmias, 225
Catheter balloon commissurotomy
 in mitral stenosis, 273–275
Cell membrane integrity testing, 360–362
Cellular cardiac electrophysiology, 188–189
Central obesity
 coronary heart disease and, 28
Children
 hypertension in, 260
Cholesterol. *See also* Lipoproteins
 dietary intake and serum levels of, 25–26
 structure of, 8
Chronic aortic regurgitation, 291–294
Chronic ischemic heart disease, 83–110
 angina in, 83–85
 bypass surgery in, 109–110
 coronary angiography in, 99–100
 echocardiography in, 94–97
 exercise electrocardiography in, 86–87
 intracoronary arterial ultrasound in, 98
 left ventricular function assessment in,
  94–98
 magnetic resonance imaging in, 98
 medical therapy in, 104–108
 myocardial perfusion imaging in, 88–93
 percutaneous transluminal coronary
  angioplasty in, 99–104
Chylomicrons
 metabolism of, 19, 30
 size and density of, 9
 structure of, 8
Coarctation of the aorta, 310–311, 323–324
Commissurotomy
 balloon
  in mitral stenosis, 273–275
Computed tomography
 single-photon emission. *See* Single-photon
  emission computed tomography
Congenital heart disease, 305–324
 anomalous left coronary artery origin as,
  312
 atrial septal defect as, 305–306
 atrioventricular septal defect as, 308–309
 balloon atrial septostomy in, 321
 coarctation of the aorta as, 310–311, 323–324
 Ebstein's anomaly as, 311
 pulmonary valve dilation in, 322
 subaortic stenosis as, 309–310
 tetralogy of Fallot as, 313–315
 transposition of the great arteries as, 318
 tricuspid atresia as, 319–320
 truncus arteriosus communis as, 316–317
 ventricular septal defect as, 307
Congestive heart failure
 diagnosis of, 130–131
 epidemiology of, 129
Constrictive pericarditis, 181–182
Contractile proteins
 normal cardiac, 113
Cor pulmonale, 327–334
 assessment of, 331–332
 natural history of, 327–328
 pathophysiology of, 328–330
 treatment of, 333–334
Cordis stents, 383–384

Coronary angiography
 in ischemic heart disease, 99–100
Coronary angioplasty
 percutaneous transluminal, 74–76, 99–104
Coronary arteries. *See also* Coronary
  artery disease
 atherosclerotic plaque formation in, 4–6
 normal circulation in, 354
 response to intervention injury of, 375–376
Coronary artery disease. *See also* Acute
  coronary syndromes
 in acute myocardial infarction, 47–53.
  See also Acute myocardial infarction
 angina in, 83–84
 central obesity and, 28
 dietary cholesterol and, 25–26
 genetic dyslipoproteinemias in, 11
 homocysteine and, 38
 low-density lipoproteins in, 23, 31
 occlusion in, 53
  reperfusion and, 62–68
 patency and survival in, 64–65
 risk of
  estrogen replacement therapy and, 36
  high-density lipoproteins and, 14
  overview of, 40
  triglyceride-rich lipoproteins in, 17–18, 22
Coronary atherectomy, 388–390
Coronary flow reserve
 ultrasound studies of, 379–380
Coronary stenting
 in ischemic heart disease, 99–104
Cortisol
 hypertension and, 241–242
Cushing's syndrome
 hypertension in, 241–242
Cutting balloon angioplasty, 390–395
Cytokines
 in atherosclerosis, 7, 39

D

Device therapy
 in advanced heart disease, 182–184
 distal protection devices in, 397–398
Diabetes mellitus
 atherosclerosis risk and, 85
Diastolic heart failure, 117–119, 131
Dietary treatment
 in atherosclerosis, 24–29
Digitalis
 in heart failure, 139–140
Dilated cardiomyopathy
 genetic causes of, 170
 idiopathic, 159–161
Dipyridamole
 in pharmacologic stress imaging, 354–358
Directional coronary atherectomy, 388
Distal protection devices, 397–398
Diuretics
 in heart failure, 134
Dobutamine
 in pharmacologic stress imaging, 354, 356
Doxorubicin therapy
 radionuclide angiography in, 368
Drug assessment
 of sinus node dysfunction, 197
Drug therapy. *See also* specific agents